Clinical Procedures in Primary Eye Care

Fifth Edition

Editor

David B. Elliott
PhD, FCOptom, FAAO
Professor of Clinical Vision Science
School of Optometry and Vision Science
University of Bradford
Bradford, Yorkshire, UK

ELSEVIER

ISBN: 9780702077890

Content Strategist: Kayla Wolfe
Content Development Specialist: Angie Breckon
Publishing Services Manager: Shereen Jameel
Senior Project Manager: Kamatchi Madhavan
Designer: Brian Salisbury
Marketing Manager: Claire McKenzie

Printed in Great Britain

Last digit is the print number: 10 9 8 7 6 5

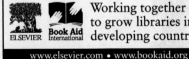

Preface

This textbook was written primarily as a teaching aid for undergraduate optometry students and for practitioners wishing to review their clinical practice.

Chapter 1, evidence-based optometry: discusses how some clinical tests seem widely used because of tradition rather than based on clinical and research evidence and the (lack of) evidence behind routine dilated fundus examinations. It also highlights the problems of screening for conditions such as glaucoma that have a low prevalence (Bayes' theorem) and discusses how this can be overcome. Chapter 1 is completed by a discussion of the lessons that need to be learned from the Honey Rose gross negligence manslaughter case.

Chapter 2, communication skills: discusses why patients might be anxious when attending for an eye examination and how to build a rapport and relax an anxious patient. It describes how to perform the case history, the cornerstone of all eye examinations and the most important (and most difficult to learn) skill.

Chapters 3-7, oculo-visual systems: Tests are subsequently grouped together in terms of which system they assess: visual function (Chapter 3), refraction and prescribing (Chapter 4), contact lens assessment (Chapter 5), binocular vision and accommodation (Chapter 6), and ocular health (Chapter 7). This layout was chosen because the organisation of the book is directed towards the assimilation of a problem-oriented approach that is built on a systems examination (section 1.4). Grouping the tests in this way, rather than in the order they are typically used in an eye examination, may also help students to better appreciate the relationship between the various tests that assess a particular system.

Chapter 8, variations in appearance of the normal eye: To develop ocular health skills in discriminating between disease and the normal eye, it is essential to know many presentations that a normal eye can make and a brief description and collection of photographs of these normal variations is presented in Chapter 8 and the accompanying website to supplement the information provided in atlases of ocular disease.

Chapter 9, physical examination procedures: completes the book with an introduction to procedures, such as blood pressure measurement, that may be used in primary care eye examinations.

What's New?

The 5th edition has been revised to reflect the increasing use of technology in optometric practice, the increasing importance of practicing evidence-based optometry, and the pandemic in myopia throughout the world:

- Sections on Ocular Coherence Tomography (OCT) and ultra-wide field imaging are substantially increased with new large banks of high-quality images.
- All procedures include a section that reviews the evidence base of when and how the procedure should be measured, using both clinical wisdom and pertinent research-based evidence.
- "A picture paints a thousand words," so the number of digital images has been substantially increased in the book and online (with the text made as succinct as possible). Video-clips have also been greatly increased.
- Dry eye assessment has been substantially updated and based on the latest international Dry Eye Workshop (DEWS II) guidelines.
- New sections on mini-scleral and scleral contact lenses.
- Changes in the eye caused by myopia at low, moderate, and high levels and the need for myopia control are highlighted, with an album of images provided.

Spotted any errors or omissions?

There is little doubt that tests and test methodologies have been included that reflect our biases owing to our particular training, research, and clinical experience. There may also be errors and omissions. We therefore welcome any comments and suggestions that would improve any further issues and editions. Please e-mail the editor, David Elliott on: d.elliott1@bradford.ac.uk

Listen to your supervisors!

There are many ways of conducting an eye examination and different ways to perform various procedures properly and some may not appear in this textbook. In particular, in university clinics it is the supervising clinician's decision as to which techniques or tests should be used in an eye examination. They are taking legal responsibility for the examination and if they indicate that a particular test needs using and in a particular way, do it! Once the patient has left and you are discussing the case with your supervisor, to further your learning, ask them about the advantages and disadvantages of their suggested technique.

List of Contributors

Brendan T. Barrett, BSc Psychol,
Dip.Optom. PhD, MCOptom, FAOI
Professor
School of Optometry and Vision Science
University of Bradford
Bradford, Yorkshire, United Kingdom

Catharine Chisholm, PhD
MCOptom FBCLA
Global Director of Education and
Training
Topcon Healthcare
Tokyo, Japan

David B. Elliott, PhD, FCOptom,
FAAO
School of Optometry and Vision Science
University of Bradford
Bradford, Yorkshire, United Kingdom

John G. Flanagan PhD, DSchc,
FCOptom, FAAO
Dean and Professor
School of Optometry
University of California Berkeley
Berkeley, California, USA

Patricia Hrynchak, OD,
MScCH(HPTE), FAAO, DipOE
Clinical Professor
School of Optometry and Vision Science
University of Waterloo
Waterloo, Canada

Alexander F. Hynes, HBSc, OD,
FAAO
Supervising Clinician
Optometry
University of Waterloo
Waterloo, Canada
Optometrist
Terri Holland Optometry
Kitchener, Canada

Konrad Pesudovs, BScOptom,
PhD, PGDipAdvClinOptom, DipWSET,
MCOptom, FACO, FAAO, FCCLSA,
FAICD
Professor
School of Optometry and Vision Science
University of New South Wales
New South Wales, Australia
Vision and Eye Research Institute
Anglia Ruskin University
Cambridge, United Kingdom

C. Lisa Prokopich, OD, MSc
Optometry and Vision Science
University of Waterloo
Waterloo, Canada

Craig A. Woods, BSc (Hons), PhD,
GradCertOcThera, FAAO, FBCLA
Professor of Optometry
School of Medicine, Faculty of Health
Deakin University
Waurn Ponds
Victoria, Australia

Additional Contributors to the Electronic Ancillary

Alexander Black, BAppSc(Optom), MPH, PhD
School of Optometry and Vision Science
Queensland University of Technology
Brisbane, Australia

Jason Booth, AM BOptom(Hons), PDOT, CO(Aviation)
Associate Professor in Optometry
College of Nursing and Health Sciences
Flinders University
Adelaide, Australia

Matthew Cufflin, PhD, MCOptom, FHEA
School of Optometry and Vision Science
University of Bradford
Bradford, Yorkshire, United Kingdom

Kelly Gibbons, BAppsSc (Orthoptics) Hons.; BOptom, PGCOT
Wodonga Eyecare
Wodonga, Victoria, Australia

Charlotte A Hazel, MSc (Optom), PhD, DipTp(IP), FACO
Bradford Teaching Hospitals National
Health Service Foundation Trust
Bradford, Yorkshire, United Kingdom

Edward Mallen, PhD, MCOptom
Professor of Physiological Optics
School of Optometry and Vision Science
University of Bradford
Bradford, Yorkshire, United Kingdom

Annette Parkinson PhD, Prof Cert LV, MCOptom
School of Optometry and Vision Science
University of Bradford
Bradford, Yorkshire, United Kingdom

Nicholas Rumney, MScOptom (Melbourne), FCOPtom DipTP(IP), ProfCertMedRet, FAAO, FEAOO, FBCLA, FIACLE, FBDO (Hon)
Professor (Hon) Clinical Optometry
University of Manchester
Manchester, United Kingdom
Professor (Adjunct) Clinical Optometry
Oulu University of Applied Science
Oulu, Finland
Chairman, BBR Optometry

Roman Serebrianik, BOptom, PGDipAdvClinOptom, PGCertOCTher, FACO
Head of Primary and Specialist Eye Care
Services
Australian College of Optometry
Melbourne, Australia
Adjunct Lecturer
Flinders University
Adelaide, Australia

Samantha Strong, BSc(Hons), PhD
Aston School of Optometry
Aston University
Birmingham, United Kingdom

Acknowledgements

I would like to thank the many friends and colleagues throughout the world who have modernised *Clinical Procedures in Primary Eye Care* in its 5th edition. Huge thanks to those who have written new sections and chapters (John Flanagan, USA; Catharine Chisholm, UK; Craig Woods, Australia; Brendan Barrett, UK; Lisa Prokopich, Canada; Alex Hynes, Canada; Konrad Pesudovs, Australia; Patty Hrynchak, Canada); provided two fantastic new online albums of optomap images (Kelly Gibbons, Australia) and OCT images (Roman Serebrianik, Australia; Jason Booth, Australia; Charlotte Hazel, UK; Nick Rumney, UK); contributed some superb new drawings, video-clips and images of clinical procedures and ocular conditions (Samantha Strong, UK; Alex Black, Australia; Bill Harvey, UK; Jason Booth, Australia; Catharine Chisholm, UK; Craig Woods, Australia; Carl Glittenberg, Switzerland; Paulo Stanga, UK; Brian Tomkins, UK; Lyndon Jones, Canada; Murray Fingeret, USA); and provided important suggestions to earlier versions of chapters (Mark Bullimore, USA; Karl Hallam, UK). I would also like to thank Karl Hallam for allowing me to observe high quality communication skills in action at the coalface of modern optometry (and introducing me to the 5 Rs) and to the large number of friends, colleagues, students, and patients involved in producing the many images and video-clips from the 4th edition that we have retained for the new edition. Last, but certainly not least, I would like to thank Mary Elliott for her skills in patiently explaining the complexities of OCT images and for her unending support and encouragement.

Table of Contents

Video Contents

Video Contents

Chapter | 1

Evidence-based eye examinations

David B. Elliott

1.1 Several tests are widely used because of tradition and not evidence

Evidence-based optometry means integrating individual clinical expertise with the best currently available evidence from the research literature.[1] For the majority of primary eye care procedures described, the evidence base for when and how they should be measured is provided. This may be from clinical experience (i.e., clinical pearls), which could be the authors' own experience or supported by citations to clinical textbooks and articles or from research evidence. What should always be avoided is the use of examination procedures based on tradition, anecdotal evidence, or habit. Three procedures that are widely used in several countries but seem principally used because of tradition are discussed below.

1.1.1 Visual acuity should not be measured with Snellen charts

The principal reason for using a Snellen chart nowadays would appear to be tradition or habit. Visual acuity (VA) charts using the logMAR system are now widely available and are much superior to Snellen charts, providing VA measurements that are twice as repeatable and over three times more sensitive to interocular differences in VA (see section 3.1.1).[2,3] VA can still be recorded and reported to others in the more familiar Snellen format of 6/6, 20/20, or 1.0.

1.1.2 The von Graefe prism dissociation test does not deserve its widespread use

The faith in this test has been such that a publication in a leading international optometry journal pronounced it as the gold standard test of heterophoria assessment[4] and used it to assess the usefulness of the cover test. The gold standard in this area should be the cover test and not the von Graefe[5–8] as it is objective and not reliant on subject responses or subject to prism adaptation and subsequent studies have shown it to be far more repeatable than the von Graefe prism dissociation test, which has been shown to be unreliable.[5–8] The study should have used the cover test as the gold standard and they would then have reported the limitations of the von Graefe prism dissociation test. Several studies have now reported that the modified Thorington test is much simpler, faster, and more reliable than the von Graefe prism dissociation test,[5-8] and if an additional test to the cover test is required, it should be the modified Thorington.

1.1.3 Lengthy tentative reading addition tests are not necessary

A final example of tests used because of tradition in phoropter-based refractions is the use of tentative reading addition tests of binocular cross-cylinder followed by negative and positive relative accommodation (NRA-PRA). These are lengthy tests given that the only study to have properly investigated the various tentative addition tests indicated that asking patients their age provided more accurate information than either of those two tests.[9] Using an ingenious study design, Hanlon et al.[9] examined patients who returned to an optometry practice because they were dissatisfied with the near vision in their new glasses. Each patient's reading addition was determined using four methods (age, binocular cross-cylinder, NRA-PRA balance, $1/2$ amplitude of accommodation). The review (recheck) examination also determined whether the near addition in the glasses the patient disliked was too low or too high. The percentage of adds for each tentative add test that gave the same result as the incorrect add or worse (higher than an improper add determined too high or lower than an improper add determined as too low) was calculated. They reported that the simplest and quickest test, asking the patient their age, accounted for the fewest errors (14%). The other techniques gave errors in 61% (binocular cross-cylinder), 46% (NRA-PRA), and 30% ($1/2$ amplitude) of cases.[9] This suggests that the tentative addition should simply be based on patient age. Subsequent research suggests that the tentative addition estimate can be further improved by considering both the patient's age and working distance and/or symptoms with their current near correction (see 4.13.1). There is little need for the lengthy binocular cross-cylinder followed by NRA-PRA.

1.2 Tips on reviewing the evidence base for clinical tests

Currently professional bodies provide clinical guidelines that are based on research evidence, and expert clinicians and researchers write review articles and books and give lectures, and this has been reported to be the preferred source of information for many optometrists.[10] Reviewing the research literature yourself should become more common in future years,[10,11] particularly for the literature pertaining to clinical procedures,

although there are clear difficulties to overcome. Medicine has been using evidence-based practice for many more years than optometry, yet numerous primary care doctors still seldom practice it because of lack of time, difficulties in searching for, appraising, and applying evidence and preference for using guidelines provided by professional bodies.[12]

1.2.1 PubMed, Google Scholar, and international optometry research journals

If you wish to review the literature,[11] two very useful free access databases are PubMed (www.pubmed.com; provided by the US National Library of Medicine) and Google Scholar. They both include the abstracts or summaries of papers from all the main optometry and ophthalmology research journals. Questions from clinicians on optometric internet/e-mail discussion groups can often be fully answered by a quick PubMed or Google Scholar search that can provide a much stronger level of evidence than anecdotal suggestions from colleagues based on one or two patient encounters.

Full access to one or more of the international optometry research journals is provided by membership of various professional bodies: *Ophthalmic & Physiological Optics* (College of Optometrists, UK), *Optometry & Vision Science* (American Academy of Optometry), *Clinical & Experimental Optometry* (Optometry Australia, New Zealand Association of Optometrists, Hong Kong Society of Professional Optometrists and the Singapore Optometric Association), *Journal of Optometry* (Spanish General Council of Optometrists), *Contact Lens & Anterior Eye* (British Contact Lens Association), *African Vision & Eye Health* (South African Optometric Association), the *Chinese Journal of Optometry & Ophthalmology*, and the *Canadian Journal of Optometry*. Some professional bodies also have their own library and provide full access to a wide range of online optometry and ophthalmology journals.

1.2.2 How do you assess the usefulness of optometric tests?

The usefulness of optometric tests is typically assessed by either comparing the test against an appropriate gold standard[13] and/or assessing its repeatability[14] and/or its discriminative ability. For example, a test that is being used as an objective measure of subjective refraction should be assessed by how closely the results match subjective refraction results[13] and new tonometers are assessed by their agreement with the results of Goldmann Applanation Tonometry (GAT, although this is not ideal when GAT has flaws, see section 7.7.1).

1.2.3 How to assess tests that are part of the subjective refraction

The use of subjective refraction as a gold standard assessment of refractive error has meant that there has been little or no comparison of the various methods used in subjective refraction. Previous studies have tended to compare the various tests against each other. For example, West and Somers[15] compared the various binocular balancing tests and found that they all gave similar results and concluded that they were therefore all equally useful. Johnson et al.[16] reported a similar finding when comparing subjective tests for astigmatism. However, the size of the differences found with the different balancing and astigmatic tests in these studies would likely have led to symptoms and patient dissatisfaction with some of the refractive prescriptions if they had been worn, so that the conclusions seem incorrect and the study design poor.[13] An inventive but underutilised approach is to use some measure of patient satisfaction[17] or dissatisfaction[9] as the gold standard. For example, Strang et al.[17] compared the refractive corrections provided by subjective refraction and autorefraction by randomly allocating glasses in a double-blind protocol. Subjects wore each prescription for 2 weeks and completed a questionnaire that assessed visual performance and ocular comfort following each period of wear.

1.2.4 Bland-Altman plots vs. correlation coefficients

In the past, test comparison studies tended to quantify the relationship between the test and gold standard using correlation coefficients. This is not appropriate for a variety of reasons,[14,18] including that correlation coefficients are very much affected by the range of values used in the analysis.[19] If a small range of values is used in calculations, the correlation coefficient is likely to be much smaller than if a larger range is used (Fig. 1.1).[19] A much better analysis, commonly known as a Bland-Altman plot, shows the 95% confidence limits of the difference between the test and gold standard (Fig. 1.2).[14,18] Bland-Altman assessments are limited in that values are in the units of measurement rather than a unitless 0 to 1 scale like correlation coefficients, so it may not be obvious what is a good result. For this reason, the extent to which the 95% Bland-Altman agreement figures are clinically acceptable should be discussed by the authors of a paper and acceptable limits should be determined prior to any assessment.[14]

1.2.5 How best to assess test-retest repeatability

Repeatability assesses the ability of a measurement to be produced consistently. It is best to assess repeatability in

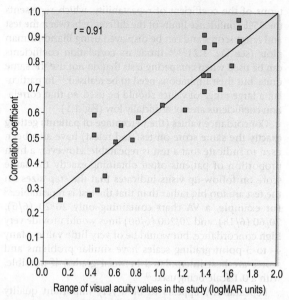

Fig. 1.1 Correlation coefficients from the literature between high-contrast visual acuity and other spatial vision measures are plotted as a function of the range of high-contrast acuities in those studies. (Redrawn with permission from Haegerstrom-Portnoy G, Schneck ME, Lott LA, Brabyn JA. The relation between visual acuity and other spatial vision measures. *Optometry and Vision Science*. 2000;77:653–62. ©The American Academy of Optometry, 2000.)

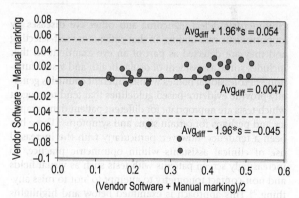

Fig. 1.2 A Bland-Altman plot of the difference (diff) between the Foveal Avascular Zone (FAZ) area (mm²) measured by the custom vendor software and manual marking as a function of the mean of the FAZ area from the two techniques. (Reprinted with permission from Arthur E, Papay JA, Haggerty BP, Clark CA, Elsner AE. Subtle changes in diabetic retinas localised in 3D using OCT. *Ophthalmic & Physiological Optics* 2018;38:477–91. ©The College of Optometrists, 2018).

terms of the coefficient of repeatability, which represents the 95% confidence limits of the difference between the test and retest scores and can be displayed using Bland-Altman plots (see Fig. 1.2).[14,18] Intraclass correlation coefficients can be used when comparing tests that do not use the same units, but their limitations need to be realised.[14] In particular, a large range of values should be used, so that correlation coefficients are not artificially low (Fig. 1.1).

Concordance values (the percentage of patients getting exactly the same score on test and retest) have also been used to indicate that a test is repeatable. However, a high proportion of patients often obtaining exactly the same score on follow-up visits indicates that the step sizes on the test are too big rather than that the test is repeatable.[20] For example, a VA chart containing only 20/20 (6/6), 20/60 (6/18), and 20/200 (6/60) lines would provide very high concordance, but would be of very little value. Many 4- to 5-point grading scales have similar problems and scores are best interpolated between grades, if possible, with a 0.1 scale being used.[21]

Repeatability appears to be a very important quality of a test, because an unreliable test is likely to correlate poorly with a gold standard and has poor discriminative ability.[22] Because these studies are also relatively quick and simple, the results of repeatability studies should be available for all clinical tests.

1.3 "Screen everybody, don't miss disease" vs. "what about false positives?"

Optometrists detect glaucoma and other eye diseases by 'opportunistic case finding' in that patients are self-selecting and they are detected as part of an eye examination that includes some assessment of ocular health and visual function.[23] Professional bodies within different countries generally provide evidence-based guidelines that tend to suggest which tests are appropriate for different patient demographics and perhaps for certain signs and symptoms. There has been a tendency, however, particularly with the increased use of clinical assistants within optometric practice, to increasingly screen patients with tests such as visual fields and non-contact tonometry to attempt to 'not to miss anything.'[24] This approach is examined below and highlights the importance of understanding diagnostic indices of optometric tests.

1.3.1 Do you really understand a test's diagnostic ability?

New diagnostic tests must have their diagnostic ability compared with a gold standard reference. The research

Table 1.1 Possible outcomes of a screening test

	Diseased eye	Normal eye
Test says diseased	True positive, TP (hit)	False positive, FP (false alarm)
Test says normal	False negative, FN (miss)	True negative, TN

study will therefore determine how well a test can correctly identify 'abnormal' or 'normal' eyes as classified independently by a gold standard test or battery of tests. For example, new instruments or techniques that attempt to identify patients with primary open-angle glaucoma (POAG) are typically assessed against classifications of patients into glaucomatous and control groups by clinical evaluation of optic nerve head assessment, anterior chamber angle, and visual fields.[25]

Please note that the following figures of sensitivity, specificity, and prevalence have been simplified to help the explanation. Imagine a POAG test that correctly detects patients with POAG 95% of the time (the sensitivity of the test is 95%); if the test indicates that a patient has POAG, what are the chances that they actually have the disease? Is it 95%? If lower, how much lower? When considering this question, you must not only consider how good the test is at identifying POAG, but you must also consider how good the test is at correctly identifying someone as normal. Unfortunately all tests provide false–positive findings: patients who have normal, healthy eyes for whom the test results suggest are abnormal. There are four possible outcomes from the results of a diagnostic test (Table 1.1), and this information is used to quantify how well the test discriminates between 'normal' and 'abnormal' eyes, by providing sensitivity and specificity values.

- Sensitivity is the ability of the test to identify the disease in those who have it.
- Sensitivity = TP / (TP + FN).
- Specificity is the ability of the test to correctly identify those who do not have the disease.
- Specificity = TN / (TN + FP).
- The false–positive rate is simply 1 minus the specificity.
- Another important term to understand is the predictive value (PV), which has positive (PPV) and negative (NPV) forms.
- PPV or +PV is the proportion of people with a positive test result who have the disease. PPV = TP / (TP + FP).
- NPV or −PV is the proportion of people with a negative test result who do not have the disease. NPV = TN / (TN + TP).

The reported sensitivity and specificity of a test will differ depending on the pool of patients examined, the gold standard used to determine the presence or absence of disease, and the cut-off criteria used. Sensitivity and specificity values and plots of one against the other for a range of cut-off values in receiver operating characteristic (ROC) curves (Fig. 1.3) are usually presented and are often quantified using the area under the ROC curve.

The ability of a diagnostic test to identify correctly those patients with disease is highly dependent on how prevalent the condition is (known as Bayes Theorem). For example, let us consider POAG and assume a prevalence in the over age 40 population of 1%, and a diagnostic test for glaucoma with 95% sensitivity and 95% specificity. The first column in Table 1.2 shows the likely outcomes from 1000 patients. Nine or all 10 patients with POAG have a positive test result, but so have 50 patients with normal, healthy eyes. Returning to the question at the beginning of this section, if a POAG test that correctly detects patients with POAG 95% of the time (95% sensitivity) indicates that a patient has POAG, the chances that they actually have the condition (given a test specificity of 95%) is 16%! Detecting disease that has a low prevalence is very difficult no matter how good your diagnostic tests are because there are so few patients with the disease and so many people who do not have that disease. This also highlights that with diseases with low prevalence, you are better off using tests (or cut-off scores for a test) that have the highest specificity (limiting false–positive results) even if this lowers sensitivity and a small number with POAG (in its early stages) are missed.

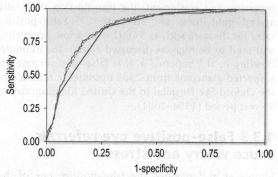

Fig. 1.3 Receiver operating characteristic (ROC) curves for prediction of high myopia in myopic children at age 11 years. (*n* = 910) Age myopia onset (*red line*); Age of myopia onset, gender, race, and school (*dashed green line*); Age of myopia onset, gender, race, school, books per week, and parental myopia (*blue line*). (Redrawn with permission from Chua et al. Age of onset of myopia predicts risk of high myopia in later childhood in myopic Singapore children. *Ophthalmic & Physiological Optics*. 2016;36:388–94. ©The College of Optometrists, 2016.)

1.3.2 The number of false–positive referrals

The number of false–positive referrals varies depending on the disease and its prevalence, the structure and funding eye care system; the level of clinical experience,

Table 1.2 Results for a 'glaucoma test' with different values of prevalence of primary open-angle glaucoma (POAG)

	SENSITIVITY 95% AND SPECIFICITY 95%		
	POAG prevalence, 1%	POAG prevalence, 10%	Repeated testing (POAG, 1%)
A. Patients with POAG	10	100	10
B. Patients without POAG	990	900	990
C. True positive (95% of A)	9.5 (i.e., 9 or 10)	95	9
D. False positive (5% of B)	50	45	2.5
E. True negative (95% of B)	940	855	47.5
F. False negative (5% of A)	0.5 (i.e., 0 or 1)	5	0.5
G. Number with positive result (C+D)	60	140	11.5
H. Number with negative result (E+F)	941	860	48
Positive predictive value: C/G	9.5/60 (16%)	95/140 (68%)	9/11.5 (78%)
Negative predictive value: E/H	940/941 (~100%)	855/860 (99.4%)	47.5/48.5 (99%)

expertise, and equipment; the introduction of locally agreed guidelines; and so forth.[26-30] False–positive rates for diseases such as POAG with a low prevalence will tend to be high, as discussed earlier. For example, Bowling et al.[31] reported a 46% false–positive rate for suspected glaucoma from 2505 optometric referrals to the Oxford Eye Hospital in the United Kingdom over a 10-year period (1994–2004).

1.3.3 False–positive eye referrals cause worry and stress

Elmore et al.[32] reported the false–positive rate of the two main breast cancer screening tests to be 6.5% and 3.7%. These translate to very good specificity values of 93.5% and 96.3%. Despite this good specificity, over a 10-year period, nearly one-third of the women screened had at least one false–positive mammogram or clinical breast examination. This highlights that if you test healthy people often enough, they will sooner or later obtain a false–positive test result. It has been shown that these false–positive results have negative psychological effects on these women and their families.[33] Similarly, considerable worry and stress are caused by a false–positive result leading to referral to a secondary eye care system.[34] Patients should not be referred to secondary eye care on the basis of a slightly high intraocular pressure using a non-contact tonometer or a single positive visual field screening result. In addition to the psychological effects on patients and their families, the costs in terms of secondary eye care staff and patient time (including the delay that other patients will suffer because of busy clinics) prompted by a positive screening result must be considered.

1.3.4 Reducing false positives 1: only screen 'at risk' patients

Owing to the high number of false–positive results when screening patients for a disease with low prevalence (Bayes Theorem), it may be better to screen only those patients who are 'at risk.' In these patients, the prevalence of the disease is higher than in the general population. The middle column in Table 1.2 considers the likely outcomes using the same test discussed earlier, on patients with a family history of POAG where the prevalence of the disease is higher and for simplicity we will assume a figure of 10%. In total, 140 patients have positive results, of which 95 have the disease (PPV = 68%). Note how much better the test performs when it is used in patients with a higher prevalence of the disease. The positive predictive value is also significantly improved if you just perform screening on all patients over 75 years of age or patients over 40 years of age who

are African American or African Caribbean or those with suspicious optic discs or high intraocular pressure. Burr et al.,[23] in their systematic review, suggested that screening of patients with 'minor' risk factors, including myopia and diabetes, did not improve the PPV sufficiently and was not cost-effective.[23]

1.3.5 Reducing false positives 2: repeat testing

Another way of keeping false–positive referrals to a minimum, and imperative if you are intending to screen more than 'at risk' patients, is to repeat positive results. For example, as part of the ocular hypertension treatment study, Keltner et al.[35] found 703 Humphrey visual field test results that showed abnormal (positive glaucoma hemifield test and/or corrected pattern standard deviation, $P < 0.05$) and reliable visual fields.[35] On retesting, abnormalities *were not* confirmed for 604 (86%)! The vast majority of visual field abnormalities were not verified on retest, and confirmation of visual field abnormalities is essential for distinguishing reproducible visual field loss from long-term variability.

If the same glaucoma diagnostic test from Table 1.2, which suggested that 60 patients had POAG (only 10 did), was repeated on these 60 patients, 9 of the 10 patients with glaucoma would be identified, but 95% of those 50 with false–positive results (47.5) would now give a normal result, with only 2.5 (i.e., 2 or 3) false positives on retest. On retesting, positive results are found for 11.5 patients, of whom 9 have the disease (PPV = 78%). Of course, you could also combine both approaches by only screening patients at risk and repeating positive tests.

1.3.6 Reducing false positives 3: mentoring inexperienced clinicians

Studies have shown that a majority of false–positive referrals are from inexperienced clinicians, typically in the first few years as a qualified optometrist.[28,30] An obvious strategy would be for newly qualified clinicians to continue to be mentored, particularly for referrals. Targeted continuing education and training for these clinicians would also likely be of benefit.[30]

1.3.7 Reducing false positives 4: intermediate/enhanced/collaborative care schemes

Given the high cost of referrals to secondary eye care, plus the burgeoning elderly population leading to ever-increasing referrals, a variety of schemes have been developed to decrease false–positive referrals. These are typically clinics intermediate between primary and secondary eye care that provide enhanced optometric services often in collaboration with ophthalmology.[27,29]

1.4 Should I perform a database, system, and/or problem-oriented eye examination?

The primary eye care examination must first and foremost adhere to the legal requirements where you are working, although these tend to be provided in very broad terms. Some professional organisations to which you may belong may also provide clinical guidelines of what your eye examination should include. These may be prescriptive or for guidance only. Three main styles for a primary eye care examination could be used singularly or in combination: (1) the database format, which uses a predetermined series of tests; (2) the systems approach, which ensures an assessment of several systems; and/or (3) the problem-oriented approach, which focuses mainly on the patient's problems.[36] In addition, some parts of the eye examination could be performed by clinical assistants.

1.4.1 The database examination

The database examination style means using essentially the same set of clinical procedures in every examination. A large 'complete' database of information is collected to ensure that most patients' problems can be addressed using the information provided. This is the style of examination that will be used by students, because they need to practice the various clinical techniques to gain technical competence. Technical competence should be

the aim for students in the early years of clinical learning. A much greater task is gaining clinical competence and understanding the tests and their results, how they interact and how they can be used in differential diagnosis, and to solve the patient's problems. Only once a student/practitioner has gained a high level of clinical competence should the database style of examination be abandoned and another approach used.

Although the database examination style is ideal for students, it is not for experienced practitioners. Often, if a large database is used, some data collected provide no useful information regarding the clinical diagnosis or treatment options. If patients require additional testing, because of the inflexibility of the database examination approach, practitioners either perform the tests at the end of the examination, which can lead to them being late for subsequent examinations, or another appointment is made at a later date. At its worst, this style of examination could be said to provide some test data which are not used and of little value and provide a bias against performing additional procedures which may be of real benefit.

1.4.2 Systems examination

A systems examination style includes an assessment of visual function, and of the refractive and binocular systems and an ocular health assessment. The optometric examination is defined not by tests used, but by the systems that are assessed (Table 1.3). This approach is much more flexible as it does not demand that a certain collection of tests be used. In such an examination style, a minimal database has been gathered when each system has been tested. In summary, think in terms of assessing systems and not of using individual tests.

Table 1.3 Classification of tests/procedures into one of four clinical oculovisual systems

Visual[a]	Binocular[a]	Refractive	Ocular Health
Case history	Case history	Case history	Case history
Visual acuity	Visual acuity	Visual acuity	Visual acuity
Disability glare	Cover test	Retinoscopy	Biomicroscopy
Photostress recovery	Convergence tests	Autorefraction	Ophthalmoscopy
Contrast sensitivity	Accommodation tests	Subjective refraction	Tonometry
Colour vision	Suppression tests	Reading add	Gonioscopy
Visual fields	Stereopsis	Keratometry	Pupil responses
	Motility		Imaging

[a]Other classifications discuss the sensory and motor systems rather than the visual and binocular systems and place suppression and stereopsis within the sensory system.

1.4.3 Problem-oriented examinations

The problem-oriented examination aligns the examination around the problems reported by the patient. However, it does not only use tests that help solve the patient's problems because it is built on a systems examination approach.[36] In addition, an array of tests are typically used as screening or 'entrance' tests,[37] which provide an initial assessment of each system. Some of the entrance tests may be part of pretesting conducted by clinical assistants, so that a period of time is required prior to meeting the patient for this information and any previous record cards to be reviewed. Clinical assistants can provide data from automated procedures including focimetry, autorefraction, fundus photography, ocular coherence tomography (OCT), ultra-widefield imaging (e.g., Optos), automated visual fields, non-contact tonometry, and pachymetry plus simple tests such as colour vision, stereopsis, and interpupillary distance (PD) measurement; the tests used may differ depending on the age of the patient.

From information from previous records (if available), the preliminary entrance tests, and the initial case history information, you will develop a mental list(s) of tentative diagnoses. These will likely lead to further questioning as part of differential diagnosis (e.g., particularly for symptoms such as red eye) and the subsequent tests used in the remainder of the problem-oriented examination will be determined by which tests best help the differential diagnosis process.

1.5 The evidence to support routine dilated fundus examinations is limited

Two main arguments are proposed in favour of the routine dilated fundus examination (DFE). The first is that a DFE increases the number of anomalies detected within the central retina.[38,39] In two studies, a non-dilated fundus examination with direct ophthalmoscopy was compared with a DFE using headband binocular indirect ophthalmoscopy and direct ophthalmoscopy.[38,39] Siegel et al.[38] also used a monocular indirect ophthalmoscope examination as part of a non-dilated examination. The poor field of view of the direct ophthalmoscope was particularly blamed for missing anomalies in the posterior pole because it is too small to examine the area quickly and easily. However, fundus biomicroscopy is now the standard of care for central fundus examination and provides a much better field of view than direct ophthalmoscopy as well as a stereoscopic view and can be conducted non-dilated (section 7.10.1).

The second argument for routine DFEs is that significant anomalies would otherwise be missed in the peripheral retina. Two studies have retrospectively reviewed record charts to determine the extent that significant fundus lesions were detected in DFEs.[40,41] Pollack and Brodie reviewed 1094 ophthalmologic records of DFEs of asymptomatic patients without risk factors and found three (0.3%) with clinically significant fundus lesions outside the vascular arcades and unlikely to have been detected using direct ophthalmoscopy.[40] Varner identified one case (0.2%) of an asymptomatic patient with a clinically significant peripheral lesion after 10 years of follow-up of 592 older (mean age approximately 70 years) patients and also concluded that the value of routine DFEs is very low.[41]

Disadvantages of routine DFEs include their inconvenience to the patient (e.g., glare and blur problems, they may not be able to drive home or return to work)[42] and the increased possibility of false–positive referrals,[43] particularly given the high prevalence of benign peripheral retina conditions in asymptomatic patients.[41] The cost of false–positive referrals must be recognised as it is not just the cost of the unnecessary secondary care appointment but the anxiety and inconvenience caused to the patient (section 1.3.3).

In summary, minimal evidence exists to support routine DFEs when compared against a routine non-dilated fundus examination with fundus biomicroscopy and DFEs in patients with pertinent signs and/or symptoms including symptoms of flashes and floaters, high myopia, recent cataract surgery, a family history of retinal detachment, and a small non-dilated pupil that would restrict the stereoscopic view of the central retina.[42]

1.6 Lessons to learn from the Honey Rose case

The potential for mistakes with overreliance on ocular imaging, particularly when taken by clinical assistants, was tragically illustrated in the United Kingdom in 2012. Details were provided in the 2016 trial of Honey Rose, a locum optometrist who was charged with gross negligence manslaughter (subsequently quashed on appeal)[44,45] owing to missing bilateral papilloedema in 8-year-old Vincent Barker who subsequently died of hydrocephalus 5 months after the eye examination. Experts agreed that his life could have been saved if the papilloedema had been spotted at the eye examination and the patient referred.[44] Although the patient had no symptoms to suggest a problem at the time of the eye examination, symptoms of a bout of unexplained headaches from a few weeks previously were reported to the optometrist.[44] Honey Rose claimed that she did not perform ophthalmoscopy because the patient closed his eyes and looked away from the bright light.[45] However, she did not make any record of this difficulty. It would also appear that the optometrist included a note on the patient's records to indicate she had viewed his inner eye.[45] Fundus images were taken at the time of the eye examination by a clinical assistant, and an expert witness indicated that they clearly showed bilateral papilloedema.[44,45] Honey Rose claimed that she had received insufficient training in the information technology (IT) systems and that she could not work the screen on the camera and asked a colleague to display it. She also claimed at different points of the trial that she viewed (1) the photograph of Vincent Barker from a previous appointment or (2) the photograph of a different patient.[44]

There are many lessons that optometry must learn from this tragic case, and these include:

- Patients can have life-threatening conditions and be asymptomatic.
- Optometrists must not rely solely on images to view the fundus.
- It is the responsibility of the optometrist to learn how to work imaging equipment and other tests usually performed by clinical assistants.

- It is the responsibility of eyecare practices to ensure that optometrists, including locum optometrists, fully understand the imaging (and other) processes used in their practice.
- It must be understood that mistakes linking images to patients (and specific examinations) can occur and great care must be taken to avoid them.

Although the evidence from this case suggests that the errors were those of the optometrist, they also highlighted other potential errors in the system, including:

- Technical problems, including a malfunctioning shutter, faulty display, and power cut on the day in question that were not dealt with in an appropriate manner.[45] Appropriate processes need to be put in place and regularly audited to ensure equipment works properly.
- Anecdotal evidence indicates that clinical assistants can fail to add patient details to images during busy clinics, thus connecting the previous patient's details to the following patient's image. This highlights the requirement for high-quality training of clinical assistants and the need for the clinician to be aware that such errors can occur and to look out for them.

References

1. Greenhalgh T. *How to Read a Paper: The Basics of Evidence-Based Medicine*, ed 3. Oxford: Blackwell Publishing; 2006.
2. Bailey IL, Lovie-Kitchin JE. Visual acuity testing. From the laboratory to the clinic. *Vision Res*. 2013;90:2–9.
3. Lovie- Kitchin JE. Is it time to confine Snellen charts to the annals of history? *Ophthalmic Physiol Opt*. 2015;35: 631–6.
4. Calvin H, Rupnow P, Grosvenor T. How good is the estimated cover test at predicting the von Graefe phoria measurement? *Optom Vis Sci*. 1996;73:701–6.
5. Rainey BB, Schroeder TL, Goss DA, Grosvenor TP. Inter-examiner repeatability of heterophoria tests. *Optom Vis Sci*. 1998;75:719–26.
6. Cebrian JL, Antona B, Barrio A, Gonzalez E, Gutierrez A, Sanchez I. Repeatability of the modified Thorington card used to measure far heterophoria. *Optom Vis Sci*. 2014;91:786–92.
7. Wong EP, Fricke TR, Dinardo C. Interexaminer repeatability of a new, modified prentice card compared with established phoria tests. *Optom Vis Sci*. 2002;79:370–5.

8. Casillas EC, Rosenfield M. Comparison of subjective heterophoria testing with a phoropter and trial frame. *Optom Vis Sci*. 2006;83:237–41.
9. Hanlon SD, Nakabayashi J, Shigezawa G. A critical view of presbyopic add determination. *J Am Optom Assoc*. 1987;58:468–72.
10. Suttle CM, Jalbert I, Alnahedh T. Examining the evidence base used by optometrists in Australia and New Zealand. *Clin Exp Optom*. 2012;95: 28–36.
11. Graham AM. Finding, retrieving and evaluating journal and web-based information for evidence-based optometry. *Clin Exp Optom*. 2007;90:244–9.
12. Hisham R, Ng CJ, Liew SM, Hamzah N, Ho GJ. Why is there variation in the practice of evidence-based medicine in primary care? A qualitative study. *BMJ Open*. 2016;6:e010565.
13. Elliott DB. What is the appropriate gold standard test for refractive error? *Ophthalmic Physiol Opt*. 2017;37: 115–7.
14. McAlinden C, Khadka J, Pesudovs K. Statistical methods for conducting

agreement (comparison of clinical tests) and precision (repeatability or reproducibility) studies in optometry and ophthalmology. *Ophthalmic Physiol Opt*. 2011;31:330–8.
15. West D, Somers WW. Binocular balance validity: a comparison of five different subjective techniques. *Ophthalmic Physiol Opt*. 1984;4:155–9.
16. Johnson BL, Edwards JS, Goss DA, et al. A comparison of three subjective tests for astigmatism and their interexaminer reliabilities. *J Am Optom Assoc*. 1996;67: 590–8.
17. Strang NC, Gray LS, Winn B, Pugh JR. Clinical evaluation of patient tolerance to autorefractor prescriptions. *Clin Exp Optom*. 1998;81:112–8.
18. Bland JM, Altman DG. Statistical methods for assessing agreement between two methods of clinical measurement. *Lancet*. 1986;1:307–10.
19. Haegerstrom-Portnoy G, Schneck ME, Lott LA, Brabyn JA. The relation between visual acuity and other spatial vision measures. *Optom Vis Sci*. 2000;77: 653–62.
20. Bailey IL, Bullimore MA, Raasch TW, Taylor HR. Clinical grading and the

effects of scaling. *Invest Ophthalmol Vis Sci.* 1991;32:422–32.

21. Chylack Jr LT, Wolfe JK, Singer DM, et al. The Lens Opacities Classification System III. The longitudinal study of cataract study group. *Arch Ophthalmol.* 1993;111:831–6.

22. Elliott DB, Bullimore MA. Assessing the reliability, discriminative ability, and validity of disability glare tests. *Invest Ophthalmol Vis Sci.* 1993;34:108–19.

23. Burr JM, Mowatt G, Hernández R, et al. The clinical effectiveness and cost-effectiveness of screening for open angle glaucoma: a systematic review and economic evaluation. *Health Technol Assess.* 2007;11:1–190.

24. Vernon SA. The changing pattern of glaucoma referrals by optometrists. *Eye (Lond).* 1998;12:854–7.

25. Dabasia PL, Fidalgo BR, Edgar DF, Garway-Heath DF, Lawrenson JG. Diagnostic accuracy of technologies for glaucoma case-finding in a community setting. *Ophthalmology.* 2015;122:2407–15.

26. Ang GS, Ng WS, Azuara-Blanco A. The influence of the new general ophthalmic services (GOS) contract in optometrist referrals for glaucoma in Scotland. *Eye (Lond).* 2009;23:351–5.

27. Baker H, Ratnarajan G, Harper RA, Edgar DF, Lawrenson JG. Effectiveness of UK optometric enhanced eye care services: a realist review of the literature. *Ophthalmic Physiol Opt.* 2016;36:545–57.

28. Davey CJ, Scally AJ, Green C, Mitchell ES, Elliott DB. Factors influencing accuracy of referral and the likelihood of false positive referrals by optometrists in Bradford, United Kingdom. *J Optom.* 2016;9:158–65.

29. Ly A, Nivison-Smith L, Hennessy M, Kalloniatis M. The advantages of intermediate-tier, inter-optometric referral of low risk pigmented lesions. *Ophthalmic Physiol Opt.* 2017;37:661–8.

30. Parkins DJ, Benwell MJ, Edgar DF, Evans BJW. The relationship between unwarranted variation in optometric referrals and time since qualification. *Ophthalmic Physiol Opt.* 2018;38:550–61.

31. Bowling B, Chen SD, Salmon JF. Outcomes of referrals by community optometrists to a hospital glaucoma service. *Br J Ophthalmol.* 2005;89:1102–4.

32. Elmore JG, Barton MB, Moceri VM, Polk S, Arena PJ, Fletcher SW. Ten-year risk of false positive screening mammograms and clinical breast examinations. *N Engl J Med.* 1998;338:1089–96.

33. Brett J, Austoker J. Women who are recalled for further investigation for breast screening: psychological consequences 3 years after recall and factors affecting re-attendance. *J Public Health Med.* 2001;23:292–300.

34. Davey CJ, Harley C, Elliott DB. Levels of state and trait anxiety in patients referred to ophthalmology by primary care clinicians: a cross sectional study. *PLoS One.* 2013;8:e65708.

35. Keltner JL, Johnson CA, Quigg JM, et al. Confirmation of visual field abnormalities in the Ocular Hypertension Treatment Study. *Arch Ophthalmol.* 2000;118:1187–94.

36. Amos JF. The problem-solving approach to patient care. In: Amos JF, ed. *Diagnosis and Management in Vision Care.* Boston: Butterworths; pp 1–8, 1987.

37. Carlson NB, Kurtz D, McGraw-Hill Education. *Clinical Procedures for Ocular Examination.* New York: McGraw-Hill Education; 2016.

38. Siegel BS, Thompson AK, Yolton DP, Reinke AR, Yolton RL. A comparison of diagnostic outcomes with and without pupillary dilatation. *J Am Optom Assoc.* 1990;61:25–34.

39. Parisi ML, Scheiman M, Coulter RS. Comparison of the effectiveness of a non-dilated versus dilated fundus examination in the pediatric population. *J Am Optom Assoc.* 1996;67:266–72.

40. Pollack AL, Brodie SE. Diagnostic yield of the routine dilated fundus examination. *Ophthalmology.* 1998;105:382–6.

41. Varner P. How frequently should asymptomatic patients be dilated? *J Optom.* 2014;7:57–61.

42. Batchelder TJ, Fireman B, Friedman GD, et al. The value of routine dilated pupil screening examination. *Arch Ophthalmol.* 1997;115:1179–84.

43. Ly A, Nivison-Smith L, Hennessy M, Kalloniatis M. The advantages of intermediate-tier, inter-optometric referral of low risk pigmented lesions. *Ophthalmic Physiol Opt.* 2037;37:661–8.

44. Mullock A. Gross negligence (Medical) manslaughter and the puzzling implications of negligent ignorance: Rose v R [2017] EWCA crim 1168. *Med Law Rev.* 2018;26:346–56.

45. Storey T. Whether 'obvious and serious' risk of death in cases of gross negligence manslaughter to be determined both objectively and prospectively: R v Rose [2017] EWCA Crim 1168. *J Crim Law.* 2017;81:343–6.

Chapter | 2

Communication skills

David B. Elliott

2.1 Turning anxious patients into satisfied ones

2.1.1 Patient satisfaction is linked to good communication skills

The research literature consistently indicates that patient satisfaction is linked with clinicians having good communication skills: being able to explain diagnoses, prognoses, treatment, and prevention using clear, non-technical terms and being honest, empathic, and able to listen well and address patient concerns.[1] Good communicators are popular with their patients, and good communication skills lead to the majority of your patients returning for future appointments; those patients inform their friends and family so that your patient base increases and you are less likely to be involved in lawsuits.[1]

2.1.2 Why are some patients anxious?

Poor patient satisfaction is linked with preconsultation patient anxiety.[2] A significant number of patients are anxious about attending an optometric examination[3,4] and particularly fear receiving 'bad news' of one form or another.[4] Patients need not display obvious signs of anxiety, and it can be useful to assume all patients have some level of anxiety prior to the examination. Anxiety reduces patient–clinician communication and causes reduced attention, recall of information, and compliance with treatment.[4] This limits the usefulness of the examination because anxious patients are unlikely to provide a full case history and reveal all their visual problems, unlikely to attend appropriately to your instructions, could provide unreliable responses in the subjective refraction, and could easily misinterpret or forget what you said about their diagnoses and management plans. To be empathic, you need to be aware of possible reasons for patient anxiety and these include:

(a) Being told they need glasses.[3] This can be a worry for both prepresbyopic[5] and presbyopic patients[3] who are concerned about the effect on their appearance.[6,7] Some younger patients report bullying at school because of wearing glasses[6] and elderly patients worry that glasses will make them appear older and more frail.[7]

(b) Fear of vision loss. Particularly true of elderly patients where eye disease is a greater risk.[3,7] There may also be an associated fear of losing their driving licence because of poor vision.[7]

(c) Cost issues. Both young and old patients are worried about the potential cost of glasses and contact lenses.[3,6,7]

(d) Fear of making a mistake. Young and old patients report worrying about making mistakes during the subjective refraction part of the examination.[6–8] This may be because they believe that a mistake on their part could lead to the provision of an incorrect refractive correction in their glasses[8] and/or are worried about feeling foolish if they make a mistake.[7]

(e) Fear of increased ametropia. Some patients worry that wearing glasses will make their eyesight worse[6] and that increasing ametropia will mean thicker and less attractive glasses.[9]

(f) Being told that they cannot wear contact lenses any more. Young contact lens wearers typically report a better vision-related quality of life than glasses wearers[9] and some may worry about being told that they cannot wear contact lenses any more.

(g) Adaptation problems. Many older patients report concerns about being able to adapt to their new glasses.[3]

(h) Fear of looking foolish. Some patients are very tentative about admitting some of their concerns about their vision in case they are made to look foolish by raising the issue. Concerns about vitreous floaters are a typical example of this.

(i) Fear of mental health problems. Charles Bonnet syndrome, in which patients suffer visual hallucinations, is not uncommon in patients with visual impairment, particularly if severe,[10] and patients are worried that they may be developing dementia or other mental health problems.

2.1.3 Building a rapport: relaxing the patient

The entire patient visit needs to be considered as otherwise the 'arrive–wait–prescreen–wait' process could add to patient anxiety prior to meeting the optometrist, particularly given the silence about data collected in prescreening. Good communication skills from reception staff and clinical assistants are hugely important to help relax the patient.

(a) Provide information about the eye examination (via websites, leaflets, pamphlets, and so forth) prior to the appointment because this can reduce anxiety and improve satisfaction with the consultation.[2]

(b) Provide a comfortable and welcoming setting in the practice waiting room. Comfortable chairs, a selection of magazines, some low level music, and so forth can all help to relax the patient. Framed copies of the qualifications of all staff, either in the waiting room or the examination room, can provide reassurance to some patients.

(c) Clinical assistants should fully explain the tests that they are performing and indicate that the test results will be discussed with them by the optometrist.

A good communicator will be able to relax an anxious patient and increase patient satisfaction with the eye examination.[1,2] There are many ways to relax a patient and build a rapport and these include:

(d) It would appear that formal attire is becoming less important than it once was. Research from medicine suggests that although some older patients prefer a formal, 'professional' appearance, there is a wide variation depending on country, setting, and context of care.[11]

(e) First impressions count and some clinicians like to greet patients by name and escort them to the examination room. Smile and make eye contact.[12]

(f) Change the chair height to ensure you are at the same eye level as the patient.[13]

(g) At the start of the case history, pay full attention to your patient and do not look at the screen (or put your pen down). Your posture and style should be relaxed but attentive.

(h) Some clinicians like to chat about non-clinical issues (e.g., weather, holidays, sports teams, parking) prior to the examination to help relax the patient. In this respect, it can be useful to make a note of any relevant information (e.g., a child's favourite sport, sports player, team, author; the patient's pets and their names, their children's successes) to allow you to start a conversation at subsequent visits.

(i) Maintain regular eye contact and use the patient's name at appropriate intervals during the eye examination. The preference for the use of the patient's first or family name can be linked with their age and it can be useful to ask which your patient prefers. Your tone of voice and intonation should match what you are saying.[12]

(j) An open question is typically used to start the case history (section 2.3.1, step 3) as this allows patients to tell you about any problems with their vision or glasses. A balance is required between allowing patients plenty of time to discuss their problems and not rushing them, but at the same time retaining control of the discussion. You need to ensure that patients feel that you have fully listened and understood their problems and you may even need to allow them to talk about information that you know is not necessary from a diagnostic viewpoint. However, you also need to develop the skill of being able to interrupt an overly talkative patient without appearing rude.

(k) Some patients are very shy, and an open question provides little information and may make the patient feel uncomfortable. Closed questions (i.e., that have a yes or no answer, such as "do you have any problems seeing the whiteboard at school?") can be useful at the beginning of the case history with such patients. An open question can be used later in the case history if the patient relaxes and conversation becomes easier.

(l) Listening is a hugely important communication skill. It is vital that you have fully listened to the patient and understood his or her problems.[2] There are a variety of cues to indicate to the patient that you are listening, and these include maintaining eye contact and demonstrating attention by nodding and/or using affirmative comments such as "I see," "I understand," "OK," and "go on,".[12] Listening is also indicated by using follow-up questions to comments, such as asking about the location, onset, frequency, and so forth of headaches when the patient indicates suffering with them. Finally, summarising the patient's problems at the end of the case history (see section 2.3.1, step 10) is a useful way of indicating to patients that you have listened to what they have to say and fully understand what problems they are having, and it also provides the patient with an opportunity to inform you if you have missed anything.

(m) Provide a brief explanation to the patient of each test that you use during the eye examination. Patient knowledge about the contents of an eye examination is poor,[6,8] and patients indicate they want to be better informed.[8] Suggested information, in lay terms, is provided for each test described in later chapters.

2.1.4 How to improve your communication skills

All students should gain adequate communication skills via lectures, reading,[13] and clinic feedback. How do you become a better communicator? A helpful quality about communication skills is that you can learn them anywhere and from anybody. Obviously observing an optometrist or another health professional who is popular with patients could be particularly beneficial. You can also learn by experience so that any summer job that involves working with the general public can be valuable. Indeed, it is obvious from the level of communication skills shown in clinics, which students have had jobs that involved working with the general public and which ones have not. Finally, recording yourself performing a case history and/or eye examination can be a valuable tool and will particularly highlight your non-verbal communication skills. Review the recording with a colleague and critique your non-verbal communications skills. Try to avoid negative non-verbal communication cues such as a blank, unresponsive face, minimal eye contact, long silences, none or few affirmative gestures, inattentive or anxious gestures such as touching your face/hair or twirling a pen, leaning backwards, using a closed body position (arm across your body, legs crossed) or a dull, quiet tone of voice with no intonation.[12]

2.2 The importance of recording

It is essential that all test results (including the 'results' from case history-taking and the discussion of diagnoses

and management plans) are recorded. If they are not recorded, subsequent legal analysis of the records will conclude that they were not performed.

2.2.1 Electronic health records

A large and increasing number of optometric records are now computer-based[14] and avoid the problem of illegible handwritten records and should reduce the likelihood of lost records (assuming appropriate backup arrangements), which were a significant problem with card-based systems.[15] Other advantages of electronic records over card-based systems include that information from a previous record can be uploaded and then amended with information from the current examination (this can also be done for the right and left eyes); they can be linked to digital ocular photographs, and referral letters are easier to produce and print.[14] Electronic health records vary widely and will continue to improve, but current disadvantages of many systems include the inability to sketch various features (e.g., cataract and fluorescein staining patterns) if digital photography of both the external and internal eye is not available; getting used to different systems can be difficult for locum optometrists; going to a complete computer system means that some companies scan old paper records which can become more illegible by that process; copying information from previous records or the other eye can lead to information overload and/or that you forget to put in details; drop-down lists can become very long and it can be difficult to get an overall picture of a patient because of the fragmented nature of the information. The latter can mean it is difficult to highlight important details as with a paper record card where you can write it in large capitals/highlighter on the front page.

2.3 Case history-taking

The case history is the cornerstone of an eye examination. It puts you in the position of detective: there are often problems to discover and you must use all your skills of observation, listening to what patients say and how they say it, and questioning to identify their problems as completely as possible. A summary is provided in Box 2.1. The case history is complicated and takes many years to learn well, so that the procedure described here begins with the simplest case of a patient without symptoms or glasses. It builds from that to a patient who wears glasses and contact lenses (CLs), but has no problems, then to a patient with oculo-visual problems, and finally discusses additional questions that should be asked of specific patients.

Box 2.1 **Summary of case history procedure**

1. Determine the chief complaint (CC). Use LOFTSEA or similar to collect all the appropriate information.
2. Refractive correction If not part of the CC, determine the type, number, and age of glasses and/or contact lenses worn, the quality of vision at distance and near with each, and the quality of vision without as appropriate.
3. Vision. If no Rx is worn, ask about the quality of vision at distance and near.
4. Symptoms. If not part of the CC, ask about symptoms of headaches, eyestrain, pain or discomfort, diplopia, and flashes and floaters.
5. Ocular history. Ask about the patient's ocular history, family ocular history, and LEE.
6. General health. Ask about the patient's general health, medications, allergies, family medical history, and LME.
7. Occupation, sports, hobbies, computer use, and driving.
8. Summarise the case history.
9. Remember that a case history continues throughout the examination.

2.3.1 The most basic case history

The case history of a patient who does not wear glasses or CLs and has no oculo-visual problems is described first because it is the simplest case history to perform. This section describes what questions you should ask (in lay terms), in what order and how to record the answers (an example of recording a basic case history is given in section 2.3.8a): It can be useful to master this case history first, before building on it with more complicated case histories described in subsequent sections.

1. Welcome the patient and introduce yourself.
2. Sit about 1 m from the patient at eye level. Your posture and style should be relaxed but attentive. Lean slightly forward toward the patient. Try to avoid long silences while writing notes and learn to type or write down answers in abbreviated form (Table 2.1) as the patient is talking, while retaining intermittent eye contact.
3. Chief complaint (CC) or reason for visit (RFV): Determine the CC by asking an open-ended question such as "Are you having any problems with your vision or your eyes?" In this example, the patient reports no vision or eye problems and has just attended for a routine eye examination.
4. Glasses/CLs. Ask "Do you wear glasses or contact lenses at all?" In this scenario, the answer is no, so ask whether the patient has ever worn glasses or CLs.
5. Last eye exam (LEE). Ask the patient when and where was their LEE. Ask if the optometrist reported any problems at that time.

6. Visual demands. Ask about the patient's distance and near vision and tailor the question to the patient's vocation and/or hobbies. For example, "How is your distance vision?" "What are the visual demands of your job?" "Can you see the white board at school?" "How about the TV?" "Do you drive?" "How is your vision for driving?"
   "How is your near vision?" "Is reading OK?" "Can you see your music sheets when playing the piano?" For presbyopic patients, you need to discover the distance used for computer use, reading, and other near tasks such as sewing, reading music, and so forth and the use of any additional reading lights (e.g., angle-poise or goose-neck lights; see section 3.2).
   It can be particularly useful to ask patients about contact sports (football, rugby, hockey), swimming, fishing, and racquet sports and whether ametropic patients wear their glasses or contact lenses for these sports and activities, so that they can be advised appropriately (see section 2.4.2).
7. Symptoms. Ask about the most prevalent oculo-visual symptoms. "Do you suffer from headaches?" "Any double vision?" "Any eyestrain?" "Any pain or discomfort in the eyes?" "Do you see flashing lights and floaters?"
8. Ocular history (OH), family ocular history (FOH):
   (a) OH: Ask an open question: "Have you ever had any problems with your eyes at all?" then more specifically: "Have you ever been to the doctor or hospital about your eyes?"
   (b) FOH: Ask an open question such as "Do any eye problems or eye diseases run in the family?" This can be clarified by providing examples of common hereditary conditions (in lay terminology) for their age, gender, and race, if pertinent. For example, for children and young adults ask "Any short-sightedness? . . Squint? . . . Lazy eyes? . . . any colour vision problems?"; for African American, African Caribbean patients over 30 years of age and all other patients over 40, ask about any family history of glaucoma; for patients over 60 ask about any family history of cataract, age-related maculopathy, and glaucoma. Do not ask about specific conditions (e.g., myopia) if you know the patient already has the condition.
   (c) If a patient reports that he or she is adopted, make sure you record this and do not ask about family history at future appointments.
9. General health information.
   (a) Ask "How is your general health?" and add a follow-up question such as "… any high blood pressure or diabetes?" If you receive a positive response, ask the patient how long he or she has had the condition because ocular effects of systemic diseases are more likely the longer the patient has had the condition. For example, the duration of diabetes is a major risk

Table 2.1 Abbreviations that could be used during the recording of a case history

Abbreviation	Stands for	Abbreviation	Stands for
CC (or PC or RFV)	Chief complaint or presenting complaint or reason for visit	Sxs	Symptoms
c/u (or C/U)	Check up	Px (or Pt)	Patient
F/U	Follow-up appointment	Hx	History
DV	Distance vision	LEE	Last eye examination
NV	Near vision	OH	Ocular history
OK	Okay	FOH	Family ocular history
↑	Increase	cat	Cataract
↓	Decrease	AMD/ARMD	Age-related macular degeneration
c̄ (or c)	With	POAG	Primary open-angle glaucoma
s̄ (or s)	Without	GH	General health
Rx	Prescription/glasses	FMH	Family medical history
CLs	Contact lenses	HBP	High blood pressure
RE (or OD)	Right eye	DM	Diabetes mellitus
LE (or OS)	Left eye	CVA	Cerebrovascular accident
B (or binoc)	Binocular	meds	Medication
BE (or OU)	Both eyes	Ung.	Ointment
1/7, 3/7	1 day, 3 days	o.d.	Once daily
1/52, 3/52	1 week, 3 weeks	b.i.d. (or b.d.)	Twice a day
1/12, 3/12	1 month, 3 months	t.i.d.	Three times a day
HA (or H/A)	Headaches	q.i.d.	Four times a day
Dip	Diplopia	p.r.n.	When needed
H	Horizontal	q.h.	Every hour
V	Vertical		
Fl & Fl	Flashes and floaters	LME	Last medical examination

A tick (✓) used to be used to indicate 'OK', 'good', or 'fine', but has been fallen out of favour owing to its misuse in other parts of the record card.

factor for vascular complications of diabetes, including diabetic retinopathy.[16] If the patient has diabetes or hypertension, ask how well the condition is controlled. The risk of diabetic retinopathy is greatly reduced with good glycaemic control in diabetic patients and by good blood pressure control in a patient with diabetes and hypertension.[16]

(b) Ask "Do you take any medications?" It is important to ask this even if patients say that their general health is good because some patients believe their general health is fine when it is controlled by

medication. Patients may also be taking medications, but are unsure why because the medical diagnosis was not properly explained or was poorly understood. Note that some drugs can have adverse ocular effects, such as beta-blockers (dry eyes) and oral corticosteroids (posterior subcapsular cataracts). If you receive a positive response, ask the patient the number and dosage of the drug and how long the patient has been taking it because this will influence the likelihood of adverse effects. Note that patients may not consider 'over-the-counter' tablets (including travel sickness pills, antihistamines, sleeping pills, and painkillers), inhalers, or eyedrops as medications, so it can be useful to ask about them specifically, particularly with patients with unexplained symptoms. Similarly, female patients may not consider birth control pills to be medication, yet the drugs in these pills can have adverse ocular effects.

(c) Ask whether the patient has any allergies.

(d) Family medical history (FMH): Ask an open question, clarified by examples, such as 'Has anybody in your family had any medical problem?' This can be clarified by providing examples of common hereditary conditions such as 'any diabetes or high blood pressure in the family?'

(e) Last medical examination (LME): Ask the patient when was your last visit to a physician and obtain the name of the physician.

10. Summary: Summarise the *pertinent* information from the case history and allow the patient to clarify any misunderstanding on your part or to add any additional information that has been missed.[17] For example, "So, Mr. Hazard, you are having no problems with your vision or your eyes and you are just here for a routine eye examination, is that correct? Are there any issues that I've missed?"

2.3.2 Case history for a patient with glasses and contact lenses but without visual problems

This builds upon the basic case history described in 2.3.1. However, at step 4, the patient indicates that they wear glasses and/or contact lenses. Step 4 is now as follows (an example of the recording is given in section 2.3.8b):

(4a) If the patient wears glasses (ask if you are unsure), you need a complete description of them.

(i) "When do you wear your glasses?"

(ii) "How is your distance vision in your glasses?" followed up by "Do you feel it is as good as it was when you first got them?" This can be adapted to suit the patient. For example, a student could be asked "Any problems reading from the whiteboard?" and "Is everything clear on the TV?"

(iii) "Any problems with reading with the glasses?"

(iv) "How is your distance/near vision without your glasses?"

(v) "How old are your glasses?"

(vi) "How many pairs of glasses do you have?"

(vii) "Where did you get these glasses?"

(viii) "How old were you when you first wore glasses?"

(ix) "Do you have prescription sunglasses?"

(4b) If you are unsure, ask if the patient wears contact lenses. If the patient does wear lenses, even if only

occasionally, then you need a complete description of them.[17]

(i) "What type of lens are they?" (e.g., soft, gas-permeable, toric, multifocal, and brand if known)

(ii) If relevant (i.e., not single use lenses): "How old are your current lenses?" "How often do you replace your lenses?" and "What care solutions do you use?"

(iii) "How long do you usually wear the lenses each day?" and "How many days per week?" The first question can be confirmed by asking when the lenses are typically inserted and when they are removed, because average wearing times are typically underestimated.

(v) "How is your vision with contact lenses and how does it compare with the vision you get with your glasses?" If the patient wears both glasses and contact lenses, you will have to ask about visual symptoms (i.e., distance blur, near blur, headaches, eyestrain) for both forms of correction.

(vi) "Are you currently having any problems with your contact lenses?"

(vii) "When was your last contact lens aftercare and when is your next aftercare check scheduled?"

2.3.3 Case history for a patient who reports a chief complaint

This further builds upon the basic case history described in section 2.3.1. At step 3, the patient indicates that they have a chief complaint. Step 3 now needs to include a series of questions aimed at obtaining a full description of the chief complaint. An example of the recording is given in section 2.3.8c. Students can be guided to which questions to ask by the mnemonic **LOFTSEA** and examples of LOFTSEA-guided questions for CCs of blurred vision, headaches or diplopia include:

(3a) L - Location/laterality

• "Is it more blurred in one eye or is it the same in both?"

• "In which part of the head is the headache located?" *For a frontal headache, ask* "Is it above one eye more than the other?"

• "Is the double vision in all directions of gaze or just one?"

(3b) O - Onset

• "When did the blurred vision/headaches/double vision start?"

(3c) F - Frequency

• "How often do you get headaches?" Prompt if the patient is unsure: "Every day? Once a week? Once a month?" "Are they any better on weekends?" "Do they tend to occur at any particular time of day? Morning mainly or evening?"

• "How often do you get double vision?" "How long does it last?" "Does the double vision occur after a lot of reading or at any time?"

(3d) T - Type
- "Did the blurred vision start suddenly or gradually?" *If sudden vision loss, ask* "Was the vision loss partial or total?"
- "Is it a throbbing, sharp, or dull headache?"
- "Is the double vision one on top of the other or side by side?"

(3e) S - Self-treatment
- "How have you coped with the blurred vision?" (e.g., possibly by squinting, sitting at the front of the class, sitting close to the TV, using ready readers, borrowing a family member's glasses).
- "Does anything make the headaches go away?" "Do you take any painkillers for the headaches?"
- "Does the double vision disappear if you close one eye?"

(3f) E - Effect on the patient
- "How is your son's school work progressing?" "Does it affect your hobbies or sports?" "Is your poor vision affecting how well you can do your job?" "Have you restricted your driving?" "How well do you manage driving at night?"
- "How badly do the headaches affect you?" "Have you been to see your GP (general practitioner/physician) about the headaches?"

(3g) A - Associated factors
- "Are there any other symptoms associated with the problem?"

6-7. Depending on the patient's chief complaint, you will have asked some questions listed in section 2.3.1's steps 6–7 and whether these symptoms occurred with and without glasses/CLs. You now need to ask about visual issues in 2.3.1's steps 6-7 not yet discussed to 'fill in the gaps'. For example, if a patient has a chief complaint of headaches, once you have a complete description of the headaches and whether they are better with or without any glasses or contact lenses, you need to ask about the patient's distance vision, near vision, eyestrain, pain or discomfort and diplopia (with and without glasses as appropriate) and flashing lights, and floaters. If a positive response to any of these questions is obtained, you then need to obtain a complete description. (See online video 2.1.)

2.3.4 Additional questions: birth history

Additional questions may be required, depending on the patient's age and/or other factors. With very young patients, you may need to ask your patient's parent/caregiver about the child's birth history because of the high prevalence of ocular abnormality (including retinopathy of prematurity, strabismus, and refractive error) in children born preterm, those with low birth weight or disorders of the central nervous system, and in children with significant birth complications (e.g., forceps delivery). Was the child a full-term baby or was the child born prematurely? What was the birth weight? (Less than 2000 g or 5 lbs is a significant risk factor for strabismus, in particular esotropia).[18] Were there significant complications at the child's birth? Is the child's current and past general health good? Since birth, has the child been investigated or received treatment for any medical condition?

2.3.5 Additional questions: patient at risk of falls

Falls are very common in the elderly, with about a third of people over 65 falling at least once per year, which can cause significant morbidity and mortality, with more than 80% of accidental deaths in this age group being caused by falls.[19] Patients with risk factors for falls should be asked: "Have you had any falls in the last year?" Risk factors include being over 75 years of age, using more than three medications (polypharmacy), antidepressant use, systemic conditions that reduce mobility, cardiac problems, diabetes, and inner ear problems. A history of falls is an important risk factor for subsequent falls and patients at high risk of falling need to be identified as they should have more regular eye examinations, earlier cataract surgery, and an altered glasses prescribing strategy (section 4.15.4).[19]

2.3.6 Additional questions: patients who smoke cigarettes

Cigarette smoking is a significant preventable risk factor for both age-related macular degeneration and cataract.[20] Patients report being comfortable being asked about cigarette smoking by their optometrist[21] and you should certainly ask patients with a family history or early signs of age-related cataract and macular degeneration: "Do you smoke?" If the patient appears uncomfortable with you asking this question (or you do), you can indicate the reason for asking: "Cigarette smoking is strongly linked with two major eye diseases" or similar. Follow-up questions of "For how long?" and "Typically how many per day?" can be used to determine whether the patient is a heavy or light smoker. These questions are probably best asked as part of the 'general health' section of the case history.

It can be very useful to ask patients who smoke whether they want to stop smoking and provide support for tobacco cessation.[21] The likelihood of optometrists asking these questions may vary across countries, and it seems likely that optometrists would be more involved in this process where there are national social marketing campaigns linking blindness and smoking. Australia became the first country to include a picture warning label on cigarettes to link blindness and smoking in 2007, and this has increased levels of awareness compared with other countries that have not yet introduced these warning labels.[22] Optometrists are in an excellent position to help people to stop smoking because fear of blindness is a potentially important motivator.[21]

2.3.7 Additional tips

Once you become more experienced, you will start the differential diagnosis process even before you begin the case history.

1. Consider the patient's age (gender and ethnicity may also be important) because this can provide useful clues to what problems the patient may have, given the known epidemiology of certain ocular problems (e.g., presbyopia in a 47-year-old patient attending a first eye examination).
2. Observe the patient's stature, walking ability, and overall physical appearance. Pay particular attention to any head tilt or obvious abnormalities of the face, eyelids, and eyes that will require further investigation, such as facial asymmetry, lid lesions, ptosis, epiphora, entropion, ectropion, a red eye, or strabismus.

2.3.8 Recording

Both positive and negative patient responses must be recorded. Remember that from a legal viewpoint, if the response was not recorded the question was not asked. Abbreviations are essential to allow a sufficiently complete case history to be recorded, while retaining intermittent eye contact with the patient, which is required for good communication and building a rapport. Use standard abbreviations (see Table 2.1) and avoid personal ones. Using the patient's own words, recorded in quotation marks, can be useful. Here are some examples:

(a) Relevant to section 2.3.1: 10-year-old boy
RFV: Routine 2-year exam. No glasses/CLs. No problems. DV & NV good. No ha, eyestrain, pain, dip, Fl & Fl or other Sxs.
OH: No probs, never been to HES. LEE: 2 years, Dr. Salah, Liverpool; no issues. No FOH, no ambly, strab, myopia, or col def.
GH. Good, no meds, no allergies. FMH: None, no DM, no HBP. LME: 2/12, Dr. Firmino, Liverpool. Hobbies: Football and Video games.

(b) Relevant to section 2.3.2: 68-year-old Asian female (retired)
RFV: Routine 2-year exam. No probs. DV & NV good c̄ Rx. Bifs, worn all time. No ha, eyestrain, pain, dip, Fl & Fl or other Sxs.
OH: 1st wore bifs age 50, this Rx 2 years old. No other OH. Never worn CLs. LEE: 2 years, Dr. Aguero, Manchester. No FOH, no cat, AMD or glauc.
GH. Type II DM for 15 years, Metformin 500 mg bid, well controlled; high BP for 15 years, Propranolol 100 mg, bid, well controlled, CU every 6/12; high cholesterol last

2 years, "statins" 40 mg od now under control; aspirin od, last 3 years to "thin blood" & "help avoid heart attack," CU every 6/12; non-smoker and no history of falls.
LME: 2/12, Dr. Sterling, Manchester. No allergies, FMH: DM type II in family. Hobbies: Walking, watching TV. No PC use. Doesn't drive.

(c) Relevant to section 2.3.3: 25-year-old Px. Caucasian. Secretary
CC: DV ↓ for driving, c̄ CLs and > c̄ specs, esp. @ night last 2/12, RE blur>LE. Better c̄ squinting. NV c̄ Cls & specs OK. No HA, no dip, no eyestrain, no Fl & Fl, no discomfort. No other Sxs.
OH: Specs ~ 4 years old – not updated LEE 2 years ago. Worn soft CLs last 6 years: 6/7 & ~10/24. Comfortable for ~8/24 then sl. gritty. Monthlies brand X, multi sol'n brand Y. Fitted by Dr Son, London. Last AC 18/12 ago. Overdue a check. No probs c̄ CLs and no other OH. FOH: parents both myopic.
GH: OK, no meds. No allergies. Non-smoker. LME: 12/12, Dr. Kane, London. FMH: pat grandfather has heart disease.
Hobbies: Tennis, climbing. Uses PC ~ 5/24, 6/7.

2.3.9 Most common errors

1. Too much writing and long silences.
2. Asking questions in a random, unorganised manner (as you remember them).
3. Using leading questions. For example, "so you wear your glasses all the time?"; as the patient may assume that you expect the answer suggested and thus respond positively.
4. Not fully investigating the patient's chief complaint. Use LOFTSEA to remind you of what questions are needed.

2.4 The 5 Rs: providing diagnoses and management plan information

Patients expect you to provide information about the cause of their visual problems, the prognoses, and any management plans, all in a clear non-technical language.[1] (See online videos 2.2 to 2.4.) The 5 Rs can be used as a reminder of the five steps involved:

1. **Repeat/Remind:** patients of the symptoms they reported.
2. **Results:** describe your results and diagnosis that explains the symptoms in lay terms.
3. **Recommend:** the best available management plans that will solve the problem
4. **Recall:** indicate when you would like to see the patient again. Link this to the prognosis of the condition.

5. **Record:** your diagnoses and management plans
   A sixth R, **Reassure**, can be used when appropriate.

2.4.1 *Remind* patients of their symptoms and link this to your *Results*

1. Indicate the eye examination has finished and you wish to discuss your findings. You may put down your pen and even turn off your chart. Make eye contact with the patient and make sure that the patient is comfortable and attentive.
2. *Remind* the patient of the patient's symptoms. Use the patient's own words here; this is why it is useful to record them.
3. Link them with your diagnosis (your *Results*).
4. Explain what the ametropia or eye disease is in simple lay terms. Give the patient time to digest the information and encourage the patient to ask questions.
5. Use photographs to help your explanation (Fig. 2.1). Most computer-based programs also include diagrams to help you with this explanation.

2.4.2 *Recommend*. Explain the best available management plans

1. Present the various options available, with their advantages and disadvantages, and involve the patient in the decision of the most appropriate management.

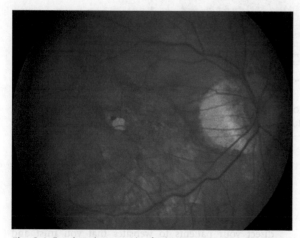

Fig. 2.1 Fundus photograph of a high myope. The thin retina could be highlighted: visible choroidal vessels beneath the retina, retinal atrophic area, and peripapillary atrophy at the disc. This could lead to a discussion of the actions to be taken should the patient suffer symptoms of retinal detachment and the need to avoid activities such as boxing or bungee jumping.

2. Demonstrate any refractive correction changes to the patient. Computerised phoropters can swiftly move from the patient's habitual correction to the new prescription. A simple approach is to show the change in distance and/or near visual acuity with appropriate spherical trial case lenses over the top of their current glasses, given that cylindrical changes from one examination to the next tend to be minor.
3. Explain when the patient should wear glasses. Do not assume that the patient will understand when to wear them. For example, if a patient's CC was distance blur when driving, it may not be enough to indicate that he or she should wear the glasses for driving and assume that the patient understands that the glasses can be worn for any other distance vision task. Indicate that the glasses could be used for TV, cinema, and theatre, watching sports, and when walking about outside if the patient wants to wear them for those tasks. In this regard, it is very important to inform patients who drives without glasses whether they are legally allowed to do so.[23]
4. If appropriate explain that progression is expected and why. For example, young myopes can be informed that because a short-sighted eye is a big eye, the myopia will tend to increase as the eye grows with age. Similarly, it can be useful to explain to hyperopes and presbyopes that a gradual reduction in unaided vision is expected with age owing to the gradual loss of their focusing ability caused by the hardening of the eye lens owing to its continual growth. These explanations can be supported by simple explanations of long and short sightedness using cross sectional diagrams (Fig. 2.2).
5. Discuss possible adaptation problems (section 4.15). If making a relatively large change in refractive correction, particularly with older patients, warn them of possible adaptation problems. This is most important when making any cylinder changes, particularly with oblique cylinders. Take note of a patient's previous reaction to refractive correction change. It is better to overestimate rather than underestimate the time that adaptation will take.
6. Occupation, sports, and hobbies: Most clinicians tailor lens information to match the patient's requirements, based on the patient's occupation and hobbies.[3] Contact lens wearers are advised not to wear their lenses for swimming and to wear prescription swimming goggles, or to wear a single use lens with standard swimming goggles, and dispose of the lens immediately after swimming.[24] Ametropes who play contact sports benefit from using contact lenses as they usually do not wear their glasses while playing, although some football/soccer players do wear glasses and should be informed of protective eyewear.[25] Contact lenses will also have benefits for many other sports and leisure activities in that they can provide a wider field of view and they are

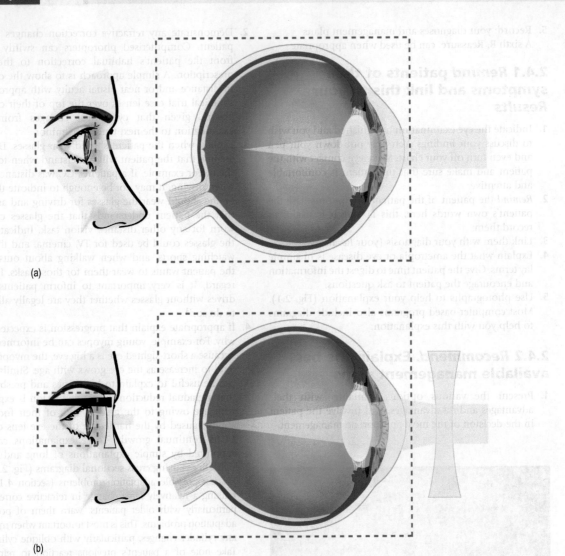

Fig. 2.2 Cross-sectional diagram showing light focusing in front of the retina in a 'large' myopic eye **(A)** and being focused onto the retina with concave lenses **(B)**. (Courtesy of Samantha Strong.)

not affected by fogging up or rain, for example. At the same time, contact lenses provide no eye protection, which can be important for sports that involve a high speed ball/puck and a stick, such as cricket, baseball, hockey (ice and field), lacrosse, and squash. [25] Finally, safety glasses may be needed for do-it-yourself (DIY) enthusiasts and keen gardeners and fishing is made easier and more comfortable with polarised sunglasses.

7. Patients increasingly obtain their health information from the internet,[26] but complementary therapies

and treatments with a poor evidence base are often presented more positively than established, evidence-based treatments[26,27] so that it can be very useful to direct your patients to websites that you trust and that provide jargon-free clearly presented material.[28] The number of optometrists recommending websites to their patients appears low and well behind other medical professions[29] and this should be improved because there are very good websites that we can refer patients to, including patient-facing websites developed by international optometry professional bodies.[30] These include:

(a) (UK) https://lookafteryoureyes.org
(b) (USA) https://www.allaboutvision.com
(c) (Australia) http://www.optometry.org.au/your-eyes.aspx
(d) The UK's National Health Service also provides a patient-friendly website (https://www.nhs.uk/conditions/) for a wide range of conditions with translations into 90 languages; the major support group agencies for eye conditions such as macular degeneration all have dedicated websites.

8. Instructions regarding contact lens care and maintenance and ocular disease management should be clear and unambiguous, with appropriate emphasis placed on the importance of procedures from a safety viewpoint.[17] Written instructions at an easy reading level (age ~8–12 years) are essential. Checking compliance, explaining the benefits of compliant behaviours, and repeating the instructions at follow-up visits can improve matters.

2.4.3 *Reassure* when appropriate

1. If the cause of the CC or other problem is not determined, then present your negative findings in a positive manner.[31] For example, nonocular headaches: "I do not believe that your headaches are caused by a problem with your eyes or vision, Mr. Aubameyang. Your eyesight is excellent and there is no need for glasses/change in glasses; your eye muscles and focusing muscles are all working normally and are working well together and there is no sign of eye disease from any of the tests that I have performed".
2. If the condition can be diagnosed, but no treatment is necessary, in addition to providing diagnosis and prognosis information in lay terms, reassure patients that they were correct in attending for examination.[31] An example would be pingueculae.
3. If a patient's attendance for an eye examination was because of increased risk of a certain condition, but you found no problems, reassure the patient that you have performed the necessary tests and confirm the reasons that the patient should regularly attend for examination. An example would be a patient with a family history of glaucoma that showed normal values for all assessments. In such a case, it can be useful to display the fundus photograph and visual field plots on your computer screen and explain what you found at and around the optic nerve head (Fig. 2.3) and what the field plot shows.
4. Reassuring patients with visual impairment and Charles Bonnet syndrome that the condition is benign and is a common response after vision loss and is not related to dementia or other mental health problems relieves concern among patients and their families.[10] Patients should be informed that, although visual

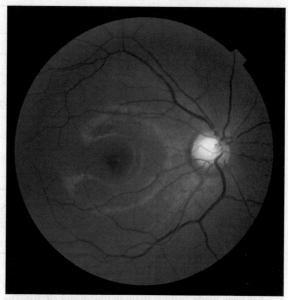

Fig. 2.3 This photograph of a British African-Caribbean fundus could be used to describe the healthy neural retinal rim on the disc and visible and healthy nerve fibre layers.

hallucinations may persist for years in some cases, they usually resolve spontaneously. Provision of a leaflet or link to an appropriate website can be useful.

2.4.4 *Recall*

1. Finally, indicate to the patient when you would like to see him or her again. This should be linked to the likely prognosis of the patient's condition(s).
2. Always inform patients that if they have any problems with their vision or their eyes before that time, they should make an appointment to see you.

2.4.5 *Record* diagnoses and management plans

It is important legally to document all your diagnoses and management plans. Similarly, it provides valuable support when dealing with patients who return with complaints that you did not provide advice regarding the management of a certain condition.

1. List each separate diagnosis in a column. Do not list the individual symptoms and signs that allowed the diagnosis. Order diagnoses with the most important first.
2. For each diagnosis, outline a plan or a series of actions to be taken in an adjoining column. This should include any advice given and supporting information provided via website links or leaflets given.

Table 2.2 Two examples of diagnosis-plan lists

No.	Diagnosis	Plan
(a)		
1	First time myope	Rx for b/board, TV, etc. Counselled to read and play s̄ Rx.
		Coun. Re typical progression and future changes in myopia. Provided link to College myopia webpage.
2	Moderate protan	Coun. Re colour vision problems and effects on career choices. Linked to NHS website.
(b)		
1	Hyperope and presbyope	Rx PALs (used previously).
		Coun. Re typical progression of presbyopia. Given leaflet.
2	High IOP and large CD ratio	Appt. made for full threshold VFs and gonio.
		Coun. Re reason for extra tests.

3. If a patient has symptoms or signs for which no diagnosis has been made, include them in the 'diagnosis' list. The management plan would be the testing required for further investigation.
4. Examples of diagnosis-plan lists are provided in Table 2.2.

2.4.6 Most common errors

1. Using technical language and jargon to explain diagnoses and treatment plans.
2. Not explaining to myopes, hyperopes, and presbyopes the likely progression of their condition.
3. Not explaining to patients when they should wear their glasses.
4. Not warning appropriate patients about possible adaptation problems.
5. Not using website links to provide patient information.

2.5 Giving bad news

2.5.1 "I find it so difficult"

There are many reasons why clinicians find it difficult to give bad news and these include:[13]

- The 'messenger' fears being blamed
- Not knowing how best to do it
- Reluctance to upset the patient
- Not knowing the patient and the patient's sources of support
- Fearing the patient's emotional reaction

Giving bad news can cause some clinicians to delay or avoid it or to provide overly optimistic information.[32] Remember that although the information will be very sad

for the patient, the patient needs understandable, personalised, accurate, and complete information, provided empathically, to properly plan for the future.[13]

2.5.2 Points to consider

In can be very useful to reflect on how you have been given bad news yourself and whether it was delivered well or poorly. Points to consider include the following:[13,32,33]

1. Indicate the eye examination has finished and you wish to discuss your findings. You may put down your pen and even turn off the chart. Make eye contact with the patient and make sure that the patient is comfortable and attentive. It can be helpful to have some tissues ready in case the patient becomes upset. It can be very useful to explain all this information to one or two family members if they are present[33] and if the patient is happy for you to do so.
2. Give an indication that bad news is coming. "I am afraid that your poor vision cannot be simply fixed." Your facial expression and demeanour should contribute to the fact that you are about to provide bad news. Pause to allow the patient to prepare for the news.[13]
3. Introduce your diagnosis by *Reminding* the patient of the symptoms and then link them with the diagnosis (*Result*). Explain what the eye disease is in simple lay terms. A photograph of the condition can be very helpful (see Figure 2.1).
4. Give the information in small chunks if possible to allow the patient time to digest the information and encourage the patient to ask questions.
5. For patients with dry age-related macular degeneration, for example, you should explain that they will not go 'blind' and should keep their peripheral vision. However, at the same time you must be honest and do

not attempt to avoid difficult questions or even 'sugar the pill.'[32] Indicate that their central, detailed vision that allows them to drive, read, and see faces is likely to get worse. Blunt statements such as "I am afraid that there is nothing more that we can do" are not helpful. This may be correct for conventional treatment with glasses, but low vision aids may be helpful for a variety of tasks. Household modifications can be made (section 3.3.7) and smoking cessation can slow progression.[21,34]

6. Empathic statements such as "I know this is not what you wanted to hear. I wish the news were better" can be helpful.[33]

7. You need to be aware of the possible emotional responses to such news. Various models have been proposed, and a common model suggests stages of denial, anger, bargaining, depression, and acceptance. These stages are not universal and some patients skip stages whereas others get 'stuck' at a particular stage. In the denial stage, patients will often seek a second opinion. You should not see this as a slight on your ability as a clinician and you may even suggest it to patients who are openly in denial when you first tell them the news.

8. Explain the prevalence of the condition. This indicates that they are not alone. It can be very useful at this point to discuss support groups and local agencies. Support groups enable patients to meet other individuals suffering from a similar problem. They can discuss their experiences with each other, provide reassurance, and offer tips that have helped them cope.

9. Discuss the availability of low vision aids and what help they could provide. In this respect, remember the stages of response to vision loss. Patients are unlikely to have the motivation to use low vision aids successfully when depressed. Do not give up on these patients. As (and when) they overcome the depression and accept their vision loss, low vision aids may usefully be provided.[34]

10. Information leaflets and/or websites are particularly useful in these situations because the patient's shock at the initial news may mean that much of the remainder of your discussion is forgotten. Make sure the leaflets and websites include links to support groups.

2.6 What should a good referral letter include?

Letters of referral to medical personnel or specialist clinicians are required to provide information regarding the reason and urgency of referral. Reports may be required to a referring colleague, teacher, general physician, and so forth. The categories of patients who require a report may be covered by legal or contractual obligations.

2.6.1 Comparison of letter types

Structured referral forms have a standardised format and various boxes to complete. These can save time and, if well designed, may reduce the possibility of the omission of pertinent information. However, non-specific optometry referral forms can lead to the inclusion of irrelevant information and a lack of required details.[35] Referral forms specifically designed for commonly referred conditions, such as cataract, glaucoma, and macular disease, particularly when supported by referral guidelines for such conditions, are likely to improve referral quality,[35] and these can be easily provided within an electronic referral system.[36] Well-written referral letters are important to help develop a good relationship with secondary eye care personnel and increase the likelihood of feedback being obtained regarding referrals. The latter is essential to improve referral quality, especially for newly qualified optometrists.[37]

2.6.2 Procedure for producing a personalised referral letter

Because completing a structured referral sheet is somewhat self-explanatory, the procedure for producing an effective personalised referral letter is described.

1. Indicate to the patient that you will be sending a referral letter/report to another person or office. You should inform the patient of the reason for the referral or report.

2. Write the letter on headed notepaper that includes your practice address and contact information. The letter should ideally not be hand written, as this will make it less legible.

3. Include the date and the recipient's name and address at the top of the letter.

4. Begin the letter with the patient's name, address, date of birth (you may need to distinguish between several people with the same name and even between two people with the same name and address), appointment date, and file number (if applicable).

5. Remember that the person you are writing to is likely to be very busy and want to read only essential information.

6. A likely outline of a referral letter would be:
   (a) Provide a diagnosis or tentative diagnosis if possible.
   (b) Indicate the relevant symptoms (these are symptoms connected to the referral diagnosis, not those connected to any uncorrected ametropia or dry eye, for example).
   (c) Include any relevant signs and provide an image if available.
   (d) Indicate if there is any urgency in the referral.
   (e) If appropriate, you might indicate what further investigations or treatment you believe to be necessary.

Box 2.2 Example of a referral letter

21 April 2020
Dr. John Smith:
Bradford Health Centre
Ilkley Road
Bradford
Re: Mrs. Mary Patient, 20 Anyold Street, Somewhere,
Bradford. DOB 21-9-35.
File No. 1234. Appointment date: 20 April 2020.
Referral for cataract surgery
    Dear Dr. Smith:
    Mrs. Patient complains of great difficulty reading
and sewing and is unable to see well when outdoors on
a sunny day. She has nuclear and posterior subcapsular
cataracts in both eyes with visual acuities of 6/9 in each
eye. However, her visual acuities in glare conditions
are 6/18 in both eyes and her Pelli-Robson log contrast
sensitivity scores are right eye 1.05 and left eye 1.10;
these latter clinical assessments represent a fairer
reflection of her functional vision. Both eyes, and
particularly both maculae, otherwise appear healthy.
I have explained the situation to Mrs. Patient and the
options open to her and she wishes to be considered
for cataract surgery.
Yours sincerely
David B. Elliott PhD MCOptom FAAO

Box 2.3 Example of a report

21 April 2020
Ms. Joan Smith
Bradford Primary School
Ilkely Road
Bradford
Re: John Young, 20 Anyold Avenue, Somewhere,
Bradford. DOB 27-8-93. File No. 4321.
Appointment date: 20 April 2020.
Colour vision deficiency
    Dear Ms. Smith
    I saw John for his first eye examination today. He
had no symptoms and his visual acuity was normal at
6/5 in both eyes. However, I found a problem with his
colour vision in that John has deuteranopia (red-green
colour deficiency) and will have difficulty differentiating
between colours such as red, orange, yellow, brown,
and green. There are no effective treatments for this
hereditary condition. I have discussed the restrictions that
this will have on his future career with his family and have
informed his GP as well as yourself. If you require any
further information, please do not hesitate to contact me.
Yours sincerely
David B. Elliott PhD MCOptom FAAO

(f) Request a reply regarding the outcome of the referral. This may require the patient's written consent.

(g) Indicate if you have copied the letter elsewhere (typically to the patient's general physician).

7. If referring a patient because of cataract (the most common referral letter; see Box 2.2) also include[38]:

(a) The effect of reduced vision on the patient's lifestyle.

(b) The patient's willingness to undertake surgery. There is no point in referring a patient who does not wish to have surgery.

8. A likely outline of a report would be:

(a) Thank the referring person (if applicable).

(b) Indicate the relevant symptoms and signs.

(c) Provide a diagnosis or tentative diagnosis if possible.

(d) If a diagnosis is not possible, indicate which tests were performed and any pertinent results.

(e) Indicate any management plan and the time of your intended follow-up appointment.

9. Make sure your spelling is accurate and grammar correct. Spelling and grammar checkers are available on all modern word processing packages.

10. Present the information at a level suitable to the recipient's knowledge. However, do not automatically assume that lay terms are appropriate in a letter to a non-medical person. It may be best to use the correct term with the lay term in brackets to avoid offence. For example, in a letter to a teacher, you may include a statement that 'David has myopia (short-sightedness) …'

11. Sign the letter with your preferred title and qualifications.

12. Keep a copy of the letter for the patient's file. If the letter or report was not to the patient's GP/physician, you may be required to send them a copy. If it is not a requirement, it is usually good practice to do so.

2.6.3 Recording

The style and content of referral letters and reports is likely to vary widely in different countries and areas within a country and because of a variety of other factors. Given this proviso, examples of a referral letter and report are given in Boxes 2.2 and 2.3.

2.6.4 Most common errors

1. In a referral of a patient with cataract, failing to include information regarding the effect on the patient's lifestyle and his or her willingness to undertake surgery.[38]

References

1. Dawn AG, Lee PP. Patient expectations for medical and surgical care: a review of the literature and applications to ophthalmology. *Surv Ophthamol*. 2004;49:513-24.

2. Court H, Greenland K, Margrain TH. Evaluating the association between anxiety and satisfaction. *Optom Vision Sci*. 2009;86:216–21.

3. Fylan F, Grunfeld EA. Visual illusions? Beliefs and behaviours of presbyope clients in optometric practice. *Patient Educ Couns*. 2005;56:291–5.

4. Court H, Greenland K, Margrain TH. Predicting state anxiety in optometric practice. *Optom Vis Sci*. 2009;86:1295-1302.

5. Pesudovs K, Garamendi E, Elliott DB. The quality of life impact of refractive correction (QIRC) questionnaire: development and validation. *Optom Vis Sci*. 2004;81:769-77.

6. Shickle D, Griffin M, Evans R, et al. Why don't younger adults in England go to have their eyes examined? *Ophthalmic Physiol Opt*. 2014;34:30-7.

7. Shickle D, Griffin M. Why don't older adults in England go to have their eyes examined? *Ophthalmic Physiol Opt*. 2014;34:38-45.

8. Irving EL, Sivak AM, Spafford MM. "I can see fine": patient knowledge of eye care. *Ophthalmic Physiol Opt* 2018; 38: 422–31.

9. Pesudovs K, Garamendi E, Elliott DB. A quality of life comparison of people wearing spectacles or contact lenses or having undergone refractive surgery. *J Refract Surg*. 2006;22:19–27.

10. Pang L. Hallucinations experienced by visually impaired: Charles Bonnet Syndrome. *Optom Vis Sci*. 2016;93:1466-78.

11. Petrilli CM, Mack M, Petrilli JJ, Hickner A, Saint S, Chopra V. Understanding the role of physician attire on patient perceptions: a systematic review of the literature—targeting attire to improve likelihood of rapport (TAILOR) investigators. *BMJ Open*. 2015;5:e006578.

12. Park KH, Park SG. The effect of communication training using standardized patients on nonverbal behaviors in medical students. *Korean J Med Educ*. 2018;30:153-9.

13. Lloyd M, Bor R, Noble LM. *Clinical Communication Skills for Medicine*, ed 4. Edinburgh: Elsevier; 2019.

14. Dabasia PL, Edgar DF, Garway-Heath DF, Lawrenson JG. A survey of current and anticipated use of standard and specialist equipment by UK optometrists. *Ophthalmic Physiol Opt*. 2014;34:592–613.

15. Steele CF, Rubin G, Fraser S. Error classification in community optometric practice–a pilot study. *Ophthalmic Physiol Opt*. 2006;26:106–10.

16. Marshall SM, Flyvbjerg A. Prevention and early detection of vascular complications of diabetes. *BMJ*. 2006;333:475–80.

17. Wolffsohn JS, Naroo SA, Christie C, et al. History and symptom taking in contact lens fitting and aftercare. *Cont Lens Anterior Eye*. 2015;38:258–65.

18. Gulati S, Andrews C, Apkarian A, et al. The impact of gestational age and birth weight on the risk of strabismus among premature infants. *JAMA Pediatr* 2014;168:850-6.

19. Elliott DB. The Glenn A. Fry award lecture 2013: blurred vision, spectacle correction, and falls in older adults. *Optom Vis Sci*. 2014;91:593-601.

20. Kennedy RD, Spafford MM, Schultz AS, Iley MD, Zawada V. Smoking cessation referrals in optometric practice: a Canadian pilot study. *Optom Vis Sci*. 2011;88:766-71.

21. Downie LE, Douglass A, Guest D, Keller PR. What do patients think about the role of optometrists in providing advice about smoking and nutrition? *Ophthalmic Physiol Opt*. 2017;37:202–11.

22. Sheck LH, Field AP, McRobbie H, Wilson GA. Helping patients to quit smoking in the busy optometric practice. *Clin Exp Optom*. 2009;92:75–7.

23. Fylan F, Hughes A, Wood JM, Elliott DB. Why do people drive when they can't see clearly? *Transp Res Part F-Traffic Psychol Behav*. 2018;56:123-33.

24. Wu YT, Tran J, Truong M, Harmis N, Zhu H, Stapleton F. Do swimming goggles limit microbial contamination of contact lenses? *Optom Vis Sci*. 2011;88:456–60.

25. Dain SJ. Sports eyewear protective standards. *Clin Exp Optom*. 2016;99:4–23.

26. McGregor F, Somner JE, Bourne RR, Munn-Giddings C, Shah P, Cross V. Social media use by patients with glaucoma: what can we learn?

Ophthalmic Physiol Opt. 2014;34:46-52.

27. Elliott DB. The Bates method, elixirs, potions and other cures for myopia: how do they work? *Ophthalmic Physiol Opt*. 2013;33:75-7.

28. Fylan F, Grunfeld EA. Information within optometric practice: comprehension, preferences and implications. *Ophthalmic Physiol Opt*. 2002;22:333-40.

29. Usher WT. Australian health professionals' health website recommendation trends. *Health Promot J Austr*. 2011;22:134–41.

30. Elliott, DB. Internet-based information about eye conditions for patients could be improved and used more. *Ophthalmic Physiol Opt*. 2015;35:463–4.

31. Blume AJ. Reassurance therapy. In: Amos JF, ed. *Diagnosis and Management in Vision Care*. Boston: Butterworths; 1987:715-18.

32. Hopper SV, Fischbach RL. Patient-physician communication when blindness threatens. *Patient Educ Couns*. 1989;14:69–79.

33. Baile WF, Buckman R, Lenzi R, Glober G, Beale EA, Kudelka AP. SPIKES-A six-step protocol for delivering bad news: application to the patient with cancer. *Oncologist*. 2000;5:302-11.

34. Binns AM, Bunce C, Dickinson C, et al. How effective is low vision service provision? A systematic review. *Surv Ophthalmol*. 2012;57:34-65.

35. Davey CJ, Scally AJ, Green C, Mitchell ES, Elliott DB. Factors influencing accuracy of referral and the likelihood of false positive referral by optometrists in Bradford, United Kingdom. *J Optom*. 2016;9:158–65.

36. Khan AA, Mustafa MZ, Sanders R. Improving patient access to prevent sight loss: ophthalmic electronic referrals and communication (Scotland). *Public Health*. 2015;129:117-23.

37. Parkins DJ, Benwell MJ, Edgar DF, Evans BJW. The relationship between unwarranted variation in optometric referrals and time since qualification. *Ophthalmic Physiol Opt*. 2018;38:550–61.

38. Do VQ, McCluskey P, Palagyi A, et al. Are cataract surgery referrals to public hospitals in Australia poorly targeted? *Clin Exp Ophthalmol*. 2018;46:364–70.

Assessment of visual function

David B. Elliott and John G. Flanagan

3.1 Distance visual acuity

Visual acuity (VA), which is a measure of the patient's ability to resolve fine detail, is the most commonly used measurement of visual function. Distance and reading VAs are used to assess the adequacy of glasses or contact lenses and as a key indicator of ocular health. Distance VA is also used to assess a person's fitness to drive or enter into some professions, such as the police force, and to enable registration as a visually impaired or blind person. However, note that VA only describes a part of how reduced vision affects how a patient functions in day-to-day activities and reductions in contrast sensitivity (section 3.3), visual field (sections 3.6 to 3.10), colour vision (sections 3.4 and 3.5), and stereopsis (section 3.11) must also be considered.

3.1.1 The evidence base: when and how should distance VA be measured

There are three principal measures of VA:

- Unaided VA, often called vision.
- Habitual ('presenting' or 'walk in') VA, with the patient's own glasses, if worn, or without glasses if not worn.
- Optimal VA, with the best refractive correction (i.e., after subjective refraction, see section 4.5).

The term best-corrected visual acuity (BCVA), although widely used in ophthalmology texts, can refer to a wide range of VA types (VA with spectacles, pinhole, autorefractor result, after a subjective spherical over-refraction, etc.) and is best avoided.[1]

Habitual VA should be measured immediately after the case history for legal reasons to document the VA level prior to your examination. Measuring unaided VA (vision) in patients who wear glasses is optional, and should be measured with patients who:

- Have lost/broken their spectacles;
- Do not wear spectacles for some distance viewing tasks (this information must therefore be obtained in the case history);
- Require the information for a report;
- Wear their spectacles all the time for distance and yet you suspect they may not need to (does the young low hyperope need to wear the spectacles for distance tasks?)

VA charts using the logMAR system are widely available on computer-based systems with flat panel displays and are much superior to Snellen charts.[2,3] These VA charts (Fig. 3.1) use the design principles suggested by Bailey and Lovie, including 0.1 logMAR progression of letter size from −0.30 to 1.0 logMAR (VAR 115 to 50; Snellen equivalents of 6/3 to 6/60; 20/10 to 20/200 and

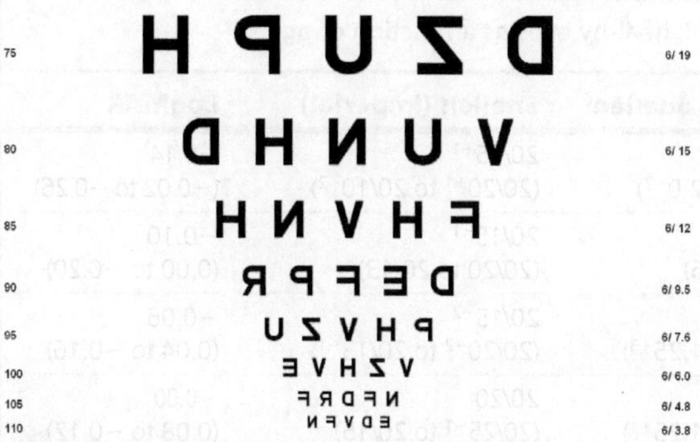

Fig. 3.1 A computer-based logMAR visual acuity chart (viewed by the patient via a mirror).

2.0 to 0.1 in decimal), five letters per line, letters of similar legibility, and per-letter scoring.[2,4] VA measurements using logMAR charts have been shown to be twice as repeatable as those from a Snellen chart and over three times more sensitive to inter-ocular differences in VA and therefore substantially more sensitive to amblyopic changes, for example.[3,5] VA measurements on computer-based systems have the advantage of allowing randomisation of letters, calculation of VA scores, and conversion of VA into different notations. The concern that patients may be worried if they are not able to see the smaller letters on a logMAR chart can be avoided by explaining that the new chart includes lines with smaller text than the old one and indicate, or even highlight, the 100 VAR line (Snellen 6/6, 20/20 or 1.0). Current computer-based VA charts are typically limited by screen sizes, so that lines of letters larger than about 70 VAR (6/24, 0.25, 20/80) have progressively fewer than five letters (Fig. 3.2) and this needs to be considered in measurement and/or recording.

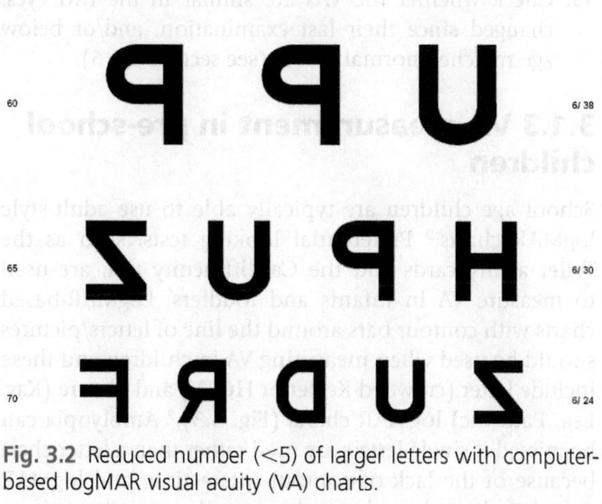

Fig. 3.2 Reduced number (<5) of larger letters with computer-based logMAR visual acuity (VA) charts.

VA is typically assessed at 6 m or 20 feet and can be described in a large variety of formats, including metric (e.g., 6/6), imperial (20/20), and decimal Snellen (1.0), log of the minimum angle of resolution or logMAR (0.0), visual acuity rating or VAR (100) and number of letters read (85).[1,2] Number of letters read is confusing and very rarely matches the actual number of letters read. For example, '85 letters read' (6/6, 20/20, 1.0) on a standard logMAR chart with five letters per line includes only 55 letters from 6/60 (20/200, 0.1) down to the 6/6, 20/20, 1.0 Snellen equivalent line.[1,2] It will not be discussed further. VAs in logMAR are non-intuitive as they get lower as VA improves and high values of VA are negative. In addition, errors can arise when subtracting 0.02 for each letter misread given that $6/9^{-1}$ and $6/7.5^{-1}$ are 0.18 and 0.08 but $6/6^{-1}$ and $6/4.8^{-1}$ are -0.02 and -0.12. Therefore, VAs will be described using VAR because it is simple, intuitive, and recommended with by-letter scoring on a logMAR-design chart[2] and equivalent values in metric, imperial, and decimal Snellen will then be provided because these are widely used and understood throughout different parts of the world.

Snellen charts were devised by the German ophthalmologist Hermann Snellen in 1862 and have been widely used ever since. There is not a standard Snellen chart and the letter size sequences, number of letters and/or numbers and varieties of letters, vary from manufacturer to manufacturer. The majority have one 6/60 (20/200, 0.10) letter, two 6/36 (20/125, 0.17) letters, and three 6/24 (20/80, 0.25) letters. They typically do not contain lines of letters at 6/30 (20/100, 0.20) or 6/48 (20/160, 0.125), and many charts have a bottom line of 6/5 (~20/15, 1.20) and thus provide truncated data given that the *average* VA of a young adult is about 107 VAR (6/4, 20/13, 1.50; Table 3.1) and many see better than this.[6] Measuring VA with a Snellen chart and a bottom line of 6/6 (20/20, 1.0) or even 6/5 (~20/15, 1.20) thus takes the approach of measuring 'distance vision adequacy' (i.e., determining whether distance VA is adequate for a patient's daily needs, similar to the approach used for reading VA) rather than distance VA (a threshold measurement). A truncated chart makes the detection of slightly reduced VA caused by eye disease or uncorrected refractive error in patients with good VA impossible. For example, if your chart (or measurement technique) is truncated to 6/6 (20/20, 1.0), you will not be able to detect the more than one line of VA loss from the average VA of a 30-year-old of 107 VAR (6/4.5, 20/15, 1.40) to 100 VAR.

3.1.2 Procedure for distance VA

(See online video 3.1.)

1. Ensure the chart is at the appropriate distance and is calibrated correctly. The luminance of the chart

Table 3.1 Average (95% limits) visual acuity data for normal, healthy eyes as a function of age.[6]

Age (yr)	VAR	Snellen (metric)	Decimal Snellen	Snellen (imperial)	LogMAR
20–49	107 (101 to 113)	$6/4.5^{+1}$ ($6/6^{+1}$ to $6/3^{-2}$)	1.25^{+2} (1.0^{+1} to 2.0^{-2})	$20/15^{+1}$ ($20/20^{+1}$ to $20/10^{-2}$)	−0.14 (−0.02 to −0.26)
50–59	105 (100 to 110)	$6/5^{+1}$ (6/6 to 6/3.8)	1.25 (1.0 to 1.6)	$20/15^{-1}$ (20/20 to 20/13)	−0.10 (0.00 to −0.20)
60–69	103 (98 to 108)	$6/5^{-1}$ ($6/6^{-2}$ to $6/4^{-1}$)	1.25^{-2} (1.0^{-2} to 1.25^{+3})	$20/15^{-2}$ ($20/20^{-2}$ to $20/13^{-1}$)	−0.06 (0.04 to −0.16)
70+	~100 (96 to 106)	6/6 ($6/7.5^{-1}$ to 6/4.5)	1.0 (0.8^{-1} to 1.25^{+1})	20/20 ($20/25^{-1}$ to 20/15)	~0.00 (0.08 to −0.12)

Note that VAs are well above 100, 6/6, 1.0, and 20/20 for many adults

should be between 80 and 320 cd/m². Leave the room lights on.

2. Seat the patient comfortably with an unobstructed view of the test chart. You should sit in front and to one side of the patient in order to monitor facial expressions and reactions.

3. Take measurements in a systematic order: (1) vision (unaided VA) of the right eye, (2) vision of the left eye, (3) binocular vision, (4) habitual VA (with spectacles) of the right eye, (5) habitual VA of the left eye, (6) binocular habitual VA.

4. Explain what measurement you are about to take. This can be as simple as "Now we shall find out what you can see in the distance."

5. Instruct the patient: "Please cover up your left/right eye with the palm of your hand/this occluder." Some clinicians prefer to hold the occluder over the patient's eye themselves to ensure it is properly occluded.

6. Ask the patient: "Please read the smallest line that you can see on the chart" or similar.

7. Continually monitor the patient to ensure they do not screw their eyes up or look around the occluder or through their fingers.

8. If the patient states they cannot see any smaller letters, push the patient to read more. Use prompts such as "Can you see any letters on the next line?" or "Have a guess. It doesn't matter if you get any wrong." Many patients will read further. Stop pushing patients to read more if they make four or more mistakes on a line of five letters.[7]

9. Score VA using a by-letter system and the VAR system (see section 3.1.5)[2] and/or an equivalent Snellen (section 3.1.5).

10. If the patient cannot see the largest letters on the chart, ask them to move closer to the letter until two or three lines can be seen (or use a printed panel chart at a reduced distance). Note the distance at which this occurs. If the patient cannot see the letters even at the closest test distance, use the following test sequence. Stop at the level at which the patient can accurately respond.

a. Hand movements (HM) @ Y cm: The patient can see a hand moving from a certain distance. Some computerised VA tests can provide accurate measurements down to the hand movements level and these should be used when available.[8]

b. Light projection (Lproj.): The patient can report from which direction the light is coming when you hold a penlight about 50 cm away. Ask the patient to point to the light and note the areas of the field in which the patient has light perception.

c. Light perception (LP): The patient can see the light but not from where it is coming. If they cannot see light, the vision is recorded as no light perception or NLP.

11. Record vision/VA.

12. Randomise the letters on computer-based systems and repeat measurements as necessary.

13. Check whether the VAs are similar in the two eyes, changed since their last examination, and/or below age-matched normal values (see section 3.1.6).

3.1.3 VA measurement in pre-school children

School age children are typically able to use adult-style logMAR charts.[9] Preferential looking tests, such as the Teller acuity cards and the Cardiff acuity test, are used to measure VA in infants and toddlers. LogMAR-based charts with contour bars around the line of letters/pictures should be used when measuring VA in children and these include letter (crowded Keeler or HOTV) and picture (Kay, Lea, Patti Pic) logMAR charts (Fig. 3.3).[9] Amblyopia can be missed if single letters are used rather than a letter chart because of the lack of contour interaction, and logMAR crowded charts have been shown to be over three times more sensitive to inter-ocular differences in VA than single letter Snellen charts and therefore substantially more sensitive to amblyopic changes. Crowded logMAR charts can be used in children who do not know their letters by providing them with a key card that includes a selection of the letters from the chart. You then point to a letter on the chart and ask the child to identify the letter on their key card. Kay pictures have been shown to over-estimate VA compared with letter charts and it may be best to use other charts for patients who are likely to use adult VA charts in subsequent visits.[10]

3.1.4 Measuring disability glare with VA

Disability glare can be simply assessed by remeasuring VA while directing a glare source, such as a penlight or ophthalmoscope, into the eye. Use a standard light source, distance and angle from the eye (e.g., from 30 cm and 30°) to ensure the glare light at the eye is repeatable.[11] A poor VA in glare conditions can provide justification for early referral of patients with cataract or posterior capsular opacification who have good VA in normal light conditions. Typically, most patients will show no change in VA or loss of up to one line. Some patients with cataract, particularly those with posterior subcapsular cataract (Fig. 3.4, section 8.4.1), can lose four lines of VA and more.

3.1.5 Recording of distance VA

VA measurements can be scored in logMAR notation, using the VAR score or converting scores to an equivalent Snellen value. VAR = 100 − 50 logMAR, but see Table 3.2 and Figs. 3.1 and 3.2 to see that it is much easier than using the formula as computerised logMAR VA charts can be set up to display the VAR score of each line. At lower levels of VA, many computer-based charts do not

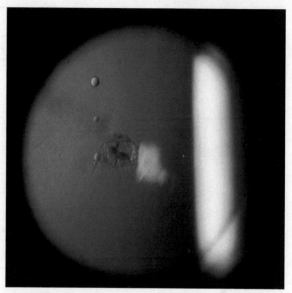

Fig. 3.4. A posterior subcapsular (PSC) cataract.

include five letters on a line (see Fig. 3.2) so that each letter is worth 5/N (VAR) and with rounding lines with four, three, and two letters per line are worth approximately 1, 2, and 2.5 VAR. VAR or equivalent Snellen can be used on your own record cards. Equivalent Snellen values should be provided when writing referral letters and reports, because currently Snellen notation is universally understood, whereas VAR is not. Comparisons of VA in VAR and Snellen (metric, imperial and decimal) plus logMAR and MAR are shown in Table 3.2.

Snellen VA is recorded as the smallest line in which the majority of the letters are seen and refined by appending plus or minus 1, 2, or 3 (e.g., $6/5^{-1}$, $20/20^{+3}$). If the patient could not see the 6/60 letter at 6 m, but could at 2 m, record 2/60. Similarly if the patient could not see the 20/200 letter at 20 feet, but could see the 20/120 letter at 5 feet, record 5/120.

Vision or 'VA s̄ Rx' or VAsc or Vsc all mean visual acuity measured without a correction.

VA c̄ Rx or VAcc mean visual acuity measured with a correction and generally refer to the VA with the patient's glasses. PH refers to pinhole VA and PHNI indicates that the pinhole provided no improvement (section 4.5.2). VA measured with the patient's contact lenses would typically be recorded as VA c̄ CLs or similar. VAs are recorded for the right eye (RE or OD), left eye (LE or OS), and binocular (BE or OU).

Examples

1. Without glasses and with the right eye, a patient reads all the letters down to the 100 VAR row but gets one

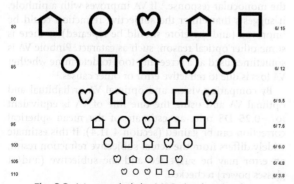

Fig. 3.3 A Lea symbols logMAR visual acuity chart.

Table 3.2 Distance visual acuity conversion table

VAR	Snellen (metric)	Snellen (imperial)	Decimal[a]	MAR[a]	LogMAR
115	6/3	20/10	2.0	0.50	−0.30
110	6/3.8	20/12.5	1.60	0.63	−0.20
105	6/4.8	20/16	1.25	0.80	−0.10
100	6/6	20/20	1.00	1.00	0.00
95	6/7.5	20/25	0.80	1.25	0.10
90	6/9.5	20/32	0.63	1.60	0.20
85	6/12	20/40	0.50	2.0	0.30
80	6/15	20/50	0.40	2.5	0.40
75	6/19	20/63	0.32	3.2	0.50
70	6/24	20/80	0.25	4.0	0.60
65	6/30	20/100	0.20	5.0	0.70
60	6/38	20/125	0.16	6.3	0.80
55	6/48	20/160	0.125	8.0	0.90
50	6/60	20/200	0.10	10.0	1.00
35	6/120	20/400	0.05	20	1.30
20	6/240	20/800	0.025	40	1.60
0	6/600	20/2000	0.01	100	2.00

MAR, Minimum angle of resolution; *VAR*, visual acuity rating.
[a]Numbers rounded to simplify sequences.

letter wrong on this row and reads none of the next row correctly. Their VA should be calculated as 99 VAR (with equivalent Snellen values of 6/6^{-1}, 20/20^{-1}, and 1.0^{-1}) and recorded as Vision RE: 99 VAR (or Vsc OD: 99 VAR).

2. With their glasses and left eye a patient reads all of the letters on the 100 VAR row correctly and three letters on the line (105) below and one letter on the following (110) line. This is equivalent to four letters after the 100 line and should be calculated as 104 VAR (with equivalent Snellen values of 6/6^{+4}, 20/20^{+4}, or 1.0^{+4}) and recorded as VA LE: 104 VAR (or VAcc OS 104 VAR).

3. With their glasses and with both eyes, a patient cannot see any letters at 6 m and can only see the top three lines at 2 m. They read the 55 row correctly at 2 m and two letters on the line (60) below. This would be calculated as 57 VAR −25 VAR (for the reduction in test distance from 6 m to 2 m; see Table 3.3) = 32 VAR.

3.1.6 Interpreting distance VA results

Any deviation from normal age-matched results, as shown in Table 3.1, should be noted. The average VA for patients less than 50 years of age is about 107 VAR (~6/4.5, 20/15,

1.3; a little more than a line better than 6/6, 20/20, or 1.0) so that 6/6, 20/20, and 1.0 represent reduced VA for the great majority of younger patients. 6/6, 20/20, and 1.0 Snellen only become the average VA for patients of about 70 years of age with healthy eyes. You must also check whether there has been any change in VA from the previous examination. In patients with normal or near normal VA, a significant change in VA is more than 5 VAR or one line.[5,12] Also note any inter-ocular asymmetry of a line (5 VAR) or more, or a binocular result that is worse than the monocular response.[5] If VA improves with a pinhole, it suggests that either the subjective refraction could be improved (and therefore should be repeated) or there is some other optical reason, such as cataract. Pinhole VA is sometimes used as a screening tool to determine whether VA loss is due to refractive error or other causes.[13]

By comparing vision and optimal VA or habitual and optimal VA and using the one line of VA is equivalent to −0.25 DS rule, an estimate of the mean spherical correction can be gained (section 4.11.4). If this estimate widely differs from the actual subjective refraction result, an error may be suspected and the subjective (and/or glasses power) rechecked.

Table 3.3 Conversion table for distance visual acuity (VAs) using charts designed and calibrated for 6 m and 4 m measured at shorter working distances for patients with visual impairment.

Chart distance	VAR	Snellen (metric)	Snellen (imperial)	Decimal*	LogMAR
(using a 6m chart)					
3 m	−15	3/x	10/x	(Calculated	+0.30
2 m	−25	2/x	~7/x	from	+0.50
1.5 m	−30	1.5/x	5/x	Snellen)	+0.60
1 m	−40	1/x	~3/x		+0.80
(using a 4 m chart)					
2 m	−15	2/x	2/x		+0.30
1 m	−30	1/x	1/x		+0.60

For example, a score of VAR 76 using a 6 m chart at 2 m would be 76 −25 = 51. X is the denominator of the Snellen line read.
For example, If a patient read the 6/24 line at 2m it would be recorded as 2/24.

3.1.7 Most common errors in distance VA measurement

1. Allowing cautious patients to decide their acuity (i.e., not pushing them to guess).
2. Permitting the patient to screw their eyes up and improve their VA.
3. Permitting the patient to look around the occluder or through their fingers and view binocularly when measuring monocular VA.
4. Not recording the result immediately and guessing the result at the end of the examination.
5. Forgetting that patients could have VA better than your bottom line (of typically 6/5, 20/15, or 1.2 with some Snellen charts).

3.1.8 Information to provide to a patient with VA loss

A discussion with a patient with VA loss should include the diagnosis, management plan, and prognosis (section 2.4) in lay terms. It may also include some of the information provided below that seems pertinent to your patient, ideally with a link to a suitable website and/or an information leaflet (see section 2.4).

Driving: The level of vision, habitual VA, and optimal VA must all be considered for drivers and advice provided as to whether they are legal to drive without glasses, with their current glasses, or with a new pair of glasses based on the latest refraction. The advice about whether they need to wear glasses to drive must be clear as a surprising number of people drive without their distance glasses.[14]

Patients with cataracts may pass the legal VA limit for driving in your office lighting conditions, but fail under glare conditions (section 3.1.4) and you may consider advising some patients to avoid driving at night (many self-restrict their driving)[15] and/or refer them for cataract surgery. Patients with VA loss close to the legal driving limit and with eye disease that has a poor prognosis may benefit from being prepared for the likelihood of losing their driving license. The loss of being able to drive can be a huge blow to many patients due to the loss of independence and, for low mileage drivers, it is useful to highlight that the savings in not having to run, maintain, and insure a car allow for plenty of trips by taxi, as well as public transport.

Blindness and low vision registration: Most high-income countries provide special assistance to people who suffer severe visual disability. Typically people can be referred to be registered as blind when VA in the better eye is either 50 (6/60, 0.10, 20/200) or 35 VAR (3/60, 0.05, 10/200) or when their visual field is greatly restricted. Some countries also provide assistance to patients with less visual impairment and clinicians must be aware of the reduced levels of VA and visual field that are used for registration purposes in the country they practice.

Reading difficulties are discussed in section 3.2.7, and problems with balance, walking, watching TV, shopping, hobbies, and leisure activities are discussed in the sections for contrast sensitivity (section 3.3.7), visual field loss (section 3.7.7; which includes discussion of Charles Bonnet syndrome; 3.6.6, 3.9.6 and 3.10.6), colour vision deficiency (section 3.4.7), and stereopsis (section 3.11.2).

3.2 Reading (or near) acuity

Near vision cards typically present sentences or paragraphs of words rather than isolated letters and some incorporate examples of near vision tasks such as sheet music, technical drawings, and telephone directories (Fig. 3.5). As individual letters are rarely used, they measure reading acuity rather than near VA. They are also now available on e-tablet and e-phones.

3.2.1 The evidence base: when and how reading acuity should be assessed

Habitual and optimal reading VA are routine measurements in presbyopes and in all patients who complain of near vision problems. Measuring unaided reading VA is optional, and should be measured in patients who are presbyopic and who do not wear spectacles for all or certain near viewing tasks (this information must therefore be obtained in the case history) or if it is required for a report.

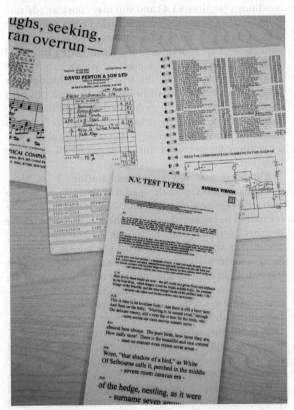

Fig. 3.5 A selection of near visual acuity charts.

Many types of charts are used to measure reading VA, including Jaeger, Faculty of Ophthalmologists (N-point), equivalent Snellen, Sloan reading cards (M-scale), Bailey-Lovie reading cards, and MNRead, Radner, and IReST charts. The latter five charts use a logMAR scale with typically well standardised sentence structure and have all the advantages of distance logMAR charts.[16,17] They should be used when:

- An accurate, non-truncated measurement of reading VA is needed
- Monitoring patients with visual impairment
- Calculating the magnification needed for a low vision aid
- Distance VA and reading VA may differ, such as with multifocal implants/contact lenses and patients with subcapsular cataract, in whom reading VA can be reduced with near pupillary constriction.

M-units are widely used in low vision clinics to allow easy calculation of magnification needs for low vision aids; they indicate the distance in metres at which the height of a lower case 'x' subtends 5 minutes of arc. A 1.0 M letter 'x' is therefore 1.45 mm high.[16]

Equivalent Snellen charts and the Faculty of Ophthalmologists N-notation charts are widely used in many parts of the world. The latter chart uses the Times New Roman font and is based on the 'point size' used by printers and word processing packages on modern computers, in which 1 point = 1/72 inch (~0.353 mm). This can be a useful aid when indicating to a patient the level of vision that would be provided for computer use by new lenses. N8 is approximately equal to 1.0 M and this eight times conversion holds for all print sizes. These charts are typically truncated as the smallest print sizes often provided are N5 (at 40 cm equivalent to ~6/9 distance VA) and 0.4 M (at 40 cm equivalent to ~20/20 distance VA)[12] so that many patients could read sentences of text smaller than this if given the chance and a threshold is not measured. 'Near vision adequacy' is a more appropriate description of these measurements than reading VA.[12] Near vision adequacy measurements have the advantage that the measurement is quicker than a threshold measurement and most patients are able to see the 'smallest line' of text. It is left to distance VA measurements, with its many advantages in this regard (e.g., fixed measurement distance, same letter format, letters of similar legibility), to provide an accurate measurement of a patient's resolution. They appear to provide adequate assessment of near vision adequacy for patients with healthy eyes and good distance VA. Cards using Jaeger notation should not be used because there is no standardisation of what J1 or J5, and so on means and different charts can give different sizes of print with the same J-value.[16,17]

3.2.2 Procedure for reading acuity

(See online video 3.2.)

The procedure is similar to the measurement of distance VA, except that:

1. Measurements should be made in similar lighting conditions to those the patient uses at home. Ask if the patient uses an anglepoise or goose-neck light at home, and if they do, use additional light during your reading VA measurements.
2. Instruct the patient to place the reading card (or e-tablet, e-phone, or e-book reader) at their normal near working distance. Measure and record this distance.
3. Measure the reading VA of the poorer eye first, if a poorer eye is known from previous records or from the case history (as memorisation of the words on the chart you use may be a problem). Otherwise, measure the right eye first.
4. Explain to the patient what measurement you are about to take. This may be a simple: "Now we shall find out what you can see at close distances. Please read the smallest paragraph you can see."

3.2.3 Adaptation for older patients and those with visual impairment

If a patient does not use additional lighting to read in their home and you subsequently find they cannot easily read N5 (or 0.4 M or 20/20) at the end of the reading addition part of the refraction, they should be encouraged to obtain an anglepoise or goose-neck or similar light for near tasks. It is very useful to demonstrate how helpful such additional light can be. The main objective of people with visual impairment is to be able to read[16] and a majority can be successfully helped in primary eye care using high reading additions, simple magnifiers, and additional lighting.[18] Note that, although reading VA levels can be associated with a range of near tasks (Table 3.4), the poorer reading VAs are threshold measurements (measurements of N5, 0.4 M, and 20/20 may be truncated and not thresholds as discussed earlier) so that patients would not be able to read print of that size comfortably for any length of time. For example, to allow somebody to read newspaper print comfortably requires a reading VA better than N8 or 1.0 M, which is the typical size of newspaper print (see Table 3.4) as a 'reading reserve' of approximately 2:1 and thus a reading VA of N4 or 0.5 M is required.[19]

3.2.4 Recording of reading VA

Note the working distance and then record the smallest paragraph size seen by the right and left eyes and binocularly. For approximate equivalents to other notations, see Table 3.4. Some clinicians do not note the working distance unless it differs from the 'norm.' However, even

Table 3.4 Near visual acuity conversion table

logMAR	N-scale	M-units	Equivalent Snellen (imperial)	Equivalent Snellen (metric)	Common usage
−0.10	2.5	0.32	20/16	6/5	
0.00	3	0.40	20/20	6/6	Medicine bottle labels
0.10	4	0.50	20/25	6/7.5	Medicine bottle labels
0.20	5	0.60	20/30	6/9	Footnotes, bibles
0.30	6	0.75	20/40	6/12	Telephone directories
0.40	8	1.0	20/50	6/15	Newspaper print
0.50	10	1.2	20/60	6/18	Magazines, books
0.60	12	1.6	20/80	6/24	Books
0.70	16	2.0	20/100	6/30	Children's books
0.80	20	2.5	20/125	6/36	Large print books
0.90	25	3.2	20/160	6/48	Large print books
1.00	32	4.0	20/200	6/60	Subheadlines
1.10	40	5.0	20/250	6/75	Subheadlines

Numbers rounded to simplify sequences.

patients with good vision present a wide range of normal working distances (22 cm to 50 cm for reading,[20] and further away for computer use), and a reading acuity is meaningless without a working distance. It can also be useful to record the working distance(s) used to determine reading VA with the patient's own spectacles to allow a comparison with the one used to determine the reading add. This can also be useful for comparison if patients return to your practice dissatisfied with the near vision in any new glasses. These cases are often due to problems with working distance determination rather than an incorrect refraction.

Reading VAs are recorded in the same format as distance VA, but should also include the near working distance in centimetres or inches. If the patient can only read a paragraph slowly or with difficulty, include this information:

Examples:

NVA c Rx.	RE: 78	LE: 83 (VAR) @ 40 cm	
Near vision.	RE: N14	LE: N12 (slowly) @ 40 cm	
NVAcc.	OD: 0.4 M	OS: 0.4 M	OU: 0.4M @ 38 cm
NVcc.	OD: 20/20 (diff.)	OS: 20/20	OU: 20/15 @ 16"

3.2.5 Interpreting reading VA results

When determining a reading addition, do not assume you have the correct add just because a patient can see the smallest text on your near chart, such as N5, 0.4 M, or 20/20, because these charts are truncated. Apart from this truncation effect, reading VA can be expected to be similar to distance VA in most cases provided that the eye is accommodating normally or that the reading addition is correct. Notable exceptions include patients with multifocal intraocular lenses or contact lenses or patients with posterior subcapsular cataract. Patients with some eye disorders, such as amblyopia, age-related macular degeneration, and macular oedema, can have significantly worse reading VA than distance VA and isolated-letter near VA.[21]

3.2.6 Most common errors in reading VA measurement

1. Not measuring or recording the test distance.
2. Measuring reading VA with an additional light rather than the light levels typically used by the patient in their home or at work.

3.2.7 Information to provide to a patient with reading difficulties

A discussion with a patient with reading VA loss should include the diagnosis, management plan, and prognosis (see section 2.4) in lay terms. It may also include some of the information provided below that seems pertinent to your patient, ideally with a link to a suitable website and/or an information leaflet (see section 2.4).

The major activity limitation reported by patients with visual impairment is typically reading[18] and improved lighting, which can significantly improve reading ability in the home, should be recommended. Furniture should be rearranged relative to windows so that daylight can illuminate newspapers and books over the patient's shoulder. In addition, anglepoise (goose-neck) lamps with the brightest bulbs recommended for the lamp should be used in favourite reading areas. Book reading can often be improved using e-book readers, such as the Kindle, because text can be increased in size to one suitable for your patient and e-books often have the capability to switch the contrast polarity (to white letters on a black background) which reduces the extent of light scatter in the eye and improves reading further for patients with slight cataract (which is often found in patients with age-related macular degeneration as the primary diagnosis).[22] Voice-activated books and apps or audiobooks can also be very helpful and are becoming more widely available. Electronic and optical low vision aids are available for letter writing and reading bills and letters and simple magnifiers can be useful for spot reading, such as for price tags, when shopping.

3.3 Contrast sensitivity

Contrast sensitivity (CS) measurements do not provide diagnostic information, but provide a much better assessment of a patient's functional vision than VA and are standard measurements in most clinical trials of ophthalmic interventions and drugs. Assessing vision using just VA measurements is analogous to assessing hearing using just the highest pitched note a patient can hear. CS measurement is analogous to providing information about hearing lower tones and the bass, without which sounds would appear 'thin' and 'tinny.' Without CS at lower frequencies, vision can similarly appear 'washed out.' To assess vision fully needs more than just VA.

3.3.1 The evidence base: when and how to assess CS

Poor CS has been shown to be a better predictor than poor VA of decrements in many activities of daily living, such as driving, reading, control of balance, likelihood of falling, and perceived visual disability.[11] The CS function of patients with visual impairment can be assessed using just two measurements: standard distance VA (section 3.1) plus a measure of CS close to the peak of the CS function, such as provided by the Pelli-Robson, MARS, or Melbourne edge-test[23] (Fig. 3.6) Fig. 3.6A shows a patient with reduced peak CS

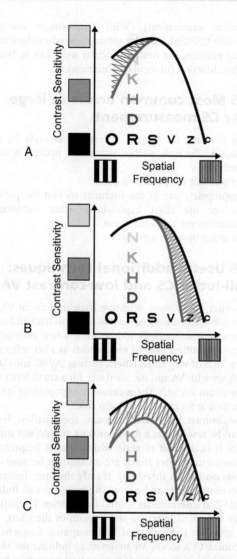

Fig. 3.6 The contrast sensitivity (CS) function of contrast threshold versus spatial frequency can be assessed by a measurement of distance visual acuity (VA) and near-peak letter CS. **(A)** Normal VA but reduced near-peak CS. **(B)** Reduced VA but normal near-peak CS. **(C)** the same reduced VA as B, but with reduced near-peak CS. (Courtesy of Samantha Strong.)

and normal VA who will complain of poor vision. The CS loss could be caused by multiple sclerosis, visual pathway lesion, refractive surgery, and diabetes.[11,24] Patients with peak CS loss and VA loss (see Fig. 3.6C), which could be caused by any eye disease, will complain of much worse visual problems than a patient with normal peak CS with the same VA (see Fig. 3.6B). CS should therefore be measured in any patient with normal or near normal VA who complains of poor vision. This could be a patient with

cataract whose symptoms suggest the need for surgery but whose VA may not and patients who have been told they have normal vision (because of normal VA) when they know they do not (see Fig. 3.6A).[24] Reduced CS can also explain a poor response to an optical aid by a patient with low vision and suggest the need for a contrast enhancing closed-circuit television (CCTV). Binocular CS that is better than best monocular, can also suggest the desirability of a binocular low vision aid over a monocular one.[11]

Pelli-Robson CS, which is quickly and simply measured, provides a reliable measurement of low spatial frequency CS (0.5 to 1.0 cycles/degree) when measured at the standard 1 m. It provides significantly more repeatable measures than sine-wave grating charts such as the Vistech[25], FACT[25], or CSV-1000 charts.[26] Other large letter CS charts, such as the MARS test, are similarly repeatable, but those provided on electronic test charts may not be because of issues with liquid crystal display screens at low contrast.[27] The Pelli-Robson chart is ideal when determining functional vision loss in patients with low vision and moderate and dense cataract; when screening for low spatial frequency loss in patients with optic neuritis, multiple sclerosis, or visual pathway lesions; when examining diabetics with little or no background retinopathy; and in patients with Parkinson's or Alzheimer's disease. The Pelli-Robson chart can be used at longer working distances such as 3 m, so that higher spatial frequencies are assessed and it becomes more sensitive to conditions such as early cataract. One disadvantage of the chart is that a variable endpoint can be gained depending on how long the patient is left to stare at the letters near threshold.[11]

3.3.2 Procedure for CS

1. Illuminate the chart (Fig. 3.7) to between 60 and 120 cd/m². If room lighting is inadequate, ensure the additional lighting provides a uniform luminance over the chart and avoids specular reflections from the surface.
2. Sit/stand the patient 1 m from the chart, with the middle of the chart at eye level. Longer distances can be used if required.
3. Patients can wear their own distance spectacles because measurements are relatively immune to moderate dioptric blur.
4. Occlude one eye.
5. Ask the patient to read the lowest letters that they can see, and encourage the patient to guess. Once the patient states that they cannot see any further, indicate where the next lower contrast triplet is on the chart and ask the patient to keep looking at this point for at least 20 seconds. Generally, if given sufficient time, at least one more triplet of letters will become visible in this manner.
6. Count the reading of the letter C as an O as a correct response to further balance the legibility of the letters.[11]

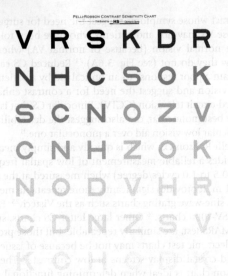

PELLI-ROBSON CONTRAST SENSITIVITY CHART

V R S K D R
N H C S O K
S C N O Z V
C N H Z O K
N O D V H R
C D N Z S V
K C H O

Fig. 3.7 The Pelli-Robson letter contrast sensitivity chart. (Reproduced with permission from Pelli DG, Robson JG, Wilkins AJ. The design of a new letter chart for measuring contrast sensitivity. *Clinical Vision Sciences* 1988;2:187–99.)

7. Score 0.05 log CS for every letter read correctly (the first triplet should be ignored as it has a log CS value of 0.00). This 'by-letter' scoring provides a more repeatable and sensitive measurement than the manufacturer's recommended scoring of the lowest line at which the patient can read two of the three letters.[11]
8. Repeat the measurements in the other eye and binocularly as required.

3.3.3 Recording of CS

Record the CS score in log units.
Examples:

Pelli-Robson. RE: 1.70 log CS, LE: 1.75 log CS, BE: 1.85 log CS
Pelli-Robson. OD: 1.70 log CS, OS: 1.25 log CS, OU: 1.65 log CS

3.3.4 Interpreting CS results

For patients between 20 and 50 years of age, monocular CS should be 1.80 log units and above; for patients less than 20 years of age and older than 50 years, monocular CS should be 1.65 log units and above. It is best to obtain your own norm values. If the monocular scores are equal, the binocular score should be 0.15 log units higher

(binocular summation). With increasingly unequal monocular CS, the binocular summation will reduce and, in some patients, the best monocular score can be better than the binocular (binocular inhibition).[28]

3.3.5 Most common errors in large letter CS measurement

1. Not allowing the patient at least 20 seconds for the letters to become visible when the patient is near threshold.
2. Not pushing the patient to guess.
3. Inappropriate use of the occluder so that the patient can see the chart binocularly when monocular measurements are being made.
4. Not using by-letter scoring.

3.3.6 Useful additional techniques: small-letter CS and low-contrast VA

Small-letter CS is more sensitive than traditional VA to several clinical conditions, such as early cataract and contact lens oedema, and should be ideal when attempting to measure subtle losses of vision such as after refractive surgery.[29] CS of very small letters, such as 20/30, correlates very highly with VA and the ideal size for a small-letter test may be about 20/50.[30] The measurement procedure is very similar to that for the Pelli-Robson chart.

Low-contrast VA charts measure the smallest letter that can be resolved at a fixed contrast and do not measure CS. It is difficult to state which spatial frequencies the low-contrast letter charts are measuring, because this depends on the VA threshold. If only the large letters at the top of the chart can be seen, the score gives an indication of CS at intermediate spatial frequencies. If a patient can see the small letters at the bottom of the chart, the score gives an indication of higher spatial frequencies. Low-contrast VA scores are believed to indicate the slope of the high-frequency end of the contrast sensitivity function (CSF). It has been suggested that they can be used to indicate the CSF when used in combination with a low-frequency or peak CS measure such as the Pelli-Robson chart and a high-contrast VA measurement. The lower the contrast of the acuity charts, the more sensitive they are to subtle vision loss. For example, for detecting subtle vision losses in aviators or subtle changes after refractive surgery, 5% to 10% charts should be used. For greater losses in vision, such as cataract, even the large letters on these very low-contrast charts cannot be seen by some patients, and a higher-contrast chart at about 25% is necessary. As with high-contrast VA measurements, charts that follow the Bailey-Lovie (logMAR) design principles should be used and the measurement procedure is the same as for high contrast VA (section 3.1.2).

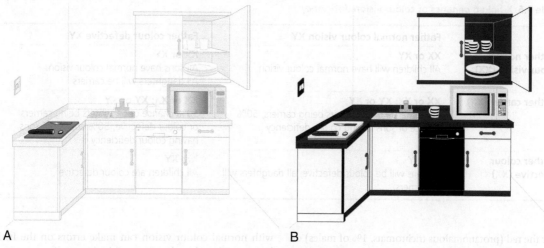

Fig. 3.8 (A) A standard kitchen with **(B)** modifications to increase contrast. (Courtesy of Samantha Strong.)

3.3.7 Information to provide to a patient with CS loss

A discussion with a patient with visual impairment should include the diagnosis, management plan, and prognosis (section 2.4) in lay terms. It may also include some of the information provided below that seems pertinent to your patient, ideally with a link to a suitable website and/or an information leaflet (see section 2.4).

Patients with good VA: Patients complaining of poor vision who have been told by other clinicians that their vision is fine because their VA is fine are relieved when a clinician agrees with them that their vision is poor and is caused by reduced CS.[24] Explain that their vision will be particularly poor in low-contrast conditions such as dim lighting, fog, and rain or looking through grubby windscreens or glasses.

Mobility and falls: Difficulties with balance control, walking, avoiding obstacles, and negotiating steps and stairs have all been linked with reduced CS more than reduced VA. They are particularly important because they can lead to falls, which is a very common and disabling problem for older people (section 4.15.4). Patients with visual impairment should be referred to the appropriate health professionals who deal with home modification strategies that can help prevent falls, such as improved lighting throughout the home, but particularly on stairs, handrails on both sides of stairs, step edge highlighters, and the removal of clutter and loose rugs.[31]

Watching TV: Position the TV to make sure that the contrast is not reduced by glare from windows and bright lights. Magnification can be provided by sitting closer to the TV, and if possible, buying a larger TV.

Improving contrast in the home: Patients with CS impairment can greatly benefit from home modifications that increase contrast. Have a selection of plain white and dark plates, which will make the stack of plates easier to see (Fig. 3.8) and can be used for pale food such as fish pie (dark plates) and darker food such as stew (white plates); the same idea can be used for chopping boards, bowls, cups, and so on. Light switches should have a white surround with a dark switch or viceversa; and similarly with doors and door handles/knobs (Fig. 3.8), stair rails with walls, and finally steps should have high-contrast edge highlighters.[32]

3.4 Congenital colour vision deficiency

Congenital colour deficiency is found in both eyes equally and does not change over time. It is virtually always a red–green deficiency and is far more common in males than females as it is an X-linked disorder (Table 3.5). Approximately 8% (1 in 12) of the male and 0.5% (1 in 200) of the female population are red–green deficient, with the great majority of females being anomalous trichromats.[33] Dichromats, with only two of the three cone photopigments, have the most severe type of colour vision anomaly. Deuteranopes (~1% of males) lack the 'green-catching' chlorolabe and protanopes (~1% of males) lack the 'red-catching' erythrolabe. Anomalous trichromats have all three photopigments, but

Table 3.5 X-linked genetics of colour vision deficiency

	Father normal colour vision XY	Father colour defective XY
Mother normal colour vision (XX)	XX or XY All children will have normal colour vision	XX or XY All sons have normal colour vision. All daughters will be carriers
Mother carrier (XX)	XX or XX; XY or XY 50% chance of daughters being carriers, 50% chance of sons having colour deficiency	XX or XX; XY or XY 50% chance of daughters being carriers or colour defective, 50% chance of sons having colour deficiency
Mother colour defective (XX)	XX; XY All sons will be colour defective, all daughters will be carriers	XX; XY All children are colour defective

either the red (protanomalous trichromats, 1% of males) or green photopigments (deuteranomalous trichromats, 5% of males) provide less discriminative colour vision than normal. Their level of colour vision anomaly ranges from near normal to near dichromat levels[33].

3.4.1 The evidence base: when and how to screen for congenital colour vision deficiencies

Because of the increased use of colour as a teaching aid in schools, it is important to test the colour vision of all children before or soon after they start school. Patients with normal colour vision can make errors on the Ishihara tests, but they do not provide the specific red–green errors[34] so that false–positive findings are not really an issue (section 1.3). However, given the much lower prevalence of congenital colour vision in females, some clinicians may prefer just screening females with a family history of the condition (see Table 3.5).

The Ishihara test (Fig. 3.9) is a very efficient screening test for red–green colour deficiency and provides quick and simple measurements.[34] It is by far the most commonly used colour vision test and is a required entrance test for several professions throughout the world, including the armed forces, and aviation and railway industries. Disadvantages include

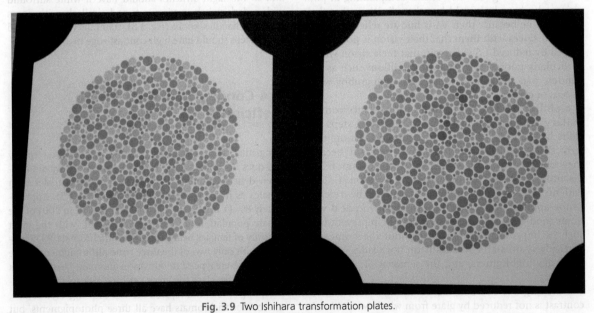

Fig. 3.9 Two Ishihara transformation plates.

that the Ishihara plates were designed as a screening test around the normal/abnormal boundary and are less useful for grading the severity of colour deficiency or for monitoring an acquired colour deficiency and they do not assess tritan (blue–yellow) colour problems.[35] For these tasks, either the City University or Farnsworth D-15 tests or similar tests are recommended. After several years, note that the colours on the Ishihara plates can fade and the test loses its validity. Tests similar to the Ishihara are available on smartphone apps, and they provide a modern, widely available, and more affordable test with fewer issues regarding colours fading.[36] However, there is currently a lack of uniformity with screen colours and size and some app tests have poor specificity and falsely identify colour normals as colour defective.[36,37] It seems likely that a Ishihara-type test will be validated for use on a tablet or similar device in future years.[37]

3.4.2 Procedure for the Ishihara test

(See online video 3.3.)

The Ishihara test is made up of several plates that present various numbers made up of coloured dots of varying size embedded in a background of different coloured dots (see Fig. 3.9). The colours of the number and background dots are chosen so that they are confused by patients with red–green colour defects (i.e., they appear isochromatic to those with colour defects), but discriminated by patients with normal colour vision. Plate 1 is a demonstration plate that should be read by all literate patients and can be used to indicate malingerers. Different designs of pseudoisochromatic plates follow, and include transformation (plates 2–9), vanishing (10–17), and hidden digit (18–21) plates. Normal trichromats can see numbers on all but the hidden digit plates. Patients with red–green colour deficiency do not see a number on the vanishing plates, see a different number than normals on the transformation plates (see Fig. 3.9), and *can* see a number on the hidden digit plates. Classification plates, which attempt to differentiate protans and deutans, are found on plates 22 to 25. Two numbers are shown on each plate. The right-hand number (blue–purple) is not seen or seen less well by deutans, and the left-hand number (red–purple) is not seen or less well seen by protans (Fig. 3.10). The rest of the plates contain pseudoisochromatic pathways and are used for patients who cannot read letters, such as young children. The patient's task is to trace the pathway (Fig. 3.11).

1. You must use the proper quantity and quality of illumination, because the colour temperature of the illuminant will affect the colours of the test. Colour vision testing is normally performed under a standard source, such as one of the Gretag Macbeth Sol-Source daylight desk lamps. This simulates natural daylight conditions provided by direct sunlight and a clear sky.

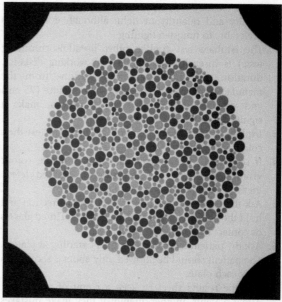

Fig. 3.10 An Ishihara classification plate.

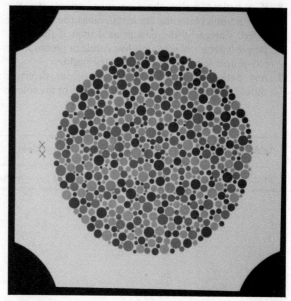

Fig. 3.11 An Ishihara pseudo-isochromatic pathway plate.

Because these desk lamps are expensive, alternative sources are also used. For example, you can use high colour rendering fluorescent lights (>5000 K) or a Kodak Wratten #78AA filter (found in camera shops) placed in front of the patient's eye in conjunction with a 100-watt incandescent light source. Natural daylight is not recommended due to its variability in both the quality and quantity of light, although even this is preferable to tungsten lighting.

2. The Ishihara test (unlike other pseudoisochromatic tests) is insensitive to changes in working distance, duration, and blur, so that deviations from the manufacturer's recommended viewing distance (75 cm) and viewing time (≤ 3 seconds) do not make a significant difference to errors.[38]

3. Explain to the patient that you are going to test their colour vision.

4. If screening for a congenital defect, measure colour vision binocularly. If screening for an acquired defect, measure colour vision monocularly.

5. Ask the patient to use their near vision correction and hold the booklet at approximately 75 cm. Tinted glasses or contact lenses should be avoided.

6. Ask the patient to read the numbers, starting at plate 1. The patient should be allowed only about 3 seconds to view each plate.

7. Use the results sheet to keep a count of any errors. Allow patients another attempt if they make mistakes that are NOT the specific mistakes that those who are red–green colour defectives make.

8. If a patient makes three or more errors, use the classification plates and attempt to categorise the colour defect. Categorise the patient as deutan if the blue–purple letter is not seen or is less visible or protan if the red–purple letter is not seen or is less visible.

9. Any patient who is diagnosed as colour defective should be counselled regarding the effects of the colour vision deficiency on their everyday life and on future career restrictions.

3.4.3 Recording of Ishihara scores

Record the number of plates correctly determined from the number of plates attempted. If a patient fails the test, attempt to categorise the defect using the result from the classification plates and record any advice given to the patient and their family.

Examples:

Ishihara 15/16 correct. Normal colour vision
Ishihara 8/16 correct. ? Deutan. Patient advised re. effects and future career restrictions
Ishihara 2/16 correct. Protan. Patient given leaflet re. colour deficiency

3.4.4 Interpreting Ishihara results

Patients with red–green colour defects will make specific errors as indicated in Table 3.6. Generally, three or more errors constitute a fail, although entrance requirements for some professions allow no errors.[34,39] Some clinicians do not present the hidden-digit plates, which are not very sensitive to colour deficiency, and just present transformation and vanishing plates.[34] Mistakes that are NOT the specific mistakes that people who are red–green colour defective make should be viewed with caution, as they are much less likely to indicate red–green colour deficiency.[39]

Table 3.6 The Ishihara 24-plates edition scoring sheet

Plate	Normal	Person with red–green deficiency	Person with total colour blindness
1	12	12	12
2	8	3	X
3	29	70	X
4	5	2	X
5	3	5	X
6	15	17	X
7	74	21	X
8	6	X	X
9	45	X	X
10	5	X	X
11	7	X	X
12	16	X	X

Table 3.6 The Ishihara 24-plates edition scoring sheet—cont'd

Plate	Normal	Person with red–green deficiency			Person with total colour blindness	
13	73	X			X	
14	X	5			X	
15	X	45			X	

		PROTAN		DEUTAN	
		Strong	**Mild**	**Strong**	**Mild**
16	26	6	(2)6	2	2(6)
17	42	2	(4)2	4	4(2)

X means that the plate cannot be read. Numbers in parentheses mean that the plate can be read, but not as easily as the other numbers.

3.4.5 Most common errors in Ishihara testing

1. Using an inappropriate light source.
2. Attempting to assess an acquired colour deficiency using only the Ishihara test.

3.4.6 Alternative procedure: standard pseudoisochromatic plates part 2

The standard pseudoisochromatic plate part 2 (SPP-2) is another very efficient screening test for red–green colour deficiency; it has the advantage over the Ishihara test in that it can also be used to screen for blue–yellow defects.[40,41] Its major disadvantage is that it is not used as a standard entrance requirement for certain professions as is the Ishihara test and, therefore, is less commonly used. Table 3.7 is a modified score sheet for the SPP-2. Place an 'X' through the figures on each plate that were missed and record the total number of blue–yellow, red–green, and scotopic errors. Asking the patient to identify which number is more distinct when two figures are seen on each page may only be helpful when testing for subtle differences between the two eyes. If the only BY error was on plate 4, then repeat the plate to rule out the error being caused by the patient's expectation of seeing only one figure. When totalling the errors, ignore any mistakes of '2' on plate 3 and '3' on plate 6. The '2' is very difficult to discern and almost everyone misses it. The '3' is a reference that can be used to compare the visibility of the two numbers on the page. A patient over 60 years of age fails the test if they make two or more errors; a patient less than 20 years of age fails the blue–yellow part of the test with two or more errors. The failure criteria for all other patients is one or more errors. Classifying an error based on a fail

Table 3.7 The SPP-2 scoring sheet

Plate	Right eye or binocular		Left eye or binocular repeat	
3	2	4	2	4
	BY	BY	BY	BY
4	6	7	6	7
	BY	BY	BY	BY
5	3	2	3	2
	BY	RG	BY	RG
6	6	3	6	3
	BY		BY	
7	5	9	5	9
	BY	S	BY	S
8	9	8	9	8
	BY	RG	BY	RG
9	5	2	5	2
	BY	RG	BY	RG
10	2	6	2	6
	BY	RG	BY	RG
11	3	5	3	5
	BY	RG	BY	RG
12	4	3	4	3
	RG/BY	S	RG/BY	S

Number of BY errors ___.
Number of RG errors ___.
Number of scotopic errors ___.

on plate 12 can be confusing because the figure can be missed by individuals with either a protan or tritan defect. In this case, errors on other plates should be considered. With other red–green errors, but not blue–yellow errors, classify the patient as a protan. With no other red–green errors, then the error should be classified as blue–yellow. With acquired defects, both red–green and blue–yellow errors can occur along with failing plate 12 and additional testing should be carried out with either the Farnsworth-Munsell D-15 or the City University test.

3.4.7 Information to provide to a patient with congenital colour vision deficiency

A discussion with the patient and family members should include the information provided below that seems pertinent to your patient, ideally with a link to a suitable website and/or an information leaflet (see section 2.4). If close family members have colour vision deficiency (see Table 3.5), your patient may be aware of some of the issues and how to cope with them and you will need to find out what they do and do not know. Protanopes and Deuteranopes (dichromats) are likely to be aware of their colour vision difficulties, whereas trichromats may not be.[33] So first ask your patient if they know anything about their colour vision problem and if anybody else in the family has it.

Depending on what they know you can:

1. Describe that the condition is hereditary and is linked to the X chromosome, so the faulty gene is passed on by the mother who is usually a carrier of the faulty gene but does not display colour vision deficiency herself (see Table 3.5). Family members who may also have colour vision deficiency are the mother's father and any brothers. Females are only colour deficient if their father has the condition and if their mother is also a carrier of the faulty gene (see Table 3.5).
2. Describe their individual condition in lay terms: that there are three types of cones and they either lack the red (protanope) or green (deuteranope) or they have all three, but either the red (protanomolous) or more likely green (dueteranomalous) does not work properly. In addition, all protans are relatively insensitive to red light.
3. Explain that although often known as 'colour blindness' or 'red–green colour blindness', colours are seen, but they are just confused and this occurs across the spectrum (Fig. 3.12).
4. Explain what colours will be confused: Dichromats (deuteranopes and protanopes) will confuse all colours from red, through orange, brown, and yellow to green, plus different shades of blue and purple (see Fig. 3.12). Anomalous trichromats can have near normal colour vision to near dichromat levels and will confuse similar colours,

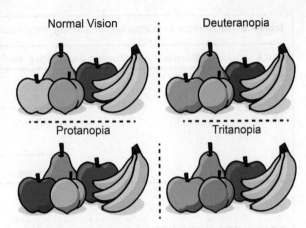

Fig. 3.12 An indication of the colours seen when viewing fruit by people with normal colour vision versus those with deutan, protan, and tritan colour vision deficiency. (Courtesy of Samantha Strong.)

particularly when they are pale or dull or seen in dim lighting. Protans will also have a very reduced sensitivity to red (many shades of red will just appear black), whereas deutans will typically confuse red with brown and green.

5. Career choices are slightly limited, in that sections of the armed forces, police, fire brigade, aviation, and railway industry may require good colour vision and the regulations that pertain to your country in this regard should be readily available. Careers that require an ability to discriminate colour, such as photography, the paint and textiles industries, interior decorating, histology, and electronics may also be best avoided.
6. Most people adapt well and have no major difficulties. The everyday problems that need to be adapted to include[42]:
   - Matching coloured objects such as clothes, and paints and materials used in crafts and hobbies
   - Differentiating differently coloured objects such as ripe and unripe fruit, school workbooks, features on maps
   - Judging when meat is cooked
   - Recognising skin rashes and sunburn
   - Difficulty with road traffic signals. Protans, because of their relative insensitivity to red light, have difficulty seeing low intensity red lights such as car and bike retroreflectors.
7. Helpful adaptations include:
   - The child's school needs to be informed, either by the optometrist or parent/guardian (Box 3.1).
   - Friends and family can be asked to help to match clothes and check on the ripeness of food and so forth.
   - Good quality lighting in the home
   - Use technology: Computers and websites have settings for colour vision deficiency and some useful apps (a current example is 'colour blind Pal') are available.

Box 3.1 **Information that could be conveyed to teachers of children with colour vision deficiencies (see colorvisiontesting.com)**

Re: John Jones

John has protanopia, a relatively severe form of congenital colour vision deficiency. He sees colours, but sees them differently than other children and will confuse some colours, particularly reds, greens, and browns, but also purples, oranges, and yellows. These colours are more likely to be confused if they are pale or dull or viewed in dim lighting. Here are some suggestions that may help John and other pupils with colour vision problems:

- Children who are colour deficient may confuse coloured workbooks or colour-coded reading schemes and make errors when making or reading colour-coded bar charts and pie charts, etc.
- Crayons, coloured pencils, and pens can more easily be identified if labelled with the name of the colour. A child who is colour deficient may prefer to use their own set of labelled coloured pencils.
- Coloured writing can be very difficult for a child who is colour deficient to see, particularly on a coloured background.

- Students who are colour deficient may appreciate help from a classmate when assignments require colour recognition, such as colour coding different countries on a world map or making colour-coded pie charts.

Particularly for young children:

- Children who are colour deficient will have difficulty with colour-matching activities.
- Most children who are colour deficient can identify pure primary colours and it is typically just different shades that give them problems. It can help them to be taught 'all' the colours.
- Label a picture with words or symbols when the response requires colour recognition.
- Make sure a child's colour vision has been tested before they have to learn their colours or colour-enhanced instructional materials are used.
- If they cannot learn certain colours, let them know you understand some colours look the same to them and it is 'OK.'

3.5 Acquired colour vision deficiency

Acquired colour vision defects are normally monocular or unequal in the two eyes, found about equally in males and females, can progress (or regress), and most often involve a loss of blue sensitivity leading to blue–green and yellow–violet discrimination loss (often described as tritanopia) accompanied by decreased vision. Compare this with the congenital condition that is binocular, the same in both eyes, does not progress, is much more common in males, and does not otherwise affect visual function. Acquired colour vision deficiency may have a similar prevalence to congenital colour vision deficiency at 5% to 15%, although this is mainly based on expert opinion rather than epidemiological data.[35]

3.5.1 The evidence base: when and how to assess acquired colour vision deficiency

In patients with acquired colour deficiencies, their colour problems can get ignored because other aspects of vision, such as VA or visual fields, are reduced and take precedent. Although these latter tests are more important

from a diagnostic perspective, colour vision is an important assessment of its impact on a patient's everyday tasks. Testing is clearly important in a patient whose occupation or hobbies include an element of colour discrimination and should be considered for any patient with the following conditions/drugs:

- Diabetes, multiple sclerosis, glaucoma, cataract, and age-related macular degeneration
- Drugs including chloroquine, digoxin, ethambutol, hydroxychloroquine, phenytoin, and sildenafil

The Ishihara test should not be used to screen or monitor acquired colour vision deficiency (see section 3.4.1) as it does not test for tritanopia and is a pass-fail screening test. The Farnsworth-Munsell D-15 test consists of 16 caps that each contains a paper of a different colour (Figure 3.13). The differences between the colours are relatively large, and the test was designed to separate patients into those with a mild colour defect who pass the test and those with a moderate to severe defect who fail the test. It can grade the severity of colour vision problems and can test for blue–yellow and red–green defects so that it can be used to detect and monitor all patients with acquired colour deficiency. It is more sensitive to protan loss than the City University test.[43]

The City University test contains 10 plates that each displays a central coloured dot surrounded by four coloured dots derived from the Farnsworth-Munsell D-15 test.[44] The patient's task is to select the peripheral coloured

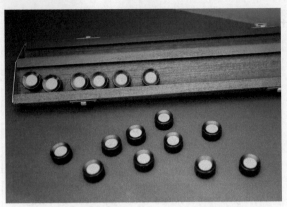

Fig. 3.13 The Farnsworth D-15 colour vision test.

dot that looks most similar in colour to the central dot. Three of the peripheral colours are chosen as typical isochromatic confusion colours for patients with a protan, deutan, or tritan deficiency, respectively. The fourth colour is very similar to the central coloured dot and is the one chosen by patients with normal colour vision. The second edition of the TCU is preferred to the third edition, which has not been independently evaluated and is substantially different from the second edition.[44] It can grade the severity of colour vision problems and can test for blue–yellow and red–green defects so that it can be used to detect and monitor all patients with acquired colour deficiency.

However, the D-15 and TCU are not as sensitive to subtle colour vision defects as is the Ishihara test and patients with a mild red–green defect could pass the D-15 and/or TCU and yet fail the Ishihara. Therefore the D-15 and TCU must never be used as screening tests, particularly given that passing the more stringent Ishihara test is a common requirement for some professions. The usefulness of any colour vision test is influenced by whether it is used as part of the entrance requirements to certain professions in the region you are working.

3.5.2 Preparation for acquired colour vision deficiency testing

(See online video 3.4.)

1. Use the proper quantity and quality of illumination as described (see section 3.4.2).
2. If grading the severity of a congenital colour vision defect, measure colour vision binocularly. If screening or monitoring an acquired defect, take monocular measurements.
3. Explain to the patient that you are going to test their colour vision.
4. Ask the patient to use their near vision correction and avoid tinted glasses or contact lenses.

3.5.3 Procedure: Farnsworth-Munsell D-15

5. Arrange the loose colour caps in a random order in front of the patient near to the box that contains the pilot colour cap.
6. Ask the patient to place the test cap that most closely resembles the colour of the pilot cap next to it in the box. This then becomes the reference cap for the next test cap, and so on (Fig. 3.13) until all caps are in place. Allow the patient time to review the ordering and make any necessary adjustments.
7. Close the box, turn it over, and open it again to determine the order that the caps have been arranged.
8. If the caps have been arranged in the correct order, or with just one or two transpositions of adjacent caps, record the result as normal.
9. If mistakes have been made in the arrangement of the caps, record the arrangement order on the D-15 score sheet (Fig. 3.14). Draw lines from the numbers on the score sheet according to the patient's arrangement of the caps. Repeat the test and plot your retest results on a different score sheet (indicate which score relates to which test).

3.5.4 The City University test

5. Hold the test in your hand or place it on the table in front of the patient, about 35 cm away with the pages at right angles to the patient's line of sight. The cap colours can become soiled with time and some clinicians use white cotton gloves (photographer's) for themselves and/or the patient.
6. Show the demonstration plate A to the patient and describe the test: "Here are four coloured spots surrounding one in the middle. Please tell me which of the four spots is nearest in colour to the one in the middle. Either point or tell me whether it is the top, bottom, left, or right, but please don't touch the pages."
7. Show the test plates 1 to 10 in turn. Allow about 3 seconds per page, with a slightly longer time for the first few pages while the patient becomes familiar with the task.
8. Record the patient's choices in the appropriate column on the record card (either right, left, or both eyes).

3.5.5 Recording of acquired colour vision tests

1. Patients with normal colour vision should make no errors and this can be recorded.
2. The D-15 score sheet should be plotted and retained for patients who make errors. It is also important to record any advice given to the patient and their family.

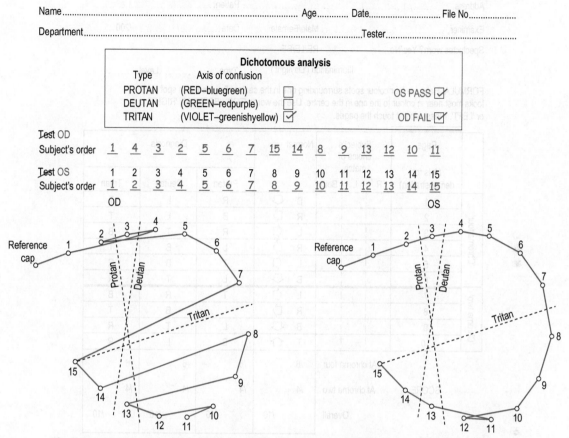

FARNSWORTH DICHOTOMOUS TEST for colour blindness–Panel D-15

Name.. Age............ Date............................. File No.................

Department...Tester...

Dichotomous analysis		
Type	Axis of confusion	
PROTAN	(RED–bluegreen)	☐ OS PASS ☑
DEUTAN	(GREEN–redpurple)	☐
TRITAN	(VIOLET–greenishyellow)	☑ OD FAIL ☑

Test OD
Subject's order 1 4 3 2 5 6 7 15 14 8 9 13 12 10 11

Test OS
Subject's order 1 2 3 4 5 6 7 8 9 10 11 12 13 14 15
                 1 2 3 4 5 6 7 8 9 10 11 12 13 14 15

Fig. 3.14 A D-15 scoring sheet showing a tritan defect in the right eye and a passed test in the left eye.

3. The TCU record form (Fig. 3.15) indicates the most likely of the four spots that will be called as most similar to the middle by colour normals, protans, deutans, and tritans. This can be used to categorise a colour defect in a patient who makes some mistakes. Score the patient's responses out of 10. The number of mistakes in the normal column indicates the severity of the colour defect. Record if the patient was unusually slow and record any advice given to the patient and their family.
Examples:

Ishihara failed; D-15 no errors: Mild R/G defect. Patient advised re. effect and future career restrictions

See attached sheet (see Fig. 3.14): D-15. OD: Acquired tritan defect. OS: No errors. Fail: patient advised re. possible effect on job as interior decorator

3.5.6 Interpreting acquired colour vision test results

Patients with normal colour vision should make no errors.

- **D-15:** Patients with mild colour vision defects may make minor errors, such as reversals of adjacent caps or one crossing of the D-15 score sheet. These errors still constitute a pass for this test. A failure, as specified by Farnsworth, is two or more crossings of the D-15 score sheet (see Fig. 3.14). These crossings should parallel one of the protan, deutan, or tritan axes marked on the score sheets.

- **TCU:** A patient fails the test if they make more than two mistakes. A patient who makes one or two mistakes is borderline and may require retesting or testing with a more extensive battery of tests. The TCU grades the severity and classifies the colour deficiency.[44]

City University colour vision test

Address... Patient...

Examiner.. Male/Female   Date .... /............ /200...........

Spectacles worn? Yes/No   RE/LE/BE

Illumination ('Daylight')   Type.................. Level.................

FORMULA: Here are four colour spots surrounding one in the centre. Tell me which spot looks most near in colour to the one in the centre. Use the words 'TOP', 'BOTTOM', 'RIGHT' or 'LEFT'. Please do not touch the pages.

	Page (A is for demonstration)	Subject's choice of match				Normal		Diagnosis		
		R	L	Both				Protan	Deutan	Tritan
'Chroma four'	1					B ⬇		R	L	T
	2					R ➡		B	L	T
	3					L ⬅		R	T	B
	4					R ➡		L	B	T
	5					L ⬅		T	B	R
	6					B ⬇		L	T	R
'Chroma two'	7					L ⬅		T	R	B
	8					R ➡		L	B	T
	9					B ⬇		L	T	R
	10					T ⬆		B	L	R

		Normal		Protan	Deutan	Tritan
	At chroma four	/6		/6	/6	/6
SCORE	At chroma two	/4		/4	/4	/4
	Overall		/10	/10	/10	/10

Probable type of Daltonism   P; PA, EPA mixed
                                 D,DA, EDA
                                 Tritan

Fig. 3.15 The City University (TCU) record form. (Reproduced with the permission of Keeler Ltd.)

Patients who fail the Ishihara and then pass the TCU have a mild red–green defect, and are unlikely to have trouble with most occupations.

3.5.7 Most common error regarding acquired colour vision testing

1. Not considering it or measuring it.

3.5.8 Information to provide to a patient with acquired colour vision deficiency

Much of the information provided for congenital colour vision deficiency (section 3.4.7) is relevant here.

For example, depending on the prognosis for the condition, young patients with an acquired colour defect should be counselled that their condition limits their career choices. Relatively common causes of acquired colour defects in the working population include diabetes and glaucoma. Note that diabetes can cause tritan-like defects even prior to the appearance of ophthalmoscopically visible retinopathy, which may be due to a higher incidence and progression of lens yellowing and/or nuclear cataract in older patients with diabetes.[45] A tritan-type defect occurs with increasing duration of diabetes due to blue light absorption by the yellow pigments building up in the lens and cataract (particularly nuclear cataract) and selective loss of the fragile S-cones.[46]

Everyday tasks, such as the appearance of clothes and tablets, can be affected (e.g., blue can appear to be black, so that a blue suit or dress may be mistakenly worn at a funeral; white and yellow tablets may be mixed up and the wrong tablets taken at the wrong time and at the wrong dosage). Hobbies that may be affected by colour defects include art, photography, interior decorating, and electronics. The famous impressionist artist, Claude Monet (1840–1926), had great trouble with acquired colour defects caused by cataract in his later life.[47]

A discussion with the patient should include the information provided in section 3.4.7 that seems pertinent to your patient, ideally with a link to a suitable website and/or an information leaflet (see section 2.4). Useful adaptations could include asking friends and family to help to match clothes, making sure the lighting in the home is high and good quality, and using technology where needed such as settings for colour vision deficiency on computers and websites and apps such as 'colour blind Pal.'

3.6 Central visual field (24°) testing

Perimetry enables the assessment of visual function throughout the visual field (VF), the detection and analysis of damage along the visual pathway, and the monitoring of disease progression.

3.6.1 The evidence base: when and how to assess the central VF

Central VF screening should *not* be performed on patients with minimal risk factors (e.g., patients over 40 years of age without other risk factors for primary open angle glaucoma, POAG) due to the problems of false–positive results when testing large numbers of healthy patients (section 1.3).[48] For example, the most commonly used screening programme for Frequency Doubling Technology (FDT) Perimetry is the N-30-5. The −5 in the programme title indicates that there is a 5% chance of a positive test being from a patient with a normal VF, so that specificity is set at 95%. With a prevalence of POAG of 2%, 20 of 1000 would have POAG, but 980 would be healthy and 5% of them (49) would have a positive test result (49 false positives, ~72% of those with a positive result).

Central VF analysis should be performed on all patients with:
- A known VF defect, risk factors for a VF defect, and when following protocols for the management of glaucoma. Significant risk factors for glaucoma include, but are not limited to, intraocular pressure (IOP) greater than 24 mm Hg, 60+ years of age, family history, narrow

angles, vertical elongation of the optic nerve head, notching of the neural rim tissue of the optic nerve head, disc haemorrhage, nerve fibre layer defect, exfoliative syndrome, pigment dispersion, and optic nerve head asymmetry (C:D > 0.2 difference between the eyes).
- Abnormal VF screening test
- Symptoms consistent with neurological disease (e.g., headache including migraine, dizziness, tingling of limbs) or neuro-ophthalmic disease
- Symptoms consistent with central field loss (e.g., non-refractive reduced vision, positive scotoma, scintillating scotoma)

The instrument should be capable of monitoring fixation, providing full threshold fields in less than 8 minutes, providing reliability indices, and analysing the results. A rapid threshold estimation algorithm, such as the Humphrey Field Analyzer (HFA)'s SITA series or the Octopus Dynamic Strategy, is recommended. These strategies take approximately 3 to 9 minutes per eye, without compromising the accuracy or repeatability of the result.[49,50] The use of faster, slightly less repeatable, thresholding strategies (e.g., HFA SITAFast or SITAFaster and Octopus TOPs) should be used for patients with a history of fatigue. Although SITA is optimised specifically for POAG, no evidence suggests a reduction in diagnostic capability for non-glaucomatous defects and it has the advantage of a reduced test time.

Central VF screening can be considered for patients who are asymptomatic with minor risk factors, such as patients with normal looking discs and intraocular pressures, but who have a primary family history of glaucoma, and who are over 75 years, or over 40 years of age and black (African Caribbean, African American) where the prevalence of POAG is higher and false–positive results less of an issue (section 1.3).[48] This is particularly true with protocols in which positive tests are repeated. The speed and accuracy of contemporary fast threshold estimation strategies have made several of the traditional suprathreshold screening techniques somewhat redundant. Fast thresholding strategies can produce an estimation of VF sensitivity in a time (2.5–4 minutes per eye) similar to single stimulus, suprathreshold screeners. All of the fast central field analysis techniques have the advantage over suprathreshold screening techniques in that they are better able to detect early VF defects, and can give an idea of defect depth and area. They have the disadvantage of taking longer than some suprathreshold techniques, although the difference in test time is marginal with SITA Faster. Those that have been independently validated (not SITAFaster to date) are similar in sensitivity and specificity for glaucoma as SITA Standard, and are better at detecting non-glaucoma VF defects than frequency doubling perimetry.[51,52] When compared with techniques for full central field analysis they are quicker but less precise and with worse test-retest characteristics.[49]

The HFA II or 3, SITAFast (Swedish Interactive Thresholding Strategy), Central 24-2 tests 58 locations over the central 25° in a 6° grid pattern that straddles the horizontal and vertical mid-lines (i.e., targets are located 3° either side of the mid-lines). In addition, there are targets located on the nasal field between 25° and 30°. The SITAFast, 24-2 programme rarely takes more than 3.5 minutes in a normal patient, and can be as quick as 2.5 minutes. Most modern perimeters have similar fast thresholding central VF programmes. Recently, the HFA 3 has added SITAFaster, 24-2. It claims to have similar accuracy and precision to SITAFast, but has a test time 30% quicker.[53] The increased speed is due to a number of modifications, including no measurement of false–negative catch trials, video gaze tracking only for the monitoring of fixation, and reduced inter-stimulus test time.

An additional new programme, SITAFaster 24-2C, tests 10 additional central locations from the 10-2 programme, in a test time that is slower than SITAFaster, but quicker than SITAFast. The programme was designed to better detect more central defects found in some patients with early glaucoma,[54] particularly those with lower initial IOP, disc haemorrhages, and vasospastic risk factors, such as hypotension, migraine, Raynaud's phenomenon, and sleep apnea[55] as well as patients with macular disease.

3.6.2 Procedure for 24° visual field testing

1. Explain the test and the reasons for performing the assessment to the patient.
2. When performing VF screening, pupils should be 3 mm or greater, whenever possible. It is considered acceptable to perform VF testing whilst a pupil is dilating, provided the pupil is at least 3 mm at the start of the test. Note the position of the upper lid (i.e., possible blepharoptosis or dermatochalasis) and consider taping if it is obstructing the field of view.
3. Reduce ambient illumination and turn on the instrument.
4. For most VF screeners: Contact lens wearers should perform the VF test wearing their lenses. This is particularly useful for aphakes and high ametropes. Full aperture trial case lenses should otherwise always be used. Reduced aperture lenses and masked cylindrical lenses (i.e., those with opaque masks running along the direction of the axis) can result in VF artefacts. Similarly bifocal and progressive addition glasses and those with small frames should be avoided. Best sphere should be used for any cylinder less than 1.50 D. If the cylinder is greater than 1.50 D, then place the appropriate spherical lens in the back cell of the lens

holder and the cylindrical lens in the cell immediately in front of the sphere. You should use a translucent occluder if the patient has latent nystagmus.
5. Seat the patient at the instrument and adjust the height of the instrument to ensure patient comfort. Over-extension of the neck and a bent back with hunched shoulders and neck should both be avoided.
6. Select 'Central 24-2' and then subsequently select 'Change Parameters' and 'Test Strategy' and choose 'SITAStandard', 'SITAFast,' or 'SITAFaster' as required.
7. Select the eye to be tested first, and unless otherwise indicated select 'Right.'
8. Enter the patient ID. Let the patient adapt to the bowl luminance while entering the data. This is a very important but frequently overlooked procedure, as it ensures a consistent level of retinal adaptation over the duration of the test. Enter as much patient data as possible, but always include patient name using the surname first, date of birth (this is often formatted as month-day-year), and patient file number if appropriate. It is often useful to enter the prescription lenses used and pupil size. It is also possible to enter a diagnostic code, VA, IOP, and cup-to-disc ratio.
9. Occlude the left eye and give the patient the response button.
10. Place the patient's head in the headrest. Explain the test to the patient: "I want you to keep looking at the yellow light in the middle of the bowl. When you see a light flashing off to the side of the yellow light, please press this button. There will be times during the test when you will not be able to see any lights flashing and this is normal. Remember to keep looking at the yellow light in the middle of the bowl all the time."
11. Align the patient using the video eye monitor.
12. Ensure that the vertex distance of the trial lens or HFA variable power lens is adjusted appropriately and the trial lens is centred in front of the eye.
13. Select 'Demo' for a naive patient. Repeat until you are happy that the patient understands the procedure.
14. Select 'Start.'
15. Some models will have a gaze monitoring feature. Once initialised, select 'Start.'
16. Monitor fixation, check that the patient's forehead has remained touching the rest, and encourage the patient throughout the test. Use phrases such as "you are doing well," "over half way now," "keep looking straight ahead . . . that's good" or "you've nearly finished.." Do not leave the patient unattended.
17. If false–negative catch trials are noted, advise the patient to rest by keeping the response button pressed down which will pause the test.
18. If false–positive catch trials are noted, pause the test by keeping the response button pressed down and re-instruct the patient.

19. When the test is completed, store the result on disc then select 'Test Other Eye.' Occlude the patient's right eye and align the left eye with the appropriate correction having been placed in the lens holder.
20. When the left eye is completed, store the results on disc and print the results if required.

3.6.3 Recording of 24° visual fields

If no test locations are highlighted on the Total and Pattern Deviation probability plots, then record 'SITA-Standard (24-2): WNL (Within Normal Limits) R and L.' Print the fields for both eyes and attach to the record card. If a new defect has been detected, particularly in a patient with no previous experience of perimetry or no history of field loss, then repeat the field measurement. Confirmation of VF abnormalities is essential for distinguishing reproducible VF loss from long-term variability (section 1.2). The single field analysis printout illustrates the data as an interpolated greyscale, raw data in decibels, and Total and Pattern deviation plots (Figs. 3.16 and 3.17AB). It also summarises the field using the Glaucoma Hemifield Test, Global Indices, Reliability Indices, and Gaze Tracking plots. When monitoring glaucoma, the Guided Progression Analysis (GPA), which is based on the Early Manifest Glaucoma Trial, is designed to identify true glaucoma progression.[56]

3.6.4 Interpreting 24° visual field results

Visual field information can usefully be interpreted using the mnemonic WANDER:

W: What instrument was used and which test parameters?
A: Accuracy. How accurate/reliable are the VF data?
N: Normal or not? What do the VF data suggest?
D: Defect? What is the type of defect? Does it obey the vertical or horizontal midlines?
E: Evaluate. What disease is suggested?
R: Review/Repeat: What do we do next?

We will now discuss each step of WANDER in more depth.

W: What was used?

As an example: the HFA 3, SITAFaster Central 24-2.

A: Accuracy.

This refers to how reliable the VF data are and consists of inspecting the following reliability indices.[57]

i) Fixation losses. The HFAII/3 employs gaze-tracking throughout the test, displayed as a bar chart on the monitor and the printout (Figs. 3.16 and 3.17AB). Upward deflections indicate eye movements and downward deflections are recorded when the position of the eye cannot be determined or there is a blink. The HFA3 has added additional video-based fixation monitoring, which is used to monitor fixation losses with SITAFaster.

Fixation losses using SITA Standard are also assessed by presenting suprathreshold targets in the blind spot (Heijl-Krakau technique). They are flagged if more than 20% occur; however, this has been found to be too stringent and 30% is a more appropriate cut-off. If fixation losses are flagged, only discard the field if you feel that the patient was struggling to fixate, or if false negatives are also flagged.

ii) False positives. False–positive errors indicate a 'trigger happy' patient who is responding when no target is presented. SITA does not use false–positive catch trials, but estimates the level of false positives by using 'listening windows,'[49] which are intervals between stimulus presentations when no patient response is anticipated. They should be less than 20%. Intervene immediately if false positives start to appear during the test and re-instruct the patient. If false positives are greater than 20%, the result should be discarded and the field repeated. For a repeat field, the test speed could be reduced.

iii) False negatives. False–negative errors accumulate when a patient fails to respond to a suprathreshold target at a given location; these are associated with fatigue and/or inattention. They should also be less than 20%. If you notice false negatives accumulating, particularly towards the end of an examination, give the patient a rest. This will often ensure that the false–negative score does not reach significance. If the false–negative rate does not improve, despite a rest, it can be better to continue on another day. There are no false–negative catch trials recorded for SITAFaster.[53] (Fig. 3.17B)

For strategies other than SITA there will also be an estimate of the intra-test variance called the short-term fluctuation, which should be within normal limits (not have a reported *p*-value).

N: Normal or not?

This can be determined using information from the single field analysis and global indices.

i) Single field analysis. The single field analysis (see Fig. 3.16) includes the following: the sensitivity level for each point in decibels; an interpolated greyscale display; the total deviation in decibels and probability of each point being normal in a non-interpolated greyscale; the pattern deviation in decibels and probability of each point being normal in a non-interpolated greyscale; and the

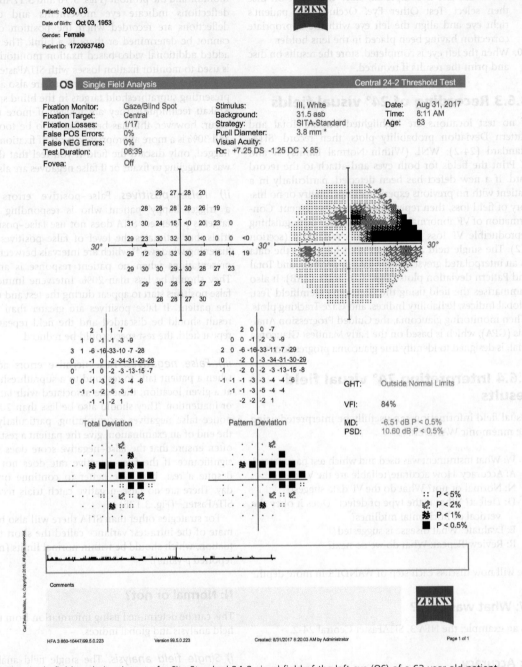

Fig. 3.16 The single field analysis printout of a Sita Standard 24-2 visual field of the left eye (OS) of a 63-year-old patient with glaucoma. It includes the sensitivity level for each point in decibels; an interpolated greyscale display; the total deviation in decibels and probability of each point being normal in a non-interpolated greyscale; the pattern deviation in decibels and probability of each point being normal in a non-interpolated greyscale; the glaucoma Hemifield test (GHT); visual field index (VFI); the gaze track plot; and global indices of mean deviation (MD) and pattern standard deviation (PSD). (Carl Zeiss Meditec, Inc. Copyright 2016. All rights reserved).

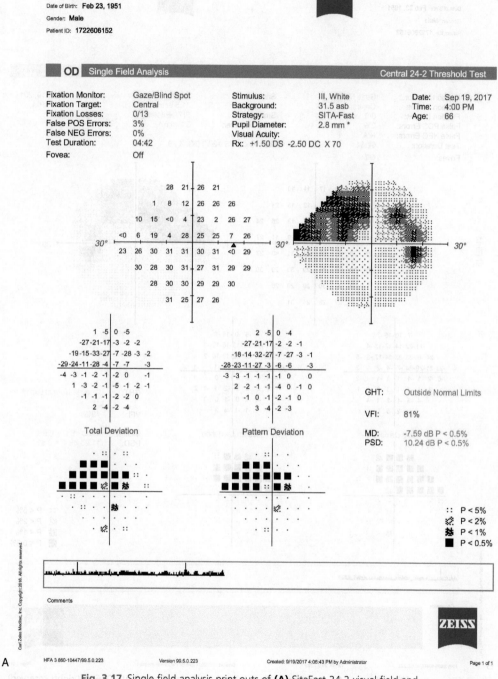

A

HFA 3 860-10447/99.5.0.223   Version 99.5.0.223   Created: 9/19/2017 4:06:43 PM by Administrator   Page 1 of 1

Fig. 3.17 Single field analysis print outs of **(A)** SitaFast 24-2 visual field and

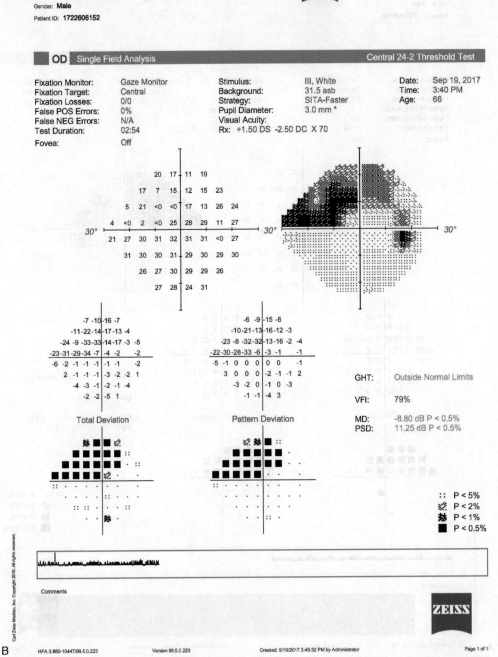

B   HFA 3 860-10447/99.5.0.223   Version 99.5.0.223   Created: 9/19/2017 3:45:32 PM by Administrator   Page 1 of 1

Fig. 3.17, cont'd (B) SitaFaster 24-2 visual field. (Carl Zeiss Meditec, Inc. Copyright 2016. All rights reserved).

glaucoma Hemifield analysis. The Octopus and Oculus perimeters also include a defect curve.

- **Total deviation (TD)** compares the result to an age-matched normal population and states the probability of each point being abnormal on a point-by-point basis.
- **Pattern deviation (PD)** compares the result to an age-matched normal population corrected for the overall level of sensitivity for the individual. The probability of any point varying from this level is stated on a point-by-point basis. This enhances the ability to observe mappable scotomata within a generalised depression, which may be induced by small pupils or poor media.
- If there are no abnormal points on the TD and PD plots, then the patient can be considered as having a normal field.
- A generalised depression most easily will be appreciated by looking for a majority of abnormal points on the TD probability chart. Clusters of two or more non-edge points together on the PD chart ($p < 0.05$) should be considered suspicious. An isolated point within the central 10° ($p < 0.05$) should also be considered suspicious. If a cluster of abnormal points exists, it should be interpreted with respect to its underlying anatomical correlate and subsequent clinical significance. Many artefacts show large jumps in sensitivity, from -1 to -28 dB, for example.
- The glaucoma hemifield test analyses the relative symmetry of five pre-defined areas in the superior and inferior field, as well as judging the overall level of sensitivity compared to age-matched normal values. The VF is then classified as being 'within normal limits,' 'outside normal limits,' (Figs. 3.16 and 3.17AB) 'borderline,' 'abnormally high sensitivity,' or to have a 'general reduction of sensitivity'. Note that some other visual defects are not picked up by the glaucoma Hemifield test, so it should not be relied on to interpret all VF losses. The defect curve ranks the test locations from most to least sensitive and plots relative to the 5% and 95% confidence interval for normal VFs.

ii) The global indices. The global indices are data reduction statistics designed to describe specific characteristics of the glaucomatous VF.[57]

In summary:

- **Mean deviation (MD)** is the mean difference in decibels between the normal expected hill of vision and the patient's hill of vision. If the mean deviation is within the normal range, a *p*-value will *not* be given. It is useful to monitor the overall change in the VF (Fig. 3.18a).
- **Loss variance (LV) and pattern standard deviation (PSD)** are measures of the extent to which the shape of the patient's field deviates from age-matched normal. A low LV/PSD indicates a smooth hill of vision, whereas a high LV/PSD indicates an irregular

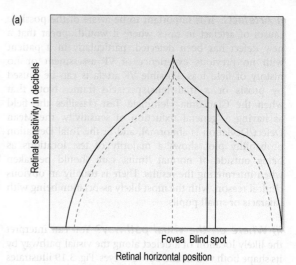

(a)

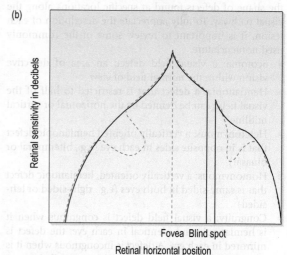

(b)

Fig. 3.18 The hill of vision, showing changes that would produce **(a)** a significant mean defect (MD) and **(b)** a significant pattern standard deviation (PSD).

hill. PSD characterises localised changes in the VF (see Fig. 3.18b). The PSD value is expressed in decibels and any value of 2 dB or greater will have a *p*-value next to it indicating the significance of the deviation (Figs. 3.16 and 3.17AB). Note that LV/PSD get better as the field defect advances to more severe stages, as the field becomes more uniform once again.

D: Defect?

What is the type of defect? Once you have established that a visual field is reliable and repeatable, then first consider artefacts.

i) Artefacts. It is important to be aware of the possible causes of artefact in cases where it would appear that a new defect has been detected, particularly in a patient with no previous experience of VF assessment or no history of field loss. Possible VF artefacts can be caused by ptosis or a trial lens/spectacle frame. Note that when the Glaucoma Hemifield Test classifies the field as having a 'general reduction of sensitivity', the Mean Defect/Deviation is abnormal, and/or the Total Deviation probability plot shows a majority of test locations as being outside of normal limits, care should be taken when interpreting the results. There is usually an obvious clinical reason, with the most likely association being with cataracts or small pupils.

ii) Where on the visual pathway? You can interpret the likely location of a defect along the visual pathway by its shape both within and between eyes. Fig. 3.19 illustrates the shape of defects found at specific locations along the visual pathway. To fully appreciate the description of each lesion, it is important to review some of the commonly used nomenclature.

- Scotoma: a visual field defect; an area of defective vision within the normal field of view
- Hemianopia: a defect that is restricted to half of the visual field; can be defined by the horizontal or vertical midline
- Heteronymous: a vertically oriented hemianopic defect that is in opposite sides in each eye (e.g., bitemporal or binasal)
- Homonymous: a vertically oriented, hemianopic defect that is same-sided in both eyes (e.g., right-sided or left-sided)
- Congruity: a visual field defect is congruous when it is hemianopic and identical in each eye; the defect is mirrored in each eye. A defect is incongruous when it is hemianopic, but not identical. Defects generally become more congruous the closer the lesion is to the occipital pole, as the visual pathway becomes more organised.
- Contralateral: from the opposite side
- Ipsilateral: from the same side

E: Evaluate

What disease is suggested? When monitoring, has the VF defect progressed?

The following are descriptions of the defects caused by lesions at the locations illustrated in Fig. 3.19.

1. A lesion or anomaly located along one optic nerve will result in a monocular visual field defect. Normally such lesions would not respect midlines, but depends on the precise location and size of the lesion. Retinal problems do not usually respect the vertical midline (e.g., central defects caused by macular degeneration, and nerve fibre layer defects causing arcuate scotomas in glaucoma).

2. When located at the posterior of the optic nerve the lesion will also affect the crossing fibres of the contralateral eye, giving a junctional scotoma. In this case, the right eye will demonstrate significant loss that is unlikely to respect the vertical or horizontal midlines, and the left eye shows a superior temporal defect.

3. A lesion at the chiasm will most usually cause a bitemporal hemianopia, mainly affecting the crossing fibres of each eye. The most common cause is a space-occupying pituitary tumor, due to the close proximity of the pituitary to the chiasm. Bitemporal hemianopias are most often incongruous. It is also possible to generate a binasal hemianopia, but such lesions are rare. It requires compression on both sides of the chiasm, as can be found when there is a space-occupying aneurysm that pushes the chiasm into the Circle of Willis on the opposite side to the aneurysm.

4. A lesion of the optic tract will create a homonymous hemianopia. If the entire tract is involved, then the defect will be congruous (as in Fig. 3.19), but it is more likely that the scotoma will be incongruous because the visual pathway is still relatively disorganised. The lesion will only affect the uncrossed fibres of the affected, ipsilateral eye and the crossed fibres from the contralateral eye.

5. A lesion of the lateral geniculate nucleus will give a sectoral, usually congruous, homonymous hemianopia. Such defects are rare and usually vascular in origin.

6. Lesions of the temporal lobe tend to damage the inferior optic radiations and give an incongruous, superior, quadrantic, homonymous hemianopia, or homonymous quadrantanopia. Such defects are sometimes referred to as 'pie in the sky.'

7. Lesions of the parietal lobe usually give a moderately congruous, inferior, quadrantic, homonymous hemianopia, or homonymous quadrantanopia. Such defects are sometimes referred to as a 'pie on the floor.'

8. A lesion of the upper bank of the right occipital lobe will result in a left-sided, congruous, homonymous, inferior quadrantanopia.

9. A lesion of the lower bank of the right occipital lobe will result in a left-sided, congruous, homonymous, superior quadrantanopia.

10. A lesion of the right occipital lobe will result in a left-sided, congruous, homonymous hemianopia, with macular sparing.

11. A lesion at the tip of the occipital lobe will result in a left-sided, congruous, homonymous, central hemianopia.

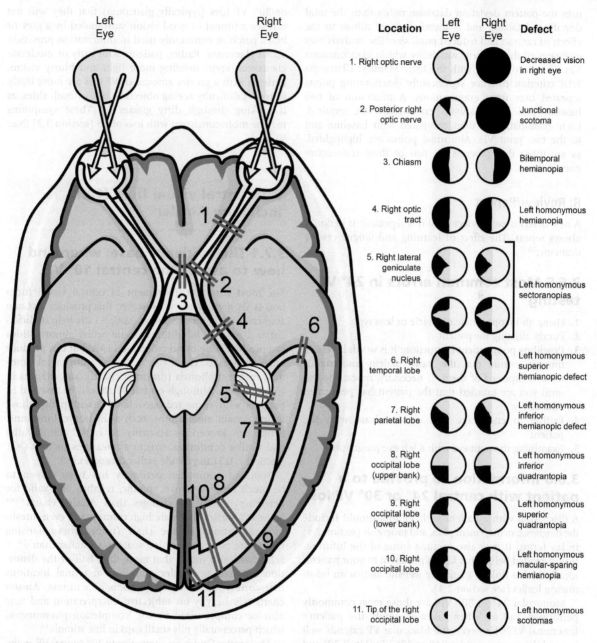

Fig. 3.19 The visual pathway, with indicative visual field scotomas caused by lesions at specific locations. (Courtesy of Samantha Strong.)

The columns of the figure are labelled:

Left Eye — Right Eye

Location | Left Eye | Right Eye | Defect

1. Right optic nerve — Decreased vision in right eye

2. Posterior right optic nerve — Junctional scotoma

3. Chiasm — Bitemporal hemianopia

4. Right optic tract — Left homonymous hemianopia

5. Right lateral geniculate nucleus — Left homonymous sectoranopias

6. Right temporal lobe — Left homonymous superior hemianopic defect

7. Right parietal lobe — Left homonymous inferior hemianopic defect

8. Right occipital lobe (upper bank) — Left homonymous inferior quadrantopia

9. Right occipital lobe (lower bank) — Left homonymous superior quadrantopia

10. Right occipital lobe — Left homonymous macular-sparing hemianopia

11. Tip of the right occipital lobe — Left homonymous scotomas

iii) Visual field progression. Change in the VF of a single patient over time is best appreciated using the Overview printout. Caution is recommended when considering change in the VF due to the high level of inter-test variability, particularly when a defect is present.[57] The mantra should be 'if in doubt always repeat.' If a glaucomatous defect is being followed, the Guided Progression Analysis (GPA) can be considered (see online figure). This is a refinement of the original Glaucoma Change Probability analysis and was developed for the Early Manifest Glaucoma Trial. GPA uses the pattern deviation database rather than the total deviation database, and is therefore more robust to the effects of cataract and reduced pupil size. The analysis uses estimates of the inherent variability within glaucomatous VFs. This is combined with the Early Manifest Glaucoma Trial criterion of three significantly deteriorating points repeated over three examinations. A minimum of two baseline and one follow-up examination are required. Each examination is then compared with baseline and to the two prior VFs. Abnormal points are highlighted, as are those that progress on two or three consecutive examinations.

R: Review/Repeat

A new defect is *not* a defect until it is repeated: 'if in doubt always repeat.' The effect of learning and fatigue can be dramatic.[58]

3.6.5 Most common errors in 24° VF testing

1. Using an inappropriate spectacle or lens type
2. Poorly aligning the patient
3. Providing poor patient instruction: It is worth investing time to ensure that the naïve patient understands what is expected of them. If necessary, repeat the test until you are satisfied that the patient has performed adequately.
4. Failing to encourage and communicate with the patient
5. Examining the right eye with a left eye programme

3.6.6 Information to provide to a patient with central 24° or 30° VF loss

A discussion with a patient with VF loss should include the diagnosis, management plan, and prognosis (section 2.4) in lay terms. It may also include some of the information provided below that seems pertinent to your patient, ideally with a link to a suitable website and/or an information leaflet (see section 2.4).

Monocular 24° or 30° VFs are those most commonly performed and are often taken to imply the patient's functional VF.[59] However, the binocular VF extends well beyond the two monocular 24° or 30° VFs (Fig. 3.20) and VF islands can occur outside the central 30° in advanced glaucoma that are not revealed by central VFs, for example.[60] To assess functional vision appropriately needs the measurement of peripheral 30° to 60° VFs (section 3.8) and/or driving VFs (section 3.9) and/or binocular confrontation testing (section 3.10).

i) Patients with glaucoma do not see 'tunnel vision': It can be useful to explain to patients who have 24°

or 30° VF loss (typically glaucoma) that they will *not* just see a tunnel of good vision surrounded by a grey or black patch as commonly used in information provision about glaucoma. Rather, patients with early or moderate glaucoma report needing more light and blurry vision. Patients with a greater amount of VF loss are more likely to report difficulty seeing objects to one or both sides, as if looking through dirty glasses.[59,61] These symptoms may be more consistent with loss of CS (section 3.3) than VF loss.

3.7 Central visual field (10°), including Amsler

3.7.1 The evidence base: when and how to assess the central 10° VF

The most common assessment of central visual function is VA measurement. However, this provides just one assessment of central vision and offers little help in differential diagnosis. In addition, some ocular abnormalities can produce little or no reduction in VA, but can produce other changes to central vision, such as centrocaecal scotomas, metamorphopsia (distorted vision), and changes in colour vision. Although central VF should be assessed in patients with suspected age-related maculopathy, those taking certain medications, such as hydroxychloroquine, which are known occasionally to cause maculopathy and similar conditions, structural measures such as OCT (section 7.11) can provide earlier diagnoses.[62]

Standard automated perimetry has been shown to be much more sensitive, specific, reliable, and valid for detecting central VF changes than Amsler charts.[63,64] Standard Amsler charts are high contrast and even threshold adaptations of the chart (using cross-polarising filters) are poor at detecting scotomas smaller than 6°.[63] Schuchard also found that more than half of the distortion reported in Amsler grids was at retinal locations that corresponded to the location of scotoma. Amsler charts rely heavily on subjective interpretation and may also be compromised by the 'completion phenomena,' which perceptually fills small gaps in line stimuli.[64]

The Amsler Grid is an alternative to 10° central VF analysis if a quick assessment of macular function is required, and it is particularly useful in cases with metamorphopsia or visual distortion. Amsler charts have the advantage that they are portable, so can be used for home visits. The recording sheets can be used for home monitoring, although compliance has been shown to be poor and it is likely that the white-on-black Amsler charts are more sensitive to macular changes than the black-on-white recording sheets.[65,66]

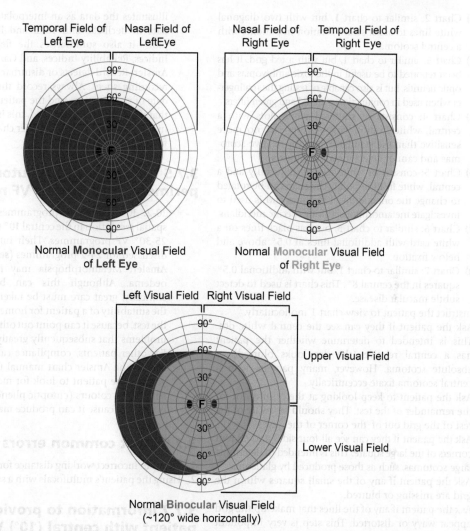

Temporal Field of Left Eye   Nasal Field of LeftEye

Normal Monocular Visual Field of Left Eye

Nasal Field of Right Eye   Temporal Field of Right Eye

Normal Monocular Visual Field of Right Eye

Left Visual Field   Right Visual Field

Upper Visual Field

Lower Visual Field

Normal Binocular Visual Field
(~120° wide horizontally)

Fig. 3.20 The full binocular visual field. Note the size compared with the diagnostic standard of 24° visual field assessment and that the far temporal fields are monocular only. (Courtesy of Samantha Strong.)

3.7.2 Procedure for the HFA 10-2 programme

The same as central VF analysis, but replace programme 24-2 with programme 10-2 (section 3.6.2).

3.7.3 Procedure for Amsler charts

1. Seat the patient comfortably in the examining chair with the appropriate near correction. As the working distance for the test is 30 cm, ideally a 3.25 D near add should be used for absolute presbyopes. However, the patient's own spectacles are usually satisfactory given

sufficient depth of focus. Use single vision glasses or trial lenses, but avoid multifocal lenses.
2. Position yourself to be able to occlude the non-viewing eye and measure the working distance. Get the patient to hold the chart at 30 cm.
3. Keep the room lights on. The method is qualitative and critical light levels are not essential; however, it is useful to be able to reproduce approximate ambient luminance levels.
4. Select the chart for testing:
   (a) Chart 1: the standard chart used in every case. Consists of a 5 mm square, white grid with each square subtending approximately 1° from 30 cm, on a black background with a central, white fixation target.

(b) Chart 2: similar to chart 1, but with two diagonal white lines to assist steady fixation in patients with a central scotoma.

(c) Chart 3: similar to chart 1, but with a red grid. It has been reported to be useful in the toxic amblyopias and optic neuritis, but is also capable of testing the malingerer when used in conjunction with red and green filters.

(d) Chart 4: consists of scattered white dots with a central, white fixation target. It appears no more sensitive than the standard chart for relative scotomas and cannot detect metamorphopsia.

(e) Chart 5: consists of white parallel lines only and a central, white fixation point. The chart can be rotated to change the orientation of the lines and is used to investigate metamorphopsia along specific meridians.

(f) Chart 6: similar to chart 5, but has black lines on a white card with additional lines at 0.5° above and below fixation.

(g) Chart 7: similar to chart 1, but with additional 0.5° squares in the central 8°. This chart is used to detect subtle macular disease.

5. Instruct the patient to view chart 1 monocularly.

6. Ask the patient if they can see the central white dot. This is intended to determine whether the patient has a central relative (the dot looks blurred) or absolute scotoma. However, many patients with a central scotoma fixate eccentrically.

7. Ask the patient to keep looking at the central dot for the remainder of the test. They should be aware of the rest of the grid out of 'the corner of their eyes.'

8. Ask the patient if they can see all four sides and all four corners of the large square. This is intended to determine large scotomas, such as those produced by glaucoma.

9. Ask the patient if any of the small squares within the grid are missing or blurred.

10. Ask the patient if any of the lines that make up the grid appear wavy or distorted. This step is very important because it detects any metamorphopsia, which is usually caused by macular oedema.

11. Repeat steps 6 to 10 with any additional chart as deemed appropriate.

12. Record any defects or disturbances on an Amsler recording sheet (see online Figure). It is sometimes useful to have the patient draw the defects on a recording chart.

3.7.4 Recording of 10° automated perimetry and Amsler VFs

- 10-2: If no test locations are highlighted on the Total and Pattern Deviation probability plots, then record 'SITA-Standard 10-2: WNL (within normal limits) R and L.' Print the fields for both eyes and attach to the record card. If a defect is evident, then consider a confirmatory field. The single field analysis printout illustrates the data as an interpolated greyscale, raw data in decibels, and Total and Pattern deviation plots. It also summarises the field using Global Indices, Reliability Indices, and Gaze Tracking plots.

- Amsler: Record defects or disturbances on an Amsler recording sheet. Always record the eye tested, the date of examination, and the patient's name. Ensure that if no defects are detected, this is recorded clearly in the patient's file (e.g., Amsler charts: central fields full R and L [OD and OS]).

3.7.5 Interpreting 10° automated perimetry and Amsler VF results

- 10-2: 10° central VF programmes provide higher spatial resolution in the central 10° than the standard 25-30° VF programmes. Their interpretation is as discussed for 24-2 programmes (section 3.6.4).

- Amsler: Metamorphopsia may indicate macular oedema. Although this can be advantageous clinically, great care must be taken when choosing the suitability of a patient for home monitoring with the test, because it can point out otherwise unnoticed problems that subsequently greatly annoy patients. For other patients, compliance can be poor.[65] The step in the Amsler chart manual that suggests that you ask the patient to look for movement of lines, shining, or colours (entoptic phenomena) has been omitted because it can produce many artefacts.

3.7.6 Most common errors

1. Using an incorrect working distance for the Amsler chart.
2. Using the patient's multifocals with a small reading area.

3.7.7 Information to provide to a patient with central (10°) VF loss

This is information beyond the standard diagnosis and management plan provision.

Patients with AMD do not see a 'black patch': It can be useful to explain to patients who have 10° VF loss (typically age-related macular degeneration, AMD) that they will not see a grey or black patch superimposed over their vision of the world as commonly used in information provision about AMD. Rather, patients report seeing patches of 'blur,' 'missing patches,' and/or 'distortion.'[67] Distortion or metamorphopsia is likely due to displacements of retinal layers in macular disease, plus top-down influences from the cortex.[68] Blur and missing patches may be binocular areas where contrast summation is relatively reduced (or contrast inhibition occurs) and where areas of the binocular VF have luminance perception levels at/near zero that cannot be perceptually 'filled in.'[69]

Charles Bonnet syndrome: Typically describes elderly patients with central vision loss, but without neurological or psychological problems, having complex visual hallucinations (e.g., people, faces, animals), which they understand are not real.[70] The prevalence has been estimated at 11% to 15% for complex hallucinations and about 50% for simple flashes and spots of light, but the former is likely higher due to a large amount of non-reporting.[70] It is thought to be caused by a combination of ageing changes to the visual sensory cortex in addition to deprivation of its normal input from the central retina, leading to spontaneous independent activity and thereby hallucinations. Social isolation and linked sensory deprivation seem to be risk factors.[70]

Not surprisingly, patients with the condition can be very worried that the hallucinations indicate impending psychiatric disease or dementia and rarely mention it without direct questioning. Given that patients experience great relief when told that their hallucinatory experiences are normal and do not signify psychiatric disease, it is very important to diagnose the condition. All elderly patients with central vision loss should therefore be asked, very sensitively and empathically, 'With reduced vision like you have, often the vision centres of the brain try to replace the reduced vision with spots or waves of light and sometimes with pictures from the brain of people or faces or animals. Have you ever had these types of hallucinations? They are not uncommon.' Regardless of the answer, it is useful to name the condition and explain it further because the patient may develop the syndrome if they do not have it at the time of your examination. Explanation and reassurance that the visions are benign and harmless, and do not signify mental illness are the main treatment.[70] Improved vision can be of benefit, so that updating glasses and referring for cataract surgery may be useful. Increased sensory stimulation, such as increased room lighting, television, music, and the company of friends and/or support groups, can also reduce the hallucinations. A large print leaflet and/or link to a website should also be provided (e.g., www.charlesbonnetsyndrome.org and www.charlesbonnetsyndrome.uk). The hallucinations can continue for weeks, months, and even several years, but typically disappear with changes in vision and/or other factors.[70]

3.8 Peripheral visual field (30° to 60°)

3.8.1 The evidence base: when and how to assess the peripheral VF

Peripheral testing is rarely indicated, other than for visual standards such as driving. However, it should be considered in some neurological cases, for example suspected

lesions of the chiasm, frontal or parietal lobes, when no central visual field defect is detected, occasional retinal conditions such as retinitis pigmentosa, and glaucoma cases when a temporal crescent is suspected on central testing or when patients report symptoms of poor peripheral vision not reflected in the central visual field. Peripheral visual field testing can also be indicated when following advanced neurological disease, peripheral retinal disease, and moderate to advanced glaucoma. Some form of VF testing outside the central 24° to 30° is recommended when monitoring the patient's functional vision.[71]

The recommended approach to peripheral field testing is to first record a fast threshold central test over the central 30° (see section 3.6.2) followed by a peripheral suprathreshold screening programme that tests between 30° and 60°. Similar programmes can be found on most modern bowl perimeters. Alternate methods would include a full field suprathreshold screening programme or combining a fast threshold central test with a fast threshold peripheral test. It should be noted that there has been no comparison of these different approaches.

Virtually all VF defects, including those caused by chiasmal or post-chiasmal lesions, are reflected within the central 30° VF. This is simply due to the anatomy of the visual pathway. There is a systematic bias towards representation of the central VF, with over 80% of the visual pathway dedicated to processing the central 30° of vision.

3.8.2 Procedure for peripheral VF

The example used is the HFA, Three-zone, Peripheral 60.
1. Following completion of the 30-2 programme, select 'Screening' test type from the 'Main Menu.'
2. Select 'Peripheral 60.'
3. Select 'Right.'
4. Select 'Change Parameters.'
5. Select 'Three Zone' test strategy.
6. Select 'Age Reference Level' test mode.
7. Follow steps 7 to 18 of section 3.6.2.
8. Print results as a merged file with the central 30° threshold result, if possible.

3.8.3 Recording of the peripheral VF

If all test locations are labelled as being 'within normal limits' on the printout, then record 'Peripheral 60, 3-zone: WNL R and L.' If there is a defect evident, then print the fields for both eyes, attach to the record card, and consider a confirmatory field. The printout illustrates the data with symbols that designate the location as 'within normal limits,' 'relative defect,' and 'absolute defect.' There is usually some indication of patient reliability (e.g., test time, catch trials, and fixation losses). The combined printout will show the threshold 30-2 result as a greyscale, surrounded by the Peripheral 60 symbols.

3.8.4 Interpreting the results

Identify any clusters of relative or absolute defect. Repeatable clusters of three or more relative defects should be noted. Look for continuity of defect from the central to peripheral field. As with all VF analysis, the position and shape of a defect, along with additional clinical findings, will dictate the management of the patient.

3.8.5 Information to provide to a patient with peripheral (30° to 60°) VF loss

(See section 3.10.6.)

3.8.6 Most common error in peripheral VF testing

Not measuring the 30° to 60° VF as it has much less diagnostic value than the 24° VF.

3.9 Visual field assessment for drivers

The Esterman test was developed for use with Goldmann perimetry as a way of assessing visual disability.[72] It expresses the VF as a percentage of seen targets, presented at a supra-threshold level of 10 dB (III3e equivalent). The monocular Esterman test uses 100 locations, and the binocular test uses 120. The stimulus pattern favours the inferior VF.

3.9.1 The evidence base: how to assess driving VFs

The binocular Esterman grid is now available on several of the automated perimeters, including the HFA, and gives an automated score. As such it has gained in popularity for the evaluation of visual impairment and visual disability.[73] It has not been validated for use with standard automated perimetry, but has become a standard of measurement in many circumstances, including the driving standard in several countries.

3.9.2 Procedure for Esterman driving VF

The example used is the HFA binocular Esterman test. Other perimeters have similar testing procedures.

Standard VF set-up applies, but in addition:

1. At the 'Main Menu' select 'Specialty Test' and select 'Esterman Binocular.'

2. Move the chin rest to the extreme right position and position the patient's chin on the left chin rest.
3. Give the patient the response button. Use the habitual prescription used for driving, and do not attempt to use trial case lenses.
4. If false–positive catch trials appear, it can be useful to pause the screening and re-educate the patient before completing the test. If false–positive catch trials get too high, the field screening will have to be repeated (see interpretation).

3.9.3 Recording of Esterman driving VF

The printout uses a non-interpolated greyscale to illustrate those grid locations that were seen (open circle) at the 10 dB screening level, and those that were missed (black box). The number of seen and missed points is also stated as a proportion of the total 120 grid locations and an efficiency score is expressed as the percentage seen. The efficiency score is then used to judge the patient's disability. At the end of the test print the result and record the efficiency score as a percentage.

3.9.4 Interpreting Esterman driving VF results

The results are interpreted as a percentage of visual function, giving an indication of visual disability. For driving standards it is often necessary to assess the extent of the horizontal binocular VF. Several jurisdictions consider 120° or more of continuous horizontal field to be the required standard. The percentage rate of false positives is an important check of the reliability of the test, because some patients can try to improve their chances of passing this driving standard test by pressing the response button when a light was not seen. Typically, a false–positive score above 20% means that the VFs are unreliable and not acceptable to a driving standards agency, so that the test must be repeated.

3.9.5 Most common errors in Esterman VFs

These are the same as for central VF analysis (section 3.6.5).

3.9.6 Information to provide to a patient with driving VF loss

Note that the Estermann test only covers a 120° binocular VF and can be easily passed by a patient with monocular vision. Patients who pass who have peripheral monocular VF loss, should be warned of the peripheral loss (see Fig. 3.20) and the need to scan this area when approaching a pedestrian crossing, for example.

3.10 Simple visual field assessments

A variety of very simple VF tests are available, which include confrontation fields, kinetic boundary testing, colour comparison fields, and oculo-kinetic perimetry. They can be used as ballpark assessments of functional VF and/or as imprecise VF screening tests.

3.10.1 The evidence base: when and how to perform simple VF screening

Binocular kinetic VF can provide assessments of functional VF loss as accurately as standard automated perimetry such as that provided by the HFA, but much more quickly.[71] However, the current availability of kinetic VF instruments seems limited and the confrontation test is the only widely available kinetic VF test in primary eye care. It can be used to obtain a ballpark estimate of the functional VF. Confrontation field testing provides a gross assessment of the patient's visual field using a comparison of the patient's VF with the examiner's field using simple targets such as a 15 mm diameter red or 4 mm white bead at the end of a stick or the examiner's fingers.

The prime use of simple VF tests in screening is during home (domiciliary) visits because they are portable and inexpensive compared with automated perimeters. The most sensitive method appears to be examination of the central VF with a red target(s).[74,75] From a VF screening point of view, all of these tests have been shown to be insensitive to all but gross field defects, such as homonymous hemianopias, when compared with automated perimetry.[74,75] It is advisable for general medical practitioners who suspect a patient may have a VF defect to refer such patients for automated field testing rather than relying on the results of a confrontation test.

3.10.2 Procedure for confrontation VF testing

The procedure below describes a monocular VF test using a bead-on-a-stick (white of ~4 mm or red 15 mm diameter), but you can assess binocular ('functional') VF and/or use your fingers as targets and ask patients to count the number of fingers (1, 2, or 4) in different VF quadrants as a check on accuracy.

1. Explain to the patients that you are going to measure the area over which they can see rather than how well they can see detail.
2. Keep the room lights on. The absolute level is irrelevant because the technique involves a comparison of the patient's and examiner's visual fields.
3. Sit between 66 cm and 1 m away from, and directly facing, the patient. You should be at approximately the same height as the patient.
4. Ask the patient to remove any glasses and occlude their left eye using the palm of their hand (not fingers).
5. You should similarly occlude your right eye.
6. Ask the patient to fixate your open eye (left) with their open eye (right). Some patients may feel uncomfortable if asked to stare into your eye directly, and you can suggest they look at the middle of your lower lid.
7. Show the patient the bead-on-a-stick and explain that you are going to move it inwards from outside the field of view and you want the patient to indicate when they can first see the target. Explain that you will continue to move the target into the centre of their vision and you want them to indicate if it disappears or fades at any point.
8. Hold the bead-on-a-stick in a plane equidistant between you and the patient and outside your field of view along one of the eight principal radial meridians. Slowly move the bead inwards until the patient reports it is just seen. Compare this point with the point when you first saw the target. Then slowly move the target towards fixation and ask the patient to indicate if it disappears or becomes less distinct.
9. Repeat this procedure for all eight radial meridians. At all times watch that the patient does not lose fixation of your eye to look towards the target. If this occurs, repeat the measurement.
10. Repeat for the other eye.

3.10.3 Recording

Record the VF type (monocular/binocular), the target used, and whether there were any significant differences between your own visual field and the patient's visual field. A normal result could be recorded as `R & L VFs grossly full to confrontation, 15 mm Red.'

3.10.4 Interpretation

Confrontation testing involves a comparison of your visual field with the patient's visual field. Providing there is no obvious abnormality in your field, the patient's field is considered within normal limits if it matches your own. It can be very useful to highlight to the patient (and family members/carers if they are present) the approximate extent of any VF loss, so that they are aware of the functional consequences.

3.10.5 Most common error

1. Using a very cluttered background (e.g., a bookcase) or a white target against a white wall.

3.10.6 Information to provide to a patient with gross VF loss

This information is in addition to diagnosis and management plan information. Describe to the patient the extent of any VF loss, any consequences of it (e.g., a monocular VF loss in the far left periphery, see Fig. 3.20, could lead to bumping into things on the left hand side, people suddenly appearing on the left as they walk past you), and any advice regarding how to deal with it (e.g., scanning to the left when approaching a pedestrian crossing). It can be particularly useful to show and then explain to a patient and their family/carergivers the binocular VF of a homonymous hemianopic VF loss after a stroke (see Fig. 3.19) and advising them to place things on the dining table (e.g., place the drinking cup on the left if the patient has a right hemianopia), next to his/her chair on the side that the patient can see.

3.11 Stereopsis

Stereopsis is typically measured in children because if children show a reasonable level of stereopisis, then they are unlikely to have amblyopia and strabismus (section 6.7). However, stereopsis tests can also provide useful information about a patient's functional vision.

3.11.1 The evidence base: when and how to assess stereopsis to provide functional information

Stereopsis should be assessed in all patients with anisometropia (including those wearing a monovision correction) or where VA or CS is different in the two eyes, such as patients with amblyopia, strabismus, and monocular eye disease (section 6.7).

There is no evidence to suggest that distance stereopsis tests are any better than near tests for the assessment of functional vision and functional tasks affected by stereopsis reductions that are at variable distances and more research is needed in this area.[76] For now, it seems best to use the stereopsis test used for screening in children (section 6.7).

3.11.2 Information to provide to a patient with stereopsis loss

A lack of or a very reduced level of stereopsis will lead to difficulties in performing everyday tasks such as driving (e.g., judging distances, changing lanes, parking), playing fast sports such as cricket and tennis,[77] chopping vegetables, pouring a drink without spilling it, walking on uneven grounds and negotiating bumps/cracks in the path, and watching 3-D movies. Reading difficulties (e.g., fine print, reading for prolonged time)[77] seem likely due to reductions in binocular CS rather than linked to stereopsis. Patients could be advised to opt for sports not involving fast 3-D decisions and taking more time and care with activities such as pouring a drink and chopping vegetables.[77]

References

1. Elliott DB. The good (logMAR), the bad (Snellen) and the ugly (BCVA, number of letters read) of visual acuity measurement. *Ophthalmic Physiol Opt.* 2016;36:355–8.
2. Bailey IL, Lovie-Kitchin JE. Visual acuity testing. From the laboratory to the clinic. *Vision Res.* 2013;90:2–9.
3. Lovie-Kitchin JE. Is it time to confine Snellen charts to the annals of history? *Ophthalmic Physiol Opt.* 2015;35:631–6.
4. Bailey IL, Lovie JE. New design principles for visual acuity letter charts. *Am J Optom Physiol Opt.* 1976;53:740–5.
5. McGraw PV, Winn B, Gray LS, Elliott DB. Improving the reliability of visual acuity measures in young children. *Ophthalmic Physiol Opt.* 2000;20:173–84.
6. Elliott DB, Yang KC, Whitaker D. Visual acuity changes throughout adulthood in normal, healthy eyes: seeing beyond 6/6. *Optom Vis Sci.* 1995;72:186–91.
7. Carkeet A, Bailey IL. Slope of psychometric functions and termination rule analysis for low contrast acuity charts. *Ophthalmic Physiol Opt.* 2017;37:118–27.
8. Schulze-Bonsel K, Feltgen N, Burau H, Hansen L, Bach M. Visual acuities 'hand motion' and 'counting fingers' can be quantified with the Freiburg visual acuity test. *Invest Ophthalmol Vis Sci.* 2006;47:1236–40.
9. Anstice NS, Thompson B. The measurement of visual acuity in children: an evidence-based update. *Clin Exp Optom.* 2014;97:3–11.
10. Anstice NS, Jacobs RJ, Simkin SK, Thomson M, Thompson B, Collins AV. Do picture-based charts overestimate visual acuity? Comparison of Kay Pictures, Lea Symbols, HOTV and Keeler logMAR charts with Sloan letters in adults and children. *PLoS One.* 2017;12:e0170839.
11. Elliott DB. Contrast sensitivity and glare testing. In: Benjamin WJ, ed. *Borish's Clinical Refraction,* ed 2. Philadelphia: WB Saunders; 2006.
12. Bailey IL. Visual acuity. In: Benjamin WJ, ed. *Borish's Clinical refraction,* ed 2. Philadelphia: WB Saunders; 2006.
13. Kumar RS, Rackenchath MV, Sathidevi AV, et al. Accuracy of pinhole visual acuity at an urban Indian hospital. *Eye (Lond).* 2019;33:335–7.

14. Fylan F, Hughes A, Wood JM, Elliott DB. Why do people drive when they can't see clearly? *Transp Res Part F Traffic Psychol Behav.* 2018;56:123–33.

15. Kimlin JA, Black AA, Djaja N, Wood JM. Development and validation of a vision and night driving questionnaire. *Ophthalmic Physiol Opt.* 2016;36:465–76.

16. Rubin GS. Measuring reading performance. *Vision Res.* 2013;90:43–51.

17. Radner W. Reading charts in ophthalmology. *Graefes Arch Clin Exp Ophthalmol.* 2017;255:1465–82.

18. Elliott DB, Trukolo-Ilic M, Strong JG, Pace R, Plotkin A, Bevers P. Demographic characteristics of the vision-disabled elderly. *Invest Ophthalmol Vis Sci.* 1997;38:2566–75.

19. Latham K, Tabrett DR. Guidelines for predicting performance with low vision aids. *Optom Vis Sci.* 2012;89:1316–26.

20. Macmillan ES, Elliott DB, Patel B, Cox M. Loss of visual acuity is the main reason why reading addition increases after the age of sixty. *Optom Vis Sci.* 2001;78:381–5.

21. Cacho I, Dickinson CM, Smith HJ, Harper RA. Clinical impairment measures and reading performance in a large age-related macular degeneration group. *Optom Vis Sci* 2010;87:344–9.

22. Legge GE. Reading digital with low vision. *Visible Lang.* 2016;50:102–25.

23. Chung STL, Legge GE, Comparing the shape of contrast sensitivity functions for normal and low vision. *Invest Ophthalmol Vis Sci* 2016;57:198–207.

24. Elliott DB, Whitaker D. How useful are contrast sensitivity charts in optometric practice? Case reports. *Optom Vis Sci.* 1992;69:378–85.

25. Pesudovs K, Hazel CA, Doran RM, Elliott DB. The usefulness of Vistech and FACT contrast sensitivity charts for cataract and refractive surgery outcomes research. *Br J Ophthalmol.* 2004;88:11–6.

26. Kelly SA, Pang Y, Klemencic S. Reliability of the CSV-1000 in adults and children. *Optom Vis Sci.* 2012;89:1172–81.

27. Thayaparan K, Crossland MD, Rubin GS. Clinical assessment of two new contrast sensitivity charts. *Br J Ophthalmol.* 2007;91:749–52.

28. Pardhan S, Gilchrist J. The importance of measuring binocular contrast sensitivity in unilateral cataract. *Eye (Lond).* 1991;5:31–5.

29. Rabin J, Wicks J. Measuring resolution in the contrast domain—the small letter contrast test. *Optom Vis Sci* 1996;73:398–403.

30. Elliott DB, Situ P. Visual acuity versus letter contrast sensitivity in early cataract. *Vision Res* 1998;38:2047–52.

31. Campbell AJ, Robertson MC, La Grow SJ, et al. (2005). Randomised controlled trial of prevention of falls in people aged > or =75 with severe visual impairment: the VIP trial. *BMJ.* 331(7520):817.

32. Foster RJ, Hotchkiss J, Buckley JG, Elliott DB. Safety on stairs: Influence of a tread edge highlighter and its position. *Exp Gerontol.* 2014;55:152–8.

33. Long JA, Honson V, Katalinic P, Dain SJ. Re: Is screening for congenital colour vision deficiency in school students worthwhile? A review. *Clin Exp Optom.* 2015;98:192.

34. Birch J. Efficiency of the Ishihara test for identifying red-green colour deficiency. *Ophthalmic Physiol Opt.* 1997;17:403–8.

35. Simunovic MP. Acquired color vision deficiency. *Surv Ophthalmol.* 2016;61: 132–55.

36. Sorkin N, Rosenblatt A, Cohen E, Ohana O, Stolovitch C, Dotan G. Comparison of Ishihara booklet with color vision smartphone applications. *Optom Vis Sci.* 2016;93:667–72.

37. Dain SJ, Al Merdef A. Colorimetric evaluation of iPhone apps for colour vision tests based on the Ishihara test. *Clin Exp Optom.* 2016;99:264–73.

38. Long GM, Lyman BJ, Tuck JP. Distance, duration and blur effects on the perception of pseudoisochromatic stimuli. *Ophthalmic Physiol Opt.* 1985; 5:185–94.

39. Miyahara E. Errors reading the Ishihara pseudoisochromatic plates made by observers with normal colour vision. *Clin Exp Optom.* 2008;91:161–5.

40. Hovis JK, Cawker CL, Cranton D. Comparison of the standard pseudoisochromatic plates–Parts 1 and 2–as screening tests for congenital red-green color vision deficiencies. *J Am Optom Assoc.* 1996;67:320–6.

41. Vu BL, Easterbrook M, Hovis JK. Detection of color vision defects in chloroquine retinopathy. *Ophthalmology.* 1999;106:1799–803.

42. Cole BL. The handicap of abnormal colour vision. *Clin Exp Optom.* 2004;87:258–75.

43. Oliphant D, Hovis JK. Comparison of the D-15 and City University (second) color vision tests. *Vision Res.* 1998;38:3461–5.

44. Birch J. Clinical use of the City University Test (2nd edition). *Ophthalmic Physiol Opt.* 1997;17:466–72.

45. Gella L, Raman R, Kulothungan V, Pal SS, Ganesan S, Sharma T. Impairment of colour vision in diabetes with no retinopathy: Sankara Nethralaya Diabetic Retinopathy Epidemiology and Molecular Genetics Study (SNDREAMS- II, Report 3). *PLoS One.* 2015;10:e0129391.

46. Cho NC, Poulsen GL, Ver Hoeve JN, Nork TM. Selective loss of S-cones in diabetic retinopathy. *Arch Ophthalmol.* 2000;118:1393–400.

47. Elliott DB, Skaff A. Vision of the famous: the artist's eye. *Ophthalmic Physiol Opt.* 1993;13:82–90.

48. Burr JM, Mowatt G, Hernández R, et al. The clinical effectiveness and cost-effectiveness of screening for open angle glaucoma: a systematic review and economic evaluation. *Health Technol Assess.* 2007;11:1–190.

49. Artes PH, Iwase A, Ohno Y, Kitazawa Y, Chauhan BC. Properties of perimetric threshold estimates from full threshold, SITA standard, and SITA fast strategies. *Invest Ophthalmol Vis Sci.* 2002;43:2654–9.

50. Budenz DL, Rhee P, Feuer WJ, McSoley J, Johnson CA, Anderson DR. Sensitivity and specificity of the Swedish interactive threshold algorithm for glaucomatous visual field defects. *Ophthalmology.* 2002;109:1052–8.

51. Liu S, Lam S, Weinreb RN, et al. Comparison of standard automated perimetry, frequency-doubling technology perimetry, and short-wavelength automated perimetry for detection of glaucoma. *Invest Ophthalmol Vis Sci.* 2011;52:7325–31.

52. Noval S, Contreras I, Rebolleda G, Munoz-Negrete FJ, Ruiz De Zarate B. A comparison between Humphrey and frequency doubling perimetry for chiasmal visual field defects. *Eur J Ophthalmol.* 2005;15:739–45.

53. Heijl A, Patella VM, Chong LX, et al. A new SITA perimetric threshold testing algorithm: construction and a multicenter clinical study. *Am J Ophthalmol.* 2019;198:154–65.

54. Hood DC, Raza AS, de Moraes CGV, Liebmann JM, Ritch R. Glaucomatous damage of the macula. *Prog Retin Eye Res.* 2013;32:1–21.

55. Park SC, De Moraes CG, Teng CCW, Tello C, Liebmann JM, Ritch R. Initial parafoveal versus peripheral scotomas in glaucoma: risk factors and visual field characteristics. *Ophthalmology.* 2011;118:1782–89.

56. Leskea MC, Heijl A, Hyman L, Bengtsson B, Komaroff E. Factors for progression and glaucoma treatment: the Early Manifest Glaucoma Trial. *Curr Opin Ophthalmol.* 2004;15:102–6.

57. Heijl A, Patella VM, Bengtsson B. *The Field Analyzer Primer: Effective Perimetry,* ed 4 Dublin, CA: Carl Zeiss Meditec; 2012.

58. Hudson C, Wild JM, O'Neill EC. Fatigue effects during a single session of automated static threshold perimetry. *Invest Ophthalmol Vis Sci.* 1994; 35:268–80.

59. Hu CX, Zangalli C, Hsieh M, et al. What do patients with glaucoma see? Visual symptoms reported by patients with glaucoma. *Am J Med Sci.* 2014;348: 403–9.

60. Nowomiejska K, Wrobel-Dudzinska D, Ksiazek K, et al. Semi-automated kinetic perimetry provides additional information to static automated perimetry in the assessment of the remaining visual field in end-stage glaucoma. *Ophthalmic Physiol Opt.* 2015;35:147–54.

61. Crabb DP, Smith ND, Glen FC, et al. How does glaucoma look? Patient perception of visual field loss. *Ophthalmology.* 2013;120:1120–6.

62. Marmor MF, Kellner U, Lai TY, Lyons JS, Mieler WF. Revised recommendations on screening for chloroquine and hydroxychloroquine retinopathy. *Ophthalmology.* 2011;118:415–22.

63. Schuchard RA. Validity and interpretation of Amsler grid reports. *Arch Ophthalmol.* 1993;111:776–80.

64. Achard OA, Safran AB, Duret FC, Ragama E. Role of the completion phenomenon in the evaluation of Amsler grid results. *Am J Ophthalmol.* 1995;120:322–9.

65. Fine AM, Elman MJ, Ebert JE, Prestia PA, Starr JS, Fine SL. Earliest symptoms caused by neovascular membranes in the macula. *Arch Ophthalmol.* 1986;104:513–4.

66. Roper-Hall MJ. The usefulness of the Amsler chart. *Eye (Lond).* 2006;20:508.

67. Taylor DJ, Edwards LA, Binns AM, Crabb DP. Seeing it differently: Self-reported description of vision loss in dry age-related macular degeneration. *Ophthalmic Physiol Opt.* 2018;38:98–105.

68. Wiecek E, Lashkari K, Dakin SC, Bex P. Novel quantitative assessment of metamorphopsia in maculopathy. *Invest Ophthalmol Vis Sci.* 2015;56:494–504.

69. Wittich W, Overbury O, Kapusta MA, Watanabe DH, Faubert J. Macular hole: perceptual filling-in across central scotomas. *Vision Res.* 2006;46:4064–70.

70. Menon GJ, Rahman I, Menon SJ, Dutton GN. Complex visual hallucinations in the visually impaired: the Charles Bonnet syndrome. *Surv Ophthalmol.* 2003;48:58–72.

71. Subhi H, Latham K, Myint J, Crossland M. Functional visual fields: a cross-sectional UK study to determine which visual field paradigms best reflect difficulty with mobility function. *BMJ Open.* 2017;7:e018831.

72. Esterman B. Functional scoring of the binocular field. *Ophthalmology.* 1982;89:1226–34.

73. Anderson DR, Patella VM. *Automated Static Perimetry.* St. Louis: CV Mosby; 1999.

74. Elliott DB, North I, Flanagan J. Confrontation visual field tests. *Ophthalmic Physiol Opt.* 1997;17: S17–24.

75. Pandit RJ, Gales K, Griffiths PG. Effectiveness of testing visual fields by confrontation. *Lancet.* 2001;358:1820.

76. Piano MEF, Tidbury LP, O'Connor AR. Normative values for near and distance clinical tests of stereoacuity. *Strabismus.* 2016;24:169–72.

77. Kumaran SE, Khadka J, Baker R, Pesudovs K. Functional limitations recognised by adults with amblyopia and strabismus in daily life: a qualitative exploration. *Ophthalmic Physiol Opt.* 2019;39:131–40.

Chapter | 4 |

Refraction and Prescribing

David B. Elliott

4.1 Focimetry (vertometry or lensometry)

The instrument used to measure lens power, optical centres, and any prism in glasses has been known by a variety of trade names including refractionometer, dioptrescope, and ultimeter, but currently the most commonly used names in different parts of the world are focimeter, vertometer, lensmeter, and lensometer.

4.1.1 The evidence base: when and how to assess lens powers and optical centres

Focimetry (vertometry/lensometry) should be used to assess lens powers and optical centres of glasses that are newly glazed (for checking they comply with the current international standard ISO 21987:2017), of unknown correction and any that patients return because they are dissatisfied with them. Ready-made reading glasses should be measured because they cannot be assumed to provide the powers suggested and the higher-powered glasses often include vertical prism.[1] Note that, although focimeters measure the vertex power, axis direction, prism, and optical centres of ophthalmic lenses, they do not provide information about other features of lenses that could cause patients problems and need to be checked, such as base curve and lens form, segment style, height, size and inset, centre or edge thickness, optical and surface quality, and the presence of a lens tint and/or surface coating (antireflection, antiscratch). Automatic focimeters are available that measure the lens powers, optical centres, and any prism automatically once the lens has been appropriately positioned and provide a printout of the results. These are very simple to use and the measurement procedure will not be explained. Their main disadvantage is that they break down more often than manual focimeters[2] and require regular calibration.

4.1.2 Procedure for focimetry (vertometry/lensometry)

See online Video 4.1 and summary in Box 4.1

1. Explain the test to the patient: "I am going to measure the power of your glasses."

65

Box 4.1 **Summary of focimetry/vertometry/ lensometry for single vision lenses**

1. Explain the test to the patient.
2. Set the power to zero and focus the eyepiece.
3. Position the middle of the ocular (back) surface of the right lens against the lens stop.
4. Adjust the lens vertically and horizontally until the illuminated target is in the middle of the graticule, then fix the lens into position using the lens retainer.
5. Turn the power wheel to bring the target into focus.
   a. Record the sphere power when the entire target is focused at the same time (lens = sphere only). Go to step 8.
   b. Record the meridian with the most plus (or least minus) power is in focus. The latter may require adjustment of an axis wheel.
6. Focus the meridian with the least plus (or most minus) power. The difference between the sphere power and the new meridian power is the cylinder power.
7. The orientation of the second meridian from the eyepiece protractor or the axis wheel is the cylinder axis.
8. Dot the lens using the marking device.
9. Repeat for the left lens.

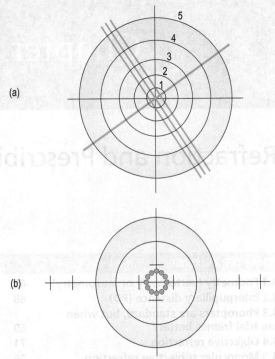

Fig. 4.1 Focimeter targets. The focimeter targets are in focus at the same time, indicating a spherical lens. The graticule scale allows measurement of prism. **(a)** A focimeter that uses a cylindrical (3-line) and spherical (1-line) target. The graticule scale is numbered 1 to 5. **(b)** A focimeter that uses a circle of dots target. The graticule scale is indicated by the intersecting lines and runs from 1–5 horizontally and 1–3 vertically in both directions from the centre. With an astigmatic lens, the dots become lines orientated along the two principal meridians.

2. Set the power to zero and focus the eyepiece (turn it as far anti-clockwise as possible, then slowly turn it clockwise until the target and graticule first come into sharp focus. The graticule is the network of circular and/ or straight lines in the focal plane of the eyepiece that allows prism measurement).
3. Measure the back vertex power by placing the glasses on the focimeter with the back (ocular) surface away from you. Position the middle of the right lens against the lens stop.
4. Adjust the glasses vertically (using the lens table) and horizontally until the illuminated target is positioned in the middle of the graticule. If the lens is high powered, you may need to turn the power wheel to bring the target into focus before it can be centred.
5. Fix the lens into position using the lens retainer.
6. Turn the power wheel to bring the target into focus.
   (a) If the entire target is focused at the same time (Fig. 4.1), the lens is a sphere and there is no cylindrical component. Record the sphere power for the right eye from the power wheel or the internal scale and go to step 8.
   (b) If parts of the target are in focus at different powers and to record in the standard negative cylinder format, turn the power wheel until the meridian with the most plus power or least minus power is focused.

   (c) With focimeters using line targets, rotate the axis wheel until the sphere line (see Fig. 4.1a) is in focus and the line is continuous without breaks. You may need to use the power wheel to gain best focus.
   (d) Record the sphere power from the power wheel or internal scale.
7. To obtain the power and axis of the cylinder:
   (a) Focus the image in the meridian at 90° from the first meridian by turning the power wheel towards the most minus (or least plus) power.
   (b) Read off the power when this meridian is in focus. With focimeters using line targets, the cylinder lines will be in focus.
   (c) Record the difference between the sphere power from step 6d and the new meridian power as the cylinder power. For example, if first (sphere) power was focused at −5.00 D and the second power at −5.75 D, the cylinder power is −0.75 DC.

(d) Record the orientation of the second meridian from the eyepiece protractor or the axis wheel as the cylinder axis. With focimeters using line targets, this will be the orientation of the cylinder lines (see Fig. 4.1a).

8. Make sure the target is centred in the graticule and dot the right lens using the marking device. This could be just one spot (the lens optical centre) or three dots (the middle is the lens optical centre, the other two indicate the horizontal line).

9. Release the lens retainer and repeat steps 5 to 8 for the left lens. Do not change the vertical position of the glasses between measurements of the right and left lenses as you need to determine if any vertical prism is incorporated in the glasses.

10. Move the lens horizontally until the target is in the same vertical plane as the centre of the graticule and dot the left lens using the marking device.

11. If the target is above or below the centre of the graticule, vertical prism is present and should be recorded to the nearest 0.5^{Δ} using the graticule scale (see Fig. 4.1).

12. Remove the glasses and measure the distance between the right and left optical centres to calculate the centration distance and record it in millimetres.

13. For front-surface solid multifocal lenses, the reading add must be measured using front vertex power. Turn the lens around so that the ocular surface faces you and reposition the glasses in the focimeter. Measure the front vertex power along one meridian in the distance portion of the glasses. Measure the front vertex power along the same meridian in the near portion of the glasses. The difference between these powers is the reading addition. Repeat the measurement in the left lens. For low-powered lenses, the front vertex power approximately equals the back vertex power, and the back vertex power add can be measured.

14. For progressive addition lenses (progressives or PALs), you need to locate the appropriate position on each lens to measure the distance and near prescription, optical centres, and any prism (Fig. 4.2). Faint symbols are etched into the nasal and temporal sides of each lens, and these must be found and marked with a non-permanent marker. The symbol may indicate the PAL manufacturer and include the power of the addition. Use the manufacturer's marking-up card to locate the appropriate distance and near centres and measure the sphero-cylindrical power and any prism at these points as previously described (see Fig. 4.2).

15. Compare the centration distance and the patient's interpupillary distance (PD). If these distances differ, calculate the induced horizontal prism using Prentice's rule (induced prism = Fc, where F is the power of the lens along the horizontal meridian and c is the difference between the centration distance and PD in

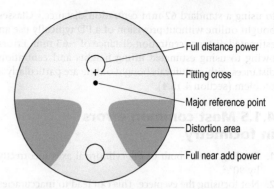

- Full distance power
- Fitting cross
- Major reference point
- Distortion area
- Full near add power

Fig. 4.2 PALs. An example of the important points and areas of a progressive addition lens.

centimetres). The direction of the prism also needs to be deduced.

4.1.3 Recording of focimetry results

Record the sphero-cylindrical correction in minus cylinder form for both lenses and the reading addition power if a multifocal. Also record any prism, the type of lens, any tints or coatings, and so forth. Use 'x' rather than the word 'axis.' Record the spherical and cylindrical power to the nearest 0.25 D, and the cylinder axis to the nearest 2.5°. The axis should be between 2.5° and 180°. Use 180 rather than 0 degrees. Do not use a degree sign as ° can look like a 0 and make an axis of 10° look like 100 degrees.

Examples:

D28 segment bifocal, CR39, MAR coat
RE: –2.00/–1.00 × 35, LE: –2.25 DS   Add +2.00 DS

NV, CR39. OD: +2.25/–0.75 × 80, OS: +2.50 / –0.50 × 105

4.1.4 Interpreting focimetry results

One of the most common errors is an axis reading incorrect by 90°.[2] Given that the cylindrical axes in the two eyes are often mirror images of each other (e.g., both axes 90° or both axes 180°; 175 with 5°; 20° with 160°; 45° with 135°), if axes are 90° different to this (e.g., 180° with 90°; 175° with 95°; 20° with 50°; both axes ~45°; both axes ~135°) then recheck the two cylindrical axes.[3] Reading additions are typically the same in both eyes, so that if they are read as different, they should be rechecked.

Patients are increasingly using ready-made reading glasses and glasses bought online and clinicians should be aware of their limitations. Ready-made reading glasses, particularly if higher powered (+3.00 and +3.50), can often include vertical prism and horizontal prism owing to using a standard 62-mm centration distance.[1] Glasses bought online without provision of a PD typically use an estimated distance centration distance of ~63 mm. Errors owing to using estimated fitting heights and centration distances with multifocals bought online are particularly a problem (section 4.15.4).[4]

4.1.5 Most common errors in focimetry

1. Reading one or both of the cylindrical axes incorrectly by 90°.[2]
2. Not focusing the eyepiece. This can lead to inaccuracies for high-powered lenses.
3. Ignoring the relative vertical position of the target between the right and left lens, thereby missing vertical prism.

4.2 Interpupillary distance

The PD (or interpupillary distance, IPD) is the distance between the centres of the pupils of the eyes.

4.2.1 The evidence base: when and how to measure PD

The PD is measured (1) prior to refraction and (2) during dispensing, so that you can place the optical centre of the (1) phoropter/trial frame lenses and (2) new glasses in front of the patient's visual axes to avoid unwanted prism and aberrations.

The anatomical PD is typically measured as it is a simple, quick measurement that just requires a millimetre ruler.[5] Inaccuracies in anatomical PD can occur owing to parallax error when there is a large difference between your PD and the patient's PD. However, the error is slight, with an 8 mm difference in the examiner's and patient's PDs leading to a 0.5 mm error in the measured patient's PD.[6] The repeatability of anatomical binocular PDs taken by an experienced clinician is approximately ± 1 to 2 mm,[7,8] slightly poorer between clinicians at about ± 1.5 to 2 mm,[8] and similar to that for a pupillometer.[7,8] Pupillometers allow monocular PDs to be measured more accurately than an anatomical measurement.[8] This is beneficial when ordering glasses for high refractive errors or for varifocals/PALs where precise centration of each lens along the patient's visual axes is necessary. In addition, pupillometers can be performed by a clinical assistant and the examiner does not need to be binocular. The PD measured with a corneal reflection pupillometer will typically be 0.5 to 1 mm smaller than the anatomical PD because it measures the

physiological PD and locates the visual axes, whereas the anatomical PD locates the lines of sight or optical axes.[7,8] Note that many pupillometers use a correction for the parallax error mentioned in the anatomical PD section.[6] Inaccuracies can occur if the pupillometer sits higher or (usually) lower on the bridge than the intended glasses frame and the nose is not straight, so that the monocular PDs can be shifted to one side.

4.2.2 Procedure for PD measurement

1. Explain the test to the patient: "I am going to measure the distance between the pupils of your eyes so that I can put your lenses in the correct position."
2. Face the patient directly at the distance desired for the near PD (usually about 40 cm).
3. Rest the PD ruler on the bridge of the patient's nose or on the patient's forehead and steady your hand with your fingers on the patient's temple to ensure that the ruler is held firmly in place.

Distance PD

4. Close your right eye and ask the patient to look at your left eye. (It is usually easiest to indicate with your finger the eye that you want the patient to fixate.)
5. Choose a point of reference on the patient's right eye. The temporal pupil margin is usually most convenient, although the centre of the pupil or the temporal limbus margin may also be used and the latter may be essential with patients with dark irides. Align the zero point on the ruler with this reference point.
6. Close your left eye, open your right, and ask the patient to change fixation to your open right eye. Take care not to move the ruler or your head position. Sight the appropriate reference point on the patient's left eye to obtain a reading for the distance PD (Fig. 4.3). This would be the left nasal pupil margin if you initially used the right temporal pupil margin.
7. Re-open your left eye, have the patient switch fixation back to it and check that the zero mark on the ruler is still aligned with the original reference point. If it is not, repeat the measurement (steps 4 to 7).

Near PD

8. Move laterally to place your dominant eye opposite the patient's nose. Ensure that you are still at a distance from the patient equal to the patient's near working distance.
9. Using your dominant eye only, choose a reference point on the patient's right eye and align the zero point on the ruler with this reference point.

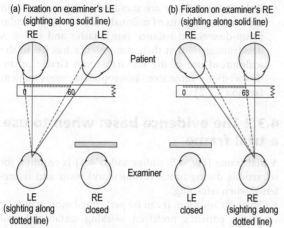

(a) Fixation on examiner's LE (sighting along solid line)

(b) Fixation on examiner's RE (sighting along solid line)

RE   LE   RE   LE

Patient

0   60   0   63

Examiner

LE   RE   LE   RE
(sighting along   closed   closed   (sighting along
dotted line)   dotted line)

Fig. 4.3 PD measurement. **(a)** Measurement of near PD. **(a and b)** Measurement of distance PD.

10. Look over to the patient's left eye and note the reading on the ruler that aligns with the corresponding reference point on the left eye (see Fig. 4.3a).

4.2.3 Recording of PD

The values are normally recorded as PD: distance/near (in mm). For example, PD: 63/60.

4.2.4 Interpreting PD results

For women the distance PD is commonly in the range of 55 to 65 mm, and for men it is 60 to 70 mm.[5] Young children may have PDs as low as 45 mm. The near PD value is usually 3 or 4 mm less than the distance PD. Glasses bought online (without a PD measurement) and ready-made reading glasses are commonly provided with centration distances of 62 or 63 mm.[1,4]

4.2.5 Most common errors in PD measurement

1. Moving the ruler during the measurement.

4.3 Phoropters are standard, but when are trial frames better?

A phoropter (Fig. 4.4; online video 4.2) is a free-standing unit that is placed in front of the patient's head and contains all the equipment necessary to measure a patient's ametropia, heterophoria, and accommodation. A trial frame is an adjustable spectacle frame that is fitted to the patient's head and includes cells into which all the various lenses required to measure a patient's ametropia, heterophoria, and accommodation can be placed.

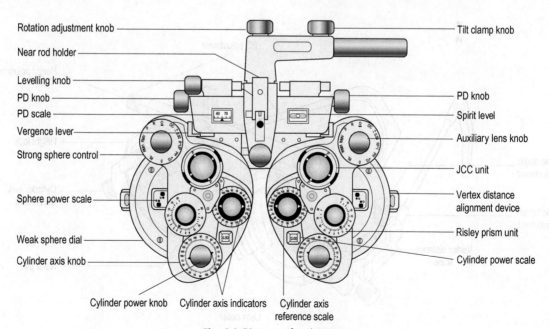

Rotation adjustment knob

Near rod holder

Levelling knob

PD knob

PD scale

Vergence lever

Strong sphere control

Sphere power scale

Weak sphere dial

Cylinder axis knob

Tilt clamp knob

PD knob

Spirit level

Auxiliary lens knob

JCC unit

Vertex distance alignment device

Risley prism unit

Cylinder power scale

Cylinder power knob   Cylinder axis indicators   Cylinder axis reference scale

Fig. 4.4 Diagram of a phoropter.

4.3.1 The evidence base: when to use a phoropter

The use of a manual or digital phoropter is the preferred technique for distance vision refraction of the majority of patients. The main advantages are:

- A quicker refraction: It is much quicker to change lens powers for both retinoscopy and subjective refraction in a phoropter compared with a trial frame.
- Less back strain: particularly with digital phoropters. This can be a problem for eye care clinicians.[9]
- Greater comfort: A trial frame containing several lenses can become uncomfortably heavy, particularly for older patients with thin skin.
- Jackson cross-cylinder (JCC) accuracy: The JCC is automatically aligned with the cylinder axis in a phoropter.
- No lens smear: Trial case lenses can become covered with fingerprints (particularly in university clinics), and require regular cleaning.
- High-tech appearance: Some patients may have more confidence in the results using phoropters, particular the digital versions, over the ancient-looking trial frame.
- Digital phoropters: These include data links to automated focimeter (vertometer/lensmeter) and/ or autorefractor and can provide easy comparison of the patient's current glasses power with the latest subjective refraction result. The refraction results can automatically be included in the patient's electronic record.

- Risley prisms: These are standard on phoropters and make measurements of fusional reserves and binocular prism-dissociated balance much faster and easier. A disadvantage is that their convenience has led to the widespread use of the unreliable von Graefe prism-dissociation subjective heterophoria measurement (section 1.1.2).

4.3.2 The evidence base: when to use a trial frame

A trial frame (Fig. 4.5, online video 4.3) is required for refractions during home (domiciliary) visits and is preferred when refracting:

- The near addition: It can be performed more naturally at the patient's preferred working distance(s) and position.
- Children and patients with binocular vision problems: Children can more easily see their parent/guardian and feel more at ease with them. The trial frame can stimulate less proximal accommodation than a phoropter and provides more repeatable results of oculomotor status.[10] In addition, it is possible to perform the cover test with large aperture lenses in a trial frame, but not with a phoropter.
- Patients with visual impairment (or poor subjective responses): Large dioptric changes in sphere and a high-powered JCC ($\pm$ 0.75 or $\pm$ 1.00 D) are required to enable patients to appreciate a difference in vision and this can easily be done

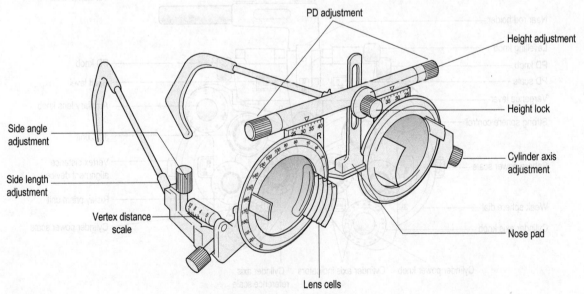

Fig. 4.5 Diagram of a trial frame.

using a trial frame. The trial frame with large aperture lenses also allows unusual head and eye positions that may be necessary for visually impaired patients using eccentric fixation.

- Patients with hearing problems: The phoropter obscures the patient's view of the examiner and therefore prevents communication with sign language or simple hand signals.
- Patients with high refractive error: The trial frame is fixed to the patient's head so that the vertex distance does not change with patient head movement and is typically 8 to 12 mm and similar to the vertex distance for glasses. One study reported vertex distances with phoropters to vary from 10 to 34 mm,[11] and vertex distances can be variable during a refraction if the patient moves behind the phoropter. In addition, the back vertex power of a combination of high-powered lenses in a trial frame can be measured in a focimeter rather than simply assume that it is the algebraic sum.
- When over-refracting patients being fitted with multifocal contact lenses: helps to keep the visual environment, binocularity, and pupil size as close to normal as possible (section 5.9.2).

4.4 Objective refraction

Objective refraction provides an assessment of refractive error that does not require subjective responses from the patient.

4.4.1 The evidence base: when to use objective refraction and which techniques

An objective measurement of refractive error, usually by retinoscopy or autorefraction, provides an initial estimate of refractive error that can be refined by subjective refraction. It is the only assessment available in patients who are unable to co-operate in a subjective refraction, such as young children and it is heavily relied on when subjective responses are limited or unreliable.

Retinoscopy provides a more accurate result of refractive error in a greater array of patients than autorefraction, although autorefraction is a useful and reliable alternative in many 'standard' adult patients and can be particularly accurate at determining astigmatism.[12] Autorefractors should not be used with young children without cycloplegia because of proximal accommodation errors producing significantly more minus results than with cycloplegia,[13,14] particularly in young hyperopes (e.g., an average 2.50 D more minus for 4-year-old children with individuals

varying from 0 up to a nearly −7.00 D difference).[13] These errors remain in children up to 18 years of age.[14,15] As the measurement of autorefraction is simple, it will not be discussed further.

Retinoscopy also provides a sensitive assessment of the ocular media (e.g., early detection of cataracts, keratoconus), can be used to determine refractive error at distance and near, measure accommodative accuracy (section 6.8), identify accommodative dysfunction, and is portable, less expensive, and less likely to break down.[2] Retinoscopy's major disadvantage is that it requires several years of training to become proficient.

There appears to be no research literature that compares the accuracy of streak or spot retinoscopes or refractions using negative or positive cylinders. The procedure will be described for streak retinoscopy, but spot retinoscopy is an acceptable alternative. Positive cylinders have the advantage of making retinoscopy easier to learn, as 'with' movement is typically easier to see than 'against' movement. However, negative cylinders are preferred as they are standard in most phoropters. In addition, there is the possibility of stimulating accommodation during subjective refraction when removing a plus cylinder from a trial frame to replace it with one of another power. For these reasons the procedure will be described using negative cylinders.

4.4.2 Procedure for retinoscopy

See online videos 4.4 to 4.7 and summary in Box 4.2. See section 4.5.3 for adaptations to this standard technique.

1. Prior to retinoscopy, it is useful to estimate the refractive correction from relevant case history (e.g., ability to read without glasses in an older patient suggests a low myope), the current glasses, and visual acuity (VA) information. (e.g., For low myopes and older hyperopes without accommodation, a one line loss of logMAR VA corresponds to approximately −0.25 DS of refractive error.[16])
2. Set the retinoscope mirror to the plano position (maximal divergence, with the retinoscope collar at the bottom of its range) and use the smaller sight hole if this option is available (Fig. 4.6; section 4.4.3, point 9c). Hold the retinoscope with your right hand.
3. Determine a comfortable working distance from the patient so that you can change lenses easily. Typically used distances are 67 cm or 50 cm (+1.50 or 2.00 DS dioptric values, respectively) and depend on arm length.
4. Switch on the duochrome (bichromatic), spotlight, or a similar distance fixation target that is easy to see when blurred and does not provide a stimulus to accommodation.

Box 4.2 **Summary of retinoscopy procedure**

1. Estimate the refractive correction from relevant case history, VA, and focimetry.
2. Ensure the retinoscope is in the plano-mirror position with the smaller sight-hole (if available) and in your right hand.
3. Switch on the duochrome, spotlight, or similar non-accommodative target.
4. Clean and position the phoropter or trial frame appropriately and set the distance PD.
5. Explain the test to the patient.
6. Dial in the working distance lenses, if appropriate.
7. Dim the room lights.
8. Align yourself with the visual axis of the patient's right eye.
9. Look across to the left eye and if 'with' movement is observed, add positive lenses until 'against' movement is obtained.
10. If the reflex is dim and the movement is relatively slow, use an appropriate lens to get nearer to neutrality.
11. If the reflex brightness, speed, and thickness are the same in all meridians, estimate the spherical lens power needed, add your estimate, and repeat until you neutralise the reflex. Then go to step 14.
12. If the reflex brightness, speed, and thickness are different across the meridians, the eye is astigmatic and you need to determine the principal meridians. Neutralise the most plus/least minus meridian first with a spherical lens.
13. Along the perpendicular meridian, add minus cylinder (with the axis aligned with the retinoscope streak) in a bracketing technique to achieve neutrality.
14. Check the neutral point by moving forward and backward slightly from your normal working distance, and check the reflex movement.
15. Repeat for the patient's left eye.
16. Remove the working distance lenses or subtract 1.50 or 2.00 D from your final result.
17. Measure the patient's visual acuities with the net retinoscopy result.

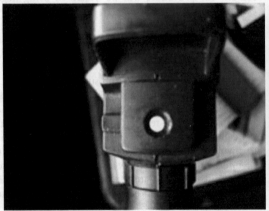 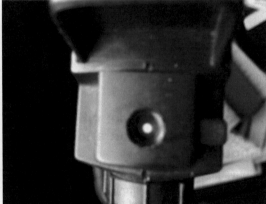

Fig. 4.6 Retinoscope sight holes. The sight hole size can be changed on some retinoscopes. Generally use the smaller sight hole to get more precise reversal. The larger one should be used when the reflex is dim and difficult to see, such as with patients with small pupils and/or cataract.

5. Clean the parts of the phoropter or trial frame that contact the patient using alcohol wipes or similar. Fit the trial frame or phoropter so that the patient is comfortable and adjust it to the patient's distance PD.
6. Explain the test to the patient: "I'm going to shine a light in your eye and get an indication of the power of the glasses you may need. Please look at the red and green target and let me know if my head blocks your view. Don't worry if the target is blurred." Ensure that your head does not block the patient's view at any time, otherwise the patient is likely to accommodate to it.
7. Either:
   (a) Dial in the +1.50 DS (or if available and preferred +2.00 DS) retinoscope lens into the phoropter or place +1.50 DS or +2.00 DS working distance lenses in the back cells of the trial frame. This technique has the advantages that all 'with' movements

indicate hyperopia and all 'against' movements indicate myopia, it avoids any calculations and provides 'fogging' lenses that will relax accommodation in a low hyperope. The disadvantage is that the working distance lens introduces two reflections, which can make retinoscopy more difficult when you are first learning the technique.

OR

(b) Do not add a working distance lens. The working distance power (+1.50 D or +2.00 D) must later be subtracted from your final retinoscope result.

8. Position yourself vertically and horizontally (Figs. 4.7a and 4.8) to align your right eye and retinoscope sight hole with the visual axis of the patient's right eye (the patient's left eye is fixating the distance target; see Fig. 4.7a), otherwise you will obtain off-axis errors.[17] If the patient is looking slightly upwards to view the target, you will need to be positioned slightly higher than the patient's eye (see Fig. 4.8).

9. Dim the room lights to provide a higher contrast view of the pupillary reflex, while providing enough light to allow easy viewing of the phoropter/trial case. Explain this to the patient: "Dimming the lights helps me to get an accurate result."

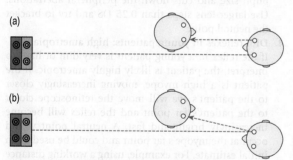

Fig. 4.7 Retinoscopist position (lateral). Plan view of the position of the examiner and patient when performing retinoscopy. **(a)** The examiner is viewing along the visual axis of the patient's right eye, while the patient's left eye fixates the duochrome target. **(b)** The examiner views off-axis in the 'good' eye of a patient with strabismus. For the strabismic eye, retinoscopy could be performed along the angle of strabismus, or the good eye could be occluded and retinoscopy performed off-axis.

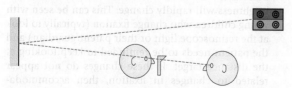

Fig. 4.8 Retinoscopist position (vertical). Side view of the position of the patient and examiner when performing retinoscopy when the target is above the patient's head.

10. Position the streak so that it is vertical. Look through the aperture of the retinoscope and direct the light at the patient's pupil and you should see the red retinoscope reflex. Sweep the retinoscope streak across the patient's pupil horizontally and compare the movement of the reflex in the pupil with the movement of the retinoscope. If the reflex moves in the same direction as the movement of the retinoscope streak, this is known as 'with' movement. If the reflex moves in the opposite direction to the movement of the retinoscope streak, this is known as 'against' movement.

11. If a patient is pre-presbyopic, ensure that the patient will not accommodate while looking at the target by quickly scoping the left eye (you do not need to be on the left eye visual axis as this does not need to be accurate) and if 'with' movement is observed, add positive lenses until 'against' movement is obtained. This will ensure that the left eye (which is viewing the target; Fig. 4.7a) is blurred by at least +1.50 D.

12. Sweep the vertical retinoscope streak across the patient's right pupil and compare the movement of the reflex with the movement of the retinoscope. Mentally note the direction of movement plus the reflex brightness, speed, and width. Then rotate the retinoscope streak so that it is horizontal and sweep across the pupil vertically and repeat the process for the two oblique meridians (45° and 135°). For all four streak positions, mentally note the direction of the reflex movement and its relative brightness, speed, and width.

13. Determine if the refractive error is spherical (the observed reflex has the same direction, speed, brightness, and thickness in all meridians) or astigmatic (the reflex differs in different meridians).

14. If the reflex seems dim and movement slow, so that any difference between the reflex speed, brightness, and thickness in different meridians is difficult to determine, the ametropia is likely high, so place an appropriate spherical lens in the phoropter/trial frame and then repeat retinoscopy along the four meridians.

15. If astigmatic, determine the principal meridians by rotating the streak axis until the angle of the reflex movement coincides with the angle of the streak in two meridians; one perpendicular to the other (Fig. 4.9).

16. Determine the spherical component by 'neutralising' (adding plus lenses to 'with' movement and minus lenses to 'against' movement until the reflex fills the entire pupil and all perceived movement stops at the 'neutral' point) the most plus/least minus meridian first (the meridian with the slowest, dullest 'with' or fastest, brightest 'against' movement). The most efficient process is to make relatively large lens changes based on estimates of the sphere change needed using the reflex's brightness and speed (see online videos) ▶

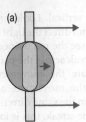 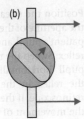

Fig. 4.9 Determining the two astigmatic meridians. **(a)** If you are scoping on axis, the reflex will move in the same direction as the retinoscopy streak. **(b)** If you are off axis, the reflex will move in a different direction than the direction of the retinoscopy streak. You should then rotate your streak to align with the reflex.

and bracketing to the final power. For example, a useful approach would be: (1) slow, dull 'with', try +4.00 DS; (2) faster, brighter 'with', try +6.00 DS; (3) fast, bright 'against', try +5.00 DS; (4) very fast and bright 'with', try +5.50 DS; (5) neutral. Result is +5.50 DS. This process will improve as you become better at judging the lens changes needed based on the speed, brightness, and thickness of the reflex.

17. Check the neutral point by moving forward slightly and observing the movement of the reflex. A bright, fast 'with' movement should be seen. If you move backward slightly from your normal working distance, a bright, fast 'against' movement should be seen. If not, recheck your result.

18. Set the minus cylinder axis parallel with the streak orientation of the least plus/most minus meridian. Move the retinoscope with the streak in this position and you should observe 'against' movement. Add minus cylinder until you achieve neutrality. As 'with' movement can be easier to see than 'against' movement, you may wish to add minus cylinder until 'with' movement is just seen and then reduce the cylinder by 0.25 D.

19. Briefly, recheck the sphere and cylinder components for neutrality.

20. Move over to the left side and align yourself with the patient's left visual axis. Repeat steps 12 to 19 on the patient's left eye.

21. Remove the working distance lenses (or subtract 1.50 or 2.00 D from your final result).

22. Measure the patient's VAs with the net retinoscopy result.

4.4.3 Adaptations to the standard procedure

1. **Determining cylinder axis using 'with' movements**
   Some clinicians prefer to determine cylinder axis by rotating the retinoscope steak until it aligns with a 'with' streak (see Fig. 4.9a). The thickness of the 'with' reflex can also be altered by slightly adjusting the sleeve position. 'With' movements are gained by moving the retinoscope collar to the top of the sleeve (concave-mirror position) as this changes all 'against' movements to 'with' movements and vice-versa.

2. **Large pupils: concentrate on the centre**
   Spherical aberration can provide a relative 'against' movement in the periphery of the pupil and a common error is to miss slight 'with' movement in the pupil centre by averaging reflex movements across the pupil (see online video 4.6). Concentrate on the central reflex and ignore the reflex at the edges of the pupil.[18]

3. **Coping with a 'scissors' reflex**
   This reflex moves like the action of a pair of scissors, moving simultaneously in opposite directions from the centre of the pupil, and accurate neutralisation can be very difficult. The reflex can be caused by optical aberrations, particularly coma in a normal eye or more rarely by abnormalities in the media, such as keratoconus or corneal scarring. Increasing the room light level can help because it reduces the patient's pupil size and cuts down the peripheral aberrations. Use larger lens steps than 0.25 DS and try to bracket the neutral point.

4. **Dim reflexes in young patients: high ametropia**
   If the reflex in a young patient is very dim or hard to interpret, the patient is likely highly ametropic. If the patient is a high myope, moving increasingly closer to the patient's eye will move the retinoscope closer to the patient's far point and the reflex will become increasingly bright and fast. A neutral point would occur at the myope's far point and could be used as an initial estimate. For example, using a working distance retinoscopy lens, if the neutral point is found at 20 cm this suggests that the patient is a −5.00 DS myope. If the reflex does not become brighter as you move closer to the patient, the ametropia is hyperopia, so add a medium to high plus lens.

5. **Fast pupil and reflex changes = accommodative fluctuations**
   During accommodative fluctuations, the pupil will be seen to vary in size and the reflex movement and brightness will rapidly change. This can be seen with young children who change fixation (typically to look at the retinoscope light or their parent/guardian) and the patient needs to be reminded to keep looking at the distance target. If these changes do not appear related to changes in fixation, then accommodative fluctuations that could be caused by latent hyperopia or pseudomyopia should be suspected and a cycloplegic refraction (section 4.12) and

assessments of accommodation (section 6.8) should be performed.

6. **Adapt retinoscopy for children**
   See cycloplegic refraction, section 4.12. Retinoscopy needs to be particularly quick because the patient's attention span can be brief.

7. **Adapt retinoscopy for a patient with strabismus**
   A strabismic eye is typically unable to fixate the target, so that retinoscopy on the 'good' eye must be performed slightly off-axis (see Fig. 4.7b) to allow the 'good' eye to fixate. This will lead to errors, so minimise the off-axis extent as much as possible.[17] Indeed, it is likely that autorefractors will be able to provide a more accurate indication of refractive error in the 'good' eye in strabismics as off-axis fixation is not required. For the strabismic eye, it can be easier to change the fixation point for the 'good' eye, so that retinoscopy along the visual axis of the strabismic eye is easier.

8. **Are you a retinoscopist with poor vision in one eye?**
   If you are unable to obtain accurate retinoscopy results in your poorer eye, you can use your better eye on both sides, but you will have to scope off-axis on one side (see Fig. 4.7b), which will provide slightly incorrect results.[17] An alternative is Barrett's method in which you perform retinoscopy of both the patient's eyes while the patient fixates the retinoscope and then checks the spherical component of this initial result with the patient fixating in the distance using your good eye. For example, retinoscopy at near gives: RE: $-1.50/-1.00 \times 10$; LE: $-2.00/-0.50 \times 170$. Retinoscopy in the distance for the right eye gives $-2.50/-1.00 \times 10$, an extra -1.00 DS. Apply this difference to the left eye so that the final retinoscopy result is: RE: $-2.50/-1.00 \times 10$; LE: $-3.00/-0.50 \times 170$.

9. **Adaptations to help cope with a dim reflex in older patients**
   A dim reflex in older patients is common owing to small pupils and some media opacity/cataract so that a reduced amount of light reaches the retina and even less returns to your retinoscope. Increasing the retinoscope light intensity may just reduce the pupil size further and a medium intensity is usually best. An autorefractor result may not be obtainable with these patients, but retinoscopy can provide a useful result if used with the following adaptations:

   (a) Perform retinoscopy at a closer distance such as 25 cm or 33 cm because this can provide a brighter reflex. You will have to subtract a larger value from your retinoscopy result to compensate for the reduced working distance (4.00 or 3.00 D, respectively, for 25 cm or 33 cm) and understand that there is a greater chance of dioptric error. For example, a 5 cm error when using a 67 cm working distance

(i.e., actually at 62 cm) causes a 0.10 D error, but the same 5 cm error when using a 25 cm working distance (i.e., actually at 20 cm) causes a 1.00 D error. There should be no error for astigmatism as long as your working distance remains constant.

(b) Use the least number of lenses in the trial frame/phoropter as you lose 8% of the reflex for each lens used owing to reflections. Do not use a working distance lens and refract each meridian using a sphere only and convert to a sphero-cylindrical combination for the subjective refraction.

(c) Use the large aperture sight hole when available (see Fig. 4.6) as this will allow more of the returning light to reach your eye.

4.4.4 Recording of retinoscopy results

Record your retinoscopy results as the sphero-cylindrical correction that neutralised the patient's refractive error after removing your working distance lenses. Do not use a degree sign as ° can look like a 0 and make an axis of 15° look like 150 degrees. Use 'x' rather than the word 'axis'. Most clinicians record the spherical and cylindrical power to the nearest 0.25 D, and the cylinder axis to the nearest 2.5° (i.e., half the step size of 5° on the axis scale). Use 180 rather than 0 degrees. Some clinicians, typically those who use autorefractors and computerised phoropters that provide refractive correction results in smaller step sizes, record to the nearest 0.125 D and 1°. Also record the monocular VA with the retinoscopy result.

Examples (with VAs in visual acuity rating (VAR), decimal, metric, and imperial Snellen)

RE: $-4.75/-1.00 \times 20$	112
LE: $-5.25/-0.75 \times 155$	114
RE: $+1.50$ DS	1.0^{+2}
LE: $+1.75/-0.50 \times 100$	1.0^{-1}
RE: $-2.00/-0.50 \times 165$	6/4.5
LE: -2.25 DS	$6/4.5^{-2}$
OD: $+2.00/-1.00 \times 105$	$20/20^{+3}$
OS: $+1.75/-0.75 \times 70$	20/25

4.4.5 Interpreting retinoscopy results

On average, retinoscopy provides a refractive result slightly more positive than subjective refraction in young patients.[19] This decreases with age, so that retinoscopy and subjective results are similar in presbyopic patients. As the stimulus to accommodation is greater in subjective refraction (the target is a line of small letters) than in retinoscopy (the target is a blurred duochrome and the eye is fogged by 1.50 to 2.00 DS), the retinoscopy result in young hyperopes can be much more positive than accepted in subjective refraction. Errors can occur in retinoscopy if it is performed off-axis (see Fig. 4.7b), which will induce spherical and astigmatic errors, or if it is performed at an incorrect working distance, which will induce a spherical error.[17] Note that cylinder axes in the two eyes are often mirror images of each other.[3,20] For example, 175° with 5°; 20° with 160°; 45° with 135°.

4.4.6 Most common errors in retinoscopy

1. Using lenses smudged with fingerprints when performing retinoscopy with trial case lenses. Student trial case lenses are notoriously smudged so try to get into the habit of cleaning lenses before using them.
2. Performing retinoscopy at an incorrect working distance, often too close as you move slightly forward to see the reflex more clearly (e.g., working at about 50 cm, while using a 1.50 D working distance lens).
3. Not concentrating on the movement in the centre of the pupil in a patient with large pupils.
4. Performing retinoscopy off-axis.[17]
5. Blocking the patient's view of the distance chart and stimulating the patient's accommodation.

4.5 Monocular subjective refraction

Binocular subjective refraction is the preferred technique for experienced clinicians (section 4.11), but it works most effectively if the starting point is close to the optimal refractive correction and this cannot be guaranteed with inexperienced retinoscopists. Therefore, monocular subjective refraction is initially the preferred technique for students. The goal should be to give the patient as few decisions as possible because patients report considerable dislike of subjective refraction testing[21-23]: some worry that they will provide wrong answers that will lead to them being provided with incorrect glasses,[21,23] whereas others become frustrated at the limited differences in the options provided.[21]

4.5.1 Procedure for monocular refraction

▶ See online video 4.8.

1. Clean the parts of the phoropter or trial frame that contact the patient using alcohol wipes or similar. Fit the trial frame or phoropter so that the patient is comfortable and adjust them to the patient's distance (PD).

2. Explain the procedure to the patient and reduce the patient's concerns about providing wrong answers[21-23]: "During this test, I will place various lenses in front of your eye to find the lenses that give you the best vision. Don't worry about giving a wrong answer because we already have a very good indication of the glasses power you need from your (old glasses/the moving light test/the autorefractor machine) and everything is double checked."
3. Sit or stand where you can comfortably manipulate the phoropter or trail frame and trial case lenses.
4. Begin with the net retinoscopy sphere and cylinder before each eye.
5. Occlude the left eye.
6. Determine the best vision sphere (BVS) (section 4.6 for phoropter-based refractions and section 4.7 for trial frame-based refractions).
7. Check that the circle of least confusion is on the retina (or behind the retina and can be brought onto the retina using accommodation) prior to the use of the JCC using the duochrome test (section 4.8).
8. Determine the cylinder axis using the JCC (section 4.9.3).
9. Determine the cylinder power using the JCC (section 4.9.3).
10. If you have changed the cylinder power or axis significantly, repeat the BVS assessment (step 6).
11. Check the final spherical endpoint using the duochrome test (section 4.8) or the +1.00 blur test as appropriate.
12. Measure VA.
13. Repeat steps 5–10 for the other eye.
14. Compare the monocular VAs with your subjective refraction result with the patient's vision or habitual VAs (as appropriate). If the VA is better with the patient's glasses, then it is likely that your subjective result is incorrect.
15. Compare the VA with the present subjective refraction with age-matched normal data (Table 4.1). If the VA is worse than expected or worse in one eye compared with the other, remeasure the VA with a pinhole aperture. If the VA improves with the pinhole, either the subjective refraction is not optimal and should be repeated or the patient has media opacity, typically cataract, which is being bypassed by the pinhole.
16. If the final refractive correction in either eye is above 5.00 D mean sphere equivalent (MSE, the sphere plus half the cylinder; e.g., −4.75/−1.50 × 180 has an MSE of −5.50 D, +5.50/−2.00 × 90 has a MSE of +4.50 D), then measure the back vertex distance. This is the distance from the back surface of the lens nearest the eye to the apex of the cornea (Fig. 4.10).

Table 4.1 Average visual acuity data for normal, healthy eyes as a function of age[a]

Age (years)	VAR	Snellen (metric)	Snellen (decimal)	Snellen (imperial)	LogMAR
20–49	107 (101 to 113)	$6/4.5^{+1}$ ($6/6^{+1}$ to $6/3^{-2}$)	1.25^{+2} (1.0^{+1} to 2.0^{-2})	$20/15^{+1}$ ($20/20^{+1}$ to $20/10^{-2}$)	−0.14 (−0.02 to −0.26)
50–59	105 (100 to 110)	$6/5^{+1}$ (6/6 to 6/3.8)	1.25 (1.0 to 1.6)	$20/15^{-1}$ (20/20 to 20/13)	−0.10 (0.00 to −0.20)
60–69	103 (98 to 108)	$6/5^{-1}$ ($6/6^{-2}$ to $6/4^{-1}$)	1.25^{-2} (1.0^{-2} to 1.25^{+3})	$20/15^{-2}$ ($20/20^{-2}$ to $20/13^{-1}$)	−0.06 (0.04 to −0.16)
70+	~100 (96 to 106)	6/6 ($6/7.5^{-1}$ to 6/4.5)	1.0 (0.8^{-1} to 1.25^{+1})	20/20 ($20/25^{-1}$ to 20/15)	~0.00 (0.08 to −0.12)

[a]The 95% confidence limits are shown in parentheses.
logMAR, Log of the minimum angle of resolution; VAR, visual acuity rating.
From Elliott DB, Yang KC, Whitaker D. Visual acuity changes throughout adulthood in normal, healthy eyes: seeing beyond 6/6. *Optom Vision Sci.* 1995;72:186–91.[24]

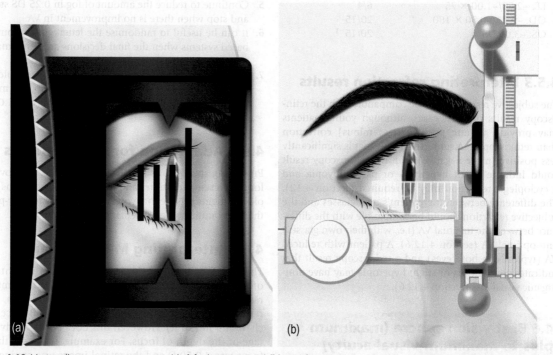

Fig. 4.10 Vertex distance measurement with (a) phoropter and (b) trial frame, when refractive correction is above 5.00 D. The standard vertex distance with phoropters is typically 13.75 mm and indicated by the long line. (Courtesy of Samantha Strong.)

4.5.2 Recording of refraction

Record the refractive correction using the same format described for retinoscopy (section 4.5.5). Record the monocular VAs. If pinhole VA is measured and reveals no improvement in VA, record PHNI ('pinhole no improvement'); otherwise record the VA with the pinhole. For refractive corrections above 5.00 D equivalent sphere, record the vertex distance. Make sure that the prescription details that you provide to patients are clearly legible. Illegible prescription forms have been reported as a surprisingly common error in optometric practice.[2]

Examples of recording (with VAs provided in VAR, decimal, metric and imperial Snellen):

(Vertex distance 10 mm)

RE: +6.00/−1.00 × 35	101
LE: +6.25/−0.75 × 145	102
RE: +2.00 DS	1.0[+2]
LE: +1.75/−0.75 × 85	0.67[(PHNI)]
RE: −3.00/−0.50 × 100	6/12[(PH 6/6)]
LE: −2.50/−1.00 × 75	6/4
OD: −2.75/−0.50 × 180	20/15
OS: −3.00 DS	20/15[−1]

4.5.3 Interpreting refraction results

The subjective results should be compatible with the retinoscopy results in most cases, although young patients may provide a more positive (less minus) correction than retinoscopy.[19] A subjective result that is significantly less positive (more negative) than the retinoscopy result could indicate latent hyperopia or pseudomyopia and a cycloplegic refraction may be required (section 4.12). The difference between the patient's own glasses and the subjective refraction should be compatible with the difference between the habitual VA (i.e., with their own glasses) and optimal VA (section 4.12.6). A patient with reduced VA (typically in both eyes) and a retinoscope result that indicates emmetropia or slight hyperopia may have non-organic visual loss (section 4.12.6).

4.6 Best vision sphere (maximum plus to maximum visual acuity)

No research literature indicates that any BVS procedure is better than another, and an experienced clinician could use a different technique for different patients or may always use a preferred approach. However, the maximum plus to maximum VA (MPMVA) technique has the advantage that

accommodation is well controlled when examining young patients. This technique is particularly easy when using a phoropter as the lens changes can be made quickly and easily.

4.6.1 Procedure for MPMVA

1. Occlude the left eye.
2. Determine the VA of the right eye.
3. Add +1.00 DS to the spherical lens determined in retinoscopy and check the VA. The VA should be reduced by about four lines. If the VA only worsens by one or two lines (or gets better), add additional positive power to the sphere until four lines of acuity are lost to ensure the eye is 'fogged.' Experienced clinicians often use a smaller fogging lens such as +0.50 DS.
4. Ask the patient: "Are the letters clearer with lens 1..." wait while you give the patient an appropriate period of time to appreciate the clarity of the letters, then reduce the amount of fog by 0.25 DS as you ask "or lens 2?" Ask the patient to read the lowest line of letters he or she can see to check that VA improves with the preferred lens.
5. Continue to reduce the amount of fog in 0.25 DS steps and stop when there is no improvement in VA.
6. It can be useful to randomise the letters on computer-based systems when the final decisions are being made to avoid problems owing to letter memorisation.
7. Remember that the *average* acuity of a 20-year-old is ~107 VAR (6/4.5, 1.40, 20/15; Table 4.1), so that most younger patients can read beyond 100 VAR (6/6, 1.0 or 20/20).

4.6.2 Adaptation for older patients

Processing speed slows significantly with age, so provide longer presentation times and repeat the presentations for older patients.[25] Note that you are more likely to over-plus than over-minus older patients (section 4.7.3).[26]

4.6.3 Interpreting MPMVA results

The MPMVA approach is designed to take advantage of a patient's depth of focus to provide the maximum range of clear vision.[27] For example, after refraction, the retinal image should be conjugate with the distance VA chart at 6 m (20 ft). However, this does not take advantage of the depth of focus. For example, if the depth of focus was +0.50 D and the retinal image was conjugate with the distance VA chart so that 0.25 D of the depth of field was in front of the VA chart at 6 m (20 ft) and 0.25 D behind it, the chart would be clear from 2.4 m (8 ft) to 'beyond' infinity. Using the MPMVA technique places the distal edge of the depth of focus conjugate with the VA chart,[27] so that with a depth of focus of

+0.50 D, the range of clear vision is from 1.5 m to 6 m (5 to 20 ft). However, using this technique does mean that patients are slightly over-plussed by 0.16 D as the distance VA chart is at 6 m (20 ft) and not infinity. This can be offset in young patients owing to a lead of accommodation (+0.25 DS) during distance refraction, but this does not occur in older patients who have lost accommodation.[27] Over-plussed/under-minused refractive corrections are common causes of unhappiness with glasses in older patients.[26] Be particularly aware of over-plussing with older patients with a large depth of focus owing to small pupils,[27] and do not use a truncated VA chart or reduce plus to just the 100, 6/6, 1.0, 20/20 line because this will aggravate the effect. An indication of over-plussing is that the measured addition is lower than expected.

4.6.4 Recording MPMVA

The results of MPMVA are not recorded because the technique is just part of the subjective refraction.

4.6.5 Most common error in MPMVA

1. Only unfogging VA to 100 (20/20, 6/6, 1.0). Given that most younger and many older patients can read 105 (20/15, 6/4.5, 1.2; Table 4.1), the patient would be slightly over-plussed/under-minused. Using the JCC when the circle of least confusion is in front of the retina, as it would be in this case, can lead to an incorrect determination of astigmatism.[28]

4.7 Best vision sphere (plus/minus technique)

▶ See online video 4.8.

The plus/minus technique for BVS (± BVS) is easier than MPMVA when using a trial frame because less lens changes are typically required. However, it does not provide as good control of accommodation in young patients as the MPMVA technique. For this reason, one or more check tests (duochrome and/or the +1.00 blur check) are typically used with the plus/minus technique in pre-presbyopic patients.

4.7.1 Procedure for ± BVS

1. Throughout the refraction, check that any lenses you are using are clean and free of fingerprints. Your patient will not be able to see through a smudged lens. For the same reason always pick lenses up using the rim and not the lens.

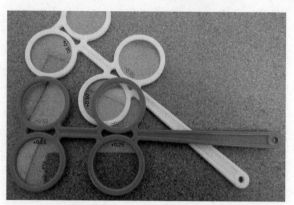

Fig. 4.11 Confirmation lenses used in subjective refraction with a trial frame.

2. Occlude one eye. Direct the patient's attention to their best VA line (or letter).
3. Ready a +0.25 DS lens (confirmation lenses can be useful in this regard [Fig. 4.11]; +0.50 DS can be used if the initial VA is relatively poor) and ask: "Are the letters clearer with the lens…" (place the lens in front of the patient's eye as you say "with the lens," then wait an appropriate period of time to allow the patient to appreciate the clarity of the letters), then ask "or clearer without it?" as you remove the lens. If the patient is hesitant, repeat the presentation (some patients feel embarrassed to ask),[22,23] but finish by asking "or is it about the same?" Some patients report that there is no difference even without the prompt.
4. If VA blurs with the +0.25 DS lens, do not add it. Go to step 9.
5. If the acuity improves or *remains the same* with the additional +0.25 DS, then exchange the spherical lens that is in the trial frame for one that has +0.25 DS added. For example, if the patient has −3.00 DS in the trial frame and the letters look clearer with +0.25 DS, then exchange the lens for a −2.75 DS lens.
6. When exchanging plus lenses in a trial frame in a young hyperope, do not remove the plus lens until the new lens has been inserted, otherwise accommodation could be stimulated. For example, if you have +2.00 DS in the trial frame and the patient indicates that additional plus power is required, insert the +2.25 DS lens first, and then remove the +2.00 DS lens.
7. Using the same approach, continue adding plus lens power in +0.25 DS steps, until the acuity first blurs. Stop at the most plus/least minus lens that does not blur the VA.
8. Regularly randomise the letters on computer-based systems to avoid letter memorisation.

9. Direct the patient's attention to their best VA line/letter. Ready a −0.25 DS (or −0.50 DS) lens and ask: "Are the letters clearer with this lens" (place the lens in front of the patient's eye as you say "with this lens," then wait an appropriate period of time to allow the patient to appreciate the clarity of the letters), then ask "or clearer without it?" as you remove the lens. If the patient is hesitant, repeat the presentation (some patients feel embarrassed to ask),[22,23] but finish by asking "or is it about the same?" Some patients report that there is no difference even without the prompt.

10. If the patient reports no change or a worsening of vision, do not add the −0.25 DS. Go to step 14.

11. If VA improves with the lens, then exchange the spherical lens that is in the trial frame for one that has −0.25 DS added. For example, if the spherical correction is −2.75 DS and −0.25DS improves VA, then remove the −2.75 DS and replace it with a −3.00 DS lens.

12. Add further minus lenses (in −0.25 D steps) *only as long as the VA improves.*

13. If a young patient (i.e., the patient is able to accommodate) reports that vision is improved with the lens, but there is no improvement in VA, ask, "Do the letters definitely look clearer, or just smaller and blacker?" If the letters just look smaller and blacker, do not add the −0.25 DS. The decision to add −0.25 DS when there is no improvement in VA is problematic, but can be supported if the VA chart is truncated so that the 'bottom line' of your VA chart is not 115 (6/3, 2.0, 20/10) as at least 25% of young adults can read beyond 110 (6/4.8, 1.25, 20/16; see Table 4.1) and up to 5% can read 115 (6/3, 2.0, 20/10). This could be supported by results from the duochrome (the additional −0.25 DS should lead to responses of "the same" or "on the red") and an increased fluency of reading the bottom line with the −0.25 DS. Ideally, use a VA chart with a bottom line of 115 (6/3, 2.0, 20/10).

14. Duochrome: Use this as a check test prior to using the JCC in younger patients (section 4.8).

15. The +1.00 blur test. Use this as a check test at the end of monocular refraction in younger patients. Place a +1.00 DS trial case lens over the final BVS correction. If the original VA is about 107 (~6/4.5, 1.25, 20/15) the average VA for a young patient, Table 4.1), then VA will blur to about 87 (~6/12, 0.5, 20/40) with +1.00 DS.[29] If VA is better than 87 with the +1.00 DS, then the patient may have been over-minused or under-plussed and the BVS should be rechecked with +0.25 DS. Note that the four-line loss of VA with the +1.00 DS blur is an average and VA loss with +1.00 DS can reliably be as small as two lines or as large as seven.[29] The vision obtained with

the ±0.25 DS is the final arbiter of the BVS and not the +1.00 blur test.

4.7.2 Adaptations to the standard ±BVS procedure

1. A variety of different instructions

There is a wide variety of approaches to the instructions provided to patients in ±BVS, but no research literature indicates whether one of these options is better than any other. Some clinicians prefer to give all three possible options of "clearer, more blurred, or the same," whereas others suggest that patients find it difficult enough to make these judgements[21–23] so that providing two alternatives rather than three is preferred. An approach used by experienced clinicians when performing refraction on young patients and close to the final correction (as indicated by an excellent VA) is to ask "is it the same with this lens... or better without?" with a +0.25 DS and "is it better or the same with this lens" with a −0.25 DS on the basis that a +0.25 DS should either blur ("worse") or relax accommodation ("same") and a −0.25 DS should either improve acuity ("better") or induce accommodation ("same").

2. Some patients provide poor responses

The subjective refraction techniques described assume that the responses provided by patients are perfect, which is seldom the case. Patients find these decisions very difficult[21–23] and some patients are embarrassed to ask you to repeat the presentation.[21] Remind the patient that you will determine the glasses' power based on several tests, including this one, and that you double check all decisions; repeat presentations using only decisions that are repeatable and attempt to keep presentations to the minimum possible. If a patient is providing unreliable responses or is unable to tell any difference with ±0.25 DS, then use ±0.50 DS or even larger steps.

4.7.3 Recording of ±BVS

The results are not recorded because ±BVS is just part of the subjective refraction.

4.7.4 Most common errors in ±BVS

1. Using trial case lenses smudged with fingerprints. A patient will report that the addition of any smudged lens makes the letters more blurred.

2. Not monitoring the VA to ensure that a change in lens power results in the expected change in VA.

4.8 Duochrome (or bichromatic) test

The duochrome or bichromatic test is based on the principle of axial chromatic aberration, where light of shorter wavelength is refracted more by the eye's optics. Duochrome tests traditionally use a red filter (peak wavelength 620 nm) and a green filter (peak wavelength 535 nm) of equal brightness and a dioptric distance between the foci of these wavelengths of around 0.44 D.[28] The targets on the red and green should look equally clear and black to a accurately corrected patient (Fig. 4.12). An eye that is slightly over-plussed will see the target on the red

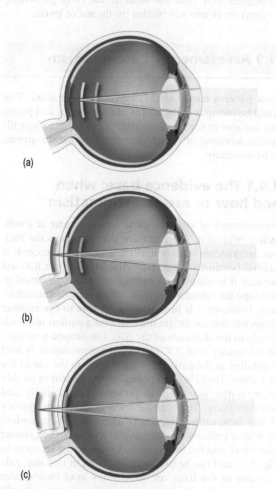

(a)

(b)

(c)

Fig. 4.12 Duochrome. Theory behind the duochrome test when reliable responses indicate that the circles look clearer and blacker on **(a)** red, **(c)** green, or **(b)** they look the same. (Courtesy of Samantha Strong.)

filter more clearly and an eye that is slightly over-minussed will see the target on the green filter more clearly (see Fig. 4.12). The test is more rarely used as a binocular balancing technique (section 4.10).

4.8.1 The evidence base: when to use the duochrome test and when to ignore the results

The duochrome is commonly used as a check on the BVS at two points during monocular refraction of younger patients. (1) Prior to the JCC test. (2) At the end of the refraction to check the final sphere result. It is used prior to JCC to ensure that the circle of least confusion is not in front of the retina because JCC works poorly in that scenario. The circle of least confusion should ideally be on the retina or otherwise slightly behind the retina, in which case a young patient can accommodate to bring it onto the retina.

Some patients give poor results with the duochrome and always prefer one colour, regardless of the changes you make to the spherical refraction, and the test gives unreliable results with blur of more than ~1.00 D. Older patients, owing to small pupils and the increased absorption of low wavelength light by the lens, tend to give more unreliable duochrome results. Colour defective patients can use the test, although the red side of the test will appear duller to protans (section 3.4). In addition, not all charts provide light of appropriate red and green wavelengths. For these reasons, only use the results of the test if the responses from the patient are clearly reliable. Otherwise, ignore the results and move on to the next step of the refraction.

4.8.2 Procedure for the duochrome test

See online video 4.8.

1. Present a duochrome target (see Figs. 4.7 and 4.8) to the patient. Some clinicians dim the room lights; this dilates the pupil and can provide more reliable responses.[30] It also reduces the veiling glare on projected charts.
2. Ask the patient: "Are the rings (or letters/dots) clearer and blacker on the red or on the green, or are they about the same?"
   (a) If they look the same (see Fig. 4.12), check whether the responses are reliable by adding +0.25 DS (this should make the rings on the red look clearer) and then −0.25 DS (now green). If the responses are appropriate, this suggests that the BVS has been obtained and the circle of

least confusion is on the retina. If the responses are not appropriate, then the duochrome is not reliable for this patient and should be ignored.

(b) If the rings on the green look clearer, add +0.25 DS and recheck which rings are clearer and blacker. If still green add a further +0.25 DS and check which rings are clearer and blacker. Note the additional spherical power required to obtain a balance or switch preference to red.

(c) If the rings on the red look clearer, add −0.25 DS until you obtain a balance. Note the additional spherical power required to obtain a balance or switch preference to green.

3. If more than ±0.50 DS is needed to balance the clarity of the rings (or letters) on the duochrome, this usually indicates that the duochrome test is unreliable for this patient and the results should be ignored.

4.8.3 Recording of duochrome results

The result of the duochrome test when used prior to the JCC is typically not recorded. However, some clinicians record the result of the duochrome at the end of the monocular refraction (e.g., R = G or R > G).

4.8.4 Interpreting duochrome results

The results of the duochrome test are used differently, depending on when they are used within the subjective refraction of a young patient:

1. Prior to the use of the JCC: JCC works poorly if the circle of least confusion is in front of the retina[28] and you need to ensure that the circle of least confusion is either on or slightly behind the retina (in this case a young patient can accommodate and bring the circle of least confusion onto the retina).

(a) If the duochrome rings appear equally clear, proceed to JCC.

(b) If the clarity of the rings changes from 'green' to 'red' with +0.25 DS or +0.50 DS, do not add plus lenses and leave the patient 'on the green'.

(c) If the clarity of the rings changes from 'red' to 'green' with −0.25 DS or (if the responses seem reliable) −0.50 DS, add the −0.25 DS or −0.50 DS and leave a young patient 'on the green.'

(d) Make a mental note of any patients left 'on the green' (they may need extra plus after JCC) or any minus lens additions (these may need removing after JCC).

2. After JCC and prior to finalising the refractive correction: If the duochrome rings appear equally clear, the duochrome suggests that the mean spherical correction is correct. Move to the next step of the refraction. Otherwise, use the additional lens power suggested by the duochrome

test and double check whether this additional power is preferred by the patient using MPMVA (section 4.6) or the plus/minus technique (section 4.7).

4.8.5. Most common errors when using the duochrome test

1. Not checking with +0.25 DS and −0.25 DS to make sure the patient's responses are reliable if the initial response is that the rings appear equally clear.

2. Relying on the result obtained with the duochrome test as the final arbiter of the spherical endpoint at the end of the refraction.

3. Asking the patient whether the red or green looks brighter. You must ask whether the rings (or letters/dots) are clearer and blacker on the red or green.

4.9 Assessment of astigmatism

Most patients have a slight degree of astigmatism. This could be owing to astigmatism of the anterior and posterior surfaces of the cornea and/or lens and/or to lens tilt and/or decentration. A high degree of astigmatism appears to be hereditary.

4.9.1 The evidence base: when and how to assess astigmatism

Measurement of astigmatism is a routine part of a subjective refraction. The literature that compares the various astigmatism tests is limited, and further research is needed (section 1.2.3). Many clinicians use the JCC test because it is simple and easy to use and is designed to fine tune the cylinder found in retinoscopy or autorefraction. However, it is important to be able to use another subjective test for astigmatism in case a patient responds poorly to the demands of the JCC. Fan-shaped tests have an advantage over JCC in that accommodation is well controlled as the patient is fogged prior to the use of the procedure. They also do not require the patient to be able to memorise two pictures presented sequentially and compare them. They can be used to determine quickly if any astigmatism is present after the BVS procedure by asking patients whether any of the lines look clearer (the block and fan looks like a clown's face if set up as in Fig. 4.13 and can be used with children in this way. Ask: "Do any of the hairs on the clown's head look clearer than the others?" However, fan-shaped tests should only be used if they include an arrow or dial to refine the precision of the axis estimation, otherwise they are significantly limited in sensitivity.[31] A very simple test to estimate the astigmatic axis is axis rotation, which

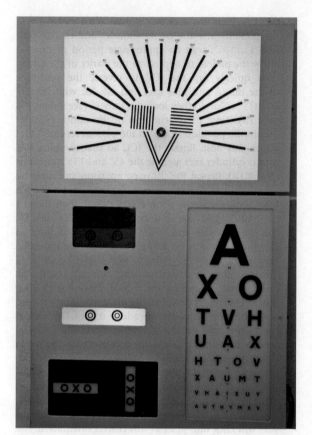

Fig. 4.13 A wall chart with the fan and block and Verhoeff ring targets illuminated.

Table 4.2 Important axis values with JCC. Recommended initial rotation of the axis and precision of bracketing for different cylinder powers when using the ±0.25 Jackson cross-cylinder based on the effective cylinder axis shift created[28]

Correcting cylinder	Initial rotation	Precision of bracketing
0.25 DC	30°	± 10°
0.50 DC	20°	± 10°
0.75 DC	15°	± 5°
1.00–2.00 DC	10°	± 5°
2.25+ DC	5°	± 2.5°

the patient, one after the other: when the correcting cylinder is incorrect, one lens increases the interval of Sturm and slightly blurs vision and the other decreases the interval of Sturm and slightly improves vision. The zero mean power of the cross-cylinder ensures that the circle of least confusion remains on the retina for both presentations. The effective axis shift is greater if the power of the correcting cylinder is low: A ±0.25 JCC will shift the effective axis by ±22.5° when combined with a −0.50 DC, but will only shift the effective axis by about 7° when combined with a 2.00 DC.[28] Therefore when making changes based on patient responses to the JCC, the amount of rotation of the correcting cylinder should consider the power of that cylinder (Table 4.2).

4.9.3 JCC Procedure

See online videos 4.9 to 4.14.

1. Ensure that the BVS is in place so that the circle of least confusion is on the retina: Use MPMVA (section 4.6) or ±BVS (section 4.7) plus duochrome (section 4.8).
2. Isolate/indicate a circular letter or a line of letters one row above the present VA (a Llandolt C from a computerised chart can be useful; Fig. 4.14c) or illuminate the Verhoeff rings or the collection of dots target (Fig. 4.14a,b)
3. Move the JCC in front of the trial frame/phoropter aperture (Fig. 4.15).
4. Instruct the patient: "I am going to show you two pictures of letter/rings/dots. Both pictures may be slightly blurred, but I want you to tell me which is the clearer of the two pictures, or whether they look the same." In all cases, repeat the presentation if the patient is hesitant or seems unsure. Patients find these decisions very difficult,[21–23] and some patients are embarrassed to ask you to repeat the presentation.[21]

involves asking the patient to view the smallest line of VA he or she can see and rotating the correcting cylinder axis first clockwise and then anticlockwise until the patient reports that the letters start to blur. The cylinder axis indicated by the technique is the midpoint between the two blur points so that if the two blur points are at 25° and 55°, the indicated cylinder axis is 40°. In patients where the subjective assessment of astigmatism is poor or not possible, it is advisable to consider multiple objective measures of astigmatism from retinoscopy, autorefraction, and (if the cylinder is large, to help determine the axis) keratometry. The astigmatism present in the patient's current glasses should also be considered.

4.9.2 The Jackson cross-cylinder

The JCC only works correctly if the circle of least confusion is on the retina so that it must follow a BVS assessment. During the test you present two lenses to

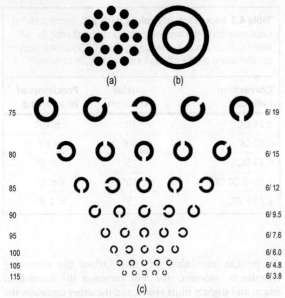

Fig. 4.14 Targets used with the Jackson cross-cylinder (JCC) include (a) circle of dots (b) rings, and a circular letter, or (c) Llandolt C one line above current VA.

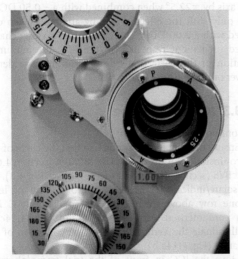

Fig. 4.15 A phoropter-based Jackson cross-cylinder set up to assess cylinder axis.

5. If cylinder was found with retinoscopy, proceed with step 7.
6. If there has been no cylinder found with retinoscopy, then set the JCC so that its minus cylinder axis (red dot) and the perpendicular plus cylinder axis (white dot) assume the 90° and 180° positions. It does not matter which dot is at 90° and which is at 180°. Ask the patient: "Are the circles rounder and clearer with lens 1 . . . ."; wait an appropriate period of time to allow the patient to appreciate the clarity of the target, then quickly flip the JCC to reverse the positions of the minus and plus axes and ask "or with lens 2" (wait) . . . "or do they look the same?" (see videos 4.8 to 4.13). Note the orientation of the minus cylinder axis in the position in which the patient reported that vision was best. Rotate the JCC so that the plus and minus cylinder axes assume the 45° and 135° positions (Fig. 4.16). Repeat the above comparison and note the orientation of the minus cylinder axis of the chosen lens. If all the lenses seem equally clear, then there is no cylinder and you have completed the JCC test for this eye. If certain lens positions are preferred, then set the phoropter cylinder axis at or between the indicated axes (e.g., if minus cylinder was preferred at 180° and 45°, then set the correcting cylinder axis to the approximate midpoint, i.e., ~25°). Place −0.25 D or −0.50 D cylinder power in the phoropter and proceed with the next step. If you add −0.50 DC in older presbyopes, you should add +0.25 DS to the spherical lens to keep the circle of least confusion on the retina (younger patients should be able to accommodate to maintain the circle of least confusion on the retina).
7. JCC axis determination: Set the JCC so that the minus cylinder axis and the plus cylinder axis straddle the correcting cylinder axis. When using a phoropter the JCC will click into place at this correct orientation. Ask the patient to compare this initial lens position "lens 1," with its flipped counterpart, "lens 2" (see Fig. 4.16) or whether they look about the same.

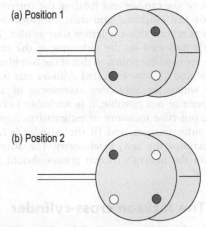

(a) Position 1

(b) Position 2

Fig. 4.16 Orientation of the cross-cylinder for axis determination in (a) 'picture or lens 1' and (b) 'picture or lens 2'.

8. Adjust the correcting cylinder axes toward the minus cylinder axis (red dot) of the preferred lens position (1 or 2). The amount of rotation typically depends on the size of the cylinder (see Table 4.2). This can be tempered by the response from the patient (see online video 4.12). For example, if the JCC response with a 1.00 DC was very strongly in favour of one lens/picture (and particularly if the VA after BVS was poor so that you suspect the astigmatism after objective refraction was incorrect by a significant amount), it may be better to rotate the cylinder by 10° or 15° rather than the 5° suggested in the table. Similarly, if the JCC response was weak and hesitant, you could make less of a change than that suggested in Table 4.2.

9. Ask the patient to compare the two presentations of the JCC at the new axis (you can use "lens 3 . . . . . or lens 4", etc., to indicate to the patient that you are not just repeating the previous presentation) and continue to adjust the axis dependent on the results. The amount of rotation of the cylinder should be reduced (approximately halved) at each change of the direction of rotation. For example, if a 0.50 DC was initially at 90°, and the JCC indicated a clockwise rotation was required, move it to 70° (see Table 4.2). If the JCC then indicates that an anticlockwise rotation was required, move the cylinder by 10° to the 80° position. Try to keep a mental note of previous decisions made with the JCC to help you 'zero-in' on the final axis. In the example above, if the JCC suggested another anticlockwise movement was required, it would be more efficient to check the correcting cylinder at 85° as the patient has already indicated a preference at 90°.

10. Use as few JCC comparisons as possible and ideally between three and seven. Many patients greatly dislike making these difficult judgements and prefer to make as few as possible.[21-23] Finalise the correcting cylinder axis when you have bracketed to approximately 2.5° (cylinders > 2.00 DC), 5° (0.75–1.75 DC) or 10° (0.25 and 0.50 DC) (see Table 4.2).

11. JCC power determination: Adjust the JCC so that either the minus axis (red dot) or plus axis (white dot) parallels the trial frame/phoropter cylinder axis (the JCC will click into place with modern phoropters; Fig. 4.17). Have the patient compare the relative clarity of lens 1 with lens 2 (Fig. 4.18).

12. If the patient reports that there is no perceived difference between the images shown, do not assume you have the correct power. Remove −0.25 D from the cylinder and repeat the comparison. Stop at the lowest cylinder power for which the patient indicates a preference.

13. Add minus cylinder (−0.25 D) if the patient prefers the minus cylinder axis (red dot) parallel to the phoropter axis. Remove −0.25 DC if the patient prefers

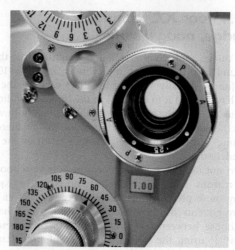

Fig. 4.17 A phoropter-based Jackson cross-cylinder set up to assess cylinder power.

(a) Position 1

(b) Position 2

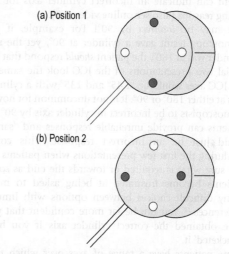

Fig. 4.18 Orientation of the cross-cylinder for power determination in **(a)** 'picture or lens 1' and **(b)** 'picture or lens 2.'

the plus cylinder axis parallel to the phoropter axis. Continue this process until no difference between lens 1 and 2 can be detected or until the power has been bracketed to less than a 0.25 D (choose the least minus cylinder).

14. For each 0.50 D change in cylinder power, change the sphere power by 0.25 D in the opposite direction (e.g., if you remove −0.50 DC, then add −0.25 DS before comparing the lens positions). This is to ensure that the circle of least confusion remains on the retina.

85

4.9.4 Poor JCC technique: 'nudge, nudge, same'

The 'nudge, nudge, same' technique requires little thinking and involves nudging the cylinder axis by ~10° to 15° (and not really knowing the exact value of the axis you have moved it to or from) in the direction indicated by the JCC until the patient first indicates that both views look the same. The cylinder axis position that first receives a 'same' response from the patient is taken as the true cylinder axis.

Do not use this technique because it is very poor for two reasons. First, it is inefficient and typically requires many more presentations than is necessary. Given that many patients dislike subjective refraction and having to choose between two very similar looking presentations[21-23] using the minimal number of presentations must be the goal. Some frustrated patients can even give up trying to make a useful decision with JCC,[21] and this needs to be avoided. Second, it can be inaccurate (occasionally extremely inaccurate) as a "same" response from a patient can indicate an incorrect cylinder axis for the following reasons (also see online video 4.9).

1. You may be *incorrect* by 90°! For example, if the retinoscopy result gave a cylinder at 90°, yet the real cylinder was at 180°, the patient *should* respond that the initial two presentations of the JCC look the same as the JCC axes would be at 45° and 135° with a cylinder axis at either 180° or 90°. It is not uncommon for novice retinoscopists to be incorrect in cylinder axis by 90°.
2. Patients can provide unreliable responses and "same" could just be an incorrect response. This could be during the first few presentations when patients are not sure what is required or towards the end as some patients become frustrated at being asked to make many difficult choices between options with limited differences.[22] You can be far more confident that you have obtained the correct cylinder axis if you have 'bracketed' it.
3. Some patients have a range of axes over which they believe that the two JCC images look the same. In these cases, the axis should be placed in the middle of the range. For example, if the patient responded "same" from 150° to 180°, the cylinder should be placed at 165°. Using the first 'same' response would likely place the cylinder axis at ~150° or 180°.

4.9.5 Examples of efficient JCC procedures for cylinder axis

Two simple examples are provided here, but there are a larger number of examples for JCC cylinder axis and power determination on the website (see online videos 4.8 to 4.13).

1. Use appropriate changes in axis and 'bracket' the final result
Cylindrical axis before JCC: -1.25×90
   (a) The JCC is set so that the minus cylinder axis (position 1: 45°, position 2: 135°) and the plus cylinder axis straddle the correcting cylinder axis of 90° and is clicked into place at this orientation. The patient choice (minus cylinder axis at 45°) indicates that the correcting cylinder should be moved clockwise. As the cylinder is -1.25 DC, it should be moved clockwise by 10° (see Table 4.2) from 90° to 80°.
   (b) The patient choice indicates that the correcting cylinder should be moved clockwise again. Move it from 80° to 70°.
   (c) The patient choice indicates that the correcting cylinder should be moved anticlockwise. This is a change in direction of movement of the JCC, so the degree of change of the correcting cylinder should be halved to 5°. The correcting cylinder should be moved 5° anticlockwise to 75°.
   (d) The patient cannot discriminate between the two lens positions (response is 'same') and the true cylinder axis position has been determined.
Four JCC comparisons were made at 90°, 80°, 70° and 75°, with the final axis of 75° bracketed at 70° and 80°.
2. An initial "same" response: make sure you bracket the axis.
   (a) The correcting cylinder is -0.75×90. The patient cannot discriminate between the two JCC lens positions and responds that they look the "same". However, there is no firm indication that the true cylinder axis position has been determined because this axis has not been bracketed (section 4.9.4).
   (b) Move the cylinder axis by 10° to 80° as the cylinder power is -0.75 (see Table 4.2) and the "same" response suggests you may be close to the final axis. The patient choice indicates that the cylinder axis is anticlockwise from 80°.
   (c) Move the correcting cylinder axis to 100°. The patient choice indicates that the cylinder axis is clockwise from 100°.
Three JCC comparisons were made at 90°, 80°, and 100°, with the axis of 90° bracketed at 80° and 100°.

4.9.6 Adaptations to the standard JCC procedure

1. Repeat presentations at the start. If a patient has provided poor responses in other parts of the eye examination, it can be useful to repeat the same JCC presentations to the patient at the start of the procedure until the patient provides the same response each time.

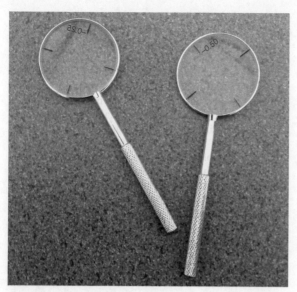

Fig. 4.19 Hand-held Jackson cross-cylinders of ±0.25 and ±0.50 D.

2. Offer only two options ("1 or 2?"): It can be difficult for some patients and particularly older patients to make a decision when there are three possible responses of "lens 1, lens 2, or the same". Some clinicians ask whether the image is "clearer and rounder with lens 1 or lens 2". The patient often indicates at some point that the two presentations look the same when this technique is used. Alternatively, after the patient has confidently provided several responses of "lens 1" or "lens 2", the patient may hesitate and appear unsure. At this point you could ask whether the two presentations look the same.

3. Use longer presentation times. This is particularly useful for older patients, given that processing speed slows significantly with age.[25]

4. Use higher powered JCCs. If accurate responses are never obtained, you may need to use a ±0.50 JCC (Fig. 4.19). This can also be useful when refracting eyes with poor VA, when even higher powered JCCs may be necessary. If a patient still cannot provide reliable answers, then you may need to use an alternative assessment of astigmatism.

4.9.7. Procedure for fan-based astigmatic tests (e.g., fan and block, Raubitschek arrow)

1. Occlude the left eye.
2. Starting with the objective refraction result, perform MPMVA or ±BVS (sections 4.6 and 4.7; keep the cylinder found during retinoscopy in the phoropter/trial frame).

3. Remove the minus cylinder estimate from retinoscopy so that the patient is fogged (techniques that suggest you measure VA to estimate the approximate cylinder power with the BVS result, assume that you do not have any estimate of the cylinder from the patient's record and/or glasses, retinoscopy, autorefraction, or keratometry, and this does not occur in practice).

4. In case the retinoscopy cylinder estimate was incorrect (and too low), add +0.50 DS to ensure that both focal lines are in front of the retina (this allows for an underestimation of the cylinder during retinoscopy of 1.00 DC). Larger amounts of additional plus can be used, but then it is likely that subsequently you will need to reduce this before the patient is able to see a difference in clarity in some of the lines on the fan.

5. Present the fan and ask the patient which lines of the fan are clearest, if any.

6. If the patient states that all the lines are equally clear, reduce the spherical correction in +0.50 DS steps and repeat the presentation of the fan. If the patient repeatedly indicates that all the lines are equally clear, then the patient has no astigmatism.

7. If the patient states that some lines are clearer than others (patients often describe this using a clock dial: "the lines at about 5 o'clock are clearest"), rotate the arrow (or 'T' or dial) to point in the same direction as the clearest lines indicated by the patient.

8. Fine-tune the arrow position by ensuring that the two sides of the arrow or dial are equally clear. This provides the cylinder axis.

9. Ask the patient to compare the two blocks (see Fig. 4.13; or lines on the different parts of the T, etc.) and the blocks/lines in line with the arrow should be clearer than those that are perpendicular.

10. Increase the cylinder power at the axis indicated in step 8 until the two blocks or two parts of the T are equally clear. Provide the lowest cylinder power if the two blocks cannot be exactly matched in clarity.

11. Reduce the plus or increase the minus power of the sphere until maximum VA is achieved.

12. Refract the left eye.

4.9.8 Recording the cylinder

The JCC or fan-based test results are not recorded individually because the techniques are just part of subjective refraction (section 4.5).

4.9.9 Interpreting cylinder results

Many astigmatic axes have mirror symmetry[3] so that the two cylinder axes should add up to approximately 180°. Both axes could be 90° or both axes 180° (i.e., 0° and 180°); one axis 175°, the other 5°; one axis 20°, the other 160°; one axis 45°, the other 135°, and so forth. You may wish to recheck astigmatic axes that do not follow this pattern, particularly if one axis has changed significantly from a previous examination or is significantly different from the retinoscopy result.

Typically, younger patients will have 'with-the-rule' astigmatism, with a steeper vertical meridian (minus cylinder axis between 160° and 20°), likely caused by pressure from the eyelids.[20] This lid tension decreases slowly with age, so that with-the-rule astigmatism slowly disappears and older patients typically have 'against-the-rule' astigmatism (minus cylinder axis between 70° and 110°).[20] Note that this change with age is slow and any significant refractive correction changes between eye examinations 1 and 3 years apart are likely to be largely spherical in nature. Significant changes in astigmatism over a 1- to 3-year period are likely to be due to refraction error at test or retest or possibly caused by ocular pathology such as keratoconus, cortical cataract or chalazion.

4.9.10 Most common errors

1. Using the 'nudge, nudge, same' technique (section 4.9.4).
2. Using too short a presentation time, particularly in older patients. Using a longer presentation time, and repeating the two views when the patient is unsure, typically provides an overall quicker JCC procedure as the responses provided are more reliable.
3. Trial frame JCC
   (a) Poor JCC alignment with the correcting cylindrical lens. Check that *both* dots (for axis) or lines (for power) are in alignment.
   (b) Believing that removal of the JCC is an option (i.e., offering 'lens 1 . . . or 2 . . . or [removing the JCC] the same').
   (c) Being unaware that some hand-held JCCs (Fig. 4.19) give the minus axis in white.

4.10 Binocular balancing of accommodation

During monocular refraction, the occluder can induce proximal accommodation, so that the eye being refracted may be accommodating.[32]

4.10.1 The evidence base: when and how to binocular balance

A binocular balance of accommodation is typically performed after a monocular refraction to relax and balance accommodation in the two eyes. The test need not be performed if the patient does not have binocular vision or accommodation (e.g., patients older than ~60 years of age or pseudophakes). Comparison of the various binocular balancing techniques in the current literature provides very limited information, and further research is needed (section 1.2.3). Some tests directly compare the vision in the two eyes (prism-dissociation balance, alternate occlusion) and are directed towards balancing accommodation whereas others are based on binocular refraction techniques (e.g., polaroid, monocular fogging, Humphriss) and determine the spherical correction in conditions close to the patient's normal viewing situation.

The alternate occlusion test continues to use an occluder, acts like a cover test, and does not allow binocularity, so that its usefulness over monocular refraction seems limited. The prism dissociated binocular balance is also fully dissociated, so that fusional vergence is not present and accommodation may not be at the same level when binocular.[32] Both these tests need the patient to have equal VA in the two eyes to be able to provide accommodative balance. Other tests, such as the polarisation balance, monocular fogging, and Humphriss immediate contrast test, are minimally dissociated and aim to determine the spherical correction in conditions similar to the patient's normal viewing situation so that vergence and pupil size are in their normal binocular state. Polaroid tests on computer-based systems are best if they include three lines of VA with a fusion lock line that is seen by both eyes. With only two lines, one seen by the right eye and one by the left, the lines may float freely and cause confusion. Fogging of one eye by a small amount in the monocular fogging technique has several advantages in that it relaxes accommodation and suppresses central vision whilst maintaining peripheral fusion. Both the polaroid dissociated (or prism-dissociated) balance tests can be used with the duochrome (section 4.8), where balance is achieved by gaining the same endpoint in both eyes (i.e. red = green in both eyes, or 'just on the red' in both eyes).[32] The duochrome and monocular fogging techniques can balance accommodation in patients with unequal monocular VA. The Turville Infinity Balance test is not described here because it requires physical movement of a septum on a mirror, making it somewhat cumbersome and it is rarely used nowadays.

4.10.2 Procedure for monocular fogging balance ('modified Humphriss')

See online video 4.15.

1. Fog the left eye until the VA is reduced by three or four lines less than the tested eye. Typically +0.75 DS or +1.00 DS is required.

2. Repeat the BVS assessment using the plus/minus technique (section 4.7).
3. If +0.50 DS or more is added, such as for some patients with latent hyperopia, it is likely that this will relax accommodation in both eyes. To ensure that the amount of fogging lens is still effective, add additional plus power to the left eye and check that VA is blurred by three or four lines.
4. Remove the fog from the left eye, then fog the right eye by three or four lines, and repeat the plus/minus BVS technique for the left eye.

4.10.3 Procedure for Humphriss immediate contrast

The following procedure is based on the technique described by Humphriss.[33]

1. Fog the left eye until VA is reduced by three or four lines less than the tested eye. Young patients with normal vision would usually require adding +0.75 DS or +1.00 DS to give a VA of 6/9 to 6/12 (0.5 to 0.67 or 20/30 to 20/40).
2. Ask the patient to look at the smallest line they can see on the letter chart (Humphriss suggested using a 6/12 [0.5 or 20/40] letter but the rationale is not clear and few clinicians use it).
3. Place a +0.25 DS lens in front of the right eye for about 1 second (or longer if the patient appears to need more time) and then replace this with a −0.25 DS for about 0.5 seconds (or half the time given to the +0.25 DS lens).
4. Ask the patient "Are the letters clearer with lens 1........ or lens 2?"
5. Examples of the situation occurring in a fully corrected, slightly over-minused, and slightly over-plussed eye are shown in Table 4.3. The image seen with each lens is determined by the clarity of the image in the clearer eye, modified by the effects of binocular summation.
6. If the patient immediately reports that the −0.25 DS is definitely clearer, repeat the demonstration of the

lenses and ask if the −0.25 DS "is definitely clearer or just smaller and blacker". Only add −0.25 DS if the patient immediately reports that the lens is definitely clearer.
7. If the patient reports after some consideration that the −0.25 DS lens is clearer, do not add −0.25 DS.
8. If the patient reports that the +0.25 DS is clearer or that there is no difference, add +0.25 DS to the refractive correction.
9. Because you have added +0.25 DS to the right eye, it is assumed that accommodation will have been relaxed in both eyes. To ensure that the amount of fogging lens is still effective, add +0.25 DS to the left eye.
10. Continue to compare the −0.25 DS and +0.25 DS until the +0.25 DS is immediately rejected.
11. Repeat the procedure on the left eye with the right eye fogged.

4.10.4 Procedure for polaroid binocular balance of accommodation

Polaroid balance tests typically include several VA lines with one (or more, dependent on the programme) line seen by the right, left, and both eyes, respectively. The line seen by both eyes provides a fusional lock.

1. Place the polarised filters before both eyes.
2. Add +0.50 DS to both eyes.
3. Ask the patient if the letters are clearer on the line seen by the right eye or left eye or if they are both the same.
4. If one line is clearer, add +0.25 DS to that eye until the two monocularly seen lines are equally blurred.
5. If a balance cannot be achieved, use the lenses that provide the best vision to the dominant eye (section 5.9.2 for dominancy testing) or the closest match.
6. Remove the polarised filters.
7. Remove the fog in binocular +0.25 DS steps until you obtain maximum VA.
8. If the patient can read the bottom line of your chart (and this is larger than 6/3, 2.0, or 20/10), you can allow

Table 4.3 The Humphriss technique. An indication of the changes made to the clearer eye and the interocular difference when either +0.25 DS or −0.25 DS is used with a +1.00 fogging lens in the Humphriss immediate contrast technique

	WITH THE +0.25 DS LENS		WITH THE −0.25 DS LENS	
	Clearer eye	Interocular difference	Clearer eye	Interocular difference
Corrected	+0.25 DS	+0.75 DS	−0.25 DS	+1.25 DS
Over-minused by −0.25 DS	Plano	+1.00 DS	−0.50 DS	+1.50 DS
Over-plussed by +0.25 DS	+0.50 DS	+0.50 DS	Plano	+1.00 DS

extra minus or less plus that makes your bottom line of letters 'clearer.' Ensure that the bottom line of letters is 'definitely clearer and not just smaller and blacker.'

4.10.5 Procedure for prism-dissociated blur balance of accommodation

See online video 4.16. Experienced clinicians often do not fog the eye (or use a smaller amount of fogging lenses) during prism-dissociated balance and use the 95 VAR (20/25, 6/7.5, 0.8) line to check accommodative balance.

1. Occlude the left eye (or ask the patient to close their eyes; the increasing diplopia produced by the prisms can be distressing) and isolate the 85 VAR (20/40, 6/12, 0.5) row of letters.
2. Introduce the Risley prisms before both eyes, so that there is 3^Δ base down before one eye and 3^Δ base up in front of the other eye. It is important that equal prism before each eye is used to equalise any image degradation by the prisms.
3. Add +1.00 DS to the right eye and check whether the 85 VAR (20/40, 6/12, 0.5) line is blurred. They should be blurred, but readable. Add further plus power in +0.25 D steps until the 20/40 is just blurred.
4. Remove the occluder (or ask patients to open their eyes) and ask if they see two 85 VAR (20/40, 6/12, 0.5) lines of letters, one above the other.
5. If the patient cannot see both lines, first check that both apertures are open. If they are, cover each eye in turn, so that the patient can see the position of the line seen by each eye. The patient should then be able to see both targets at the same time. If the patient still cannot see two lines, then one eye is likely suppressing and a binocular balance is not required.
6. Add plus lenses in +0.25 DS steps to the left eye until both eyes have equally blurred images.
7. If a balance cannot be achieved, use the lenses that provide best vision to the dominant eye (section 5.9.2 for dominancy testing) or the closest match.
8. Remove +0.25 DS from both eyes, and ask whether the two images remain equally blurred (you may need to isolate the 90 VAR, 20/30, 6/9, 0.67 line for this comparison). If one image is clearer, add +0.25 DS to the eye with the clearer image until both eyes have equally blurred images. If a balance cannot be achieved, use the lenses that provide the closest match.
9. Remove the Risley prisms (ask the patient to close their eyes while this is done) and display the bottom part of the VA chart. Check the VA to ensure that the best acuity line *has not* been achieved.
10. Remove the fog in binocular 0.25 DS steps until you obtain maximum VA. If the patient can read the bottom line of your chart (and this is larger than 115 VAR, 20/10, 6/3, 2.0), you can allow extra minus or

less plus that makes your bottom line of letters 'clearer.' Ensure that the bottom line of letters is 'definitely clearer and not just smaller and blacker.' This should be no more than −0.50 DS extra than the refractive correction used to see 100 VAR (20/20, 6/6, 1.0).

11. Measure monocular and binocular VAs, especially if the binocular difference is more than 0.25 D from the monocular subjective. If monocular VA is reduced in one eye following this procedure, recheck the results.

4.10.6 Recording of binocular balance

The monocular subjective refraction result and the correction after binocular balance can both be recorded with the accompanying VA results. Alternatively, the change in spherical power made with the binocular balance can be recorded. The binocular VA is also measured after binocular balancing. For example:

Monocular subjective
RE: −0.50/−0.50 × 170   107
LE: −0.75/−0.50 × 15   106

Monocular fogging
RE: −0.50/−0.50 × 170   107
LE: −0.50/−0.50 × 15   106
BE: 109

Monocular subjective
RE: −1.50/−1.25 × 160   1.33
LE: −1.25/−1.00 × 20   1.33

Monocular fogging: +0.25 DS RE
BE: 1.33

Monocular subjective
RE: +2.75/−0.75 × 175   6/3.8^{-2}
LE: +1.75/−0.50 × 10   6/4.8^{+2}

Humphriss balance
RE: +3.00/−0.75 × 175   6/3.8^{-1}
LE: +2.00/−0.50 × 10   6/4.8^{+2}
BE: 6/3.8

Monocular subjective
OD: −3.25/−0.75 × 20   20/15^{+1}
OS: −3.50/−0.75 × 170   20/15^{+1}

Prism balance: +0.25 DS RE
OU: 20/15^{+3}

4.10.7 Interpreting binocular balance results

Typically, binocular balance tests either find no change in refractive correction from the monocular refraction result or find a small amount of additional positive lens power in one eye, or more rarely, both. However, with latent hyperopia there can be a significant increase in the amount of plus accepted with this technique. This is because monocular subjective refraction can lead to possible over-minusing or under-plussing, particularly in patients with hyperopia, pseudomyopia, and antimetropia, because the occluder can stimulate accommodation in the non-tested eye and thus an equivalent increase in accommodation in the eye being tested.

4.10.8 Most common errors in binocular balancing

1. Attempting to balance the accommodation in patients who do not have binocular vision or accommodation (e.g., patients over 60 years of age and pseudophakes).
2. Monocular fogging and Humphriss immediate contrast: Failure to modify the fogging lens when +0.50 DS or more has been added to the fellow eye.
3. Humphriss immediate contrast: Presenting the +0.25 DS and −0.25 DS for an equal amount of time.
4. Prism dissociated blur: Using a truncated VA chart and not allowing extra minus or less plus that makes your bottom line of letters 'clearer.' This can lead to an over-plussed or under-minused refractive correction, particularly when associated with a MPMVA technique in older patients.[26]

4.11 Binocular subjective refraction

Binocular refraction techniques are performed under conditions that are as close to the patient's normal distance viewing situation as possible.

4.11.1 The evidence base: when and how to refract binocularly

Most experienced clinicians perform binocular subjective refraction whenever possible because it provides better control over, and greater relaxation of, accommodation, and it is slightly quicker than monocular refraction because no binocular balancing is required. The reduced number of subjective decisions to be made is appreciated by patients.[21-23] It also provides better control over latent nystagmus as the occluder used in monocular refraction manifests the nystagmus and makes subjective refraction difficult. Binocular refraction is not possible with patients who do not have binocular vision and a small number of patients with highly dominant eyes find it very difficult to give good subjective responses with their non-dominant eye during binocular refraction. Refraction can be performed binocularly using monocular fogging (modified Humphriss), Humphriss immediate contrast, and polaroids (section 4.10). Monocular fogging refraction can only be used with ±BVS (section 4.7)

and JCC, because MPMVA and fan-based tests of astigmatism require the tested eye to be blurred. Polaroid refraction uses a chart that has letters on one-half polarised at, say, 45° and letters on the other half polarised orthogonally (in this example at 135°). The patient views the chart with polaroid filters that transmit the letters from one-half of the chart to one eye and the other half of the chart to the fellow eye. Light from the background of the chart and a central vertical bar is transmitted to both eyes. Disadvantages include that the light transmitted by the polarising filters is reduced by 50%. This makes the letters of slightly lower contrast than normal and this can be a problem when refracting patients with some conditions such as cataract. Another problem is that it can be difficult economically to produce polarised letters in very small sizes below 20/20 or 20/15.[31] Students should only use binocular refraction once they have mastered monocular refraction and its components and the various adaptations that can be used for different patients.

4.11.2 Binocular refraction procedure

1. Clean the parts of the phoropter or trial frame that contact the patient using alcohol wipes or similar. Fit the trial frame or phoropter so that the patient is comfortable and adjust it to the patient's distance PD.
2. Begin with the net retinoscopy sphere-cylinder before each eye.
3. Explain the procedure to the patient and reduce any concerns about providing wrong answers[21-23]: "During this test, I will place various lenses in front of your eye to find the lenses that give you the best vision. Don't worry about giving a wrong answer as we already have a very good indication of the glasses power you need from your (old glasses/the moving light test/the autorefractor machine) and everything is double checked."
4. The subjective refraction traditionally begins on the right eye (or the poorer eye if you determine there may be a poor eye from the case history).

Monocular fogging

5. Occlude the right eye and fog the left eye until the VA is reduced by three or four lines less than the tested eye. Typically +0.75 DS or +1.00 DS is required. Remove the occluder from the right eye.
6. Determine the BVS (sections 4.6 or 4.7) and cylinder power and axis using the JCC (section 4.9). Check the end result sphere using the duochrome (section 4.8) and measure VA.
7. Remove the fogging lens from the untested eye and fog the right eye. Determine the optimal subjective refractive correction in the left eye using the plus/minus technique and JCC and measure VA.

8. Remove the fogging lens and measure binocular VA.
9. Compare the monocular VAs with the habitual VAs and age-matched norms and measure the vertex distance, if required (section 4.11.3; Fig. 4.10).

Polaroid binocular refraction

10. Place the polarised filters before both eyes and direct the patient to the chart that is seen by the right eye
11. Determine the optimal subjective refractive correction in the right eye using your preferred techniques for BVS and astigmatism assessment (sections 4.6 to 4.9) and measure VA.
12. Repeat for the left eye after directing the patient to the chart that is seen by the left eye.
13. Remove the polarised filters and measure binocular VA.
14. Compare the monocular VAs with the habitual VAs and age-matched norms and measure the vertex distance, if required (section 4.11.3).

4.11.3 Check tests after refraction

1. Compare monocular VAs after your refraction with the patient's vision or habitual VAs, as appropriate. If the VA is better with the patient's glasses, then it is likely that your subjective result (or VA) is incorrect.
2. Compare the VA with the present subjective refraction with age-matched normal data (see Table 4.1). If the VA is worse than expected or worse in one eye compared with the other, remeasure the VA with a pinhole aperture. If the VA improves with the pinhole, either the subjective refraction is not optimal and should be repeated or the patient has media opacity, such as cataract, that is being bypassed by the pinhole.
3. If the final refractive correction in either eye is above 5.00 D spherical equivalent (SE, the sphere plus half the cylinder; e.g., $-4.75/-1.50 \times 180$ has an SE of -5.50 D, $+5.50/-2.00 \times 90$ has an SE of $+4.50$ D), then measure the vertex distance (see Fig. 4.10). This is the distance from the back surface of the lens nearest the eye to the apex of the cornea. Back vertex distance can be read from the millimetre scale or periscope on the sides of the trial frame or phoropter, respectively, or by using a vertex distance gauge. The standard vertex distance in phoropters (the long line in Fig. 4.10a) is 13.75 mm.

4.11.4 Recording and interpreting binocular refraction results

See sections 4.5.2 for recording results. A subjective result that is significantly less positive (more negative) than the retinoscopy result or a subjective result more minus than suggested by unaided VA could indicate latent hyperopia

or pseudomyopia and a cycloplegic refraction may be required (section 4.13).

The difference between the patient's own glasses and the subjective refraction should be compatible with the difference between the habitual (with own glasses) and optimal VAs. For example, if patients have a VA of 85 (6/12, 0.5, 20/40) in their glasses and 105 ($\sim$6/4.5, 1.25, 20/15) after subjective refraction, you could expect the subjective refraction to be 1.00 DS more myopic than the glasses correction ($-0.25 \approx 1$ line of log-MAR VA). Thus, a 6/12 VA with a glasses correction of $-1.00/-0.50 \times 180$ would suggest a refractive correction of $-2.00/-0.50 \times 180$. If the subjective refraction was $-2.50/-0.50 \times 180$ or even $-3.00/-0.5 \times 180$, this suggests you may have over-minused the subjective refraction. Changes in hyperopic refractive errors are more difficult to explain in this way; they are dependent on the amount of accommodation the patient has (and therefore the patient's age). Changes in astigmatism that are not caused by pathology are usually small.[20] Patients with refractive error change that is a result of cataract or other eye disease will not typically follow the same rules for improvement in VA (e.g., nuclear cataract can cause a 1.00 D myopic shift with only a one- to two-line improvement in VA).

A patient with reduced VA (typically in both eyes) and a retinoscope result that indicates emmetropia or slight hyperopia may have non-organic visual loss (also called functional or psychogenic visual loss).[34,35] It may be accompanied by visual field defects, which are often tubular.[35] In young children, this is often because the child wishes to wear glasses (perhaps a best friend or a parent wears glasses), but can be caused by social problems at home or school and can include sexual abuse.[34,35] In adults, non-organic visual loss is linked with trauma (typically head trauma), chronic pain conditions including migraine, and underlying minor psychiatric problems that include feelings of stress, anxiety, and depression.[35] A useful test, particularly with children, is to perform a subjective refraction using a variety of lenses that have no effect on VA (e.g., a combination of +0.25 DS and –0.25 DS in a trail frame) and encourage the patient to read further down the VA chart. In many cases, the patient can be encouraged to read normal or near normal VA in this way and if ocular health appears normal, a diagnosis of non-organic visual loss can be made and reassurance given to the child and parent.

4.11.5 Most common error in binocular refraction

1. Using binocular refraction without having mastered monocular refraction and getting into difficulties.

4.12 Cycloplegic refraction

This involves a determination of the refractive error when the patient's accommodation has been totally or partially paralysed using a cycloplegic drug.

4.12.1 The evidence base: when to perform cycloplegic refraction and using which drugs

The following can indicate the need for a cycloplegic refraction[36]:

- Young children (especially < 7 years) where subjective refraction is very limited and 'dry' (i.e., non-cycloplegic) retinoscopy can be difficult, particularly at their first eye examination and in repeat examination for younger patients (< 4 years)
- A suspected latent hyperope (i.e., a dry subjective result significantly less positive [< 1.00 DS] than retinoscopy): accommodative problems suggested in the case history (e.g., difficulty changing focus) or by a fluctuating pupil size and/or reflex during retinoscopy. Pseudomyopia is also caused by spasm of accommodation, but results in myopia (and thus blurred distance vision) rather than hyperopia. Symptoms might include distance vision blur after a lot of near work, a myopic subjective with an emmetropic, or hyperopic non-cycloplegic retinoscopy, more myopia than suggested by unaided VA, and possibly esophoria on cover test.
- A suspected accommodative disorder: similar symptoms as latent hyperopia or pseudomyopia and/or problems suggested by amplitude of accommodation, dynamic retinoscopy, or accommodative facility testing.
- Unexplained poor vision and/or a poorly co-operating young patient.
- Children with special educational needs.

The key disadvantages of cycloplegia are the initial stinging when the drop hits the eye (this can lead to difficulties in instilling the drops in some children) and the blurred vision and photophobia that can last several hours. The slight degradation of distance vision is caused by the increase in ocular aberrations as a result of dilated pupils and near vision is greatly reduced by the large decreases in accommodation. Adverse reactions to two drops of cyclopentolate 1% are common, particularly in younger children (< 6 years) and those with a low body mass index; they include drowsiness, excitation and hyperactivity, and behavioural changes,[37] and one drop of cyclopentolate 1% is preferred as it leads to less adverse reactions.[36,37] Adverse reactions to tropicamide are rare.[37] In all cases, choose the drug with the least possible adverse effects and the lowest concentration that will allow you to efficiently attain the cycloplegia that you require.

Note that eyes with darker irides will need stronger dosages. Research has suggested that cyclopentolate 1% is sufficient to produce good cycloplegia, with an effect similar to atropine 1%, in patients with accommodative esotropia[38] and that tropicamide 1% is as effective as cyclopentolate 1% for the measurement of refractive error in low hyperope, non-strabismic infants,[39] although children with dark irides may need higher dosages.

4.12.2 Procedure for cycloplegic refraction

1. Ask the patient (and/or parent/carer) whether the patient has had any allergic reaction to drugs or medication and record the response. If the patient's record card indicates an allergic reaction to eyedrops previously, you should consider near retinoscopy (section 4.12.6) or referral for cycloplegic refraction under hospital care.
2. Using patient age, body mass index (i.e., be more careful if the child is small and/or thin for their age), and iris colour information, choose the drug/combination with the least possible adverse effects and the lowest concentration that will allow you to efficiently attain the cycloplegia that you require.
3. Obtain informed consent: Explain why you want to use a cycloplegic drug and explain the visual effects (near vision blur, pupil dilation, and increased light sensitivity) and their duration (dependent on the drug used and the dosage). Also inform the patient that the drops will sting a little initially for a few seconds, but that the stinging will disappear. Some clinicians prefer to use topical anaesthetic drops initially as they sting less than cycloplegic drops.[35]
4. Unless indications suggest the possibility of a narrow anterior angle (e.g., high hyperopia or anterior segment abnormality), it may be unnecessary to conduct a full examination of the anterior angle prior to cycloplegic instillation. Cycloplegia is typically performed on young children who will have wide anterior angles owing to the thin nature of the lens in childhood.
5. Instil the drug(s) using drops or spray (see instillation of drops, section 7.8).
6. Ask the patient to sit in the waiting room for about 20 (tropicamide) to 30 minutes (cyclopentolate) until the drug has obtained maximal or near maximal effect. Check that sufficient reduction in accommodation has been obtained by quickly checking the patient's amplitude of accommodation. Add another drop if sufficient accommodation reduction has not been obtained. Also check for anisocoria (usually less mydriasis in the eye receiving drops last), which could indicate unequal cycloplegia and the need for another drop in the eye with the smaller pupil.

7. Perform retinoscopy and/or autorefraction in the usual way. When performing retinoscopy, you must concentrate on the central 3 to 4 mm of the pupil. The peripheral part of the pupil may show a different reflex motion owing to aberrations and these should be ignored.
8. Subjective refraction should be attempted if possible.

4.12.3 Recording of cycloplegic refraction results

Record the cycloplegic used, its dosage, the number of drops, the drug batch number (BN) and expiry date, and the time of instillation. Then record the refraction results (retinoscopy and subjective if both used) in the standard manner, with the approximate time of the refraction. As an alternative to noting the times of instillation and refraction, you could note the period of time the refraction was performed after instillation of the cycloplegic.

For example:

10:00 am: 1 drop cyclopentolate 1%,
dark iris, BN 54321, expiry 2/2022
Retinoscopy, 10:30 am:

RE: +2.25 /−0.50 × 180 98 VAR
LE: +1.75/−0.75 × 180 101 VAR

Tropicamide 0.5% × 2, blue iris, BN 86421
Expiry 8/2022, ref'n 20 mins post instill'n.
Retinoscopy:

OD: +1.25/−0.50 × 170   1.0⁻²
OS: +1.25/−0.50 × 10   1.0⁻¹
Subjective:
OD: +1.00/−0.50 × 175   1.0⁻¹
OS: +1.00/−0.50 × 5   1.0

1 × cyclopentolate 1%, dark iris, BN 12345,
expiry 11/2021. ref'n 30 mins post instill'n.
Retinoscopy.

RE: +2.00 DS   6/6⁻²
LE: +1.75/−0.50 × 180   6/6⁻³

2:30 pm 1 drop tropicamide 1%, blue iris,
BN 12468 expiry 11/2021,
Retinoscopy, 2:50 pm:

OD: +1.75/−1.00 × 170   20/20⁻²
OS: +1.25/−0.50 × 5   20/20⁻¹
Subjective:
OD: +1.50/−1.00 × 170   20/20⁻¹
OS: +1.00/−0.50 × 10   20/20

4.12.4 Interpreting the results

Clearly there are limitations to many of the measurements made in 'dry' (non-cycloplegic) refractions of patients with excessive or fluctuating accommodation, but there are also limitations in 'wet' (cycloplegic) refractions and all must be considered when prescribing and deciding on the best patient management. During cycloplegic retinoscopy it is vital to concentrate on the reflex in the central 3 to 4 mm and ignore the reflex in the periphery that is influenced by peripheral aberrations. Both autorefraction[15] and retinoscopy[40] provide accurate assessments of refractive correction under cycloplegia in children. Also note that the cycloplegic VA is likely to be slightly reduced compared with the VA after a dry refraction owing to the peripheral aberrations. Cyclopentolate 1% does not require an allowance for muscle tonus (unlike atropine) so that the full cycloplegic refraction result can be prescribed if required. Alternatively, the hyperopic correction could be reduced to aid adaptation (section 4.16.3). The non-cycloplegic or dry retinoscopy result (which can be quite accurate owing to the nonaccommodative target and fogged vision) can give an indication of the distance VA likely with the full hyperopic correction prior to adaptation.

4.12.5 Most common error in cycloplegic refraction

Neutralising the retinoscopy reflex seen for the whole of the pupil. The periphery of the reflex should be ignored; you should concentrate on the centre of the pupil when interpreting retinoscopy reflex movements.

4.12.6 Alternative procedure: Mohindra near retinoscopy

Mohindra near retinoscopy was developed as an alternative to cycloplegic refraction in children and infants.[41] It may be used in countries in which cycloplegic drops are restricted and in patients in whom cycloplegic drops are contraindicated or when it is extremely difficult to instil the drops. A dim retinoscope light is used as a fixation target; seen in complete darkness it provides little stimulus to accommodation, so that patients assume their resting focus due to tonic accommodation. This is typically +0.75 DS, so that when working at 50 cm, −1.25 DS rather than the standard −2.00 DS (i.e., the working distance lens) is added to the final retinoscopy result.[41] You need to dim the retinoscope light as low as possible while ensuring it still provides you with an easily visible retinoscopy reflex. Turn off all room lights and perform retinoscopy using a lens rack or individual trial case lenses. An infant will only hold a steady gaze for a short period of time, so that you need to perform the test quickly. The standard technique is to occlude the nonfixating eye using your hand or the parent's hand. However, this can cause infants to become agitated and even begin to cry, so that performing the test binocularly may be preferable in some cases.[42] Some studies that have compared

Mohindra near retinoscopy with cycloplegic retinoscopy have indicated that the test is variable and should not be used, whereas others have suggested that the test is comparable to cycloplegic retinoscopy.[42,43] It would appear that to become competent with the technique, it needs to be performed regularly[41] and this is a disadvantage for the primary care optometrist who only occasionally examines an infant.[42] Saunders and Westall recommend adding −0.75 DS for infants (< 2 years) and −1.00 DS for children (> 2 years) rather than the original −1.25 DS.[43]

4.13 The reading addition

About the age of 40 to 45 years (earlier for some ethnic groups, people with short arms, or working distances and hyperopes; later for people with long arms/working distances and myopes) most people become presbyopic.[44,45] This means that they do not have enough accommodation to be able to read or perform other near work clearly and comfortably. These patients require a positive lens addition to the distance refractive correction. This is called the reading or near addition. With increasing age and further losses in accommodation, the power of the reading addition needs to be increased. At 55 to 60 years of age, objective tests indicate that accommodation is zero (what can be measured clinically is probably depth of focus).[46] Although the average reading addition continues to increase after age 60 years, it does so at a slower rate (Fig. 4.20). This is likely caused by the increases in add needed by some older subjects with reduced VA who use a reduced working distance to provide some magnification to offset the VA loss.[44,45,47,48]

4.13.1 The evidence base: when and how to determine a reading addition

A reading add is determined for all presbyopic patients. An incorrect reading addition is a common cause of patients' unhappiness with new glasses,[26,49,50] and to avoid such complaints it is important to determine the range of clear near vision required by the patient and prescribe glasses that fulfill those requirements. It is difficult to determine appropriate near working distances and ranges in a phoropter, and an addition determination using a trial frame with trial case lenses is recommended.

A determination of the reading addition begins with a tentative addition being determined prior to refinement. This is similar to using an objective measurement of refractive correction (retinoscopy, autorefraction) as a starting point for subjective refraction of the distance correction. In a very useful study, Hanlon et al. determined the required reading addition of 37 dissatisfied patients who returned

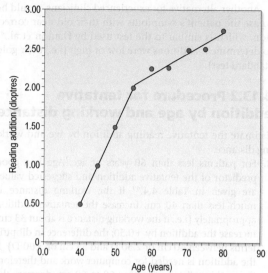

Fig. 4.20 The near addition as a function of age from the data of Pointer[45] and Blystone.[47]

to a university clinic because of improper add power.[49] From the case history information in the review (recheck) examination, it was determined whether the improper addition was too low or too high. For each patient, their reading addition was then determined using four methods (age, ½ amplitude of accommodation, negative relative accommodation/positive relative accommodation (NRA/PRA) balance, and binocular cross-cylinder). The percentage of additions for each test that gave the same result as the improper addition or worse (higher than an improper addition determined too high or lower than an improper addition determined as too low) was determined. They reported that the simplest and quickest test, asking the patient their age, accounted for the fewest errors (14%). The other techniques gave errors in 61% (binocular cross-cylinder), 46% (NRA/PRA), and 30% (½ amplitude) of cases. This suggests that for most patients the tentative addition should simply be based on age. Over the age of about 55 years, the patient's working distance appears to determine their addition as accommodation is zero.[48]

The tentative add estimates based on accommodation tests provide an estimate for both eyes. Unequal estimates of the tentative addition in the two eyes can indicate that the distance refractive correction has not been adequately balanced and needs to be rechecked. This 'double-checking' of the spherical powers of the distance refraction in presbyopes may be an advantage to inexperienced refractionists. Note that for patients over 60 years of age, these tests are measuring depth of focus and not accommodation, which objective tests indicate is zero.

Another alternative for experienced clinicians, would be to use the patient's symptoms with their old near correction, which is similar to the test used by Hanlon et al.,[49] to determine if additions were low or high (i.e., their gold standard test).

4.13.2 Procedure for tentative addition by age and working distance

Estimate the tentative reading addition by age and working distance.

1. For patients less than 60 years of age: Age is a good predictor of the tentative addition and suggested values are given in Table 4.4.[49] If the working distance is much less than 40 cm, increase the tentative addition appropriately (i.e., if the working distance is about 33 cm, increase the addition by +0.50; the difference in dioptric terms between 40 cm or 2.50 D and 33 cm or 3.00 D). If the addition is needed for computer work and therefore the working distance is about 50 to 60 cm, decrease the tentative addition by about +0.50 DS.
2. For patients over 60 years of age: Estimate a tentative reading addition from the patient's working distance, with a small reduction made to allow for depth of focus.[48] In this way, working distances of 50, 40, or 33 cm (dioptric values +2.00, +2.50, and +3.00) indicate tentative additions of +1.75, +2.25, or +2.50 DS, respectively, with higher additions allowing slightly more for depth of focus.[48]

4.13.3 Procedure for tentative addition as a proportion of the amplitude of accommodation

This procedure is most useful for presbyopes less than 55 years of age when patients still retain some accommodation.

1. Measure the amplitude of accommodation (section 6.9).
2. Calculate the tentative reading addition from the following calculation:

Tentative reading addition = working distance in dioptres − ½ of the amplitude of accommodation in dioptres (some clinicians subtract ⅔ of the amplitude).

Table 4.4 Tentative near addition estimates as a function of age up to the age of 55 years[a]

Patient age (years)	Tentative add (D)
45	+1.00
50	+1.50
55	+2.00

[a]These estimates should be adjusted for working distances significantly different from 40 cm (16"). Patients with longer working distances will need a slightly smaller add and vice versa.

4.13.4 Procedure for binocular or fused cross-cylinder

1. Adjust the phoropter to the near PD, occlude the untested eye (typically the left eye), and position the cross-hatch target at the patient's working distance (or 40 cm).
2. If the patient has significant astigmatism (more than approximately 1.50 DC), check that the horizontal and vertical lines of the target appear equally clear. If they do not, the astigmatic correction should be rechecked at distance. If equal clarity can still not be achieved, the astigmatic correction should be checked at near.
3. Dial the cross-cylinder (+0.50/−1.00 × 90) into the phoropter.
4. If the expected addition is high (> +2.00 DS), add +1.00 DS to the distance correction. Ask the patient to close their eyes while you dial the extra power into the phoropter.
5. Ask the patient: "Are the lines running up and down or those running from side-to-side clearer?" The presbyopic patient should report that the horizontal lines are clearer.
6. Add plus lenses in +0.25 DS steps until the patient reports that the vertical lines are just clearer than the horizontal.
7. Repeat steps 2 to 6 for the other eye.
8. If the tentative addition for each eye differs, recheck the results. If they remain different, the binocular balance of the distance refractive correction should be rechecked.
9. Allow both eyes to see the target and reduce the plus power in both eyes until the horizontal and vertical targets appear equally clear.

4.13.5 Procedure for balancing negative and positive relative accommodation

1. Adjust the phoropter to the near PD and attach the near point card. Make sure that the optimal distance refractive correction is in place and that both eyes can view the near point card.
2. Direct the patient's attention to letters one or two lines larger than their best near VA on the near point card. Ask the patient if the letters are clear. If they are not clear, add plus sphere power, +0.25 D at a time, until the patient reports that the letters are clear. This becomes the 'initial tentative near addition.'
3. Negative relative accommodation (NRA): Add plus lenses binocularly, +0.25 D at a time, until the patient reports the first sustained blur. 'First sustained blur' means that the patient notices that the letters are not as sharp and clear as they were initially, even if the patient

Table 4.5 Tentative addition based on patient symptoms and habitual near correction from example 1

	Symptoms regarding near vision	Tentative addition	Tentative addition
1	Difficulty reading and blurred near vision; easier if near work held further away than would prefer	One that provides NV Rx of +2.75 DS	+1.25 DS
2	No problems (and happy with current near working distance)	One that provides NV Rx of +2.25 DS	+0.75 DS
3	Difficulty reading, has to hold too close to be able to read easily	One that provides NV Rx of +1.75 DS	+0.25 DS

NV Rx, Near vision correction.

can still read them. The total amount of plus added is the NRA.

4. Return the lenses in the phoropter to the 'initial tentative near addition' found in step 2.

5. Positive relative accommodation (PRA): Add minus lenses binocularly, −0.25 D at a time, until the patient reports the first sustained blur. The total amount of minus added is the PRA.

6. Adjust the 'initial tentative near addition' that would provide equality for NRA and PRA. The adjusted figure is the 'final tentative addition'. For example, if the 'initial tentative near addition' was +1.00 and sustained blur points were found with a +2.00 and a +0.50 add, the NRA would be +1.00 (2.00–1.00) and the PRA would be −0.50 (0.50–1.00). A 'final tentative near addition' of +1.25 DS would equalise the NRA and PRA (they would both be 0.75 DS). The change suggested by the NRA/PRA is their algebraic sum divided by two. In this example, that would be 0.50/2 = +0.25 DS.

4.13.6 Procedure for tentative addition using the patient's symptoms and habitual correction

This technique is best described by using some examples.
Example 1: 50-year-old patient, wearing bifocal glasses:

RE +1.00 DS   95 (6/7.5, 0.8, 20/25)
LE +1.00 DS   95 (6/7.5, 0.8, 20/25)
Reading addition +1.25D. N5 (0.4 M) with difficulty R and L.

Remember that patients read through their near vision correction (distance refractive correction + reading addition) and NOT their reading addition. The refractive correction for near is RE: +2.25 DS, LE +2.25 DS. Given that the average change in distance spherical refractive correction with age in presbyopes is a hyperopic shift,[51] a

common change for the patient in the example above is for the distance correction to change to:

RE: +1.50 DS   105 (~6/5, 1.2, 20/15)
LE +1.50 DS   105 (~6/5, 1.2, 20/15)

With the new distance correction of +1.50 DS, the tentative addition would be estimated as shown in Table 4.5.

Note that for the most common case (namely, a patient finding difficulty reading and easier if near work held further away), the most appropriate tentative add is the same as the habitual add (+1.25). Because the distance correction has increased by +0.50 DS, the near vision refractive correction has increased to +2.75 DS and would likely alleviate the symptoms.

Example 2: Some patients develop nuclear cataract with age, and this can lead to a myopic shift to the refractive correction.[52] For example, 72-year-old patient; present glasses and habitual VA:

RE: +0.25/−0.50 × 95   90 (6/9, 0.67, 20/30
LE: +0.25/−0.50 × 85   90 (6/9, 0.67, 20/30)
Reading addition +2.25 D. R & L at 30 cm.

(The mean sphere equivalent of the *near* correction is therefore +2.25 DS.)

If the distance refractive correction undergoes a myopic shift and the new distance correction is:

RE −0.25/−0.50 × 100   98 (6/6^{-2}, 1.0^{-2}, 20/20^{-2})
LE −0.25/−0.50 × 90   97 (6/6^{-3}, 1.0^{-3}, 20/20^{-3})

The mean sphere equivalents of the distance refractive correction is −0.50 DS, so that appropriate tentative additions would be estimated as shown in Table 4.6.

Note that an increased tentative add (compared with their habitual add) is suggested if the patient has no symptoms to counteract the minus shift in the distance correction. This situation is not uncommon because these

Table 4.6 Tentative addition based on patient symptoms and habitual near correction from example 2

	Symptoms regarding near vision	Tentative addition	Tentative addition
1	Difficulty reading and blurred near vision; easier if near work held further away than would prefer	One that provides NV Rx of +2.75 DS	+3.25 DS
2	No problems (and happy with current near working distance)	One that provides NV Rx of +2.25 DS	+2.75 DS
3	Difficulty reading, has to hold too close to be able to read easily	One that provides NV Rx of +1.75 DS	+2.25 DS

NV Rx, Near vision correction.

patients are under-minussed at distance in their habitual glasses and over-plussed at near, and they adapt by using a slightly closer reading distance, which provides a little magnification to help counteract reduced VA caused by the cataract.

Leaving the reading addition the same at +2.50 DS, under the misapprehension that this would provide the same near correction as in the old glasses, would leave the patient under-plussed by +0.75 DS. An under-plussed near correction, particularly in patients with nuclear cataract, has been shown to be a cause of patient dissatisfaction and returning new glasses.[26]

4.13.7 Procedure: final reading addition and range of clear vision

See online video 4.17 and summary in Box 4.3.

1. If you have determined the distance refractive correction in a phoropter, add the distance correction to the trial frame using trial case lenses.
2. Ask the patient if they read in normal room lighting or with an additional 'reading' light and only use additional lighting if the patient indicates they use such lighting at home.
3. It can be useful to use a chair without arm rests or tilt the arm rests out of the way when measuring the patient's near working distance as they can influence the measurement.
4. Ask the patient to hold the reading card at their preferred near working distance(s) and measure this distance(s). For example, depending on the patient's occupation and hobbies (as determined in the case history), you may need to determine at what distances a patient sews, reads, and uses their computer. Instruct a patient who has complained that they habitually have to place their near work too close or too far away than they would like, to hold the near VA chart at the distance they would like to read/work at rather than the distance they may have adopted to be able to see clearly in their current glasses.

5. Explain the procedure to the patient: "I am now going to determine the power you need for your reading glasses/bifocal/progressive lens."
6. Tentative addition determination: From one or a combination of the techniques obtain an estimate of the reading addition for the indicated working distance (sections 4.13.2 to 4.13.6) and add these lenses to the trial frame.

Box 4.3 Summary of the near addition procedure

1. Add the distance correction to the trial frame using trial case lenses.
2. Explain the procedure to the patient.
3. Ask the patient if he or she reads in normal room lighting or with an additional 'reading' light and use additional lighting if indicated.
4. Determine the near visual tasks the patient would like to perform (if not already known) and the relevant working distances.
5. Ask the patient to hold the near VA chart at the distance with which the patient would like to read/work.
6. Determine a tentative addition. This is most easily obtained from the patient's age (if less than 60 years of age) or from their working distance (if over 60 years).
7. Determine the final addition by the preferred working distance or trial lens method.
8. Determine the range of clear vision with the binocular reading add.
9. If you are unable to obtain a range that encompasses all the required near working tasks, consider a progressive addition lens, compromise near addition or an intermediate addition.
10. Record the final addition(s), acuity, and range of clearest vision obtained with the addition(s).

7. Determine the final addition for the required near working distance(s). This can be performed in one of two ways:
   (a) Preferred working distance method. Ask the patient to hold the near VA chart where the lenses in the trial frame provide the best vision. Ask the patient if this distance corresponds to their preferred near working distance. If it does not, then change the reading addition appropriately: increase the addition power if you wish to decrease the working distance and decrease the addition power if you wish to increase the working distance provided. Continue this process until the working distance obtained with the trial case lenses equals the patient's preferred working distance.
   (b) Trial lens method. Direct the patient's attention to the best acuity paragraph of text on the near chart, which is held at the patient's preferred working distance. Add −0.25 DS and ask if the letters become clearer, more blurred, or are unchanged. Confirmation lenses (±0.25 DS flippers) are useful for this task (Fig. 4.11). If the acuity improves with the additional minus, then continue adding −0.25 DS until the near acuity or clarity does not improve with the additional −0.25 D. If the vision is unchanged or decreased with −0.25 DS lenses, then do not add them. Add +0.25 DS. If the VA is unchanged or decreased, then do not add the lens. If VA improves with the lens, then add further plus lenses (in 0.25 D steps) only as long as the near VA or its clarity improves.

8. Determine the range of clear vision with the binocular reading add. This is important as the range decreases with higher add powers (Table 4.7). It is particularly important if you are intending that the reading addition will be used for tasks at more than one working distance.
   (a) To determine the near endpoint of the addition's range, ask the patient to move the reading card slowly in until first noticing blur for the best acuity paragraph. Measure this distance.
   (b) Determine the far endpoint of the addition range by asking the patient to move the card slowly away until the best acuity paragraph just blurs.

9. If you are unable to obtain a range that encompasses all the near working tasks that patients have indicated they perform, you may consider that some form of progressive addition lens will provide the range of clear vision required. Alternatively, you could determine whether a compromise near addition would work. For example, the patient may have a preferred reading distance of 40 cm, but the addition that provides best clarity at this distance does not provide adequate clarity for their computer at 67 cm. A compromise addition providing best clarity at 50 cm, but adequate clarity at 40 cm and 67 cm may work. Alternatively, you may need to determine individual additions for their different working distances that could be provided in several pairs of single vision glasses or multifocals.

10. Record the final addition(s), acuity, and range of clearest vision obtained with the addition(s).

Note that if this assessment ends with the patient unable to read the smallest print on your chart (e.g., N5, 0.4 M, 20/25) with their optimal near refractive correction and

Table 4.7 Calculations of the range of clear vision with increasing add powers

Age (years)	Amplitude of accommodation (D)	Near add (D)	Working distance (cm)	Range of clear vision (cm)
45	3.50	+0.75	40	133–24
		+1.25	33	80–21
50	2.50	+1.25	40	80–27
		+1.75	33	57–24
55	1.50	+1.75	40	57–31
		+2.25	33	44–27
60+	1.00	+2.00	40	50–33
		+2.50	33	40–29
		+3.00	29	33–25

Depth of focus effects are included in the amplitude of accommodation measurements and are therefore included in these calculations. The near add was calculated from the equation: near add (D) = working distance (D) − 1/2 amplitude of accommodation. The far point of clear vision (m) was calculated from the inverse of (working distance [D] − 1/2 amplitude), and the near point of clear vision (m) was calculated from the inverse of (working distance [D] + 1/2 amplitude). Note the significant reductions in the range of clear vision with increased add.

the patient does not have an additional 'reading' lamp at home they should strongly be advised to obtain one.

4.13.8 Recording the reading add

Record the final addition(s), reading acuity in each eye, and the range of clear vision.

Examples:

Add +1.50 DS N5 R and L, range 25 to 67 cm
Near add +2.25 DS 0.4M R & L, range 25 to 50 cm

4.13.9 Interpreting reading add results

Most additions are equal for the two eyes. Unequal additions require further testing: either a retest of the near addition endpoints used for each eye or a recheck of the distance binocular balance. The prescribing of unequal additions between the eyes is the exception and is rarely satisfactory. Assuming no accommodative insufficiency, the power of the addition usually increases with age in patients above 40 to 50 years of age. Patients in poor general health can ask for a higher addition than is normal for their age and working distance. In some cases a reading addition that is low for a patient's age and working distance can indicate that the distance refraction has been over-plussed/under-minused.[26] Clinicians rarely give additions greater than +3.00 D in patients with normal VA. It is prudent to keep the addition as weak as possible to keep the range of clear vision as long as possible (see Table 4.7).

4.13.10 Most common errors in reading add values

1. Estimating the tentative addition of patients over 60 years of age based on their age and not their working distance.
2. Not determining the patient's near vision needs and subsequently prescribing an addition that gives an inadequate range of clear near vision for those needs.

4.14 Myopia control

4.14.1 The myopia pandemic

The worldwide prevalence of myopia has been increasing rapidly in recent years and has reached pandemic levels in East Asia, with over 90% of East Asian children in Singapore exhibiting myopia.[53] Predictions suggest that the worldwide prevalence of myopia will increase from about 23% to 50% by 2050 at current progression rates, with high myopia (> 5.00 D of myopia) increasing dramatically from 2.7% (163 million) to 9.8% (938 million).[54]

4.14.2 Pathological myopia[55]

Higher levels of myopia are linked with greater risk of visually disabling conditions, including myopic maculopathy, retinal detachment, and glaucoma, so that this pandemic increase in prevalence is a major public health concern.[56] Lower levels of myopia also carry a risk of pathological changes, so that reducing the level of myopia as well as the number of myopes would produce public health benefits.[56] Indeed, Bullimore and Brennan have shown that reducing myopia by 1.00 D could reduce the risk of myopic maculopathy by 40% regardless of the level of myopia.[57]

4.14.3 What is causing these increases

The rapid increase in myopia suggests that the cause lies with environmental factors rather than genetic. Living in a crowded urban environment rather than rural and greater emphasis on education and thus close work at an early age have been shown to be important risk factors,[53] with circadian disruptions owing to modern lighting and its patterns being another likely factor, whereas an accommodative mechanism for myopia seems increasingly unlikely.[58] The aetiology is complex and likely multifactorial.[55]

4.14.4 The evidence base: when and how to provide myopia control strategies

This is a hugely active research area and regular checking of the research literature is required to keep up to date. Currently the clearest evidence for successful myopia control has been shown in children between 6 and 16 years of age with low to moderate myopia. However, initiating myopia control in patients identified as at high risk prior to them becoming myopic is also recommended.[55,59] A number of myopia control options have been shown to have a strong evidence base and include low dose (0.05%) atropine drops, multifocal soft contact lenses, executive bifocals and orthokeratology, plus increased time outdoors and breaks from near vision activities.[60]

The mechanisms by which these myopia control strategies work is not fully understood,[55,58,60] but the current leading theory of myopia progression suggests that it is caused by relative peripheral hyperopia leading to signals being sent to the peripheral retina to elongate to align with the hyperopic focus (Fig. 4.21). This may be a side effect of the emmetropisation process that attempts to guide eye growth from the hyperopia of youth to emmetropia. One theory suggests that emmetropisation is guided by peripheral oblique astigmatism, which requires a consistent relationship between the peripheral astigmatic images and the retina as provided by outdoor scenes

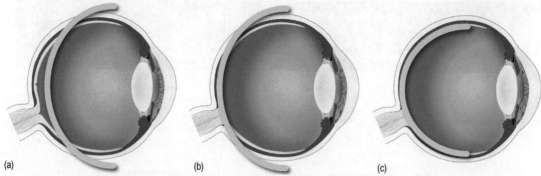

Fig. 4.21 Cross sectional images of a myopic eye with its image shell from a distance object when **(a)** uncorrected, **(b)** corrected with spectacles but showing relative peripheral hyperopia, and **(c)** corrected with multifocal peripheral add contact lenses. (Courtesy of Samantha Strong.)

(i.e., a uniform dioptric field of view) and that cluttered indoor scenes, close working distances, and head tilts all disrupt this process.[61] Elongation of the peripheral retina leads to elongation of the whole posterior globe and thus increased axial length and myopia. Treatments such as soft multifocal and orthokeratology contact lenses, with the plus addition provided in the periphery of the lens, are thought to work by correcting the relative peripheral hyperopia (Fig. 4.21). Outdoor activity perhaps provides the visual scenes necessary for the emmetropisation process to work effectively.[56,61]

4.14.5 Procedure for myopia control

In all examinations of school aged children:

1. Determine any family history of myopia in the case history. Note that children of East Asian descent are more likely to be myopic, become myopic earlier, and the myopia progresses faster.
2. Determine how much near work (including books, computer, gaming, tablet, and smartphone use) they do on a daily basis.
3. Determine their levels of outdoor activity in hours per week. Minimal values of 1 to 2 hours per day on average have been suggested as providing clinically useful protection.[59]
4. Measure their near working distances for reading and smartphone/tablet use. Working distances less than 20 cm are a risk factor for myopia.[59]
5. Consider the results of the subjective refraction and if the patient was already wearing glasses, determine the myopic progression.
6. Identify young children with low to moderate myopia.
7. Identify 'premyopes': young children who are emmetropic or slightly hyperopic with high risk factors for myopia—a strong family history (one or both biological parents are myopic) and/or a myopic lifestyle (high levels of near

work, coupled with low levels of outdoor activity): age 6 ($\leq$ +0.75 DS), 7 to 8 ($\leq$ +0.50 DS), 9 to 10 ($\leq$ +0.25 DS), and 11+ years (emmetropia).[55,59]

8. Use the myopia calculator from the Brien Holden Institute (https://calculator.brienholdenvision.org) and input your patient's age, ethnicity, and current mean sphere refractive error. The calculator provides estimates of the future level of myopia given no treatment or after using any one of a range of myopia control management strategies (multifocal soft contact lenses, peripheral defocus glasses, executive bifocals, orthokeratology, atropine at various doses, and combined treatments) that are based on the best current available evidence (Fig. 4.22).
9. If this is a first examination, describe myopia and its treatment in lay terms (section 2.4). Also discuss myopia progression using the results from the Holden Institute calculator and its possible long-term consequences (maculopathy, glaucoma, retinal detachment; Table 4.8). This is best achieved with supporting leaflets and/or provision of website information. Currently many children and their parents (East Asian parents may be an exception) are not aware of the potentially damaging effects of myopia and believe it is merely an 'optical inconvenience,' 'expense,' and 'cosmetic inconvenience.'[62]
10. The following recommendations appear useful for all but moderate to high hyperopic children, but should be strongly recommended to patients at higher risk of myopia and their families.[59]
    (a) Increase their outdoor activities. A extra hour/day outside appears a useful target.[63]
    (b) Take regular breaks from near vision activities (including smartphone and tablet use). The 20-20-20 rule, originally developed to help prevent eye strain when using a computer, is easy to remember: every 20 minutes, take a 20-second break and look in the distance (20 feet away to those who understand distances in feet).

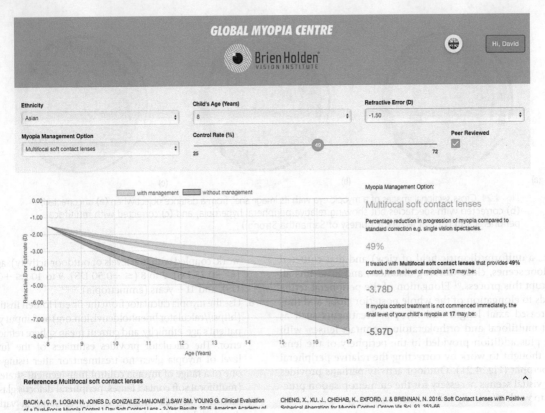

Fig 4.22 A screen shot from the Brien Holden Vision Institute myopia calculator showing the predicted myopia progression for an Asian 8-year-old child with −1.50 DS of myopia with and without myopia control.

Table 4.8 Approximate odds ratios for the risk of eye diseases as myopia increases

Degree of myopia	Maculopathy	Retinal detachment	Glaucoma
−1.00 to −2.99	2	4	2
−3.00 to −4.99	10	9	3
−5.00 to −6.99	41		
−7.00 to −8.99	127	~ 21	
9.00 +	349	~66	

Adapted from Flitcroft DI. The complex interactions of retinal, optical and environmental factors in myopia aetiology. *Prog Retin Eye Res.* 2012;31:622–60.

(c) Ensure high illumination levels when reading.[64]

(d) Read further away than currently.

11. This advice should be supported by leaflets and/or links to suitable websites.

12. Consider what myopia control strategies you can provide yourself and what are available by referral locally. Multifocal soft contact lenses and orthokeratology are briefly discussed in section 5.11. They have the potential adverse effects of infection, with greater risks for orthokeratology because of overnight wear,[65,66] and these should be discussed with the patient and their parents/carers. The risks seem no greater than for adults, may be improved in younger children owing to careful parental supervision,[65,66] and seem far outweighed by the risk of visual impairment owing to higher levels of myopia.[67] Myopia control strategies can slow myopia progression by the following extents[59]:

(a) Orthokeratology: 30% to 60%. This has the advantage that lenses do not have to be worn during the day. However, progression can be difficult to monitor and axial length measurements are needed.

(b) Multifocal soft contact lenses: 30% to 50%.

(c) Atropine: 30% to 80%, with greater effectivity with stronger dosages, but also greater side effects of photophobia and reduced near vision.

4.15 Guidelines for prescribing glasses

Patients returning to their optometrist because they are unhappy with their new glasses occurs in about 1% to 3% of cases.[50,68] One way that experienced clinicians keep this figure as low as possible is to use various guidelines for prescribing glasses. Note that these guidelines are for certain cases and must NOT be used in prescribing decisions for young children, for example, which must consider the normal refractive error for their age and the need to encourage emmetropisation and prevent amblyopia.[69]

4.15.1 Should you prescribe a small refractive correction?

Should you prescribe a small correction, such as +0.50 D, of hyperopia or hyperopic astigmatism? This can be a very difficult question. Here are some points to consider:

1. If there are no symptoms related to the use of the eyes and no other indications from other tests in the eye examination, then glasses are not needed.
2. Consider other ocular causes of the symptoms, such as inadequate convergence, accommodative facility or vergence facility, and decompensated heterophoria. Also consider nonocular causes of headaches, including tension, migraine, nasal sinusitis, and hypertension. Tension headaches, which are common, can be difficult to differentiate from ocular-related headaches because they are often frontal or occipital, get worse towards the end of the day, and are better over the weekend.
3. If a patient has symptoms that are related to detailed vision tasks, you are more likely to prescribe a small correction if the patient does a lot of detailed work and/or if the patient has a personality that is detail-oriented, precise, or intense.[70]
4. If glasses with a small correction are to be of any value, the responses during subjective refraction should be very certain, appropriate, and repeatable.
5. Usually small corrections make little change to the VA (particularly if a truncated Snellen chart is used) and so basing decisions on VA improvements is usually not helpful.
6. The effect of the Rx on binocular vision tests can be helpful.[71] For example, if binocular vision tests suggest

that a heterophoria is decompensated with no refractive correction and compensated with it, then the glasses are likely to help and should be prescribed.[71]

7. You can view prescribing glasses as a diagnostic tool. Often the only way to be certain whether the symptoms are caused by the uncorrected refractive error is to prescribe it and see if the symptoms disappear. You could offer the patient a pair of basic loan glasses to determine whether the refractive correction will relieve the symptoms. This approach is often used in medicine. However, be aware that glasses can provide a placebo effect[72] and relieve the symptoms for a short period before they return.

4.15.2 The evidence base: when to partially prescribe a change in correction

For some patients experienced clinicians tend to consider both the patient's current glasses and the subjective refraction result and prescribe a correction somewhere between these two using a selection of clinical maxims or pearls (of wisdom).[68,73,74] Prescribing partial refractive changes commonly occurs when patients are (1) very happy with their current glasses and (2) when changes in refractive correction are large, and should be particularly used with older patients and younger patients known to have difficulty adapting to new glasses.

If patients are very happy with their current glasses, making a change risks making the patient unhappy. Given that the subjective refraction results can vary by up to 0.50 D for individual clinicians and up to 0.75 D between clinicians,[75,76] and research has shown that small spherical and cylindrical errors (of 0.25 DS and 0.50 DC) can cause symptoms and dissatisfaction to some patients,[77,78] any individual subjective refraction might not be correct for the patient. This is particularly true if the responses during subjective refraction were poor (and remember that many patients find subjective refraction judgements very difficult).[21-23] On the other hand, if a patients say that the glasses they are wearing provide very good vision with no symptoms, then that is an excellent indicator that the correction in their glasses is correct for the patient.

Partial prescribing is also used when refractive changes are large. Although new glasses typically provide improved vision, they also provide changes in magnification. These alter the vestibulo-ocular reflex (this makes your eyes move at exactly the same speed, but in the opposite direction to your head movements to make sure that your surroundings do not appear to move when your head moves) so that surroundings can seem to 'swim' for some patients with new glasses that include a large change in correction. Cylinder changes alter magnification in different meridians, which may be different in the two eyes, and these can make floors and walls appear to slope and round objects appear oval until the patient adapts to the new glasses. Older people tend to have greater problems adapting to new glasses[74] with oblique cylinder changes causing dizziness[79] and changes in correction of over 0.75 D can increase falls (section 4.15.4).[80,81]

4.15.3 Clinical maxims (or pearls)

1. 'If it ain't broke, don't fix it.' Making changes of 0.50 D or more in patients with no symptoms who have good VA is a very common cause of patient dissatisfaction and glasses needing remaking.[82] If patients are happy with their glasses, but would like a new frame, prescribe the old correction with which the patient is happy, not your subjective refraction result.
2. 'If it ain't broke, don't fix it' (distance specific). For example, if patients have good distance VA and are very happy with their distance vision in their glasses, but have difficulties reading, 'needs longer arms' and a +0.50 D increase in their near add (which is not uncommon), prescribe the old distance correction that the patient is happy with and not your subjective refraction result and increase the old near addition by +0.50 DS.
3. 'If it ain't broke, don't fix it much.' If a patient wants new glasses but has no symptoms and reasonable VA and you find a change of 0.50 D or more (particularly if spherical) that the patient appreciates when shown the comparison, prescribe about half the change in spherical power.[82] It is likely in such cases that the patient would start to develop symptoms in the following months, so that a small change seems sensible.
4. Be careful of reducing a myopic correction. Myopia can decrease, particularly in patients aged 25 to 35 years, but be extremely careful of reducing a myopic correction in these patients, especially if there are no symptoms. Remember that if you are refracting at 6 m or 20 ft, this is not infinity, so that patients are likely to be over-plussed by +0.17 D with a 6 m (20 ft) refractive correction. Also some low myopes tend to wear their glasses only for driving and especially at night, and 'night myopia' may be an additional problem. Depending on the patient you may wish to prescribe the correction in their current glasses ('if it ain't broke, don't fix it') or half the reduction in myopia ('if it ain't broke, don't fix it much').
5. Avoid big cylindrical changes. Cylinder power and axes changes can be particularly hard to adapt to for some patients, yet improvements in vision can be relatively small. When cylinder changes are moderate to large, generally make partial changes in cylinder power and axis (~half-way between the habitual correction and subjective result). Be particularly wary of making large changes in cylinder power and/or axis if the axes are oblique. It can be useful to trial frame the partial correction you are going to prescribe and even ask the patient to walk around in them.

6. 'Cut the plus.' Consider prescribing a partial hyperopic correction that is sufficient to remove the symptoms in a young patient. Just as you would not prescribe glasses to a young, asymptomatic low hyperope because they have sufficient accommodation to cope with slight hyperopia, why prescribe the full amount of hyperopia? It makes adaptation more difficult and can make it more difficult for the patient to see when they take off their glasses. Over-plussing the distance correction has been reported as the most common reason for failure of acceptance of glasses.[26]

4.15.4 Guidelines for elderly patients at risk of falls

Falls are common in elderly people with a third of people over 65 years reporting a fall in the previous year and this rises to 50% in people aged 80+.[81] They can have devastating consequences, with falls being the leading cause of accidental death in the elderly in addition to causing hip and other fractures and 'long lies.' Although visual impairment is an important risk factor for falls, correcting visual impairment does not always reduce falls rate. For example, large changes in refractive correction have been shown to *increase* the falls rate in older patients because some find adaptation to large changes in correction difficult,[80] likely owing to changes in hyperopic/myopic magnification and distortion caused by astigmatism.[81]

In addition, multifocal glasses increase falls risk because of blur in the lower visual field (e.g., beyond 40 cm and thus blurring step edges) plus peripheral distortion in varifocal/PALs (see Fig. 4.23a) and both diplopia and image jump in bifocals.[81,83]

To help prevent falls, you first need to recognise patients who are at moderate to high risk of falls (see Table 4.9). The more risk factors the patient has, the more likely the patient is to fall.[84]

The following are recommended for all patients who are at moderate to high risk of falls:

1. Ask the patient if they have fallen in the last year.
2. Ask the patient if they wear their glasses when walking outdoors and if they take off their multifocals when ascending/descending stairs.
3. Do not make large changes in refractive correction because these increase the risk of falls.[80] Limit changes to 0.50 D and keep cylindrical axis changes to a minimum, particularly oblique axes, which can cause dizziness.[79,81] For this reason, suggest more regular eye examinations for patients at risk of falls and make regular, small changes as needed.

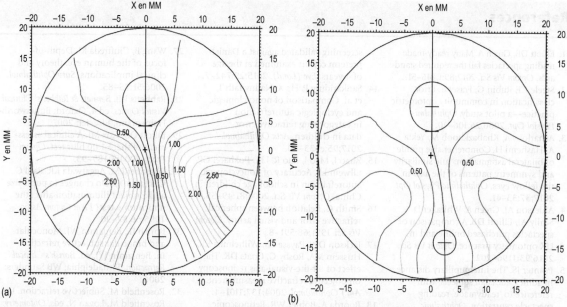

Fig 4.23 PAL blur and distortion. In addition to extensive lower visual field blur of the floor, steps, and stairs with high adds **(a)**, varifocals/PALs include peripheral areas of aberrational astigmatism (distortion), which are greater with higher-powered adds **(a)** +2.50 add, **(b)** +1.00 add. (Courtesy of Essilor R&D.)[86]

Table 4.9 Intrinsic risk factors for falls[a]

Increasing older age
Female
Poor balance and/or gait
Systemic conditions, including diabetes, arthritis, hypotension, stroke, dementia, Parkinson disease, and arthritis
Taking more than 4 tablets per day (polypharmacy)
Taking sedatives or antidepressants
A history of falls
Visual impairment

[a]The more risk factors the more the patient is at risk of falling.[87]

4. Do not prescribe PALs/varifocals or bifocals unless the patient has successfully worn them previously. These lenses double the risk of falls.[85]

5. With patients who have worn PALs, varifocals, or bifocals for many years, but have become at moderate to high risk of falls as they have become older, you have several options:

   a. Patients who rarely leave the home and are in-active should continue to wear their usual PAL, varifocal, or bifocal.[83] Try to keep changes as minimal as possible and this includes lens type

as well as refractive correction. The need to fit these higher add varifocal/PAL lenses accurately is clear from their distortion patterns (see Fig. 4.23a), which highlight the small margins for error. Online purchasing of such lenses which are often glazed using 'average' estimates of the optical centre positions seems dangerous and wholly inappropriate.[4]

   b. For fit and active patients, prescribe an additional pair of single vision distance lenses for walking outside the home. This has been shown to reduce falls risk.[83] Alternatively, if the patient is a low myope you could recommend that they walk outside the house without their multifocal.

   c. For patients who do not want to forego their multifocal glasses when walking outside the home, suggest a low add multifocal (~ +1.25 D) that provides reasonable spot reading (of price tags, menus, smartphones etc) with safer walking owing to minimal blur for the floor, steps, and stairs and reduced peripheral distortions (see Fig. 4.23b).[86]

6. Be wary of a monovision approach because of the loss of stereoacuity.[81]

7. Refer patients earlier than usual for first eye cataract surgery.[81,87]

8. Refer patients with low vision to appropriate health professionals who can provide home modification advice to help prevent falls.[88]

References

1. Elliott DB, Green A. Many ready-made reading spectacles fail the required standards. *Optom Vis Sci.* 2012;89:E446–51.

2. Steele CF, Rubin G, Fraser S. Error classification in community optometric practice—a pilot study. *Ophthalmic Physiol Opt.* 2006;26:106–10.

3. Asharlous A, Khabazkhoob M, Yekta A, Hashemi H. Comprehensive profile of bilateral astigmatism: rule similarity and symmetry patterns of the axes in the fellow eyes. *Ophthalmic Physiol Opt.* 2017;37:33–41.

4. Alderson AJ, Green A, Whitaker D, Scally AJ, Elliott DB. A comparison of spectacles purchased online and in UK optometry practice. *Optom Vis Sci.* 2016;93:1196–202.

5. Pointer JS. The interpupillary distance in adult Caucasian subjects, with reference to 'readymade' reading spectacle centration. *Ophthalmic Physiol Opt.* 2012;32:324–31.

6. Brown WL. Interpupillary distance. In: Eskridge JD, Amos JF, Bartlett JD, eds. *Clinical Procedures in Optometry.* Philadelphia: JB Lippincott; pp 39–52, 1991.

7. Osuobeni EP, al-Fahdi M. Differences between anatomical and physiological interpupillary distance. *J Am Optom Assoc.* 1994;65:265–71.

8. Holland BJ, Siderov J. Repeatability of measurements of interpupillary distance. *Ophthalmic Physiol Opt.* 1999;19:74–8.

9. Kitzmann AS, Fethke NB, Baratz KH, Zimmerman MB, Hackbarth DJ, Gehrs KM. A survey study of musculoskeletal disorders among eye care physicians compared with family medicine physicians. *Ophthalmology.* 2012;119:213–20.

10. Casillas E, Rosenfeld M. Comparison of subjective heterophoria testing with a phoropter and trial frame. *Optom Vis Sci.* 2006;83:237–41.

11. Weiss RA, Berke W, Gottlieb L, Horvath P. Clinical importance of accurate refractor vertex distance measurements prior to refractive surgery. *J Refract Surg.* 2002;18:444–8.

12. McCaghrey GE, Matthews FE. Clinical evaluation of a range of autorefractors. *Ophthalmic Physiol Opt.* 1993;13:129–37.

13. Fledelius HC, Bangsgaard R, Slidsborg C, la Cour M. The usefulness of the Retinomax autorefractor for childhood screening validated against a Danish preterm cohort examined at the age of 4 years. *Eye (Lond).* 2015;29:742–7.

14. Sankaridurg P, He X, Naduvilath T, et al. Comparison of noncycloplegic and cycloplegic autorefraction in categorizing refractive error data in children. *Acta Ophthalmol.* 2017;95:e633–40.

15. Zhao J, Mao J, Luo R, Li F, Pokharel GP, Ellwein LB. Accuracy of noncycloplegic autorefraction in school-age children in China. *Optom Vis Sci.* 2004;81:49–55.

16. Smith G. Relation between spherical refractive error and visual acuity. *Optom Vis Sci* 1991;68:591–8.

17. Jackson DW, Paysse EA, Wilhelmus KR, Hussein MA, Rosby G, Coats DK. The effect of off-the-visual-axis retinoscopy on objective refractive measurement. *Am J Ophthalmol.* 2004;137:1101–4.

18. Roorda A, Bobier WR. Retinoscopic reflexes: theoretical basis and effects of monochromatic aberrations. *J Am Optom Assoc.* 1996;67:610–8.

19. Millodot M, O'Leary D. The discrepancy between retinoscopic and subjective measurements: effect of age. *Am J Optom Physiol Opt.* 1978;55:309–16.

20. Read SA, Vincent SJ, Collins. The visual and functional impacts of astigmatism and its clinical management. *Ophthalmic Physiol Opt.* 2014;34:267–94.

21. Irving EL, Sivak AM, Spafford MM. "I can see fine": patient knowledge of eye care. *Ophthalmic Physiol Opt.* 2018;38:422–31.

22. Shickle D, Griffin M. Why don't older adults in England go to have their eyes examined? *Ophthalmic Physiol Opt.* 2014;34:38–45.

23. Shickle D, Griffin M, Evans R, et al. Why don't younger adults in England go to have their eyes examined? *Ophthalmic Physiol Opt.* 2014;34:30–7.

24. Elliott DB, Yang KC, Whitaker D. Visual acuity changes throughout adulthood in normal, healthy eyes: seeing beyond 6/6. *Optom Vision Sci.* 1995;72:186–91.

25. Woods DL, Wyma JM, Yund EW, Herron TJ, Reed B. Corrigendum: age-related slowing of response selection and production in a visual choice reaction time task. *Front Hum Neurosci.* 2015;9:193.

26. Hrynchak P. Prescribing spectacles: reason for failure of spectacle acceptance. *Ophthalmic Physiol Opt.* 2006;26:111–5.

27. Wang B, Ciuffreda KJ. Depth-of-focus of the human eye: theory and clinical implications. *Surv Ophthalmol.* 2006;51:75–85.

28. Rabbetts RB. *Bennett & Rabbetts' Clinical Visual Optics*, ed 4. Oxford: Butterworth-Heinemann, Elsevier; 2007.

29. Elliott DB, Cox MJ. A clinical assessment of the +1.00 blur test. *Optom Pract.* 2004;5:189–93.

30. Rosenfield M, Aggarwala KR, Raul C, Ciuffreda KJ. Do changes in pupil size and ambient illumination affect the duochrome test? *J Am Optom Assoc.* 1995;66:87–90.

31. Borish IL, Benjamin WJ. Monocular and binocular subjective refraction. In: Benjamin WJ, ed. *Borish's Clinical Refraction.* Philadelphia: WB Saunders; 2006.

32. Rosenfield M. Subjective refraction. In: Rosenfield M, Logan N, eds. *Optometry: Science, Techniques and Clinical Management.* Edinburgh: Elsevier; pp. 209–28, 2009.

33. Humphriss D. Binocular refraction. In: Edwards K, Llewellyn R, eds. *Optometry.* Oxford: Butterworths; 1988.

34. Mondok L, Traboulsi EI. Nonorganic vision loss in children. In: Traboulsi E, Utz V, eds. *Practical Management of Pediatric Ocular Disorders and Strabismus.* New York, NY: Springer; 2016.

35. Lim SA, Siatkowski RM, Farris BK. Functional visual loss in adults and children patient characteristics, management, and outcomes. *Ophthalmology.* 2005;112:1821–8.

36. Doyle LA, McCullough SJ, Saunders KJ. Cycloplegia and spectacle prescribing in children: attitudes of UK optometrists. *Ophthalmic Physiol Opt.* 2019;39:148–61.

37. van Minderhout HM, Joosse MV, Grootendorst DC, Schalij-Delfos NE. Adverse reactions following routine anticholinergic eye drops in a paediatric population: an observational cohort study. *BMJ Open.* 2015;5:e008798.

38. Celebi S, Aykan U. The comparison of cyclopentolate and atropine in patients with refractive accommodative esotropia by means of retinoscopy, autorefractometry and biometric lens thickness. *Acta Ophthalmol Scand.* 1999;77:426–9.

39. Yazdani N, Sadeghi R, Momeni-Moghaddam H, Zarifmahmoudi L, Ehsaei A. Comparison of cyclopentolate

versus tropicamide cycloplegia: a systematic review and meta-analysis. *J Optom*. 2018;11:135–43.

40. McCullough SJ, Doyle L, Saunders KJ. Intra- and inter-examiner repeatability of cycloplegic retinoscopy among young children. *Ophthalmic Physiol Opt*. 2017;37:16–23.

41. Deng L, Gwiazda J. Birth season, photoperiod, and infancy refraction. *Optom Vis Sci*. 2011;88:383–7.

42. Twelker JD, Mutti DO. Retinoscopy in infants using a near noncycloplegic technique, cycloplegia with tropicamide 1%, and cycloplegia with cyclopentolate 1%. *Optom Vision Sci*. 2001;78:215–22.

43. Saunders KJ, Westall CA. Comparison between near retinoscopy and cycloplegic retinoscopy in the refraction of infants and children. *Optom Vision Sci*. 1992;69: 615–22.

44. Millodot M, Millodot S. Presbyopia correction and the accommodation in reserve. *Ophthalmic Physiol Opt*. 1989;9:126–32.

45. Pointer JS. The presbyopic add I, II and III. *Ophthalmic Physiol Opt*. 1995;15: 235–54.

46. Charman WN. The path to presbyopia: straight or crooked? *Ophthalmic Physiol Opt*. 1989;9:424–30.

47. Blystone PA. Relationship between age and presbyopic addition using a sample of 3,645 examinations from a single private practice. *J Am Optom Assoc*. 1999;70:505–8.

48. MacMillan ES, Elliott DB, Patel B, Cox M. Loss of visual acuity is the main reason why reading addition increases after the age of sixty. *Optom Vis Sci*. 2001;78:381–5.

49. Hanlon SD, Nakabayashi J, Shigezawa G. A critical view of presbyopic add determination. *J Am Optom Assoc*. 1987;58:468–72.

50. Freeman CE, Evans BJ. Investigation of the causes of non-tolerance to optometric prescriptions for spectacles. *Ophthalmic Physiol Opt*. 2010;30:1–11.

51. Guzowski M, Wang JJ, Rochtchina E, Rose KA, Mitchell P. Five-year refractive changes in an older population: the Blue Mountains Eye Study. *Ophthalmology*. 2003;110:1364–70.

52. Pesudovs K, Elliott DB. Refractive error changes in cortical, nuclear and posterior subcapsular cataract. *Br J Ophthalmol*. 2003;87:964–7.

53. Rudnicka AR, Kapetanakis VV, Wathern AK, et al. Global variations and time trends in the prevalence of childhood myopia, a systematic review and quantitative meta-analysis: implications

for aetiology and early prevention. *Br J Ophthalmol*. 2016;100:882–90.

54. Holden BA, Fricke TR, Wilson DA, et al. Global prevalence of myopia and high myopia and temporal trends from 2000 through 2050. *Ophthalmology*. 2016;123: 1036–42.

55. Flitcroft DI, He M, Jonas JB, et al. IMI—defining and classifying myopia: a proposed set of standards for clinical and epidemiologic studies. *Invest Ophthalmol Vis Sci*. 2019;60:M20–30.

56. Flitcroft DI. The complex interactions of retinal, optical and environmental factors in myopia aetiology. *Prog Retin Eye Res*. 2012;31:622–60.

57. Bullimore MA, Brennan NA. Myopia control: why each diopter matters. *Optom Vis Sci*. 2019; 96:463–5.

58. Chakraborty R, Ostrin LA, Nickla DL, Iuvone PM, Pardue MT, Stone RA. Circadian rhythms, refractive development, and myopia. *Ophthalmic Physiol Opt*. 2018;38:217–45.

59. Gifford KL, Richdale K, Kang P, et al. IMI—clinical management guidelines report. *Invest Ophthalmol Vis Sci*. 2019;60:M184–203.

60. Wildsoet CF, Chia A, Cho P, et al. IMI—interventions for controlling myopia onset and progression report. *Invest Ophthalmol Vis Sci*. 2019;60:M106–31.

61. Charman WN. Myopia, posture and the visual environment. *Ophthalmic Physiol Opt*. 2011;31:494–501.

62. McCrann S, Flitcroft I, Lalor K, Butler J, Bush A, Loughman J. Parental attitudes to myopia: a key agent of change for myopia control? *Ophthalmic Physiol Opt*. 2018;38:298–308.

63. Xiong S, Sankaridurg P, Naduvilath T et al. Time spent in outdoor activities in relation to myopia prevention and control: a meta-analysis and systematic review. *Acta Ophthalmol*. 2017;95:551–66.

64. Hua WJ, Jin JX, Wu XY, et al. Elevated light levels in schools have a protective effect on myopia. *Ophthalmic Physiol Opt*. 2015;35:252–62.

65. Bullimore MA. The safety of soft contact lenses in children. *Optom Vis Sci*. 2017;94:638–46.

66. Bullimore MA, Sinnott LT, Jones-Jordan LA. The risk of microbial keratitis with overnight corneal reshaping lenses. *Optom Vis Sci*. 2013;90:937–44.

67. Tideman JWL, Snabel MC, Tedja MS, et al. Association of axial length with risk of uncorrectable visual impairment for Europeans with myopia. *JAMA Ophthalmol*. 2016;134:1355–63.

68. Howell-Duffy C, Scally AJ, Elliott DB. Spectacle prescribing II: practitioner

experience is linked to the likelihood of suggesting a partial prescription. *Ophthalmic Physiol Opt*. 2011;31:155–67.

69. Leat SJ. To prescribe or not to prescribe? Guidelines for spectacle prescribing in infants and children. *Clin Exp Optom*. 2011;94:514–27.

70. Woods RL, Colvin CR, Vera-Diaz FA, Peli E. A relationship between tolerance of blur and personality. *Invest Ophthalmol Vis Sci*. 2010;51:6077–82.

71. Dwyer P, Wick B. The influence of refractive correction upon disorders of vergence and accommodation. *Optom Vis Sci*. 1995;72:224–32.

72. Elliott DB. The placebo effect: is it unethical to use it or unethical not to? *Ophthalmic Physiol Opt*. 2016;36: 513–8.

73. Hrynchak PK, Mittelstaedt AM, Harris J, Machan CM, Irving EL. Modifications made to the refractive result when prescribing spectacles. *Optom Vis Sci*. 2012;89:155–60.

74. Werner DL, Press LJ. *Clinical Pearls in Refractive Care*. Boston: Butterworth-Heinemann; 2002.

75. Goss DA, Grosvenor T. Reliability of refraction—a literature review. *J Am Optom Assoc*. 1996;67:619–30.

76. MacKenzie GE. Reproducibility of sphero-cylindrical prescriptions. *Ophthalmic Physiol Opt*. 2008;28: 143–50.

77. Miller AD, Kris MJ, Griffiths AC. Effect of small focal errors on vision. *Optom Vis Sci*. 1997;74:521–6.

78. Atchison DA, Schmid KL, Edwards KP, Muller SM, Robotham J. The effect of under and over refractive correction on visual performance and spectacle lens acceptance. *Ophthalmic Physiol Opt*. 2001;21:255–61.

79. Supuk E, Alderson A, Davey CJ, et al. Dizziness, but not falls rate, improves after routine cataract surgery: the role of refractive and spectacle changes. *Ophthalmic Physiol Opt*. 2016;36: 183–90.

80. Cumming RG, Ivers R, Clemson L, et al. Improving vision to prevent falls in frail older people: a randomized trial. *J Am Geriatr Soc*. 2007;55:175–81.

81. Elliott DB. The Glenn A. Fry award lecture 2013: blurred vision, spectacle correction, and falls in older adults. *Optom Vis Sci*. 2014;91:593–601.

82. Howell-Duffy C, Hrynchak PK, Irving EL, Mouat GS, Elliott DB. Evaluation of the clinical maxim: 'If it ain't broke, don't fix it'. *Optom Vis Sci*. 2012;89:105–11.

83. Haran MJ, Cameron ID, Ivers RQ, et al. Effect on falls of providing single lens

distance vision glasses to multifocal glasses wearers: VISIBLE randomised controlled trial. *BMJ.* 2010;340:c2265.

84. Tinetti ME, Speechley M, Ginter SF. Risk factors for falls among elderly people living in the community. *N Engl J Med* 1988; 319:1701–7.

85. Lord SR, Dayhew J, Howland A. Multifocal glasses impair edge-contrast

sensitivity and depth perception and increase the risk of falls in older people. *J Am Geriatr Soc.* 2002;50:1760–66.

86. Elliott DB, Hotchkiss J, Scally AJ, Foster R, Buckley JG. Intermediate addition multifocals provide safe stair ambulation with adequate 'short-term' reading. *Ophthalmic Physiol Opt.* 2016;36:60–8.

87. Palagyi A, Morlet N, McCluskey P, et al. Visual and refractive associations with falls after first-eye cataract surgery. *J Cataract Refract Surg.* 2017;43:1313–21.

88. Campbell AJ, Robertson MC, La Grow SJ, et al. Randomised controlled trial of prevention of falls in people aged > or =75 with severe visual impairment: the VIP trial. *BMJ.* 2005;331:817.

Chapter | 5 |

Contact lens assessment

Catharine Chisholm and Craig A. Woods

Patient preference for contact lenses over glasses is common owing to perceived conveniences (i.e., no spectacle fogging, can see better in rain, can wear off-the-shelf sunglasses) as well as improvements in appearance and abilities in sports.[1] There is a relatively high discontinuation of contact lens wear (~16% United States, ~30% Europe),[2,3] but patients are more likely to succeed when fitted with lenses that suit their eyes and lifestyle. They tend to achieve better compliance with lens care when you manage their expectations.[4] Worldwide, the majority of new fits are soft lenses, with rigid lenses accounting for around 11% of new fits, (4% UK and US, 7% Canada

and Australia, >23% Austria, Netherlands, and France.[5] Despite the small proportion of new fits, it is important to maintain rigid gas permeable (RGP) lens fitting skills because they remain the first choice of lens for a proportion of patients, as well as a significantly higher proportion of refits. It is not uncommon to fit a patient with more than one lens type (e.g., RGP lenses for day-to-day use with a small supply of soft single-use lenses for swimming with goggles and other sporting activities). In addition, there is a growing interest in the use of contact lenses in the management of myopia progression, multifocal lenses as well as orthokeratology designs.[6] Recently, there has been a resurgence in the use of scleral lenses, both full haptic and reduced sized (mini) scleral lenses, principally for patients requiring complex lenses for therapeutic purposes, corneal irregularity, and protection (i.e., dry eyes).[7] These lenses are briefly considered in section 5.12, but a detailed discussion of fitting such lenses falls outside the scope of this book.

5.1 Contact lens fitting

The purpose of the preliminary contact lens fit examination is to:

1. Quantify ocular parameters to aid selection of the first trial lens.
2. Confirm the normality of the ocular tissues and to record for future reference, any acceptable abnormality (e.g., a corneal scar resulting from a historical eye injury).
3. Discover issues that potentially preclude or limit contact lens wear (and manage or refer as necessary), or indicate the need for a particular type of contact lens.

4. Allow the recording of baseline data against which to judge possible contact lens-induced changes.

In general, the patient needs to trial the contact lenses and return for the first follow-up check before the fitting is concluded and a lens specification can be issued. The preliminary examination includes the following, which are further described in the next sections:

1. A pre-fit case history to determine what the patients want from contact lenses, what they know about lenses, and to help determine whether they are a suitable candidate.

2. Measurements to help determine lens parameters: horizontal visible iris diameter, pupil diameter (average and mesopic), palpebral aperture (PA) and lid position, corneal curvature and regularity, and subjective refraction (unless a recent refraction has taken place).

3. Assessments to help determine suitability for lens wear: anterior eye health and tear film quality. Examination of the posterior segment is only included in the pre-fit examination if any new symptoms or signs indicate that further investigation is warranted, or if there has been a significant time period since the last posterior segment assessment.

4. Selection of the trial lenses: The findings from the preliminary assessment and how they influence lens choice should be discussed with the patient. There may be a clear indication for a particular lens type, such as single-use lenses for a patient who only wants to wear lenses two or three times a week; or there may be a range of possible options requiring the pros and cons of each lens type, including cost and impact of lens care use, to be discussed with the patient to enable the patient to make an informed decision.

5. Post-trial assessment: Assess the performance of the trial lenses in terms of fit, compatibility with the eye/tear film, and visual acuity (lens power verification).
   (a) It may be necessary to trial more than one lens to meet the patient's needs.
   (b) Remove the lenses and check the eyes using the slit lamp.
   (c) Discuss your findings with the patient and, in the case of disposable soft lenses, consider providing them with lenses for a prolonged trial.

6. Teach the patient to handle and care for the lenses: Ensure the patient fully understands the do's and don'ts of lens wear and the importance of lens and lens case maintenance.

7. Final check of trial lenses: Allow the patient to trial the lenses for a few days. Undertake the first check-up when the lenses have been *in situ* for a few hours; if everything is satisfactory, order the final lenses and provide the patient with a copy of the contact lens specification. Further changes to the lens(es) and an extended trial may be required before the fitting can be considered

complete, particularly for some toric, multifocal, or complex lens fits.

5.2 Pre-fitting case history

5.2.1 The evidence base: the importance of the pre-fitting case history

Many of the issues covered in section 2.3 also apply during a contact lens examination, such as the importance of communication and putting the patient at ease. Trying contact lenses for the first time can be a very daunting process for some patients; a common worry is that the lenses will cause pain when they are placed on their eyes. Encourage them that, at worst, the sensation is similar to having an eyelash in their eyes and at best they are simply not aware the lens has gone in.[8] Also, reassure the patient that any discomfort will have significantly reduced within a week of starting wear.[9] Spending sufficient time to fully understanding a patient's wants from contact lenses, determining what they know about them, explaining the issues, and managing their expectations, are important factors to limit contact lens drop outs.[10] Make it clear from the start that a successful fit may require more than one appointment, particularly in the case of complex lenses—correcting astigmatism, presbyopia, controlling myopia, or more complicated lens designs.[11] Finally remind the patient that regular aftercare is essential. It is often useful to make your answers to questions more of a tutorial embracing areas, such as lens types and designs, hygiene, and wearing times, thereby increasing information exchange. Suitability may be determined by clinical, social, or financial constraints. Motivation may depend on social, occupational, sports, refractive, visual, or psychological factors.[12] In the case of myopia progression management, a careful consideration of balancing the needs of patient and that of the parents' expectations is required.[13]

5.2.2 Procedure for pre-fitting contact lens case history

1. Observe your patient; their ability to speak and articulate, intellectual capacity, emotional state, cleanliness, length of fingernails, use of eye make-up, size of fingers, roughness of skin, and dexterity.

2. Consider their age and gender. For example, older females are more likely to have poorer tear quality, requiring careful lens material selection and perhaps the use of ocular lubricants.[14] For myopia progression management, the maturity of the wearer and their

ability to wear lenses independently from their parents should be considered.[13]

3. Ask the following questions:

(a) Why do you want to wear contact lenses? What has sparked their interest in contact lenses? Any previous history of contact lens wear should be investigated thoroughly to determine previous lens types worn or trialled, and reasons for discontinuing use. Do not be afraid of refitting a former lens wearer because many contact lens dropouts are owing to poor compliance, or associated with older lens designs and materials, rather than a lack of patient suitability.[15]

(b) What would you like to wear the lenses for? This will range from complete replacement for spectacles to occasional social wear. Some may wish to sleep in lenses for convenience or practical reasons (e.g., travelling abroad, antisocial working hours).[8,11] Most people need lenses that allow for the occasional nap in lenses, for example, on the train home from work.[16] Reportedly, over 60% of single-use soft lens wearers had napped or slept in their lenses.

(c) What do you know about lenses? This is an opportunity to explain the different types of lenses, their pros and cons. Include the cost of the different types of lenses and their maintenance. For those who wear their lenses four or more days a week, monthly, or fortnightly disposable lenses are more cost effective than daily disposable lenses.[17] It is important that the patient understands from the start, the cost of the lenses, fitting and aftercare appointments, along with the importance of regular aftercare, maximising healthy and successful contact lens wear.[8] Outline the risks involved in contact lens wear and that compliance with instructions is important to minimise them.[4] Direct patients to a website that provides unbiased, generic information on contact lenses, such as the *British Contact Lens Association, American Academy of Optometry*, or the *Cornea and Contact Lens Society of Australia* or *Contact Lens Update*.

(d) How do you feel about inserting lenses and touching your eye? Patients may be motivated, but fearful of touching their eye! If the patient is nervous, demonstrate how they can gently touch the lower forniceal conjunctiva with their finger, while they look up and suggest they do this a few times prior to the fitting visit. This will give them confidence. Those who habitually wear cosmetics are not likely to be as nervous.[18]

(e) You do understand that you will need to clean the lenses after each wearing episode, or is convenience a major factor? You will have to outline what is involved in lens care, even for those with a lens-wearing family member. Any reluctance is an indication for the use of single-use daily disposable lenses.

4. Medical and ocular history. If the patient has recently undergone an eye examination in your practice, ask open questions to verify that nothing has changed since. For those who attend for a contact lens fit with a spectacle prescription from elsewhere, a full history routine is required with a modified examination to take account of previous or potential contact lens wear. Questions should cover:

(a) General health, including whether the patient suffers from cold sores that may periodically have an impact on contact lens handling. The medical history may reveal contraindications to contact lens wear, the need for a particular type of lens, or more regular aftercare check-ups (e.g., diabetes). Ask about smoking because it is known to increase the risk of contact lens inflammatory events[19] and is therefore a contraindication to extended wear lenses.

(b) Use of systemic medication particularly long-term treatment, such as steroids, beta-blockers, psychotropic agents (antidepressants), and regular use of over-the-counter pain medication. The main way in which medication can affect contact lens wear is through changes to the tear film and is summarised in the TFOS DEWS II report by Stapleton et al.[20]

(c) Ocular history covers whether the patient has had previous ocular treatment or surgery or contact lens problems in the past. A history of an ocular abnormality requires you to look for the manifestations of the disorder that may have an impact on suitability for contact lenses or direct you towards a particular type of lens (e.g., RGP for an irregular cornea associated with a previous corneal injury). Previous surgery may dictate the lens type to be used (e.g., RGP lenses post corneal refractive surgery). Are they susceptible to hordeolums or chalazion that might be associated with recurrent blepharitis? Is the patient's refraction stable? Are they interested in a better control of their myopia progression? With these last two, the patient should be advised that frequent changes to their contact lenses may be needed, with financial implications depending on the type of lens.

(d) Family history information determines if there are any hereditary ocular and/or medical conditions that may be relevant. A strong family history of myopia can indicate the need to consider lens designs that limit the progression of the patient's myopia.

(e) Information regarding the patient's occupation and hobbies is very useful, particularly when the patient is presbyopic because you need to ensure the lens chosen will give the patient good vision for the required working distances. Patients who spend a lot of time looking at a display screen are more likely to suffer from dryness associated with a reduced blink rate and tear film instability.[21] Ask specifically about water sports because the patient may require the use of full scleral lenses or additional, single-use lenses if they swim regularly, and should be advised regarding the use of goggles over the top.[22] Contact sports also require careful lens selection with single-use soft lenses most commonly providing the best option or no daytime lens wear as is provided by orthokeratology lenses.

(f) Environmental factors include regular exposure to a smoky atmosphere; an environment that is dusty, contains fumes, is of low humidity (associated with heating or air conditioning), or is unhygienic in some other way.

5.2.3 Recording

Both positive and negative patient responses must be recorded. Remember, from a legal viewpoint, if the response was not recorded, effectively the question was not asked. Use standard abbreviations (see Table 2.1) and avoid personal ones. Using the patient's own words recorded in quotation marks can be useful.

Example of a Patient Record

32-year-old Px. Caucasian, teacher.

RFV: Wants CLs for rugby & occ. social use. Girlfriend wears SCL which she cleans daily. Happy to clean lenses. No previous CL wear. Happy c Rx for work. Good DV and NV with Rx. No HA. No other Sxs.

OH: Wears Rx constantly. This Rx 2 years old. Blunt rugby injury to RE 1/12 ago, seen by HES – all clear. No other OH. LEE: 1/12, Mr. Klopp, Emery Opticians, Liverpool. FOH: none.

GH = OK, occ. cold sores, no meds. No allergies. LME: 4 years, Dr. Duggan, Didsbury. FMH: mat grandfather has type II DM.

Hobbies: rugby (no Rx worn), hiking, swimming 1/7. Uses PC ~ 4 /24, 6/7. Driver.

Observations: large fingers, sl. squeamish?

5.2.4 Interpreting the results

Interpretation of the data collected relies on an understanding of why questions are asked and a good knowledge of lens characteristics, such as wettability and lubricity (smoothness).

Selecting the most suitable lens modality, replacement schedule, and lens type depends on:

- The patient's requirements, including lifestyle (i.e., daily vs. extended wear, daily disposable vs. regular replacement)
- The patient's ocular characteristics (i.e., lens design, small vs. large, spherical vs. toric)
- The financial position of the patient (i.e., soft vs. RGPs, daily disposable vs. regular replacement)
- The lenses you have available in your clinic (i.e., 3–4 types of single-use lenses covering a range of materials and prices is useful)
- Purpose of lens correction (i.e., distance vision only vs. presbyopia, control of myopia; consider specific designs)

Interpretation of the case history as shown in the example of a patient record above suggests that the patient wants lenses for occasional use only, specifically for contact sports (rugby), and therefore a single-use lens would be the best option if available in their prescription. This will avoid the issue of lenses sitting in solution for extended periods between wearing episodes. In addition, mud in the eye and lens loss are common in rugby and therefore single-use lenses are preferred for hygiene reasons. Regular swimming is yet another indicator for single-use lenses, and tight-fitting goggles over the top will reduce the risk of complications from swimming in lenses. The patient will need to be advised not to wear their lenses when they are suffering from a cold sore or at least to take extra precautions in terms of hygiene before handling the lenses. This patient may need more time spent with them for insertion/removal training owing to their large fingers and possible squeamishness.

5.2.5 Common errors

1. Not gaining a full understanding of what the patient wants from contact lenses.
2. Not recording all information obtained from the patient.
3. Assuming the same information is still current from the last eye examination.
4. Not applying all the information gathered to the selection of trial lens.
5. Agreeing to undertake a contact lens fit when the patient does not have a valid spectacle prescription (within recall date)

5.3 Determining contact lens diameter

PA height is the vertical distance in millimetres between the upper and lower lid margins at the widest point.

Horizontal visible iris diameter (HVID) is a surrogate measure of actual corneal diameter. HVID aids the selection of lens total diameter for both RGP and soft lenses. PA in relation to lens size determines whether an RGP fit will be interpalpebral or lid attached, and has an influence on the stability of soft toric lenses.[23] Pupil size has an impact on the selection of optical zone diameters for RGP lenses and when considering which presbyopic lens option to select.

5.3.1 The evidence base: corneal diameter, pupil and lid aperture measurement

PA height, HVID, and pupil size can be measured using a corneal topographer (Fig. 5.1), or a contact lens rule (Fig. 5.2). Many topographers allow a measurement of 'white-to-white' or HVID based on an anterior photograph.[24] The measurement can simply be read off the screen, along with the photopic and

mesopic pupil diameters, so it is not described further. Pupil measurements under low illumination can be made easily with a topographer, but are difficult with a contact lens (CL) rule.[25]

Pupillometers, an expensive alternative, can provide pupil measurements at very low light levels, but the accuracy at higher light levels is similar to simple rulers.[25] and they are generally restricted to refractive surgery clinics, where pupil diameter measurements under controlled scotopic conditions are critical.

5.3.2 Contact lens rule measurement procedure

1. Ask the patient to remove any spectacles.
2. Ask the patient to look directly at your dominant eye or an object held just below your eye.
3. **PA height.** Hold the CL rule vertically and align the zero on the millimetre rule with the lower lid margin. Estimate the PA height by reading off the average position of the upper lid with the patient looking in the primary position of gaze.
4. **HVID.** Position the CL rule on the patient's forehead so that the semicircles are facing downwards and the rule bisects the iris. Move the rule horizontally until the semicircle on the rule and the visible semicircle of the iris match to create a continuous circle. It is often easier to judge when the diameter is slightly too large or small and take the HVID value as the reading in between.
5. **Pupil size.** Ask the patient to fixate an unlit distant object. Ensure that you do not get in the way of this fixation.
   (a) **Maximum pupil size.** Best measured with a topographer or pupillometer using the dynamic or low light/mesopic setting (Figs. 5.3 and 5.4). Significant pupil decentration can also be quantified. If a topographer or pupillometer is not available, a Burton lamp on the blue light setting is useful for providing sufficient illumination to view the pupil with less pupil constriction, and the crystalline lens fluoresces under the UV light.[11]
6. **Minimum pupil size.** Additional local lighting directed towards a near reading chart can be used to measure the minimal pupil size at near, which is of interest when considering lens options for a presbyopic patient.

5.3.3 Interpreting the results

The average HVID value is 11.75 mm with a range of 10.8 mm to 13.6mm.[24] The rule of thumb for calculating lens diameters: corneal RGP, total diameter is at least 2 mm smaller than HVID; larger RGP lenses can be as large as the HVID; mini sclerals and soft lenses

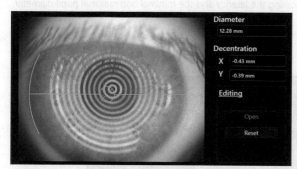

Fig. 5.1 Measurement of the horizontal visible iris diameter (HVID) captured using a topographer.

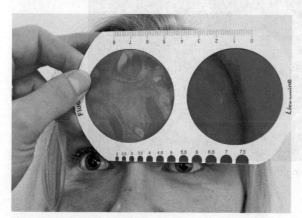

Fig. 5.2 Pupil size measurement with a contact lens rule.

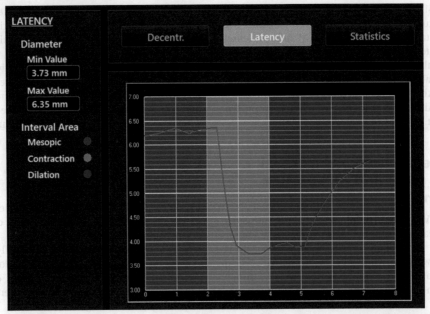

Fig. 5.3. Dynamic pupillometry captured using a topographer, showing the latency and the minimal and maximal pupil diameter as it responds to light.

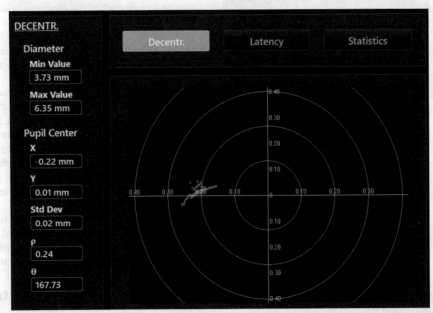

Fig. 5.4. Results of pupil assessment using a topographer, showing the maximal and minimal pupil size along with the position of the pupil centre in relation to the visual axis.

are at least 2 mm greater than HVID. It is also useful to consider the corneal diameter when selecting the first trial lenses for larger lens sizes (RGPs, mini sclerals and soft lenses), because these lens fits are most closely related to the sagittal height of the cornea, which in itself is dependent on a number of factors, including curvature and diameter. Larger corneas generally need a flatter base curve, and smaller corneas, and steeper base curve.[26]

The maximal pupil diameter under low illumination is of interest when selecting an RGP trial lens. To minimise the risk of flare and halos at night, particularly in someone who drives for a living, the back optic zone diameter of the contact lens should be at least 1 mm larger than the maximal pupil diameter, or larger still for a lid-attached lens.[11]

The average PA height is around 9.75 mm, commonly ranging from 9.0 mm to 10.5 mm. The size of the PA influences the fit for corneal RGP lenses. A particularly large PA will result in an interpalpebral fitting corneal RGP lens. A smaller PA means that a larger proportion of the superior cornea is covered by the lid so that lid attachment is likely. The position of the lower lid has an effect on the success of translating multifocal RGP designs.[8] Such lenses require interaction between the lower lid and lens in down gaze, in order to displace the lens upwards so that the near portion lies over the pupil. With a lower lid that is 1 mm higher or lower than the inferior limbus, translating designs are less likely to work. Such designs also require reasonable tension of the lower lid to facilitate translation.[18]

The angle of the lids, both in the stationary position and with a blink, should also be noted because this can influence the rotation of toric soft and front surface toric RGP lenses. An eye with oblique lid alignment or an unusual lid movement on blink is more likely to suffer from rotational instability if fitted with a soft toric lens.[23]

5.3.4 Most common errors

1. When using some corneal topographers, pupil diameters and PA measures may be influenced by the measuring process (i.e., not all devices offer mesopic measurements) and a bright light source results in pupil constriction or the patient may be forcing their PA to be wider for the measurement.
2. When using a CL rule:
   (a) Poor alignment resulting in a parallax error.
   (b) Failing to notice that the patient is narrowing their PA by squinting to see a blurred distant target.
   (c) Positioning yourself between the patient and target so the patient focuses on you, resulting in pupil constriction.

5.4 Corneal topography

Corneal topography is a method of assessing the corneal profile or curvature.

5.4.1 The evidence base: when and how to assess corneal topography

You will measure corneal topography in the initial assessments and monitoring of contact lens, orthokeratology, and refractive surgery patients.[11] Tear film assessment using Placido disc-based topographers is a useful adjunct. Initial assessments will screen for keratoconus, surgically induced irregularity, and other diseases that change corneal shape.[11] Topography also provides baseline data for monitoring purposes and indicates appropriate initial fitting parameters for RGP contact lenses.[11] It is minimally needed in the fitting of soft contact lenses because the fit of a soft lens is more closely related to the sag of the cornea rather than the curvature at its apex, plus the limited range of soft lens radii and diameters means that the use of topographers for the determination of soft lens fit is not necessary. The traditional method to assess corneal topography used to be a keratometer. This is an instrument that projects a symmetrical image onto the corneal apex, using it as a reflective surface and the application of the optical principles of a convex mirror to estimate the radius of curvature at two assumed perpendicular principal meridians. The keratometer is increasingly being replaced in clinical practice by the corneal topographer (or videokeratoscope). To collect more data points from the corneal surface, these instruments project a Placido image (series of concentric rings) onto the cornea (Fig. 5.5) or utilise the Scheimpflug principle. The image is captured by a high-resolution CCD Charge-coupled device camera, and data are processed by a computer. In addition to providing more detailed information, the area covered by these projected rings in the case of the more common Placido disc-based topographers is wider than that of a keratometer, up to 10 mm compared with 3.0 to 3.5 mm. Topographers also calculate nominal primary meridian values for the two principal meridians for RGP lens fitting, negating the need to use a keratometer (Fig. 5.6). Depending on the topographer, other assessments can be made, such as corneal thickness, non-invasive tear break-up time (NIBUT), effect of tear film on aberrations, interblink interval, and meibography (see videos 5.1 and 5.2). Anterior segment optical coherence tomography (OCT) (section 7.11) provides valuable information about the real sagittal height of the cornea, which is more predictive of soft contact lens fits than either keratometry or topography measurements.[27] Knowledge of the profile of the corneo-scleral junction is

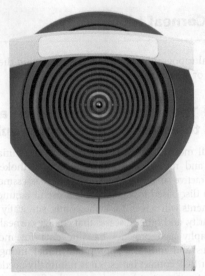

Fig. 5.5 Placido disc rings used by many corneal topographers.

helpful when fitting gas permeable scleral and mini-scleral lenses, which are used for both irregular and regular corneae. OCT is likely to become more widely used in the future, particularly for the rapid assessment of apical clearance in scleral and mini-scleral lens fits (Fig. 5.7).[28]

5.4.2 Procedure with corneal topographers

Although many different makes of corneal topographers exist, the following is a guide that is applicable to most. You should also refer to the user manual for your specific device.

1. Explain the procedure to your patient: "I am going to measure the shape of the front of your eye, the cornea." You may add: ". . . so that I will know the size of contact lens to fit" and so forth.

2. Ask the patient to remove their glasses or contact lenses. If a contact lens wearer keeps their lens in place, then you will measure the topography of the contact lens front surface rather than the cornea.

3. Most topographers hold patient information on their self-contained database, so complete these details before measurements begin.

4. The next prompt screen will have a selection of options: to review existing data or to collect data. Once you have selected *collect new data* the camera will turn on and the Placido rings will illuminate (see Fig. 5.5).

5. Ask the patient to place their chin on the chin rest once the rings have illuminated to avoid unnecessary photophobia; the patient will have already adjusted to the light level. Alignment is automatic for some devices, but if not, follow the on-screen instructions to align the camera. The fine focusing to align the alignment targets will allow you to capture the image, either manually

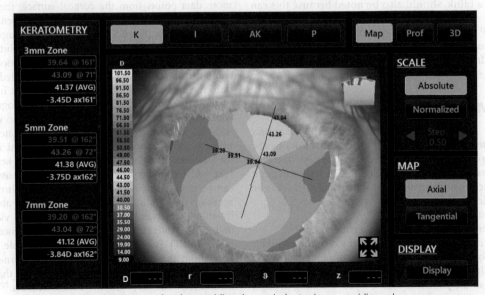

Fig. 5.6 Topography plot providing the equivalent primary meridian values.

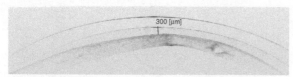

Fig. 5.7 Anterior segment optical coherence tomography (OCT) image showing 300 μm apical clearance of a scleral contact lens fitted to a keratoconic cornea treated with Intacs.

(pressing the button) or automatically. Before the image is captured, ask the patient to blink a few times and then hold. Some instruments have a chin rest that encourages a slight head turn, which helps remove the nose shadow from the captured images.

6. Switch eyes: again this may be automatic or manual. Usually the instrument moves rather than the patient. Align and focus the targets and capture the image of the second eye.

7. The patient can now rest their head back while you confirm the captured images are acceptable and the instrument processes the data and generates the colour maps.

5.4.3 Procedure for one-position keratometer

1. Ideally, before the start of the clinic, focus the instrument eyepiece by observing a distant object (e.g., the room wall). First turn the eyepiece anticlockwise as far as it will go and then back clockwise until the black cross hair just comes into sharp focus.

2. Seat the patient comfortably at the keratometer and ask the patient to remove any spectacles or lenses. Dim the room lighting.

3. Explain the procedure to the patient as with the corneal topography procedure.

4. Adjust the height of the patient's chair and the keratometer to a comfortable position. Ask the patient to place their chin on the chin rest and forehead against the headrest. Occlude the eye not under test by swinging the keratometer's occluder into place. Adjust the chin rest so that the outer canthus aligns with the headrest marker.

5. Ask the patient to look at the reflection of their own eye in the centre of the keratometer and to open the eye wide after a full blink. If a high refractive error prevents the patient seeing their own eye, then ask the patient to look down the centre of the keratometer. Make vertical adjustments of the keratometer if the patient is unable to see into the centre, or shine a pentorch through the observation eyepiece on to the patient's face and adjust the keratometer's height until the light shines on the patient's eye.

6. Align the keratometer so that the lower right mire image is centred on the crosshairs and lock it into place.

7. Adjust the focusing of the keratometer by turning the focusing knob until the mires are clear and the lower right mire is no longer doubled. Keeping one hand on the focusing knob, constantly adjust it to exclude doubling of the lower right mire.

8. Measure the principal meridian that is closest to the horizontal first. Rotate the instrument so that the plus signs are set 'in step' (Fig. 5.8b) and the minus signs are parallel. This ensures that the instrument is aligned precisely on a principal meridian. This is easier to judge when the mires are adjusted to be relatively close to the endpoint. Continue adjusting the focusing knob to ensure a single, clear plus sign. Note that you will need to adjust the keratometer's position constantly to maintain image focus, so keratometric measurements are always a two-handed operation. Note the radius of curvature (or dioptric power) and orientation of this meridian.

9. Measure the second principal meridian, which is theoretically 90° to the primary meridian. Adjust the focusing knob to give the best focus for the minus signs and then adjust the vertical alignment wheel until the minus signs are superimposed (see Fig. 5.8). Note the radius of curvature (or dioptric power) and orientation of this meridian. On a toric cornea, the plus signs will be out of focus and not superimposed, but this does not matter as you have completed your measurement of the first principal meridian.

10. Repeat the measurements on the other eye.

5.4.4 Procedure for two position variable doubling type keratometer

1. Set up the patient and the instrument as described in steps 1 through 8 above.

2. Move the telescope forward by adjusting the focusing knob or joystick appropriately. You may need to make minor adjustments both horizontally and vertically to centre the mire images and achieve a view as depicted in Fig. 5.9. If the blocks and staircase are in step (see Fig. 5.9a), then the orientation of the instrument arc is aligned to one of the two principal meridians and you can now proceed to step 4.

3. If the mires you see are similar to those in Fig. 5.9c where the blocks and staircase are out of step, then the angle of the instrument arc is not aligned along a principal meridian. Rotate slowly until the staircase and block mires are aligned as in Fig. 5.9d. This is easier to judge when the mires are relatively close together.

4. Ask the patient to blink and then keep their eyes as wide open as possible. Turn the knurled knob until the

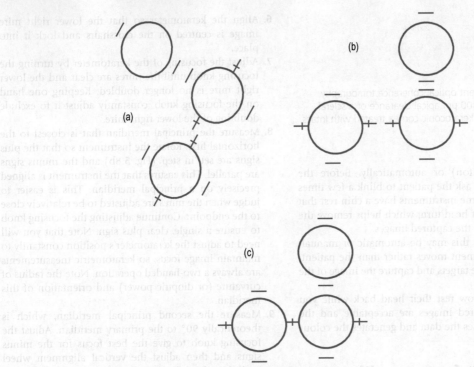

Fig. 5.8 Alignment of the mires on a Bausch and Lomb keratometer. **(a)** The view when the mires are off the principal meridians. **(b)** The view when the mires are on the principal meridians. **(c)** The view when the plus and minus signs are overlapping to measure the 'horizontal' and 'vertical' radii of curvature/equivalent power.

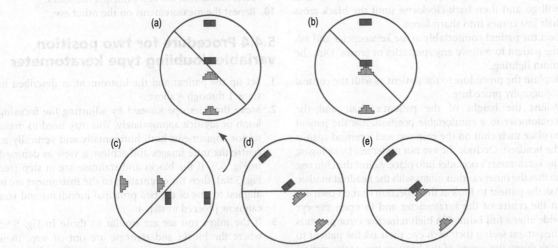

Fig. 5.9 The mire images as seen on a Javal-Schiotz keratometer. **(a)** Aligned mire images along the horizontal. **(b)** Mires from 'a' touching with no overlap. **(c)** Non-aligned mire images. **(d)** Mire images from 'c' brought into alignment along an oblique meridian. **(e)** Mires from 'd' touching with no overlap.

staircase and block mires are just touching. You must simultaneously adjust the instrument position with your other hand to maintain focus of the mire images. If you turn the knob too much and the mires overlap, a yellow/white area of overlap will be seen. Adjust the position of the mires until they are just touching with no overlap. If the hair wire does not pass through the middle of the touching mires, make final horizontal and vertical adjustments to achieve this.

5. Record the angle of the arc from the degree scale of the instrument and the corneal curvature along this meridian from the millimetre scale.

6. Rotate through 90° and make adjustments as in steps 4 and 5 to achieve a picture similar to those in Figs. 5.9b and 5.9e. Record angle and curvature values for this second meridian.

5.4.5 Recording

Increasingly practice management software will link with your corneal topographer and transfer the results to the patient records. Many topographers display the corneal curvature data in a variety of ways:

a. **Absolute colour map.** The colour codes on the map represent fixed values relating to specific radii of curvature. Typically, steep areas of the cornea are shown as red, average areas as yellow through to green, and flatter areas as blue. The colour scale covers the whole range of curvature values for the instrument's normative dataset (Fig. 5.10). Fixed values allow comparison of corneal curvatures between eyes or between visits, and give an idea of how steep or flat a patient's cornea is in comparison to the population. The disadvantage is that the intervals are large, so the map may lack sensitivity to small differences in curvature.

b. **Relative or normalized colour map.** The colour codes are distributed across the range of curvature values for that specific eye measurement. This reduces the step interval so that colour maps have increased sensitivity and provide more detail on shape variations for that individual cornea (Fig. 5.11). Be cautious when comparing relative colour maps between eyes or between visits, because the same colour will not necessarily represent the same curvature value. A relative colour map may show an area of curvature as red, because it is the steepest part of that cornea, but the absolute colour map may show the same area as green or blue, because in comparison to the normative dataset, that area is relatively flat.

c. **Difference colour maps.** These compare two measurements (absolute maps) and allow a visualisation of the difference, which is helpful to observe change over time (i.e., the impact of wearing orthokeratology lenses or the progression of keratoconus).

d. **Indices of symmetry.** Different topographers have different names for indices that quantify the coefficient of variability of a cornea (e.g., Regularity Index or Keratoconus Indices). They quantify measures such as how symmetrical a cornea is, the curvature of the steepest

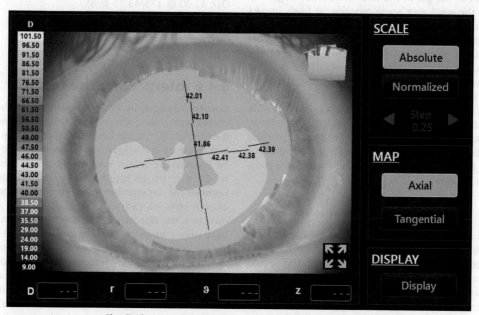

Fig. 5.10 A topography plot using the absolute colour map.

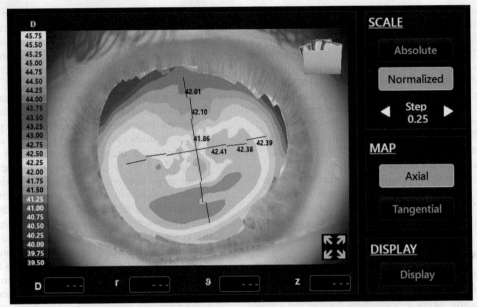

Fig. 5.11 A topography plot using the relative or normalized colour map.

point, and how quickly the curvature changes away from that steep point—all early indicators for the development of conditions such as keratoconus.

e. **Quality of vision indices.** Most topographers assess the position of the pupil, the level of corneal irregularity within the pupil area; some quantify the likely impact of corneal shape on the patient's vision. Often this is expressed in terms of the level of higher order aberrations relating to the anterior surface of the cornea, the principal refracting surface of the eye. This helps you decide how likely it is that a patient's reduced vision is caused by corneal irregularity (Fig. 5.12).

Both topography and traditional keratometry provide keratometry measurements for the principal meridians, usually over a similar area around the centre of the cornea. The results can be recorded with the radius of curvature of the most horizontal meridian first followed by the most vertical as follows:

R 7.75 @ 175/7.60 @ 85
L 7.70 @ 180/7.60 @ 90

The @ nomenclature can be replaced by 'along' or 'al.' The millimetres and degree sign (^{0}) need not be used. With a keratometer, if the mires are distorted, this should also be recorded.

Alternatively, the results can be recorded in dioptres (equivalent power), in which case the amount of corneal astigmatism is usually calculated and recorded. It can be useful to consider the amount of corneal astigmatism in relation to the spectacle astigmatism, when deciding whether a spherical RGP lens can be used to correct astigmatism.

OD: 42.00 @ 175/43.75 @ 85,
   total corneal astigmatism −1.75 × 175
OS: 43.50 @ 180/44.25 @ 90,
   total corneal astigmatism −0.75 × 180

5.4.6 Interpreting the results

Corneal topography has the advantage of showing the corneal curvature over a wide range of locations, making it easier to differentiate between symmetrical astigmatism and asymmetrical astigmatism. This can be easily observed by viewing the colour map. Astigmatism is represented on the map by the appearance of a bow-tie pattern. For symmetrical astigmatism, this bow-tie pattern is seen as even bows on each side (Fig. 5.13). As the asymmetry increases, the disparity in the size of the bows increases. Increasing asymmetry in the pattern could be an indicator for correcting the astigmatism with soft toric lenses or larger diameter RGP lenses, rather than corneal RGP lenses which may decentre owing to the profile asymmetry (Fig. 5.14). An exaggerated asymmetrical bow-tie pattern is indicative of early keratoconus, particularly if the apex is decentred inferior nasal. However, keratoconus

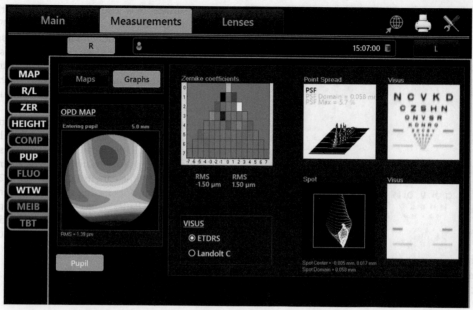

Fig. 5.12 The quality of vision indices calculated from the topography map.

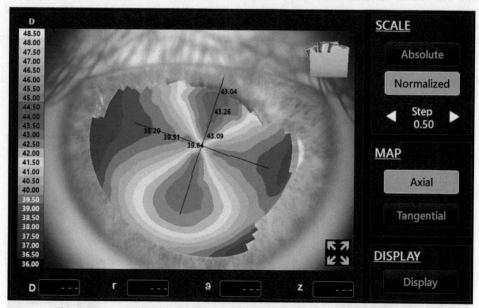

Fig. 5.13 A sagittal or axial curve plot of the front surface of an astigmatic cornea.

can produce a range of different topographical patterns (Fig. 5.15). Large changes in the degree of astigmatism within a short time can be indicative of keratoconus, lid neoplasms, pterygium, or a chalazion.

Large changes in spectacle astigmatism without corneal astigmatic changes in the elderly are likely caused by a cortical cataract. Corneal curvature measurements can also be used to help indicate whether ametropia is refractive or axial. For example, a patient with increasing myopia but no change in corneal curvature probably has axial myopia. An anisometrope with different curvature readings probably has refractive anisometropia, whereas an

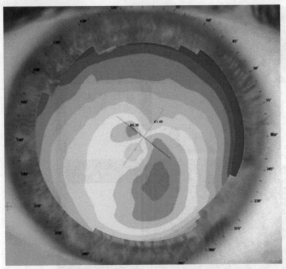

Fig. 5.14 A sagittal curve plot of the front surface of an asymmetric astigmatic cornea.

anisometrope with similar curvature readings probably has axial anisometropia.

Keratometer readings: The power of the anterior corneal surface (Fc) is estimated from the radii measurements (r) using the equation Fc = (n-1)/r. The refractive index (n) of the cornea is about 1.376, but most instruments use a value for n of 1.3375. The lower value for n is intended to compensate for the negative power of the posterior

corneal surface. It is assumed that the posterior surface reduces the overall corneal power by about 10%, but this amount varies among individuals. This also assumes that the two surfaces have the same proportion of astigmatism. Other factors that lead to errors in keratometry readings include the assumption that the cornea is spherical (most are elliptical) and that the visual axis runs through the corneal apex, which it usually does not.

Small radius values mean a steep corneal surface, which is more powerful and more myopic (or less hyperopic). Larger radii mean flatter surfaces, which are less powerful and more hyperopic (or less myopic). The anterior radii of curvature of the cornea are usually between 7.25 mm and 8.50 mm, with myopes having steeper (smaller) radii and hyperopes having flatter (larger) radii. Dioptric powers generally range between 46.50 D and 40.00 D, and the anticipated corneal astigmatism is usually less than 2.00 D.

5.4.7 Most Common Errors

Corneal topography

1. Poor centration: not aligning the visual axis with the instrument's camera which also displaces the Placido ring image (less of an issue with automated and semi-automated devices).
2. Poor focusing of the corneal reflection resulting in blurred ring edges.
3. Not ensuring that the patient keeps their eyes wide apart, resulting in part of the Placido ring image being obscured by the shadow from the lids.

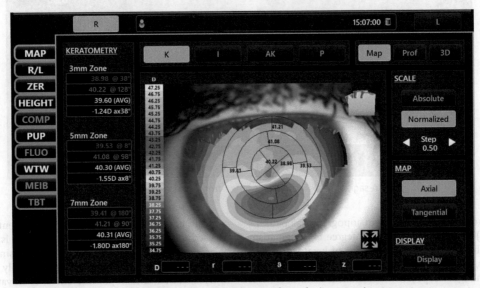

Fig. 5.15 A topography plot of the front surface of a keratoconic cornea.

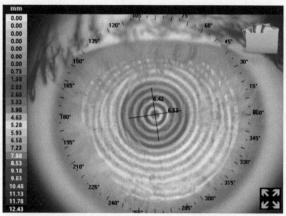

Fig. 5.16 Missing data points from the Placido disc topography image as a result of a poor tear film quality.

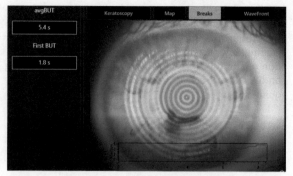

Fig. 5.17 Image of tear film NIBUT.

4. Not checking quality of the Placido disc image. Data can be missing owing either to tear break-up in patients with dry eye (solved by instilling drops) or to poor instructions to the patient (Fig. 5.16)
5. Taking measures with the room lights on is likely to increase these errors and the time taken to take the measures, which results in a smaller pupil measurement.

Keratometry

1. Failing to maintain mire image focus when attempting superimposition of the mire image.
2. Not ensuring the patient keeps their head against the headrest.
3. Forgetting to focus the eyepieces.
4. Not centering the mire images.
5. Forgetting to calibrate the instrument regularly.

5.5 Assessment of ocular physiology

An assessment of the health of the anterior portion of the eye and adnexa is necessary to identify issues that potentially preclude or limit contact lens wear or indicate the need for a particular type of contact lens. The assessment also allows the recording of baseline data so that changes over time, contact lens induced or otherwise, can be monitored.

5.5.1 The evidence base: preliminary tear film assessment

The tear film and the way it interacts with the lens surface is very important in successful contact lens wear. Contact lenses have been reported as one of the modifiable factors that lead to symptoms of dry eye.[20] A large proportion of contact lens wearers cite discomfort and symptoms of dryness as reasons for reducing their wearing time or ceasing lens wear.[29,30] The tests shown to best predict contact lens-induced dry eye in new wearers are symptoms such as late-in-the-day dryness. These symptoms can be reliably quantified using questionnaires.[31-33] The signs useful as predictors are NIBUT (Fig. 5.17) and surface staining.[33] A thorough assessment of the tear film and its impact on the ocular surface allows the practitioner to select a more suitable lens material, such as one with low water content (to limit dehydration) and high lubricity (to minimise friction). It also allows better management of the patient's expectations.

5.5.2 Procedure for preliminary slit lamp and tear film assessment

For a detailed description of slit lamp examination and tear film assessment, see sections 7.1 and 7.2. These sections describe the procedures for assessing the tear film, which are generally undertaken as an additional component in the slit lamp biomicroscopy and/or topography examination.

5.5.3 Recording

See recording sections for slit lamp biomicroscopy (7.1.4) and tear film (7.2.10). It is useful to record and grade everything seen to provide baseline information. For example, grade 1 papillae on the lateral margins of the superior lid (video 5.3) would not be considered abnormal, but it is invaluable to note this prior to contact lens fitting. A number of grading scales are available, but the most commonly used scales are from the Brien Holden Vision Institute (http://www.contactlensupdate.com/wp-content/uploads/2011/05/Grading_Scales_web.pdf) and the Efron grading scales,[34] which are standardised images of common complications at different levels of severity. Try to stick to just one grading scale, as this will improve your grading accuracy and repeatability over time. The detection of clinical differences can be improved by recording findings in 0.1 steps[35] because these scales are generally quite coarse.[34]

5.6 Soft contact lens fitting

5.6.1 Soft lens application

Patients may be anxious about lenses being applied to their eyes for the first time and you need to try to put the patient at ease (section 2.1). Patients need to be comfortable and feel part of the process, which must involve an appropriate informed consent process, where explaining what you do at each stage and answering any questions they may have is key.[18]

1. Wash your hands thoroughly as per the World Health Organization guidelines (WHO) (http://www.who.int/gpsc/clean_hands_protection/en/): rubbing both sides of the hands, in between the fingers and the fingertips. Rinse thoroughly and dry with a lint-free towel.
2. Check the lens specification on the container and the expiry date.
3. Remove the lens from the container, place on your index finger (finger next to the thumb) tip and check whether the lens is inside out or the correct way round by:
   (a) Checking the lens profile, which should be slightly bowl-shaped (Fig. 5.18a) rather than saucer-shaped (Fig. 5.18b).
   (b) Gently nipping the lens should result in the edges curving inwards rather than outwards (Fig. 5.18c).
   (c) Using the crease test, which involves placing the lens in the palm of your hand along the main crease, cupping the hand slightly so that the lens is partially folded and looking to see if the edges roll inwards (correct) or outwards (incorrect). There is an alternate inversion test where by the lens is pinched between thumb and index finger (see videos 5.4 and 5.5).
   (d) Some lenses have inversion indicator engravings. Make sure you know from which side of the lens the engraving should be correctly viewed.
   (e) If incorrect, simply pick up the lens and turn it over, repositioning it on your fingertip.
4. Check for debris or defects. Any debris should be rinsed off with saline or multipurpose solution. Dispose of defective lenses.
5. Make sure you have your three key fingers reasonably dry; the index finger where the lens is resting, the

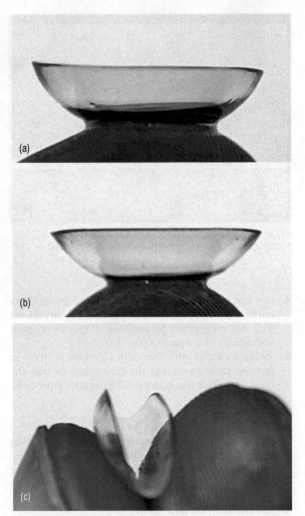

Fig. 5.18 Profiles of contact lenses **(a)** the correct way round (bowl shaped); **(b)** inside out (saucer shaped); and **(c)** edges curving inwards when gently pinched.

middle finger of the same hand, and the index finger (or thumb) of the other hand. These two 'extra' fingers will hold the eyelids apart during the application of the lens. If the lens or finger is too wet, there will be too much contact between the two and it will not be easy to apply the lens. Too little contact, usually as a result of lens dehydration, may result in the lens falling off the finger during application.[11]

6. Stand slightly to the side of the patient on the side where you are going to apply the lens first. This may necessitate rotating the patient's chair away from you. The following instructions assume that the practitioner will apply the right lens first using their right hand.

7. Ask the patient to rest their head against the headrest of the chair, turning their head slightly away from you for the right eye application to make the process easier.

8. Explain that you are going to gently hold the lids apart and place the lens on the eye. Make it clear that once the lens is on, the patient will hardly feel it.

9. Ask the patient to look down and use the thumb (or index finger) of your left hand to lift their superior eyelid from just behind the lashes. Hold it firmly against the brow bone; do not push into the orbital cavity.

10. Ask the patient to look straight ahead and use the middle finger of your right hand to pull the lower lid down from just behind the lashes.

11. Gently place the lens on the eye in one of the following ways[11]:
   (a) Directly on the cornea whilst the patient looks straight ahead
   (b) On the inferior conjunctiva whilst the patient looks up
   (c) On the temporal conjunctiva whilst the patient looks nasally
   The preferred procedure is usually determined by practitioner preference influenced by the patient's compliance.

12. The lens will often have a bubble of air underneath it when first applied, particularly if the lens has been placed on the conjunctiva, which is flatter than the cornea. Keep your finger in position initially and ensure that the lens has adhered to the surface of the eye rather than sticking to your finger. A very gentle massaging motion will help this. Slowly withdraw your finger, asking the patient to gradually look straight ahead to centre the lens.

13. Release the lower lid then ask the patient to look down before slowly releasing the top lid to cover the lens.

14. The patient should now be encouraged to make slow, gentle blinking movements whilst looking down.

15. Repeat for the left eye, standing on the other side of the patient and using your left hand to apply the lens.

16. These instructions assume that the practitioner is able to use both their dominant and non-dominant hand for lens application and will therefore use their right hand for the right eye, and left hand for the left eye. If this is not the case, the practitioner will have to use their dominant hand for one eye and reach over the patient, taking care not to touch the patient's nose, in order to apply the lens to the other eye.

The different insertion techniques are shown in the online videos (see videos 5.6 and 5.7).

5.6.2 Problem solving

1. If lens application produces a sensation of grittiness or discomfort, ask the patient to look up, displace the lens down and/or temporal with your index finger and allow it to recentre. If the grittiness persists, remove the lens, check for debris and defects, rinse and reapply or replace as appropriate (see video 5.8).

2. If lens application results in a stinging sensation and watering of the eye, remove the lens, rinse with saline, and reapply. Profuse watering on lens application can be indicative of something on the lens, such as soap from handwashing, or a difference in tonicity or pH of the patient's tears and the solution on the lens. Significant lacrimation tends to give an apparently tight-fitting lens on assessment; the hypertonic tears cause the lens to adhere to the surface of the eye, especially lenses of ionic material.[18]

3. If a patient is very motivated to wear contact lenses, but is very unsure about someone else placing a lens on their eye, teach them to apply and remove the lenses themselves during the fitting appointment.[11]

5.6.3 Removal procedure

1. Wash your hands thoroughly as per the WHO guidelines.

2. Position yourself and the patient as for lens application (section 5.6.1).

3. Explain that you are going to gently hold the lids and slide the lens off the eye.

4. Ask the patient to look down and use the thumb (or index finger) of your left hand to lift their superior eyelid from just behind the lashes and hold it firmly against the brow bone. Do not press into the orbital cavity.

5. Ask the patient to look up and nasal and use the middle finger of your right hand to pull the lower lid down from just behind the lashes.

6. Gently place the index finger of your right hand on the lens, slide it firmly down and temporal until it is completely clear of the cornea.

7. Bring your right thumb in and pinch the lens between thumb and index finger.

8. Release the lids.

9. Repeat for the left eye, standing on the other side of the patient and using your left hand to displace the lens and pinch it off.
(See video 5.9)

5.6.4 Most common errors
Preparation

1. Having fingernails that are too long and/or dirty.

2. Not thoroughly drying the hands, leading to a risk of infection.

3. Approaching the eye from the front rather than the side, resulting in less contact between fingers and lids and therefore poorer lid control.

4. Not holding the lids firmly enough or too far from the lid margin, therefore allowing the patient to blink during the application process (see video 5.7).
5. Holding the lids right at the base of the lashes, or in front of the lashes, causing discomfort to the patient and increasing the risk of touching the cornea and/or conjunctiva.
6. Not ensuring that both your fingers and the patient's lids are dry before trying to handle them. The patient's eye may water during the procedure and the lids may need to be dried with a tissue before reattempting application.
7. Not positioning the lens on the very tip of the finger. This is particularly important for practitioners with large fingers.
8. Lens too wet so that surface tension draws it to the finger rather than the ocular surface.

Lens application

1. Allowing the patient to blink while there is still a large bubble under the lens. The lens is likely to be squeezed out of the eye.
2. Not instructing the patient to blink slowly and gently once the lens has been applied. A hard, quick blink is more likely to squeeze the lens out of the eye if it is not completely in apposition with the cornea.

Lens removal

1. Pinching the lens off the eye whilst it is still on the cornea, risking damage to the cornea.
2. Putting insufficient pressure on the lens whilst sliding it off the cornea, resulting in little or no movement.

5.7 Selecting a soft trial lens

Having discussed with your patient the option of contact lenses to correct their vision and answered any questions they may have (informed consent process), select a lens that you think is suitable for the patient.[18] Deciding which lens is best requires consideration of lens options and parameters in the following order:

1. Lens replacement frequency: The majority of soft lenses are disposable and replaced either daily, twice weekly, or monthly. Deciding the replacement frequency starts the process of restricting your choice of lens design and material.
2. Lens material: Owing to their increased oxygen transmissibility silicone hydrogel lenses are now the preferred option, except for occasional wear. When a silicone hydrogel lens material is not selected, this is

usually because a parameter needed to fit that patient is not available. It may be that the best option is a daily disposable lens and a parameter is only available in a hydrogel material.
3. Lens power: This will be based on the patient's refraction. The back-vertex distance (BVD) needs to be considered for moderate to high ametropes ($> \pm 4.00$ D). This is determined by the equation ocular refraction $= F/(1-dF)$, where F is the spectacle refraction at a vertex distance of d (in metres; i.e., a vertex distance of 12 mm, means that d = 0.012). An approximate vertex distance factor can be added to the spectacle refraction as follows: For ± 4.00 to 5.75 add $+0.25$; ± 6.00 to 7.75 add $+0.50$; for ± 8.00 to 9.75 add $+0.75$. Myopic prescriptions therefore become less myopic and hyperopic prescriptions become more hyperopic.
4. For soft lens fitting to a patient with astigmatism, the power of the trial lens should be the mean spherical correction (i.e., sphere + half the cylinder). For example: spectacle prescription $= -2.00/-0.50 \times 180$; the power of trial lens should be $-2.00 + (-0.50/2) = -2.25$ DS. For levels of astigmatism of 0.75 D or more, consider a soft toric lens design.
5. Base curve: Despite keratometry results traditionally being used as a guide to lens base curve selection, keratometry has now been shown to have limited value for lens selection.[36] In addition, most soft lenses are available only with one or two base curves. For soft lens fitting, keratometry is therefore only really useful to establish normality, as the lens with the flattest base curve is trialled first. You should change to the steeper base curve only if the lens fit was not acceptable or if the patient complains of lens awareness.
6. Total diameter: The lens edge must always rest on the conjunctiva beyond the limbus. Lens edges that align with the limbus will result in complications, reduced wearing times, and discomfort. This parameter is theoretically determined by measuring the horizontal visible iris diameter, although lenses are rarely available in more than one diameter. If the lens you have selected is too small you are likely to have to select another lens brand. Lenses that are too large may simply be too hard to remove.[11]
7. Having selected the best lenses, place them on the patient's eyes. The different insertion techniques are shown in the online videos (see videos 5.6 and 5.7).

5.8 Assessment of the soft lens fit

Lens assessment has two phases, an initial brief phase followed by a later, detailed assessment (see videos 5.10 through 5.16).

5.8.1 Initial brief assessment of lens fit

1. Initial gross observation: The first assessment is observational. Soft lenses are comfortable devices, even to the naïve wearer. If the patient has comfort issues, follow the problem-solving procedure in section 5.6.2.
2. Initial patient assessment: Ask how the patient feels and if they can see, anticipating a positive response.
3. Closer inspection: The next step is to assess the fit, either with the naked eye or the slit lamp. The basic need is to make sure the lenses are in the correct position, not decentred, and that this continues between blinks.
4. First vision assessment: Lens centration can also be confirmed by assessing the patient's visual acuity.

At this point the lens has probably not settled sufficiently to make an accurate assessment and it is often preferable to send the patient out of the consulting room to let them try the lens. If a risk assessment determines that the patient is wearing a well-centred lens with acceptable acuity, say 6/9 (20/30, 0.66) or better, then send the patient out for a walk. If the vision or fit is questionable, let the patient have a seat in the waiting room. The settling period should be at least 10 minutes,[37] but may be longer if it fits better with your appointment schedule and the patient.

5.8.2 Detailed assessment of lens fit

As part of the detailed assessment you will need to carefully measure the vision and assess how the lens is fitting. As both of these are interlinked, the order will be determined on how the patient is doing (see videos 5.10 through 5.16).

1. Ask the patient how the lenses feel and how their vision is.
   (a) If patient's response to both is positive, then assess the vision first followed by an assessment of fit.
   (b) If the patient is uncomfortable, assess the fit first and then the vision.
   (c) If the patient complains that the vision has deteriorated, this could be owing to an adjustment needed to the lens power or to the fit and the order of assessment is your choice. Degraded vision may also indicate a poor wetting surface. Poor wettability can be assessed using a topographer, Placido ring image, or slit lamp. Alternatively, a retinoscope gives a quick impression over the pupil region, with shadows developing between blinks.
2. Gross assessment of lens fit: While the patient is sitting in the chair, observe the lens on the eye without magnification. You want to make sure the lens is still correctly centred and see if you can observe lens movement on a natural blink. Next, using your index

finger, push the lower lid over the lens edge while the patient looks straight ahead, again observing to see if you can see lens movement.
3. Slit lamp assessment of lens fit: The slit lamp should be set up for direct illumination with low magnification ($\times 10$):
   (a) With the patient looking straight ahead, observe how the lens moves during two to three blinks, which should take only 15 to 20 seconds. Sweep the observation microscope across the lens to observe movement temporally and nasally. You should also observe the lens size in relation to the HVID. Look for good, even coverage of the cornea and limbus.
   (b) Post blink movement: Ask the patient to look slightly up so you can see the inferior edge of the lens. Observe lens movement in this position with continued blinking because this is a good determination of overall lens movement.[38]
   (c) The push up: Place your thumb or index finger against the lower lid and use it to displace the lens, again observing the lens movement. It should displace easily and return to its former position in a smooth and rapid manner.[38] This is the single most valuable assessment of the fit of a soft lens.[39] (see video 5.17).
   (d) With the eye back in the primary position ask the patient to look left and right, again observing the lens movement.
   (e) During all of these assessments, the lens should demonstrate movement over the surface of the eye and the lens edge should not encroach the limbus. The patient's blinks should appear natural and not as if they are experiencing discomfort.
4. Assess lens movement: Most slit lamps allow you to generate a very small circular spot of light that is 1.0 mm in diameter. You can use this spot of light as an indicator of size when you are making observations through your slit lamp using moderate magnification ($\times 16$ to $\times 20$). While the patient is either in the primary position of gaze or looking up, place the edge of the spot on the outer edge of the limbus or the inner edge of the lens and ask your patient to blink and observe the lens movement, estimate the amount of movement in relation to the size of the spot of light and record it in millimetres. You should expect to record movement of no more than half of the spot's diameter (i.e., 0.5 mm) (see video 5.18).
5. Assess lens centration: While the patient is in the primary position of gaze, observe the lens with low magnification ($\times 10$ or less) while using a diffuse light source. This will allow you to gauge the lens position in reference to the centre of the pupil or the HVID. Record whether the lens is centred or has decentred and the direction of that decentration (i.e., superior, nasal,

inferior, temporal). The grading system could simply record centration as ideal (0), good (+1), acceptable (+2), or poor (+3), with all except ideal having a direction indicator (e.g., +1T is good with temporal decentration).

5.8.3 The ideal lens fit

In the primary position the lens should be well centred with an even lip of lens extending beyond the limbus. The centration is graded with reference to the centre of the pupil (or the HVID). A grade of +3 (poor) is not acceptable; this is only likely to be seen during an unsuccessful initial lens trial. A natural blink should induce movement that is observable but does not move the lens edge to encroach on the limbus. If a lens moves excessively where the edge abuts the limbus, a tighter lens is needed. If no movement is observable but the lens moves easily during the push-up test, then the fit is acceptable. When a lens does not move during the push-up test, then it is considered too tight and needs to be replaced with a looser fitting lens.

5.8.4 The extended trial

If the lens is well centred, shows good movement, and the patient is comfortable, you have a lens that can be used for an extended trial. This should be over at least a couple of days, so would require the patient to have been taught how to handle and care for the lenses. The length of the extended trial should fit in with your appointment schedule as well as be convenient for the patient and therefore varies from 3 days to 2 weeks. When the patient returns, treat the visit as the first aftercare visit. As the lens will have demonstrated good vision and good fitting before being dispensed, the likely issues will relate to adaptation, lens handling, and care.

5.8.5 Solving lens fitting problems

1. Too tight, loose, or decentred: A tight lens shows no movement with the push-up test. A loose lens can be seen to move in the absence of a provocative test, such as the push-up test, and/or it decentres on upward gaze alone or it does not smoothly recentre. Generally tight lenses start with good initial comfort that degrades markedly during wear, whereas a loose lens has significant initial discomfort that may (or may not) improve with wear. A lens with excessive decentration encroaches the limbus with the lens edge. Lens centration is usually assessed in the primary position of gaze, but excessive decentration on upward gaze should also be a cause for concern and indicate that a change in fit is needed. You can alter the fit by:
   (a) Changing the base curve—flatter if the fit is steep and steeper if too flat or decentred

   (b) Changing the lens diameter—smaller if too steep and larger if too flat or decentred
   (c) Altering the lens thickness—thicker if too steep and thinner if too flat or decentred
   (d) Switch to a silicone hydrogel material if your initial hydrogel lens was too flat, and to a hydrogel lens if the initial silicone hydrogel lens was too steep or decentred.

   In order for you to make any of the above changes, you generally have to change brand, because most lenses are only available in one or two different base curves with no option to change lens diameter or thickness.
2. Difficulty with lens removal: If the patient is having difficulty removing the lenses despite good technique and short finger nails, either flatten the lens fit and/or reduce the lens diameter. Also consider the lens material.
3. Too small: If the lens is encroaching the limbus, you should reduce the lens sagittal height by either increasing the lens diameter or flattening the base curve.
4. Variable vision following a blink: You should anticipate the appearance of non-wetting areas (Fig. 5.19) observable with a slit lamp or topographer. The greatest challenge to manufacturers of silicone hydrogel lenses is to fabricate the surface of the lens and ensure good wettability. Any defects usually present as non-wetting areas will have an impact on vision and comfort. Also consider that excessively steep or flat fits also result in variable vision with the blink (see section 5.8.6).

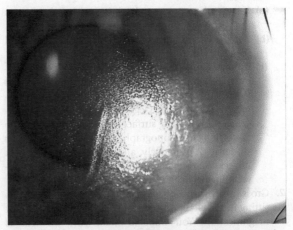

Fig. 5.19 The non-wetting surface of a silicone hydrogel soft contact lens. (Courtesy of CORE, University of Waterloo.)

5.8.6 Over-refraction, VA, and ocular motor balance

1. Over-refraction (See video 4.14): In the majority of cases the trial contact lens power is selected to be as close as possible to the spectacle prescription leaving a small over-refraction if any. In a patient with good binocularity, this allows a quick binocular over-refraction (section 4.11). Refraction is generally restricted to spheres only because patients with small degrees of astigmatism (< 0.50 DC) in their spectacles are likely to be fitted with spherical soft contact lenses (leaving their astigmatism uncorrected) or spherical RGP lenses (correcting corneal astigmatism using the tear lens behind the contact lens). Measurement of astigmatism should be undertaken only if the visual acuity does not reach the expected level.

2. Visual acuity (See videos 3.1 and 3.2): With the over-refraction (OR) in place, distance and near VA should be assessed (sections 3.1 and 3.2). Also record the stability of VA after a blink. Vision that blurs immediately after a blink and then clears suggests that the lens is loose; the blink causes lens movement. Vision that clears briefly immediately following a blink suggests the lens is tight or drying out; the blink flattens the lens against the cornea for a moment or there are areas of non-wetting on the lens surface. Visual instability is less obvious for hydrogel soft lenses even when the fit is very poor, because the lenses are so thin and flexible.

3. Muscle balance (See videos 6.1 through 6.10): The ocular muscle balance should be checked for comparison with the preliminary measurement, particularly in patients known to have a heterophoria at distance and/or near. Control of a heterophoria may differ between spectacles and contact lenses (section 6.2). A cover test at distance and near is usually sufficient. Higher myopes may complain of asthenopia during the adaptation phase owing to a transitory associated exophoria.

4. Recording example:

RE: CL −3.00 DS   OR +0.25DS   1.2 VAR, stable c blink
LE: CL −3.00DS   OR +0.50DS   1.2 VAR, stable c blink
Lens powers to be ordered: R) −2.75 DS, L) −2.50 DS

5.8.7. Post-fitting health check

See videos 5.19 through 5.21.

Having removed the trial lenses, the final act before writing the lens order is to check the eyes for unwanted side effects of contact lens wear. This involves a slit lamp biomicroscope examination of the cornea and conjunctiva, looking for fluorescein and lissamine green staining (section 7.2.1). The findings should be recorded in a diagram and graded using the Cornea and Contact Lens

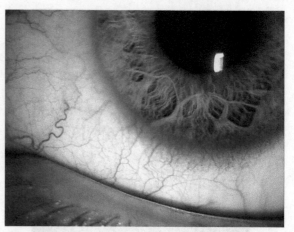

Fig. 5.20 Circumlimbal staining (lissamine green) as the result of interaction between the soft lens edge and the conjunctiva. (Courtesy of CORE, University of Waterloo)

Research Unit (CCLRU) or other grading scale, and compared with the preliminary assessment prior to lens insertion. Very occasionally the findings of the post-fitting check indicate that the lens fitting process must begin again; circumlimbal staining of the conjunctiva indicates an interaction between the lens edge profile and the conjunctiva (Fig. 5.20).[40] Lens edge designs vary significantly, and swapping to a rounder edge profile can eliminate the staining. Alternatively, the high modulus of the lens may be the cause and a less stiff material can be trialled. A tight-fitting lens can also cause such staining, but this should have been identified during the fit assessment.

Another finding that would indicate the need to refit would be signs of corneal (punctuate fluorescein staining) and conjunctival (lissamine green staining) dessication, as the result of a lens material incompatible with a poor quality tear film. Do not confuse solution-induced corneal staining (SICS) (Fig. 5.21)[41] with a lens fitting staining appearance (see Fig. 5.20) as the management of each differs (i.e., change the lens care system or change the lens material or design). SICS is characterised by having a superficial punctate staining appearance that often appears in a donut pattern around the peripheral cornea, although it can cover all of the cornea. SICS is also transitory, with a maximal observable appearance at 2 to 4 hours of lens wear and diminishing with increased lens wearing time.[42] If SICS is observed, the intensity may be reduced by introducing or improving the technique of a rub and rinse of the lenses before their overnight soak in the disinfecting solution.[43] Staining associated with a poor lens fit is likely to have a more intense staining pattern or

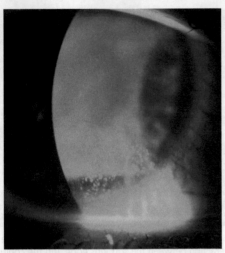

Fig. 5.21 Fluorescein punctate staining under cobalt blue illumination and a yellow barrier filter of the typical appearance during soft lens wear of dehydration staining. This should not be confused with the staining appearance for solution-induced corneal staining (SICS), which generally has a symmetrical donut appearance.

resemble a dehydration staining pattern (i.e., within the interpalpebral aperture) and increasing with lens wearing time. With careful history-taking and a thorough ocular and tear assessment informing the trial lens choice, these should be avoided.

5.8.8 Most common errors

1. Allowing the wearer to look up too high when assessing post-blink movement.
2. Push-up test: Positioning your thumb or fingers such that the lower lid rolls out during the push-up test, resulting in minimal contact between the posterior lid margin and lens edge and hence little or no movement on push up.
3. Overestimating lens movements: Use a small 1-mm spot to judge sizes.
4. Using the slit lamp to assess lens fit with the rheostat set too high, such that the patient's eyes water, affecting the lens fit.

5.9 Toric soft lens fitting

(See videos 5.22 through 5.24.) When a patient has 0.75 DC or more of astigmatism in their spectacle prescription, they will most likely need this correcting in order to have

optimised visual acuity with contact lenses. Around 47% of patients are estimated to have 0.75 DC or more of astigmatism in at least one eye.[44] Correction can be achieved using a toric soft contact lens regardless of the origin of the astigmatism. A spherical RGP lens (section 5.11.6) can also be used if the astigmatism is corneal in nature. A soft toric lens corrects the astigmatism by having a different lens thickness in each principal meridian. The lens must then be stabilised to prevent it from rotating. This is achieved using a number of different techniques, including prism ballast and various forms of dynamic stabilisation, in which raised areas of the lens interact with the eyelids.[18] Modern soft toric designs generally work very well and provide stable vision. There are some patients in whom rotational stability with soft torics can be challenging, including those with particularly angled eyelids or unusual lid movements on blink, or an oblique axis of astigmatism.[18]

5.9.1 Trial lens selection

The majority of off-the-shelf toric lenses are available only in one base curve and diameter; therefore, trial lens selection is simple. However, if the lens does not provide an adequate fit, a different brand must be trialled. These lenses are generally not available in every cylinder power and axis combination, with many brands offering between two and four different power options (e.g., 0.75 DC, 1.25 DC, and 1.75 DC).[11] The practitioner must select the nearest astigmatic power with the rule of thumb that it is better to under correct than over correct (section 4.15). This is because a smaller cylindrical correction gives less induced astigmatism if the lens does rotate, leading to more stable vision. Custom-made toric lenses with any power, axis, and dimensions are also available in a wide range of materials, but they are more expensive and therefore tend to be offered on a less-frequent replacement schedule and never as a single-use lens.

The trial lens power will require the spectacle prescription to be adjusted for BVD if one or both meridians have a power greater than 4.00 D. To do this, the power of each meridian is calculated, the BVD adjustment is applied to each meridian, and the resulting powers are recombined (see section 5.7, point 3). For example, a correction of $-6.00/-2.00 \times 180$ at a vertex distance of 12 mm has powers of -6.00 D along 180 and -8.00 D along 90, so that powers are approximately -5.50 and -7.25 at the cornea, giving an ocular refraction of $-5.50/-1.75 \times 180$. The initial trial lens is selected in much the same way as a spherical trial lens with the frequency of replacement determined by the initial discussion of patient needs, the lens material determined by the history and preliminary examination (section 5.2), the diameter determined by the HVID measurement (section 5.3), but also the availability of a suitable cylinder power and axis. The method of stabilisation is also a factor; in patients with a similar prescription in each eye, it can be informative to trial lenses with a different stabilisation mechanism in each eye.

5.9.2 Toric lens fit assessment

(See videos 5.22 through 5.24.) The fit of a soft toric lens is assessed in the same way as a spherical soft lens (section 5.8.2). The only differences are that the lens should be left to settle for around 10 to 15 minutes before assessing[45] and the orientation of the lens must also be examined. Rotational stability is essential for good vision with toric lenses, and the lens must remain reasonably stable as the eye moves around to avoid inducing astigmatism and blurring vision. It can be worth examining the fit and orientation before over-refraction as there is no point in checking the power of a lens that has poor rotationally stability. To check the orientation:

1. Identify the location of the orientation marker or markers using diffuse light. The markings vary with lens brand and can be a single line at 6 o'clock, three lines centred on 6 o'clock, or markers at 3 and 9 o'clock.
2. Note the position of the marker(s) as the patient blinks and with eye movements in a number of different directions of gaze.
3. Narrow the beam to a wide optic section (1 to 2 mm), position it straight ahead and rotate it until it lines up exactly with the marker(s) on the lens. On a Haag-Streit type slit lamp this is done by rotating the top of the illumination tower.
4. Read off the degree of rotation and note the direction and stability of rotation.

Rotational stability should be assessed once the lens has settled for at least 10 to 15 minutes. If the rotational stability of the lens is poor and varies with eye movements or between assessments, a lens brand that uses a different stabilisation mechanism should be trialled instead. A lens that consistently rotates by the same amount in the same direction is perfectly acceptable; the axis of astigmatism can be adjusted using two possible methods:

- LARS (Left Add, Right Subtract): As you observe the patient, if the rotation is toward your left, add the degree of rotation to the cylinder axis. If the rotation is toward your right, subtract the degree of rotation to the cylinder axis.
- CAAS (Clockwise Add, Anticlockwise Subtract): As you observe the patient, if the rotation is clockwise, add the degree of rotation to the cylinder axis. If the rotation is anticlockwise, subtract the degree of rotation to the cylinder axis.

Whether you use LARS or CAAS, the result is the same. This allows a contact lens to be ordered with an

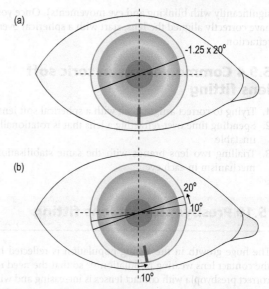

Fig. 5.22 CAAS (Clockwise Add, Anticlockwise Subtract) rule drawing showing how the lens order can be altered to compensate for consistent rotation of a soft toric lens.

axis of astigmatism that differs from that of the spectacle prescription, knowing that this lens design will rotate to position the astigmatic power correctly.

For example: (Fig. 5.22).

- Lens specification: Brand X 8.50:14.50/−2.00/−1.25 × 20
- On the eye the lens orientation marking consistently rotates 10° anticlockwise from the 6 o'clock position (where it should be), taking the cylinder power of the lens from the planned axis of 20° to 30°.
- Rotation of the marker from 6 o'clock in an anticlockwise direction indicates subtraction, so the following lens is ordered:
  - Brand X 8.50:14.50/−2.00/−1.25 × 10
- On the eye, the new lens is expected to rotate by 10° anticlockwise, taking the axis of the cylinder from 10° to the intended 20°.

5.9.3 Over-refraction of toric soft lenses

If a lens is not orientated correctly, the astigmatism of the lens will combine with the uncorrected cylinder of the eye and the resultant astigmatism will have an axis part way between the two—there is no point in trying to measure this. A different lens should be trialled that either has a different axis of astigmatism (if the orientation is wrong and consistently at the wrong axis) or has a different stabilisation mechanism (if the orientation varies significantly with blinking and eye movements). Once you have correctly aligned the lens, start with a spherical over-refraction.

5.9.4 Common errors in toric soft lens fitting

1. Trying to correct astigmatism with a spherical soft lens.
2. Spending time over-refracting a lens that is rotationally unstable.
3. Trialling two lens brands with the same stabilisation mechanism in each eye.

5.10 Presbyopic soft lens fitting

The huge growth in the ageing population is reflected in the contact lens wearing population[5,46] so that the need to correct presbyopia with contact lenses is increasing and will continue to do so. Fitting contact lenses that correct presbyopia can be challenging and you must adopt a philosophy of precision, as the smallest level of uncorrected ametropia or miscalculation in reading addition will likely lead to a higher level in symptoms than expected. Be precise. As with non-presbyopes the preferred choice is to fit them with disposable lenses to avoid the disadvantages associated with continued use of ageing lenses. As the required reading addition increases, the visual compromise needed to provide function distance and near vision increases and it is very likely you have to change the correction type you use.

5.10.1 The evidence base: comparison of correction options

Using distance contact lenses with reading spectacles (known as over-readers in this situation) is probably the most commonly used option and as long as the patient accepts wearing reading spectacles, it is very successful. Morgan et al.[5] reported about half of presbyopes wearing contact lens were wearing a multifocal contact lens, with the remainder wearing spherical lenses or monovision. Wearers do not have to be refitted with new contact lenses, just provided with over-readers, in the form of reading spectacles or half eyes (both of these can be in the form of ready readers and thus at relatively little cost), or spectacle multifocals (i.e., with a plano distance portion). There is no additional visual compromise unlike other contact lens corrections for presbyopia and this is the obvious choice for patients who have a high visual demand, whether for distance or at near (e.g., a patient who drives at night for a living). However, some patients will not appreciate the 'ageing' appearance and/or inconvenience

of wearing over-readers and will prefer other options. Monovision provides correction for distance viewing in one eye (the dominant eye) and near viewing in the other and is simple to fit. Current contact lens wearers only need a change in lens power in one eye and no refitting into a new design or material is required, and lens costs are the same as distance only contact lenses. Patients who wear toric lens designs are ideal for monovision because, although there are some custom designed soft lenses that provide correction for both astigmatism and presbyopia, these are not available as daily disposable contact lenses. Monovision is successful so long as the patient can tolerate the induced blur, reduced stereopsis, and possible retinal rivalry.[47] As the reading addition increases this blur increases and particularly when above +2.00 D may lead to symptoms, especially when driving at night, where it is difficult to suppress the bright myopic blur circles seen by the non-dominant eye.[48] Introducing modified monovision may solve these problems or refitting with a pair of distance contact lenses with over-readers. Monovision used to be the preferred option for correcting presbyopia mainly owing to the poor optical designs and poor reproducibility of multifocal contact lenses, but significant improvements in design and manufacture of multifocal contact lenses have changed that preference.[5]

Because monovision has been successfully used for many years to correct presbyopia, a modified version has been developed that incorporates multifocal lenses, by correcting the dominant eye with a distance bias multifocal and the non-dominant eye with the near bias multifocal or various combinations of single vision lenses and multifocal lens designs. The suggestion is that these multifocal lenses provide functionality for both distance and near and thus reduce the disparity between the eyes as well as the blur. You are likely to need to try different combinations to get the correct visual balance and so this may consume more chair time.

Studies comparing multifocal lenses with monovision now report patient preference toward multifocals and away from monovision[49,50] The most commonly used multifocal lenses use a simultaneous lens design and are typically distance biased lenses, where the central portion of the lens contains the distance power and is surrounded by an increased relative positively powered region providing the near element. When a high reading add is required, near biased designed lenses (the central portion contains the near power and is surrounded by an increased relative negatively powered distance vision region) will need to be used, resulting in a marked reduction in distance correction and explains why a multifocal design has a reduction in performance for distance vision as the reading addition increases.[48]

These optical portions can be formed by two distinct spherical zones, but are usually aspheric and create a multifocal progression from the distance portion to the near portion. The majority of lens designs are the latter: aspheric and centre distance. Another multifocal approach uses multiple concentric rings of alternating distance and near powers and are available in low, medium, and high reading additions. Situ et al.[51] reported on the success of this lens design when refitting existing monovision wearers with 53% still wearing the multifocal contact lens after 1 year. Multifocal contact lenses have high levels of subjective preference and are very successful for lower reading adds, but there is a greater compromise in vision as the reading addition increases.[52] As a consequence, it is likely that distance contact lenses and over-readers become the preference as the reading addition increases. Disadvantages include the increased cost compared with single vision lenses and the fact that the multifocal design that works best for the patient may not be available in the ideal material for that patient.

An additional method to correct presbyopia with contact lenses uses translating designs where the contact lens has a distance correcting area and a near correcting area. In the primary position of gaze, the distance vision area aligns with the primary visual axis and on downward gaze the lens translates such that the near vision area aligns with the visual axis of the eye. Translating soft lenses are only available in one design,[53] which is not available as a disposable contact lens. This limited availability restricts their usefulness and possibly reflects the limited success achieved with them; they are not frequently fitted owing to their poor translation (limited unpredictable movement), increased discomfort (lenses are thicker and usually prism ballasted), and they are only available as custom designs. These lenses are complex to fit and beyond the scope of this book. However, translating designs lend themselves well to being manufactured in gas permeable materials.

5.10.2 Fitting contact lenses for presbyopia

When assessing the performance of multifocal or monovision contact lenses, it is important to let the patient have an extended trial with the lenses, taking them away for a few days. The optimum trial length need not be longer than 2 to 3 days. Papas et al.[54] It also concluded that the reliability of clinical measures to determine success was limited and subjective responses were more reliable; ask the patient what they think about their vision. Do they think the fitting is successful? The assessment of static visual acuity is used to optimise the lens power and to act as a safety measure (i.e., the driving standard.)[54]

Fitting the lenses is otherwise the same as described in sections 5.7 and 5.8. In addition, note that:

1. Over-readers: A reading addition (section 4.13) should be determined with the distance contact lenses in place.

Do not use the reading addition determined with the spectacle prescription.

2. Monovision: You need to determine which eye will wear the distance contact lens and which will wear the reading lens; generally more success is found when the non-dominant eye wears the near powered lens.[47] There are several methods to determine ocular dominance; two are recommended here:

   - Hole in the card technique.[55] A card is fabricated with a hole in the middle; the patient is asked to hold the card with both hands and to look through the hole at a distant target. They then close the right eye; if they adjust the position of the card, their right eye is distant dominant, if they do not their left eye is dominant.
   - Blur acceptance.[56] With the patient corrected for distance, get the patient to observe the small letters of the distance acuity chart and place a +0.75 D lens over the right eye and then the left. Ask which they prefer and when they can see the letters more clearly? They will prefer to have the +0.75 D trial lens placed over their non-dominant eye.

   For example:
   RE: $-2.00/-0.25 \times 180$ LE: $-2.50/-0.25 \times 170$ Reading add $+1.50$ Dominance test: Right eye dominant
   Trial soft lens powers selected: R -2.00 D; L -1.00D.
   Result is distance power in the dominant right eye and near in the left, with the small cylinders ignored.

3. Monovision: When you explain to the patient how monovision works, the patient may start covering one eye to see the difference in vision. Ask the patient not to do this because it increases their awareness of the one aspect that results in monovision failing: the unacceptable blur from the near lens when looking in the distance. Remind the patient that they had never done that before wearing monovision.

4. Multifocal soft lenses: These are available in a variety of designs, but all have the same fitting requirement of precise centration. As these lenses are generally aspheric in nature, a decentred lens will induce visually compromising aberrations, such as astigmatism, coma, and curvature. Decentred lenses can be assessed using the slit lamp. A decentred lens is likely to result in poor distance visual acuity that cannot be improved. It is recommended that you follow the fitting guide developed by the manufacturer; all of the designs have subtle variations and one universal fitting philosophy will not work. The following guide to supplement manufacturers' instructions is recommended to increase fitting success.[57] It is summarised by the acronym RISONS:

R. Refraction: Do not use a current contact lens prescription as the starting point; perform a binocular refraction with the reading addition determined at the patient's habitual working distance.

I. Initial trial lens: Base the lens power on the new ocular refraction, adjusting for any cylinder as necessary; select the reading addition using the manufacturer's guideline.

S. Settling time: This should be at least 15 to 20 minutes (i.e., longer than the time for single vision lenses).

O. Over-refraction: Use full aperture lenses in a trial frame with the monocular fogging technique (section 4.11) in a trial frame to keep the binocularity, pupil size, and gaze position (i.e., downgaze when checking near vision) as close to normal as possible. If the initial over-refraction is greater than 0.50 D, do not order the lenses, but try a different diagnostic lens and repeat the over-refraction.

N. Near vision: Do not assess monocularly; maintain binocularity and only make unilateral adjustments when assessing distance vision.

S. Send away: Once the final trial lens is selected, allow an extended wearing trial of up to 4 days.

5. Modified monovision: The key is to find a balance in the vision that satisfies the patient's visual needs. The following stepwise approach, incorporating both straight multifocals and modified monovision, could be followed:

Lens Combinations

Reading addition	Dominant eye	Non-dominant eye
Near symptoms, pre-presbyope	Distance contact lens	Low add multifocal
< 1.00 D	Multifocals (low add)	
< 1.50 D	Low add multifocal	Mid add multifocal
< 2.00 D	Multifocals (mid add)	
> 1.75 D	Mid add multifocal	High add multifocal
> 1.75 D	Multifocals (high add)	

5.10.3 Solving problems

Remember that patients with presbyopic contact lenses can suffer with all the problems of standard lenses. For example, symptoms of fluctuating vision should lead you

to reassess the patient's tear film stability and the lens fit. In addition:

1. Over-readers.

   Poor near vision: Check to make sure the distance vision is correct and then assess whether the reading addition power is appropriate for the patient's habitual working distance(s).

2. Monovision

   (a) Poor distance vision: Make sure the distance vision is optimised, including the correction of small cylinders. An increase in the distance power (−0.25 D) may improve the distance vision; however, this is likely to have a significant effect on near vision. This could be tried in the dominant eye alone. Reducing the reading addition in both eyes or in the dominant eye alone may improve distance vision, but again at the expense of reducing the vision at near. You may need to consider refitting with multifocals or modified monovision.

   (b) Poor near vision: Again make sure the distance vision is optimised. A reduction in the distance power (−0.25 D) may improve near vision with a marginal change in distance vision. This could be tried in the non-dominant eye alone. Increasing the reading addition in both eyes or only in the non-dominant eye may improve near vision, but possibly at the expense of reducing vision in the distance.

   (c) Distance ghosting: This may be owing to uncorrected astigmatism or the patient may have weak or variable dominance and not be able to suppress their non-dominant eye. It is more likely to occur when the reading add is high, less so when aspherical designs are used and more so for the alternating concentric ring design. Different lens designs can be tried, along with a reduction in the disparity between the two eyes, but this may have an impact on the clarity of the distance or near vision.

3. High reading additions

   If you have a patient who has had success with either monovision or multifocal lenses but subsequent to an increase in reading addition has developed symptoms, refitting with modified monovision may resolve those symptoms. Ultimately refitting with distance contact lenses and over-readers may be the final solution.

5.11 Fitting corneal RGP contact lenses

Corneal lenses are also known as hard contact lenses, RGP lenses, or simply GP lenses. For convenience and consistency, we will refer to them as RGP lenses. RGP lens use diminished with the introduction of soft lenses in the 1980s and has remained at around 10% of lenses fitted, although this varies among countries.[5] This reduction is thought to be owing to their significantly longer adaptation period compared with soft lenses characterised by discomfort, possible vision fluctuations, and the need to increase wearing time gradually during this adaptation period. They can be used to correct simple refractive error, including corneal astigmatism, but because of their rigid nature and hence their ability to form a tear reservoir behind the lens, they can also be used for more complex conditions such as irregular astigmatism, keratoconus, post keratoplasty, and refractive surgery as well as orthokeratology.

5.11.1 Comparison of lens types

Corneal RGP lenses: All have posterior (back surface) curves that are classified as follows (Fig. 5.23):

- Back Optical Zone Radius (BOZR): This is the primary central curve of the lens that establishes a relationship with the cornea to optimise vision.
- Mid-peripheral radii: These curves create the area of the lens (mid periphery) that establishes the lens fitting relationship with the cornea and controls lens stability.
- Final edge radius, the edge lift: The final peripheral curve forms the outer portion of the lens that creates a band of edge clearance. The curves are significantly flatter than the cornea. The purpose of this area is to optimise the tear pump and aid lens removal.
- Total diameter: Standard corneal lenses have a range for their total diameter from 8.50 mm to 10.50 mm. Large

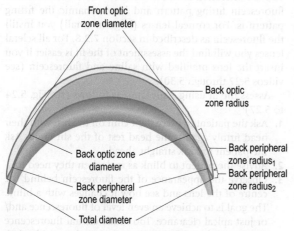

Fig. 5.23 A schematic diagram showing the parameters for a rigid gas permeable (RGP) contact lens.

diameter RGP lenses have a larger size with a range from 11.00 mm to 13.00 mm. The purpose of the large size RGP lenses is to ensure the edge clearance area rides over, but does not touch, the limbus. The larger diameter corneal lenses offer increased protection for the peripheral cornea, improved centration, reduced lens movement, and a reduction in lens awareness.

The cornea has a shape that is similar to a prolate ellipse; the curvature progressively flattening from the corneal apex out to the peripheral area at the limbus. Corneal RGP lens back surface designs try to mimic this shape change and do so generally using one of two approaches:

Spherical designs: A spherical optical curve followed by spherical peripheral curves progressively increasing in flatness. These designs usually have three or four zones: the optical zone, mid-peripheral zone (one or two curves), and the edge band (one curve).
Aspheric designs: True aspheric designs have the aspheric progression starting at the apex of the lens. The rate of flattening of the peripheral portion of the lens may have a consistent degree of eccentricity or a progressively increasing degree of eccentricity.

Alternately the BOZR starts as a spherical curve and transitions through an aspheric curve of increasing asphericity. Regardless of the design, the edge band is a flatter spherical curve. The edge band will appear narrow for aspheric designs compared with a spherical lens design.

Spherical designs have the advantage that you can alter any curve to change the fit of the lens. This allows the practitioner greater control in designing the lens, for example: changing the optical area of the lens, or increasing or reducing the edge lift, width or height. It is not possible to change an aspheric design other than the BOZR or the lens total diameter. However, the differing zones of a spherical design will have visible demarcations and these may present problems for patients with larger pupil diameters, as the edge of the optical zone may lie within the pupil area and result in symptoms of blur or glare. The junctions between the different zones may compromise corneal physiology and leave concentric rings or compressions where lens and cornea touch. These do not occur with aspheric lenses unless the lens itself is too small. These lenses also generally show a closer alignment fitting relationship between the back surface of the lens and the cornea, which some consider to be desirable, although too close alignment in fit may cause the lens to bind.

5.11.2 Observing how an RGP lens fits

The fitting relationship between the posterior surface of a contact lens and the front surface of the cornea can be observed by instilling fluorescein into the tear film and illuminating the eye with ultraviolet/blue saturated light from a Burton lamp, slit lamp, or some topographers, using low magnification. Changing various aspects of the RGP lens can change the fitting pattern seen.

Some lens materials contain a UV inhibitor and so appear 'black' under UV light. This prevents observations of the fluorescing tears behind the lens and thus an assessment of the lens-to-cornea fitting relationship. When using materials that contain a UV inhibitor, observations can only be made with a slit lamp, which provides a significant amount of blue light, but not a Burton lamp because it has a predominantly UV light source.

The basic goal when fitting an RGP lens is to ensure:

1. The central apex of the cornea and lens either fit in alignment or demonstrate marginal apical clearance; an even, low level of fluorescence or a very slight gradual reduction in fluorescence centrally to the mid periphery of lens will be visible.
2. The mid region of the lens should be aligned with the corneal surface, an even lower level of fluorescence compared with the BOZR area.
3. The edge of the lens has a band of high fluorescence, the edge lift.

5.11.3 Simplified fitting approach

The starting point when fitting a corneal RGP lens is to determine three parameters: The BOZR, Back Optic Zone Diameter (BOZD), and total diameter (TD). The following can be applied to either a standard spherical lens design or an aspheric design:

1. **BOZR**: This should either equal or be 0.05 mm flatter than the flattest corneal meridian (keratometry value—real or simulated), for example:

    7.80 mm along 180; 7.90 mm along 90 - BOZR selected 7.90 mm or 7.95 mm

    It is a personal choice whether you find it easier to assess the fit of an RGP lens that has apical clearance or apical alignment. If you prefer assessing definite clearance as your starting point, start with a trial lens with a BOZR of 7.85 mm. Some aspheric designs are only available in 0.10 fitting steps, in which case the starting point would be 7.90 mm.
2. **BOZD**: This should be larger than the maximal (mesopic) pupil diameter of the patient (not needed if fitting aspheric lens designs). For a pupil diameter measuring 7.0 mm the required BOZD should be 7.50 mm, not 6.50 mm. Some lens designs link the BOZD to the TD and so you may need to increase the TD to achieve the desired BOZD. This would obviously not be the case if you vary the parameters yourself—a level of complexity beyond the scope of this book and standard lens designs.

3. **TD**: This should be about 2 mm smaller than the HVID (section 5.3). It is common for lens designs to offer three lens diameter options, such as 9.50 mm, 9.80 mm, and 10.20 mm, or 9.00 mm 9.40 mm, and 9.80 mm. One approach is to assess the patient's eye and decide if the patient has a small, medium, or large HVID and select accordingly. For larger corneal RGP lenses the TD should match the HVID with the resultant fit giving coverage of the limbus by the edge clearance area of the lens.

Once these parameters have been determined for both eyes, you have your first pair of trial lens to assess. The following procedure is suggested for corneal and large diameter RGP lenses:

1. Advise the patient you are going to place a lens on their eye. This first lens allows you to decide what changes will be needed so that the lens fits their eye more accurately.
2. Instill a local anaesthetic into both eyes (section 7.8), and wait 1 to 2 minutes before proceeding.
3. Place the selected trial lens on the tip of the index finger of your right hand. If you want to prewet the lens, place a small drop of saline on the lens, but do not use a lens conditioning drop because these drops can affect how easily the fluorescein spreads in the tears.
4. The different lens insertion methods are shown in the online videos (see videos 5.25 and 5.26).
5. Allow the lenses to settle. The lens should settle in 3 to 5 minutes.
6. Instil fluorescein and assess the lens fit using a Burton lamp or slit lamp.

5.11.4 Assessment of lens fit

You are interested to know whether you have the desired fluorescein fitting pattern and how dynamic the fitting pattern is. For corneal lenses (large or small) you instill the fluorescein as described in section 7.2.8. For all scleral lenses you will find the assessment of the fit is easier if you insert the lens prefilled with saline and fluorescein (see videos 5.27 through 5.30).

Assess the fit using a slit lamp as follows (see Fig. 5.24 to 5.27):

1. Ask the patient to place their chin on the rest with their head firmly against the head rest of the slit lamp. Ask the patient to look straight ahead.
2. Advise the patient to blink as and when they need to.
3. Observe the appearance of the fluorescein behind the centre of the lens and see how it changes with a blink. The goal is to achieve an even level of fluorescence and/ or just apical clearance. Too much central fluorescence indicates a steep fit (or clearance) and unstable dark areas within the optical area are suggestive of a flat fit (or touch).

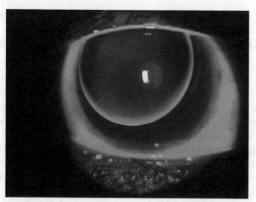

Fig. 5.24 Good lid attachment fit. Superior edge of the lens inherently rests under the upper lid. Slight fluorescein appearance at the corneal apex and in the mid periphery with an increasing edge clearance inferiorly.

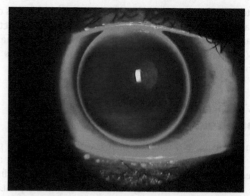

Fig. 5.27 Good alignment fit for an aspheric lens design. There is a slight fluorescein haze at the corneal apex and in the mid periphery with an even narrow edge clearance.

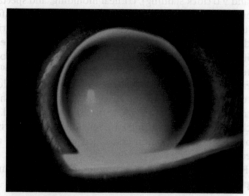

Fig. 5.25 Fluorescein tear film pattern with cobalt blue illumination and a yellow barrier filter for a steep fit for an RGP lens; marked apical clearance, mid peripheral bearing, narrow edge clearance.

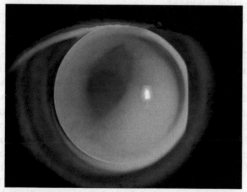

Fig. 5.26 Fluorescein tear film pattern with cobalt blue illumination and a yellow barrier filter for a flat fitting RGP lens; apical bearing, mid peripheral pooling, irregular excessive edge clearance associated with decentration.

4. The fluorescence in the mid periphery of the lens should be darker than in the centre and appear even. A steep lens will have touch in the mid periphery of the lens and a flat fit will have too much fluorescein spilling from the optical area in to the mid periphery. Changing the BOZR will change the mid peripheral fit. There should be a bright band of fluorescence around the edge of the lens. If you consider it to be too wide or bubbles are visible in this area, you will need to try a design with a reduced edge lift; the ideal width is 1 mm. Changing the design to aspheric will have that effect. Absence of an edge band of fluorescein is very uncommon, but it can be increased by changing from an aspheric design to a C4 (4 curve) spherical design or to a design of known increased edge lift.

5. Observe the lens movement on blink. This should be smooth and vertical. If the lens does not move very well, it may be a steep fitting. If the lens appears to rock around the corneal apex after a blink as it drops, it may be too flat.

6. Decide about the lens fit and adjust one of the three parameters accordingly. BOZR: a lens that is too steep, increase by 0.1 mm. A lens that is too flat reduce it by 0.1 mm. BOZD: increasing the BOZD increases the sagittal depth on the lens and makes the fit steeper, reducing this makes the lens flatter. TD: if the lens looks too small go bigger. Bigger lenses are likely to be more comfortable and more stable.

7. You can now repeat steps 2 to 4 for the left eye.

Interpalpebral fit or lid attachment fit

The fit of an RGP lens can be described either as an interpalpebral fit or a lid attachment fit and is determined more by the characteristics of the patient's cornea/lid relationship than by the lens design. The factors that lead to a lid attachment fit are narrower PAs, smaller HVIDs, and tighter lids. Larger corneal RGP lenses are more likely to adopt an interpalpebral fit.

5.11.5 Assessment of lens (and tear film) power

Once you have a lens for each eye that appears to give an acceptable fit, perform a spherical over-refraction and measure VA (sections 4.5 or 4.7). Alterations in the fit of an RGP lens can cause very subtle changes to the patient's vision and you may find two fits that you think work, but the patient reports a preferable visual performance with one. Where you find this, opt for the lens of optimal fit and preferred vision, alternatively select the lens giving the steeper or increased corneal clearance fit.

Tear lens power: When you change the fitting relationship between an RGP lens and the cornea, the tear film behind the lens (the tear lens) will change; a steeper fitting RGP lens results in increased separation between the lens and the cornea and creates a more positive tear lens. Generally increasing the sagittal depth of an RGP lens increases the positive tear lens power and the follow rule of thumb applies:

Increase BOZR by 0.05 mm, changes tear lens power by −0.25 D
Increase BOZD by 0.50 mm, changes tear lens power by +0.25 D

For aspheric designs, increasing the TD by 0.5 mm, changes tear lens power by +0.25 D.

For example:

7.80 (BOZR): 7.50 (BOZD) C4 design 9.80 -3.00, over refraction of −0.50 D

if you modify the fit to:

7.75:7.50 C4 design 9.80 −3.00, the over-refraction will now be −0.75 D

(tear lens power increased by +0.25 D)

5.11.6 Correcting astigmatism with corneal RGP lenses

Variations in corneal shape can be neutralised by the tear lens and a spherical RGP lens can mask corneal astigmatism. However, as the astigmatism increases, the fit of the lens becomes increasingly compromised resulting in decentration, instability, or increased discomfort. To compensate for this, it is common practice to steepen the BOZR of the RGP lens very slightly:

BOZR is steeper than the flattest keratometry value by one-third of the difference between the keratometry

values (e.g., K readings: 7.80 mm along 180 7.50 mm along 90.

BOZR selected is 7.70 mm (i.e., 0.10 mm steeper than flattest 'k' reading.

This adjustment generally allows a corneal RGP lens to mask up to 1.50 D of corneal astigmatism. Levels higher than this need alternate strategies of either fitting a corneal toric lens design or opting to fit semi-scleral lenses. A semi-scleral lens simply vaults the corneal toricity by aligning with the conjunctiva. In severely toroidal eyes, the sclera may also be toroidal and the semi-scleral lens will need to have a toroidal periphery to enable an even and aligned fit across the landing zone.

Toric corneal RGP lenses: Compromising the fit of a spherical RGP lens by more than that suggested above to enable centration on an increasing toroidal cornea is likely to result in corneal physiological compromise (3 and 9 o'clock staining), corneal moulding, and spectacle blur.[58,59] Compromised fits can also increase discomfort, so that fitting a toric RGP lens may be more appropriate and is recommended once corneal astigmatism exceeds 1.50 D. Some authors recommend using toric lenses only when the corneal astigmatism is greater than 2.00 D[60], or even greater than 3.00 D.[8] However be aware as the level of corneal astigmatism increases you are likely to have increasing issues associated with the compromised fit, such as a poor lens fit, increase lens discomfort, corneal moulding, variable vision associated with the blink, and spectacle blur.

Fitting toric lenses can be complex, but here is a simple approach:

Refraction: −2.00/−1.50 × 180
Transpose to cylindrical form: −2.00 × 90/−3.50 × 180
K readings: 7.50 mm (or 45.00 D) along 90; 7.80 mm (or 43.25 D) along 180
Lens trial selection:
7.55/7.85 (BOZR): 7.80 (BOZD) C4 design 9.80 (TD) −3.50/−2.00

The fit of a toric lens is likely to be steeper than an equivalent spherical lens design because both meridians should be in close alignment. Consequently, start with a slighter flatter BOZR compared with the keratometry readings, as shown in the example above. This diagnostic lens would need to be ordered for a trial because it is very unlikely you would have a toric RGP lens trial set unless you specialise in contact lenses. Note that placing a toroidal lens that matches the toroidal shape of the cornea on the eye should give a fluorescein fitting pattern that appears spherical with spherical tear lens profile behind the lens.

Modifying a toric lens should be kept simple; keep the difference in the BOZR the same as that of the cornea. For example, if the fit of the lens in this example is thought to be too steep:

7.55/7.85 is too steep; change BOZR to:7.60/7.90

Ordering an RGP toric design on the back surface of a lens to improve the fit of a lens will induce astigmatism. If the lens is ordered as shown above, the manufacturer will automatically supply you with a bitoric lens to correct for this induced astigmatism. Greater complexity than this simplified approach is beyond the scope of this book.

Irregular corneas: Fitting irregular corneas is very challenging and requires a high level of skill and experience. Low levels of irregular astigmatism or early keratoconus can be fitted using conventional RGP lens designs and you can try progressing to these fits as you gain confidence. Be aware that at some point, standard designs will not work and specialist designs will be needed. Before you get to that stage, you need to attend specific courses on fitting complex lenses. Early keratoconics should be assessed for corneal cross-linking treatment before lenses are considered, with the referral and suitability criteria varying among countries.[61]

5.11.7 Material choice

RGP lens are available in a range of materials. Reasons for selecting a specific material might include:
- The lens design chosen has a restricted material choice (i.e., aspheric designs)
- Need for a material of higher permeability to reduce or minimise hypoxia
- A compromised fit needs a material of increased rigidity to reduce flexure.

When fitting large diameter lenses, consider using a material that optimises oxygen permeability. Increasing lens diameter reduces the tear pump efficiency.

5.11.8 Ordering lenses

On completion of a successful trial, the RGP lens can be ordered. The details required for standard or aspheric designs are as follows: BOZR, TD, BVP, and lens design. Most lens manufacturers will allow you to exchange lenses if you need to modify the fit or adjust the lens power for a period of up to 3 months. RGP lens manufacturers understand the complexity of fitting RGP lenses and are very knowledgeable, especially about their own lenses. They can support you to get it right. If something does not make sense, ask them and listen to their advice because it is in their interest for you to achieve a successful lens fit for your patient.

5.11.9 Common problems

1. **Adaptation**: The biggest problem when fitting corneal RGP lenses is encouraging the patient to persevere through the adaptation phase. You should optimise the fit of the lens as soon as possible and continue to encourage the patient. The initial wearing time may need to be shorter than is desirable and then gradually increased. If adaption is hard, keep the wearing time reduced. Be prepared to accept that some patients cannot adapt to corneal RGP lenses and that semi-scleral, full scleral, or soft lenses may be better alternates.
2. **Glare at night**: When a patient presents with the symptoms of glare at night with corneal RGP lenses, they are most likely wearing a spherical lens design. The BOZD is probably too small and should be increased. If you cannot increase the BOZD further, you should consider changing the design to an aspheric design. This rarely occurs with larger diameter RGP lenses as the BOZDs are generally larger.
3. **Fluctuating vision with blink**: When vision fluctuates after a blink, the corneal lens is likely to be fitting too steep. If it continuously changes and is corrected by a blink, the fit is likely to be too flat. Confirm this by reviewing the fit of the lens with fluorescein on the slit lamp and reordering the lens with the corrected BOZR. For larger lenses this variable vision may be more indicative of a poor wetting surface.
4. **Lenses dislodge**: If a blink causes the corneal lens to dislodge occasionally, the lens could be too small (so increase the TD), too steep (so flatten the fit), or the edge lift is too high (so reduce it or refit with an aspheric lens). Larger RGP lenses provide increased stability and rarely become dislodged.

5.12 Scleral RGP lenses

More recently there has been a resurgence of larger diameter RGP lenses, larger corneal RGPs, mini-scleral lenses, semi-scleral lenses, and full scleral lenses.[7] These lenses are of increasing size and are designed for a different purpose—eyes where standard lenses have failed. Note this chapter offers a simplified approach to fitting these different types of RGP contact lenses and assumes you will be fitting these lens designs to healthy normal eyes.

5.12.1 Comparison of lens types

Semi- and mini-scleral lenses (Fig. 5.28)

- BOZR: This is the primary central curve of the lens that vaults the corneal apex and optimises vision.
- Mid-peripheral radii: These curves are designed to continue the same corneal vault as is found

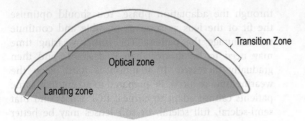

Fig. 5.28 A schematic diagram showing the parameters for a scleral contact lens.

at the corneal apex over the peripheral cornea and limbus.

- Final radius, the landing zone: This area of the lens rests on the conjunctiva beyond the limbus. The final peripheral area aligns with the shape of the conjunctiva and forms the outer portion of the lens that incorporates a band of edge clearance. The purpose of this area is to establish a stable platform for the lens design to generate the corneo-limbal vault.
- Total diameter: Semi-scleral lenses have a total diameter range from 13.00 mm to 15.00 mm and mini-scleral lenses from 15.00 mm to 18.00 mm. The goal for semi-scleral lenses is to have a narrower landing zone between 1.5 and 2.5 mm beyond the limbus.

Full scleral lenses (see Fig. 5.28)

- The optical zone, BOZR: This is the primary central curve of the lens that vaults the corneal apex and optimises vision.
- The transition zone, mid-peripheral radii: These curves are designed to continue the same corneal vault as is found at the corneal apex over the peripheral cornea and limbus.
- The haptic zone (landing zone), final radius: This area of the lens rests over the conjunctiva beyond the limbus. The final peripheral area aligns with the shape of the conjunctiva and forms the outer portion of the lens that incorporates a band of edge clearance. The purpose of this area is to establish a stable platform for the lens design to generate the corneo-limbal vault.
- Total diameter: Scleral lenses have a range for their total diameter from 18.00 mm to 23.00 mm. The goal for scleral lenses is to have a haptic zone well beyond the limbus and to cover the majority of the exposed bulbar conjunctiva.

5.12.2 Observing how a scleral lens fits

1. The central apex of the lens is generally 150 μm clear from the cornea with this clearance continuing over the peripheral cornea and limbus. It may need to be larger in corneas with pathology (see Fig. 5.7).
2. The transition zone, the mid peripheral region of the cornea and limbus should not have any lens contact.
3. The landing zone should align with the conjunctiva beyond the limbus with the edge of the lens aligned or showing some edge clearance and definitely not so tight as to result in vascular blanching.

5.12.3 Simplified fitting approach

The starting point when fitting a scleral RGP lens is based on the total diameter and how that will create the lens clearance over the limbus and cornea with the BOZR based on lens size, not necessarily the keratometry value. To fit a scleral, consider these four fitting steps:

1. **The total diameter:** Lenses that require greater corneal clearance need to be larger in diameter. Generally larger lenses are for more severe disease, mini-sclerals for normal eyes and where VA requirements outweigh any therapeutic requirement. Scleral lenses with diameters over 20 mm may require an offset optical zone to compensate for the flatter nasal scleral.
2. **Corneal clearance:** The goal is to generate 100 to 150 μm of clearance above the cornea and limbus. The sagittal height for the corneal clearance needs to be assessed with the standard measuring point being for a chord of 15 mm and assessed using an anterior OCT. As with the total diameter, an increasing corneal clearance is needed with increasing disease severity, up to a maximum of 600 μm. Note that as the corneal clearance increases, the expected visual acuity reduces.
3. **The landing zone:** The landing zone can influence the corneal clearance—too steep and the corneal clearance is increased. The goal is an aligned fit, which is assessed using a slit lamp. Any blanching areas indicate an incorrect fit; mid peripheral blanching indicates a flat fit; and peripheral blanching indicates a steep fit.
4. **The lens edge lift:** This is to aid lens removal only and can be observed as a shadow under white light with a slit lamp. Unlike corneal RGP lenses, this edge lift does not aid or support tear exchange behind the lens.

The procedure for placing a scleral lens onto the surface of the eye differs somewhat from that used for smaller diameter lenses (see video 5.31).

1. Advise the patient you are going to place a lens on their eye.
2. Instill a local anaesthetic into both eyes waiting, 1 to 2 minutes before proceeding.
3. The patient is best seated on a chair with space to tip their head forward and for you to position yourself lower than their head.
4. Hold the selected trial lens balanced between your thumb, and first and second fingers of your right hand.
5. Fill the lens with saline solution to the top and stain the saline with fluorescein.
6. Ask the patient to bend forward so that their face is parallel to the floor. Bend or kneel down beside the patient.
7. Use the fingers of your left hand to lift the upper lid of their right eye, while using the third finger of your right hand to pull back the lower eyelid.
8. Without tipping the lens, move it up to make contact with the surface of the eye and release the lids over the lens edge.
9. Gently dab the eye as excess saline will spill out.
10. Check no large bubbles are trapped beneath the lens, which would require the lens to be removed and reinserted.
11. Allow the lens to settle for 2 to 3 minutes before making an initial assessment of the fit using a slit lamp and anterior OCT.

5.12.4 Assessment of lens fit

Assess the fit as follows (Figs. 5.29 to 5.32):
1. Ask the patient to place their chin on the rest and their head against the slit lamp headrest. Get them looking straight ahead.
2. Advise the patient to blink as and when they need to.
3. Observe the appearance of the fluorescein behind the centre of the lens and see how it changes with a blink. The goal is to get an even level of fluorescence over the corneal and limbal regions. Too much clearance will likely result in the appearance of bubbles behind the lens; insufficient clearance will result in darkened areas.
4. For the landing zone it is important to assess the status of the vasculature of the conjunctiva. Blanching of vessels is to be avoided, blanching in the periphery indicating a steep fit, and blanching toward the limbus a flat fit. Fluorescence should be apparent toward the edge of the landing zone. Steep or flat fitting on the landing zone will influence the fit of the optical zone accordingly and should be adjusted to modify the optical zone fit.

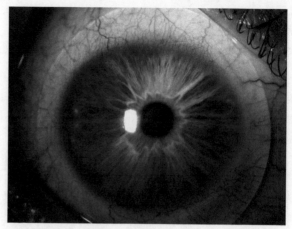

Fig. 5.29 A good fitting mini-scleral contact lens. (Courtesy of Brian Tompkins.)

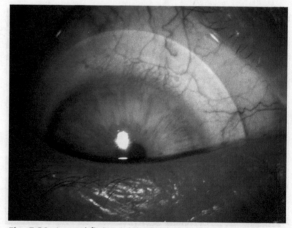

Fig. 5.30 A good fitting mini-scleral contact lens. Sodium fluorescein stain shows the tear lens clearance behind the lens. (Courtesy of Brian Tompkins.)

5. Observe the lens movement on blink. This should be smooth and minimal, decreasing with increased total lens diameter. The lens movement on blink should mimic that of a soft lens.
6. You can now repeat steps 3 to 5 for the left eye.

5.12.5 Assessment of lens (and tear film) power

See section 5.11.5.

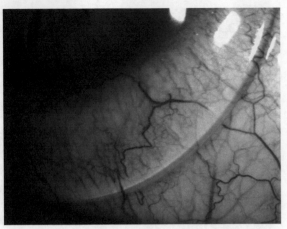

Fig. 5.31 A tight fitting mini-scleral contact lens demonstrating slight vessel blanching along lens edge. (Courtesy of Brian Tompkins.)

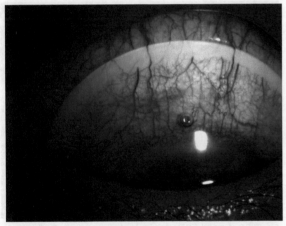

Fig. 5.32 A tight fitting mini-scleral contact lens demonstrating significant vessel blanching along lens edge. (Courtesy of Brian Tompkins.)

5.12.6 Correcting astigmatism with scleral RGP lenses

See section 5.11.6, in addition, semi-scleral and full scleral lenses become more of a consideration with increasing corneal complexity. The fundamental fitting philosophy is to vault the area of complexity, allowing the posterior tear lens to mask the irregularity and to ensure the landing zone clears the limbal region and offers fitting stability for the lens.

5.12.7 Material choice

For full scleral lenses the tear pump can be considered equivalent to that of a soft contact lens (i.e., negligible). For this reason, it is critical to select a material with high oxygen permeability.

5.12.8 Ordering lenses

See section 5.11.8.

5.13 Management of myopia progression

Growing evidence indicates that the prevalence and intensity of myopia is increasing and with this an increased need to control the progression of a patient's myopia, not just correct it optically.[62] A variety of options are available, including contact lens options based on the evidence that modification of the peripheral optics results in myopic peripheral blur, which has been shown to slow axial length progression.[63] This peripheral modification can be achieved in a number of ways:

Soft and rigid multifocal contact lenses: These designs are generally centre distance designs with the peripheral relative increase in plus power (reduction in minus power) generating the peripheral myopic blur. Some myopia researchers have advocated the use of centre distance multifocal lens designs labelled for correcting presbyopia, for off-label use in myopia management.[64] Specific designs for myopia control are available in some countries, including a daily disposable option.

Orthokeratology: The original purpose of RGP orthokeratology lenses was to mould the cornea overnight and consequently allow vision free from optical aids during waking hours. A coincidental side effect from the use of these lens designs has been a relative increase in peripheral corneal power owing to a relative reduction in peripheral corneal flattening. This has been shown to have a potential role in myopia management.[65] The fitting of orthokeratology lenses is outside the scope of this book, but benefits from corneal topography. The overnight wear that is a fundamental part of orthokeratology requires candidates to be carefully selected.

Practitioners need to be prepared to have the conversation with parents and their myopic children using tools such as the myopia calculator (www.brienholdenvision.org/translational-research/myopia/myopia-calculator).

5.14 Patient instruction for contact lens care

5.14.1. Lens care and maintenance

Other than single-use lenses, all other contact lenses need a cleaning solution, a disinfecting solution, and a conditioning or wetting solution to prepare the lens surface. These requirements are usually combined as a multipurpose lens care system. As RGP lenses are not replaced as frequently as soft lenses, patients must be educated on the need for supplemental cleaning processes. With age, lenses increasingly deposit, and deposit removal may be needed on an ongoing basis. Lenses will also become scratched. You may consider introducing a planned replacement scheme whereby RGP lenses are replaced on an annual basis.

5.14.2 Contact lens application and removal training

Spending the necessary time to teach a patient to handle their lenses correctly is an important part of the lens fitting procedure, an activity that may be delegated to well-trained support staff. Contact lens handling should be taught under good quality diffuse lighting and away from the communal areas of the practice to avoid putting pressure on the patient to perform in front of others. Lenses should not be taken away by the patient until the patient can demonstrate safe application and removal, as well as a full understanding of the importance of hygiene,[66] the cleaning regimen, and how to minimise the risk of complications. To aid compliance, it is important the patient understands why certain steps should be included and never dropped from their routine.[67] Do not simply give them a list of instructions; talking through and annotating a checklist (www.bcla.org.uk) can be useful. Areas to cover include handwashing, lens inspection, lens application and removal techniques, lens and case cleaning, lens and case replacement, recommended wearing times, minimising risks (i.e., contact with water, napping, illness), and when to seek advice.

The lens application procedure for a patient is almost identical to that for the practitioner (section 5.6.1), with the patient leaning over a flat mirror or using a mirror stood on a clean surface; for their right eye, position the lens on the very tip of the right index finger and use the right middle finger to pull down the lower lid and the left hand to lift the upper lid. It is generally easier to place the lens directly on the cornea rather than on the conjunctiva and sliding the lens.

5.14.3 Cleaning lenses

With the exception of single-use lenses, all contact lenses require cleaning after each wearing period. Lenses should be rubbed and rinsed with the cleaning fluid prior to storage, so as not to leave the storage solution with too great a microbial load on the lens surface.[68] Specific instructions vary between brands and types of lens solution but are summarised below:
1. Wash hands and dry thoroughly.
2. Remove one lens, placing it in the palm of the hand and, using a fingertip, gently rub the lens surface with the cleaning solution (multipurpose or specific cleaning solution). Cupping the hand stops the lens from sliding around.
3. Turn the lens over and rub the other side.
4. Transfer the lens to the palm of the opposite hand and rinse thoroughly.
5. Place the lens in a dry case and fill with solution (multipurpose, hydrogen peroxide, or other specific storage solution).
6. Secure case lids tightly and leave for 4 to 6 hours, depending on the manufacturer's instructions.
7. Before applying lenses, the solution should be neutralised, if required (hydrogen peroxide). In the case of multipurpose solutions, rinse the lenses with fresh solution prior to insertion.

5.14.4 Case cleaning and replacement

Case cleaning is just as important as good lens care, but frequently overlooked.[69] The patient should be shown how to clean their case and the importance of removing the biofilm from the inside surfaces should be explained.
1. Following lens application, empty the case and rinse it out with fresh solution.
2. Rub the case thoroughly with a clean, lint-free tissue.[70]
3. Rinse the case again to remove any debris and leave to air dry, upside-down in a room other than the room containing the lavatory.
4. Replace the case at least every 3 months.
5. Never reuse old solution.

5.15 Contact lens aftercare

The contact lens fitting procedure can be considered complete once a new patient has completed the first aftercare visit and the lenses are deemed successful. For new patients, a number of aftercare visits might be undertaken during the first 6 months of wear, but after this period, the frequency of appointments is a matter of practitioner judgement and depends on the characteristics of the patient. Those with a higher risk of complications (e.g., poor compliance, extended wear, diabetic, smoker, history of problems) should be seen more frequently, as should those who are more likely to exhibit ocular changes that may require a change in lens power, fit, or material (e.g., unstable refraction, medication that may lead to tear film changes). For other patients, a recall period between 6 and 12 months is the norm in clinical practice.

The purpose of a contact lens aftercare examination is to:

- Identify any difficulties the patient may have with their eyes and lenses
- Ensure that the patient's needs are met by the current contact lenses
- Consider the lens parameters and make changes where indicated
- Ensure that the lenses are not having an adverse effect on the eyes and manage where necessary
- Check patient compliance with lens wear and care instructions and re-educate, where required, to maximise healthy, successful lens wear and reduce the risk of future complications.

Summary of aftercare routine

---

1. Patient discussion: reason for visit, details of current contact lens wear, medical history, compliance, needs from contact lenses
2. Assessment of vision
3. Over-refraction and ocular motor balance with lenses
4. Assessment of lens fit and condition using slit lamp
5. Observe patient removing lenses
6. Slit lamp assessment of the anterior segment, including tear assessment
7. Assessment of corneal shape: corneal topography or keratometry to monitor changes in curvature and regularity
8. Ophthalmoscopy and/or other supplementary investigations, if indicated
9. Refraction if indicated
10. Summary of outcomes and re-education of patient regarding lens care and wear

---

5.15.1 Patient discussion—aftercare history taking

1. Determine the reason for the visit (chief complaint if any). Using the same form of questioning as used in the eye examination and involve the use of LOFTSEA

to gather all the appropriate information about the complaint (section 2.3.3). It is also important to determine whether lens removal is associated with cessation of the complaint or whether symptoms persist. Remember, it is possible that the complaint is completely unrelated to contact lens wear.

2. Question the patient specifically about other symptoms, which may or may not be related to contact lens wear: distance vision, near vision, eyestrain, headaches, ocular pain, discomfort, dryness, and diplopia.
3. A complete description of the contact lenses currently worn is needed. This may just be a matter of confirming that the practice notes are correct:
   (a) "What type of lens (or lenses) do you use?" (e.g., soft, gas permeable, toric, multifocal), brand and specification if known, and recommended frequency of replacement (e.g., single use, two weekly, monthly). Note that some patients may use more than one type, for example, monthly disposable toric lenses for general use and single-use lenses for swimming. A presbyope might wear single vision lenses with reading glasses for work and single-use multifocal lenses socially.
   (b) "Who prescribed the lenses?"
   (c) "How long have you been wearing this type of lens?
   (d) "How old is your current pair of contact lenses?"
   (e) "How often do you replace your lenses?" (as opposed to how often are you *supposed* to replace your lenses)
4. Contact lens history:
   (a) "How long have you worn contact lenses in total and have you tried any other lens types in the past?" If other types have been worn or trialled, it is important to ask further questions to ascertain why a particular lens type was abandoned, to avoid wasting time retrialling a lens type in the future that has failed to provide satisfaction.
   (b) "Have you ever had to stop contact lens wear for any reason, even for a short time?" If a positive answer is given, further questioning will be required to ascertain the reason for ceasing lens wear.
5. Wearing habits:
   (a) "When did you put your contact lenses on today?"
   (b) "How many days per week do you tend to wear your lenses?"
   (c) "How many hours of comfortable lens wear do you achieve on average in a day?" "When do you generally take your lenses out at night?" and "For how long would you like to wear them?" If there is a mismatch between these two periods of time, the current lenses are not meeting the patient's needs and another lens should be trialled.

(d) "What is the longest time that you wear your lenses?"

(e) "How often do you sleep or nap in your lenses?"

(f) "Do you ever shower in your lenses or use them for water sports, including swimming?"

6. General questions:

(a) "When was your last contact lens aftercare?"

(b) "When was your last eye examination?"

(c) "Do you have an up-to-date pair of spectacles that you could wear should you be unable to wear your lenses for a few days?"

7. Questioning should cover more general aspects of ocular and systemic health (section 2.3) because these issues can have an impact on contact lens wear. In addition, practitioners should remember that they remain responsible for the health of the whole eye, even during a contact lens aftercare, and they should not assume a particular symptom is contact lens related. It is particularly pertinent in contact lens wearers to ask "Do you smoke?" since this significantly increases the risk of microbial keratitis.[19]

8. During a contact lens aftercare appointment, you will also need to ascertain how compliant the patient is. Studies show that up to 90% of patients are non-compliant.[16] In some cases, this is because they do not understand or have forgotten how they should look after their lenses, whereas in other cases, they know but do not follow the full instructions owing to laziness or a lack of understanding of the purpose of a particular stage. They will tend to give the correct answer if they know they are being tested. Questioning should cover:

(a) "What cleaning solutions do you use?" (assuming the lenses are not single-use lenses)

(b) "How do you clean your lenses?" If time allows, it is generally more informative to ask the patient to demonstrate lens handling and cleaning.

(c) "Do you always wash your hands and dry them thoroughly prior to handling your lenses and/or case?"

(d) "How do you store your lenses if you are not wearing them?"

(e) "How frequently do you replace your lens case?" and "What do you do with your lens case once you have applied your lenses" and "How do you clean your case and how often?"

(f) With all patients, it is essential to re-enforce instructions regarding lens and case care, along with healthy wearing habits, explaining why certain steps are included, to improve compliance.

9. Occupation, hobbies, computer use, and driving (section 2.3): Practitioners should ask specifically about water sports because of the increased risk of microbial keratitis associated with allowing lenses to come in to contact with water.[71]

> **Example case history: Miss Pernille Harder, Graphic designer, Driver**
>
> CC: "Eyes become gritty during the day at work" c̄ CLs since starting new job 6/12 ago. Affects OU equally and gives gen. feeling of eyestrain. VDU all day. Becomes a problem after ~ 5 hours. Eases when CLs removed. DV and NV c̄ CL and specs OK. No H/A. No other Sxs.
>
> OH: SCLs for last 6 years. 6/7 for ~8 hours, 16 hours. max. Monthly disp hydrogel, brand X. No previous CL wear. Fitted by Dr. Pep Guardiola. CLs replaced ~1/12. Current 5 weeks old! Lenses in for 6 hours. today. Never sleeps in CL. No previous probs c̄ CL.
>
> Last AC 11/12 ago. Last LEE: 18/12. Has up to date specs – good DV and NV. No other OH. FOH: parents both myopic.
>
> GH: OK, no meds. No allergies. Non-smoker. LME: 12/12, Dr. Lucy Bronze, Bradford. No FMH: Hobbies: Football, swimming 2x/week (monthly CL c̄ goggles), climbing. Uses PC ~ 7/24.
>
> Soln: multipurpose brand Y. Washes hands superficially. Rubs lens each side for 30 seconds and rinses with so'ln each time worn. Rubs lens case with tissue and leaves to air dry each day. Replaces case every 2/12.

In this case, the areas of interest are the discomfort after 5 hours of wear and some aspects of compliance. The patient cannot wear her lenses comfortably for as long as she would like, and it is important to determine the reason for this dryness and manage it appropriately (e.g., look for conditions such as meibomian gland dysfunction that frequently cause dry eye, try ocular lubricants, refit with a lens material with lower water content and better lubricity). The eyestrain is probably related to the dryness, but an association with refractive error and/or binocular vision problems should be ruled out. Lens and case care appear to be good, but handwashing needs intervention and additional single-use lenses for swimming should be considered in addition to goggles in a regular swimmer.

5.15.2 Over-refraction, acuity, and ocular motor balance

See section 5.8.6.

5.15.3 The evidence base: assessment of lens and lens fit

Assess the fit as described in sections 5.8 (soft lenses) and 5.11 (RGP lenses). An unacceptable fit requires the practitioner to trial a different lens as a matter of urgency. (See videos 5.32 through 5.34.)

Whilst the patient is on the slit lamp biomicroscope, the integrity of the contact lens and the condition of the lens surface can be examined. Specular reflection off the prelens tear surface can be very informative (section 7.1.3) and using the Placido disc from a topographer is also useful to assess the global impact surface deposits have on the tear film stability as well as measuring the NIBUT (see video 5.1) (section 7.2.3). All lenses need to interact with the tear film, and it is inevitable that there will be deposit on the lens surface; in fact some of the interactions and depositions are desirable because they help condition the lens and contribute to its wettability. Clinically observable lens surface deposition has been shown to occur within minutes of wear[72] and significant amounts after just one day of wear.[73] The level, composition, and appearance of deposition on the lens surface are influenced by the tear film,[74] environmental variables such as air quality, lens care products used, cosmetic and skin care products, and industrial environments (particles and vapours), the replacement frequency of the lens, and the lens material.[74,75]

5.15.4 The evidence base: management of deposition

If a patient presents with lens surface deposition that is clinically significant, the following strategies should be considered:

1. Change lens material: Hydrogel materials Group II (ISO system of contact lens materials classification BS EN ISO 18369-1: 2006/DAM1) tend to have increased levels of lipids and Group III the least.[76] Silicone hydrogels have an increased level of lipid deposition (least on lotrafilcon A and B, moderate level with asmofilcon A, and most with galyfilcon A and balafilcon A.[77]
2. Change lens care system: If patients are not rubbing and rinsing their lenses on removal, instruct them on this procedure. Newer dual disinfecting multipurpose solutions contain ingredients to increase surface hydrophilicity, which should reduce deposition. The introduction of a peroxide system may also be effective.[78]
3. Change frequency of replacement: Increasing the frequency of lens replacement will reduce the level of deposition. Whereas daily disposable contact lenses do get deposits, the level of deposition is much reduced compared with two-weekly or monthly replacement contact lenses.[78,79]

5.15.5 Observation of lens removal

The point in the routine where the lenses need to be removed provides an opportunity for the practitioner to observe the patient's contact lens handling skills. It is also useful to ask the patient to demonstrate their lens cleaning technique at this point. Check:

1. Is their handwashing technique adequate?
2. Did the patient dry their hands sufficiently before handling the lenses?
3. Do they have a safe lens removal technique and are they confident, or do they need some pointers?
4. Do they have a good lens cleaning technique and was it undertaken long enough?
5. Do they rinse the lenses thoroughly?
6. What is the condition of their lens case?
7. At the end of the examination, do they wash their hands before lens insertion?
8. Do they have a safe lens application technique and are they confident, or do they need some pointers?

Deficiencies should lead to re-education (section 5.15.7).

5.15.6 Check ocular health

Following removal (see videos 5.35 through 5.37) of the lenses, perform a slit lamp biomicroscope examination of the anterior segment (section 7.1), including staining with fluorescein sodium and lissamine green, lid eversion (see video 5.38), and tear assessment.[14]

Topography or keratometry (section 5.4) should be undertaken to assess the corneal shape to look for changes, particularly in terms of regularity. Unlike the days of hard polymethylmethacrylate lenses and thick hydrogel soft lenses, corneal warpage is now rare, but it occasionally occurs with RGP and tight-fitting, high-modulus silicone hydrogel lenses.[80]

Examine the posterior segment of the eye (section 7.10) unless it has been undertaken during a recent eye examination and there is nothing in the symptoms to raise suspicion, such as unexplained visual acuity loss. Be mindful of the possibility of pathology in patients wearing contact lenses. For example, do not make protracted changes to a patient's contact lens specification over a period of weeks in response to a symptom like 'vision not quite right,' without checking the whole eye for signs of pathology.

5.15.7 Summary of outcomes and re-education of patient

Finally, you need to create an action plan to discuss with the patient. This summary must include the importance of regular aftercare visits and should cover the following:

1. The assessments performed during the examination and what has been found, if anything.
2. Any actions in light of what has been found.
3. Re-enforce healthy lens wearing, good hygiene, and lens care habits. Talking through a written check list and indicating to patients where they are doing well

and where they could improve is a useful way of communicating such information (www.bcla.org.uk and www.aoa.org/x8024.xml).

4. Give the patient a new, dated lens prescription.

5. Ensure the patient has a new supply of lenses of the correct specification. Patients may wish to buy the lenses online, in which case highlighting the importance of regular aftercare is particularly crucial.

6. Inform the patient when their next aftercare and eye examinations are due.

7. Remind the patient to remove their lenses and contact you if their eyes no longer 'see good, feel good, look good.'

References

1. Pesudovs K, Garamendi E, Elliott DB. A quality of life comparison of people wearing spectacles or contact lenses or having undergone refractive surgery. *J Refract Surg.* 2006; 22:19–27.

2. Rumpakis J. New data on contact lens dropouts: an international perspective. *Review of Optometry.* 2010. Available at: http://www.revoptom. com/content/d/contact_lenses_and_ solutions/c/18929/.

3. Sulley A, Young G, Hunt C, McCready S, Targett MT, Craven R. Retention rates in new contact lens wearers. *Eye Contact Lens.* 2018;44:S273–82.

4. Dumbleton KA, Woods CA, Jones LW, Fonn D. The relationship between compliance with lens replacement and contact lens-related problems in silicone hydrogel wearers. *Cont Lens Anterior Eye.* 2011;34:216–22.

5. Morgan PB, Woods CA, Tranoudis Y, et al. International contact lens prescribing in 2017. *Cont Lens Spect.* 2018;32:28–33.

6. Wildsoet CF, Chia A, Cho P, et al. IMI—Interventions for controlling myopia onset and progression report. *Invest Ophthalmol Vis Sci.* 2019;60:M106–31.

7. Vincent SJ. The rigid lens renaissance: a surge in sclerals. *Cont Lens Anterior Eye.* 2018;41:139–43.

8. Gasson A, Morris J. *The Contact Lens Manual: A Practical Guide to Fitting,* ed 4. Philadelphia, PA: Butterworth Heinemann Elsevier; 2010.

9. Morgan PB, Maldonado-Codina C, Efron N. Comfort response to rigid and soft hyper-transmissible contact lenses used for continuous wear. *Eye Contact lens.* 2003;29(suppl 1): S127–30.

10. Bennett ES, Stulc S, Bassi CJ, et al. Effect of patient personality profile and verbal presentation on successful rigid contact lens adaptation, satisfaction and compliance. *Optom Vis Sci.* 1998;75:500–5.

11. Phillips A, Speedwell L, eds. *Contact Lenses,* ed 6. Philadelphia, PA: Elsevier; 2019.

12. Gupta N, Naroo SA. Factors influencing patient choice of refractive surgery or contact lenses and choice of centre. *Cont Lens Anterior Eye.* 2006;29: 17–23.

13. Jones L, Drobe B, González-Méijome JM, et al IMI—Industry guidelines and ethical considerations for myopia control report. *Invest Ophthalmol Vis Sci.* 2019;60: M161–83.

14. Efron N, Morgan PB. Rethinking contact lens aftercare. *Clin Exp Optom.* 2017;100:411–31.

15. Young G. Why one million contact lens wearers dropped out. *Cont Lens Anterior Eye.* 2004;27:83–5.

16. Dumbleton K, Richter D, Woods CA, Jones L, Fonn D. Compliance with contact lens replacement in Canada and the United States. *Optom Vis Sci.* 2010;87:131–9.

17. Efron SE, Efron N, Morgan PB, Morgan SL. A theoretical model for comparing UK costs of contact lens replacement modalities. *Cont Lens Anterior Eye.* 2012;34:28–34.

18. Efron N, ed. *Contact Lens Practice,* ed 3. Philadelphia, PA: Elsevier; 2018.

19. Stapleton F, Edwards K, Keay L, et al. Risk factors for moderate and severe microbial keratitis in daily wear contact lens users. *Ophthalmology.* 2012;119:1516–21.

20. Stapleton F, Alves M, Bunya V, et al. TFOS DEWS II Epidemiology Report. *Ocul Surf.* 2017;15:334–68.

21. Willcox M, Argueso P, Georgiev G, et al. TFOS DEWS II Tear Film Report. *Ocul Surf.* 2017;15:369–406.

22. Wu YT, Tran J, Truong M, Harmis N, Zhu H, Stapleton F. Do swimming goggles limit microbial contamination of contact lenses? *Optom Vis Sci.* 2011;88:456–60.

23. Young G, Hunt C, Covey M. Clinical evaluation of factors influencing toric soft contact lens fit. *Optom Vis Sci.* 2002;79:11–9.

24. Alfonso JF, Ferrer-Blasco T, González-Méijome JM, et al. Pupil size, white-to-white corneal diameter, and anterior chamber depth in patients with myopia. *J Refract Surg.* 2010;26: 891–8.

25. Twa MD, Bailey MD, Hayes J, Bullimore M. Estimation of pupil size by digital photography. *J Cataract Refract Surg.* 2004;30:381–9.

26. Young G. Ocular sagittal height and soft contact lens fit. *J Brit Cont Lens Assoc.* 1992;15:45–9.

27. Hall LA, Young G, Wolffsohn JS, Riley C. The influence of corneoscleral topography on soft contact lens fit. *Invest Ophthalmol Vis Sci.* 2011;52: 6801–6.

28. Rathi VM, Mandathara PS, Dumpati S, Sangwan VS. Change in vault during scleral lens trials assessed with anterior segment optical coherence tomography. *Cont Lens Anterior Eye.* 2017;40:157–61.

29. Richdale K, Sinnott LT, Skadahl E, Nichols JJ. Frequency of and factors associated with contact lens dissatisfaction and discontinuation. *Cornea.* 2007;26:168–74.

30. Dumbleton KA, Richter D, Woods CA, et al. A multi-country assessment of compliance with daily disposable contact lens wear. *Cont Lens Anterior Eye.* 2013;36:304–12.

31. Simpson TL, Situ P, Jones LW, Fonn D. Dry eye symptoms assessed by four questionnaires. *Optom Vis Sci.* 2008;85:692–9.

32. Chalmers RL, Begley CG, Moody K, Hickson-Curran SB. Contact lens dry eye questionnaire-8 (CLDEQ-8) and opinion of contact lens performance. *Optom Vis Sci.* 2012;89:1435–42.

33. Nelson JD, Craig JP, Akpek EK, et al. TFOS DEWS II introduction. *Ocul Surf.* 2017;15:269–75.

34. Efron N, Morgan P, Katasara S. Validation of grading scales for

contact lens complications. *Ophthalmic Physiol Opt.* 2001;21:17–29.

35. Bailey IL, Bullimore MA, Raasch TW, Taylor HR. Clinical grading and the effects of scaling. *Invest Ophthalmol Vis Sci.* 1991;32:422–32.

36. Young G, Schnider C, Hunt C, Efron S. Corneal topography and soft contact lens fit. *Optom Vis Sci.* 2010;87:358–66.

37. Maldonado-Codina C, Efron N. Impact of manufacturing technology and material composition on the clinical performance of hydrogel lenses. *Optom Vis Sci.* 2004;81:442–54.

38. Wolffsohn JS, Hunt OA, Basra AK. Simplified recording of soft contact lens fit. *Cont Lens Anterior Eye.* 2009; 32:37–42.

39. Young G. Evaluation of soft contact lens fitting characteristics. *Optom Vis Sci.* 1996;73:247–54.

40. Maïssa C, Guillon M, Garofalo RJ. Contact lens-induced circumlimbal staining in silicone hydrogel contact lenses worn on a daily wear basis. *Eye Contact Lens.* 2012;38:16–26.

41. Bandamwara KL, Garrett Q, Cheung D, et al. Onset time course of solution induced corneal staining. *Cont Lens Anterior Eye.* 2010;33:199–201.

42. Luensmann D, Moezzi A, Peterson RC, Woods C, Fonn D. Corneal staining and cell shedding during the development of solution-induced corneal staining. *Optom Vis Sci.* 2012;89:868–74.

43. Peterson RC, Fonn D, Woods CA, Jones L. Impact of a rub and rinse on solution-induced corneal staining. *Optom Vis Sci.* 2010;87:1030–36.

44. Young G, Sulley A, Hunt C. Prevalence of astigmatism in relation to soft contact lens fitting. *Eye Contact Lens.* 2011;37:20–5.

45. Richdale K, Berntsen D, Mack C, Merchea MM, Barr JT. Visual acuity with spherical and toric soft contact lenses in astigmatic eyes. *Optom Vis Sci.* 2007;84:969–75.

46. Morgan PB, Efron N, Woods CA. An international survey of contact lens prescribing for presbyopia. *Clin Exp Optom.* 2011;94:87–92.

47. Evans BJ. Monovision: a review. *Ophthalmic Physiol Opt.* 2007;27: 417–39.

48. Woods J, Woods CA, Fonn D. Visual performance of a multifocal contact lens versus monovision in established presbyope. *Optom Vis Sci.* 2015;92: 175–82.

49. Richdale K, Mitchell GL, Zadnik K. Comparison of multifocal and

monovision soft contact lens corrections in patients with low-astigmatic presbyopia. *Optom Vis Sci.* 2006;83:266–73.

50. Woods J, Woods CA, Fonn D. Early symptomatic presbyopes—what correction modality works best? *Eye Contact Lens.* 2009;35:221–6.

51. Situ P, duToit R, Fonn D, Simpson T. Successful monovision contact lens wearers refitted with bifocal contact lenses. *Eye Contact Lens.* 2003;29: 181–4.

52. Gupta F, Naroo SA, Wolffsohn JS. Visual comparison of multifocal contact lens to monovision. *Optom Vis Sci.* 2009;86:98–105.

53. Ezekiel DF. A 'genuinely' new bifocal lens design. *Optom Today.* 2002;17: 34–5.

54. Papas E, Decenzo-Verbeten T, Fonn D, et al. Utility of short-term evaluation of presbyopic contact lens performance. *Eye Contact Lens.* 2009;35:144–8.

55. Robboy MW, Cox IG, Erickson P. Effects of sighting and sensory dominance on monovision high and low contrast visual acuity. *CLAO J.* 1990;16: 299–301.

56. Schor C, Erickson P (1987). Patterns of binocular suppression and accommodation in monovision. *Am J Optom Physiol Opt* 64: 723-30.

57. Woods J, Woods CA, Fonn D. Fitting soft center-near design multifocal lenses. *Cont Lens Spectr.* 2010;24:44–6.

58. Edwards KH. The calculation and fitting of toric lenses. *Ophthal Optician.* 1982;22:106–14.

59. Yamane SJ. Are hard lenses superior to soft? The advantages of soft lenses. *Cornea.* 1990;9:S12–4.

60. Meyler JG. Fitting and calculating toric corneal contact lenses. *J Brit Cont Lens Assoc.* 1989;12:7–14.

61. Shajari M, Kolb CM, Agha B, et al. Comparison of standard and accelerated corneal cross-linking for the treatment of keratoconus: a meta-analysis. *Acta Ophthalmol.* 2019;97: E22–E35.

62. Holden B, Sankaridurg P, Smith E, Aller T, Jong M, He M. Myopia, an underrated global challenge to vision: where the current data takes us on myopia control. *Eye (Lond).* 2014;28:142–6.

63. Benavente-Perez A, Nour A, Troilo D. Axial eye growth and refractive error development can be modified by exposing the peripheral retina to relative myopic or hyperopic

defocus. *Invest Ophthalmol Vis Sci.* 2014;55:6765–73.

64. González-Méijome JM, Peixoto-de-Matos SC, Faria-Ribeiro M, et al. Strategies to regulate myopia progression with contact lenses: a review. *Eye Contact Lens.* 2016; 42:24–34.

65. Cho P, Tan Q. Myopia and orthokeratology for myopia control. *Clin Exp Optom.* 2018;102:364–77.

66. Campbell D, Mann A, Hunt O, Santos LJR. The significance of hand wash compliance on the transfer of dermal lipids in contact lens wear. *Cont Lens Anterior Eye.* 2012;35: 71–6.

67. McMonnies CW. Improving contact lens compliance by explaining the benefits of compliant procedures. *Cont Lens Anterior Eye.* 2011;34:49–52.

68. Rosenthal RA, Henry CL, Schlech BA. Contribution of regimen steps to disinfection of hydrophilic contact lenses. *Cont Lens Anterior Eye.* 2004;27:149–56.

69. Hickson-Curran, S, Chalmers RL, Riley C. Patient attitudes and behaviour regarding hygiene and replacement of soft contact lenses and storage cases. *Cont Lens Anterior Eye.* 2011;34: 207–15.

70. Cho P, Cheng SY, Chan WY, Yip WK. Soft contact lens cleaning: rub or no-rub? *Ophthalmic Physiol Opt.* 2009;29:49–57.

71. Carnt N, Stapleton F. Strategies for the prevention of contact lens-related Acanthamoeba keratitis: a review. *Ophthalmic Physiol Opt.* 2016;36:77–92.

72. Bontempo AR, Rapp J. Protein and lipid deposition onto hydrogel contact lenses in vivo. *CLAO J.* 2001;27:75–80.

73. Leahy CD, Mandell RB, Lin ST. Initial in vivo tear protein deposition on individual hydrogel contact lenses. *Optom Vis Sci.* 1990;67:504–11.

74. Luensmann D, Jones L. Protein deposition on contact lenses: the past, the present, and the future. *Cont Lens Anterior Eye.* 2012;35:53–64.

75. Ng A, Heynen M, Luensmann D, Jones L. Impact of tear film components on lysozyme deposition to contact lenses. *Optom Vis Sci.* 2012;89: 392–400.

76. Lorentz H, Jones L. Lipid deposition on hydrogel contact lenses: how history can help us today. *Optom Vis Sci.* 2007;84:286–95.

77. Teichroeb JH, Forrest JA, Ngai V, Martin JW, Jones L, Medley J. Imaging protein

deposits on contact lens materials. *Optom Vis Sci.* 2008;85:1151–64.

78. Brennan NA, Coles ML. Deposits and symptomatology with soft contact lens wear. *Int Contact Lens Clin.* 2000; 27:75–100.

79. Maïssa C, Franklin V, Guillon M, Tighe B. Influence of contact lens material surface characteristics and replacement frequency on protein and lipid deposition. *Optom Vis Sci.* 1998;75:697–705.

80. Alba-Bueno F, Beltran-Masgoret A, Sanjuan C, Biarnés M, Marín J. Corneal shape changes induced by first and second generation silicone hydrogel contact lenses in daily wear. *Cont Lens Anterior Eye.* 2009;32:88–92.

Chapter 6

Assessment of binocular vision and accommodation

Brendan T Barrett

CHAPTER OUTLINE

Tests of accommodation and binocular vision are presented together in this chapter because, from a problem-oriented examination viewpoint, it is frequently not obvious whether a patient's signs and symptoms are primarily accommodative or binocular in origin. Core or 'entrance' tests[1] act as screening tests in patients without symptoms that suggest a binocular vision or accommodative problem and are performed after the case history and before refraction. These are followed by additional, supplementary tests that may be performed in patients whose symptoms or results of screening tests suggest that they may prove useful.

Note that symptoms may not be present in patients with a binocular vision or accommodative anomaly[2] because tasks that are difficult (e.g., near-work) are avoided, or because the patient may not know what is 'normal' and so does not report difficulties (more likely in children) or suppression (section 6.6) may be present. Of course, visual symptoms can also exist without an associated accommodative or binocular defect.

It is especially important that testing is conducted in a rigorous and systematic fashion because many of the tests rely heavily on subjective responses, which often involve the concepts of blur and diplopia; these are difficult for children in particular to understand and for this reason, clear instructions are crucial. Even when the tests are appropriately conducted and carefully explained, it is becoming clearer there is a very wide variation in test results obtained in patients who are apparently visually normal.[3] To circumvent this problem, it is important to look at the results from more than one test rather than placing too much emphasis on a single, abnormal test result. In the final section of this chapter (section 6.18), a brief overview is provided of how the results from different tests can be considered in combination in order to aid diagnosis and thus inform management.

6.1 Adaptations when testing younger patients

When it comes to testing younger patients, a number of adaptations can help to engage the child to ensure that the best possible test results are obtained: (1) use the simplest methods available, (2) try to present the test in the format of a game, and (3) remember that the testing needs to be complete in as short a time as possible. Thus, when the near point of convergence (NPC) (section 6.5) is being measured, for example, an interesting target (e.g., a colourful cartoon character) should be used rather than the RAF rule or pen target. It is not appropriate to use a phoropter in children and, wherever possible, even the use of a trial frame should be avoided. Free space methods are preferred. By turning the test into a game (e.g., 'finding the ball' during stereopsis testing with the Frisby test, or by playing a matching game, for example during stereo-testing with the Lang test; section 6.7), the child's attention can, with luck, be captured and retained until at least a good clinical impression about the normality or otherwise of the test result can be gained. Indeed, it is often more appropriate to think of results in terms of pass/fail (e.g., accommodative amplitude and facility, sections 6.8 and 6.15) rather than as absolute measures. Sometimes alternative approaches are called for. For example, rather than measuring fusional reserves (section 6.12) using a prism bar or rotary prisms, an acceptable alternative in younger patients is to use the 20 base-out prism test (section 6.12). It is of course vitally important to make the child feel at ease so young children will want to sit on their parent's lap and it is better if testing room is suitably configured (e.g., bright colours, toys).[4] As soon as co-operation has been lost, bring the testing to a close and try again on a separate occasion. Adaptations to testing in older (presbyopic) patients are not considered separately here but rather are described in the test sections where appropriate.

6.2 The cover test: detection and assessment of strabismus and heterophoria

The only currently available test that can differentiate between a strabismus and heterophoria (phoria) is the cover-uncover test. The test has the advantage of being an objective test, because while it requires co-operation from the patient, it does not require a verbal response. In strabismus, the test can indicate the constancy, laterality, direction, and magnitude of a deviation. In phoria, the test allows the direction and magnitude to be determined and it provides information on whether or not the phoria is compensated or decompensated. The test is simple to perform, requires only an occluder and a suitable fixation target. With phoria, the cover-uncover test is usually supplemented by the alternating cover test, which is useful because the deviation observed will usually be considerably larger (and therefore more obvious) than that seen with the cover-uncover test.[5] This is because binocular vision is suspended altogether during the alternating cover test, whereas binocular vision is merely interrupted and then restored during the cover-uncover test. To conduct the cover test, it is crucial that you are systematic in your approach (Box 6.1). First, search for a strabismus using the cover-uncover test. If one exists, then by definition, a phoria cannot be present simultaneously. Second, if there is no strabismus, search for a phoria using the cover-uncover and/or the alternating cover test. Finally, if you cannot see any phoria, perform a subjective cover test.

6.2.1 The evidence base: when and how to detect and assess strabismus and phoria

As the detection of strabismus and phoria is a fundamental part of any assessment of the binocular vision system, a cover-uncover test assessment should be part of every eye examination. It is used to detect these two conditions in the habitual state (i.e., with and/or without glasses in the pre-refraction part of the eye examination). A limitation of the cover test is that it requires a good view of your patient's eyes, so that it is not possible to accurately perform the test in a phoropter or trial frame with reduced aperture lenses. For this reason, when subjective refraction indicates that a non-strabismic patient's refractive correction has altered substantially, changes in the oculomotor status are typically estimated using subjective tests such as the modified Thorington or Maddox rod and wing tests (section 6.11) rather than using the cover test.

A limitation of the cover test is that even experienced clinicians cannot detect very small deviations (up to 2–3$^\Delta$).[6] Thus when no movements are detected on the objective test, the alternating cover test can also be run in a subjective fashion, where the patient is asked to say if the target being viewed appears to move when the cover is transferred from one eye to the other. The subjective test is particularly useful for identifying small vertical deviations, which can otherwise be missed and can cause significant visual problems.[5]

6.2.2 Procedure for the cover test

The online videos 6.1-6.10 show a variety of cover test movements with strabismus (exotropia, esotropia, hypertropia,

Box 6.1 Cover test procedure

Step 1: Check for strabismus.
Strabismus present (Y/N)?
Procedure: Cover one eye whilst observing fellow eye.

RE moves when LE covered	LE moves when RE covered	RE moves when LE covered and LE moves when RE covered	Neither eye moves when fellow eye covered
Dx. RE strabismus	Dx. LE strabismus	Dx. Alternating strabismus	Dx. No strabismus is present, now check for phoria

Step 2: If no strabismus is present, check for phoria.
Step 2a: Procedure: cover-uncover test.
Cover one eye, then observe that eye as it is uncovered.

Previously covered eye moves IN when cover is removed	Previously covered eye moves OUT when cover is removed	Previously covered eye moves UP when cover is removed	No movement seen when previously covered eye is uncovered
Dx. EXOphoria	Dx. ESOphoria	Dx: hypophoria of that eye[a] Previously covered eye moves DOWN when cover is removed Dx: hyperphoria of that eye[a]	Dx: No phoria present[b]

[a]Note that hyperphoria of one eye is equivalent to hypophoria in the other eye (i.e., R hyperphoria = L hypophoria; L hyperphoria = R hypophoria).
[b]Sometimes the eye moves when it is covered but it does not move back to retake fixation when the cover is removed. Thus, after the cover test, a strabismus is present. This is easily confused with 'no phoria present.'

Step 2b: Procedure: alternating cover test.
Observe each eye as it is uncovered when the cover is transferred to the fellow eye.

Eyes move IN when cover switched to fellow eye	Eyes move OUT when cover switched to fellow eye	Eyes move UP/DOWN when cover switched to fellow eye:	No movement seen when cover switched but Px. reports shift in apparent target position.	No movement seen when cover switched and Px. reports no shift in apparent target position when cover switched to fellow eye.
Dx. EXOphoria	Dx. ESOphoria	Dx. Vertical phoria (i) If R moves down and L moves up: Dx: R hyperphoria (ii) If R moves up and L moves down: Dx: L hyperphoria	Dx. Phoria present (WITH movement in EXOphoria, AGAINST in ESOphoria)	Dx. ORTHOphoria

Dx: diagnosis; Px. Patient. RE: right eye (or OD); LE: left eye (for OS)

---

alternating) and heterophoria (exophoria, esophoria, Hering's movements and Phi movements). Videos 6.11 and 6.12 show heterophoria measurement using a prism bar. A summary of the procedure is shown in Box 6.1.

1. Prior to performing the test, be aware of possible strabismus from indicators in other parts of the eye examination, which could include simple observation of your patient; symptoms of diplopia when tired; an ocular or family history of an eye turn, patching or strabismus surgery; premature birth; reduced visual acuity in one eye suggesting possible amblyopia, and strabismic risk factors such as anisometropic hyperopia.[7]

2. Similarly, be aware of possible signs and symptoms of decompensated heterophoria, such as symptoms of

blurred vision, headaches, or asthenopia at distance and/or near; poor reading ability (or reading avoidance); poor progress at school. It is important to note that a lack of symptoms does not mean that the binocular system is normal as the patient may have suppression.[8]

3. Keep the room lights on and, if necessary, use localised lighting so that you can see your patient's eyes easily without shadows.

4. Explain the purpose of the test to your patient: "I am now going to find out how well your eye muscles work together."

5. Use the following targets:

    (a) For the distance cover test, isolate a single letter of a size one line larger than the patient's worst visual acuity. For example, if monocular visual acuities are 105 VAR (6/4.8, 20/16 or 1.25) and 90 VAR (6/9.5, 20/32 or 0.63), use an 85 VAR letter (6/12, 20/40 or 0.50) as a target. The patient must be able to see the letter easily with both eyes, but it should be a target that requires accurate fixation and stable accommodation. If you cannot present an isolated letter, ask the patient to look at a letter at the end (or beginning) of a line. If the monocular visual acuity in either eye is 75 VAR (6/19, 20/63 or 0.32) or worse, use a spotlight for fixation.

    (b) For the near cover test, a fixation stick should be used that contains letters or pictures of various sizes (Fig. 6.1). A single letter of a size one line larger than the patient's near visual acuity of the poorer eye should be chosen. The fixation stick should be held at the patient's typical near working distance. This may be at an intermediate distance (e.g., 60 cm) if you wish to assess the binocular status at a distance corresponding to the distance from which the patient views a computer screen.

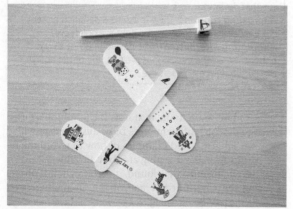

Fig. 6.1 Fixation sticks used for the near cover test and other tests requiring near fixation.

6. Sit directly in front of your patient, at a distance of 33–40 cm away, so that you are close enough to be able to critically note eye movements. Make sure you do not block the patient's view of the target.

    (a) For the distance cover test, make sure that the patient has their head held straight with the eyes in the primary position of gaze.

    (b) For the near cover test, make sure the patient's eyes are in a slight downward gaze to replicate their viewing position when reading.

7. Instruct your patient: "I would like you to look at the letter* at the other end of the room (or the letter * on this stick). If the letter moves when I cover one eye, please follow it and try to keep it as clear as possible at all times".

8. Perform the cover-uncover test to look for a strabismus (Box 6.1, Fig. 6.2):

    (a) Place the cover before the left eye and observe the right eye. Repeat this procedure two or three times. If the right eye moves when the left is covered, then a strabismus is present in the right eye. You should allow the eye time to take up fixation, which may be as long as 2–3 seconds. If the eye moves OUT to take up fixation, then in the binocular situation it must have been directed inwards and so an ESOtropia is present. If the eye moves IN to take up fixation, an EXOtropia is present. If the eye moves UP to take up fixation, then in the binocular situation it must have been directed downwards and so a HYPOtropia is present. If the eye moves DOWN to take up fixation, a HYPERtropia is present.

    (b) Repeat the cover-uncover test by placing the cover over the right eye and look for a strabismus in the left eye. Once again, repeat the procedure two or three times. If neither eye moves when the other is covered, there is no strabismus and you should go to step 8 below.

    (c) In a unilateral strabismus, when the deviating eye is covered and then uncovered, the 'normal' eye will continue to fixate and will not move. Reduced visual acuity (e.g., caused by amblyopia) will often be present when there is unilateral strabismus. For this reason, eyes with strabismus and amblyopia may not take up fixation immediately when the normal eye is covered, particularly if the visual acuity is poor in the deviating eye. Give them time to fixate and actively encourage them to do so. Note and record any fixation instability or tremor (nystagmus).

    (d) If strabismus was detected, repeat the test to confirm your diagnosis.

    (e) Estimate or measure the size of the strabismus. The lowest prism power that eliminates movement of the strabismic eye to take up fixation using the cover-uncover test indicates the strabismus size. The base direction should be IN for exotropia, OUT for esotropia, DOWN in front of a hypertropic eye, and

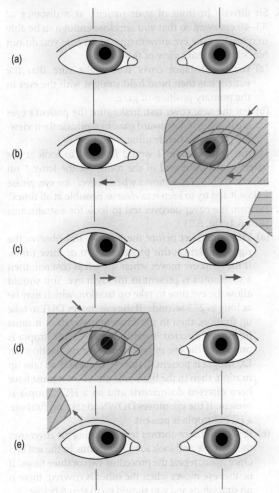

Fig. 6.2 Cover test in a patient with a right esotropia.(a) The right eye deviates inwards slightly, but this may not be obvious depending on its size and your experience. (b) As the left eye is covered, the right eye is seen to move out to take up fixation. Behind the cover, the left eye moves to the right, obeying Hering's law. (c) As the left eye is uncovered, it moves out to take up fixation as it is the non-strabismic eye. (d) When the right eye is covered, the left eye does not move. (e) When the right eye is uncovered, neither eye moves. (Reprinted with permission from Pickwell D. *Binocular Vision Anomalies*. Oxford: Butterworth-Heinemann; 1989.)

UP in front of a hypotropic eye. Although it does not matter which eye receives the prism, it is easier to place the prism in front of the fixating (i.e., the non-deviating) eye as you then have an unobstructed view of the movement of the strabismic eye.

(f) If a strabismus is present, it is not appropriate to search for a phoria. You should record your result

Table 6.1 Cover test strabismus diagnoses

Unilateral: the deviation (strabismus) is only ever present in one eye (e.g., esotropia of the right eye).	**Alternating:** the deviation can exist in either eye. Only one eye deviates, but it can be the right eye or the left eye.
Constant: the deviation is present all of the time.	**Intermittent:** The deviation is present only some of the time (e.g., an esotropia may appear only when the patient is tired).
Comitant: The size of the strabismus does not vary with the angle of gaze.	**Incomitant:** The size of the strabismus varies with the angle of gaze; the strabismus may only be present in one gaze direction or it may not be present in some gaze directions.
Distance: The strabismus is present when viewing distant targets (e.g., whilst watching TV).	**Near:** The strabismus is present when viewing near targets (e.g. when reading).
Affected by refractive correction: The presence and size of strabismus is not affected by the wearing of appropriate refractive correction.	**Not affected by refractive correction:** The presence and size of strabismus is affected by the wearing of appropriate refractive correction (e.g., the strabismus is smaller or absent altogether when spectacles are worn).

Unilateral constant: One eye deviates all of the time and it is always the same eye.
Unilateral intermittent: The deviation is only present some of the time. When it is present, it is always the same eye that deviates.
Alternating constant: There is always a deviation present but the deviating eye can be the right eye or left eye.
Alternating intermittent: The deviation is not always present. When the deviation is present, the deviating eye can be the right eye or left eye.

and move on to the next test. The terminology used to describe different types of strabismus is provided in Table 6.1, and examples of how to record the results from cover testing are given in Table 6.2.

9. If no strabismus was found, now search for phoria using the cover-uncover and/or the alternating cover test[1,5,8,9] (see Box 6.1, Fig. 6.2).

(a) Cover-uncover: Place the cover before the left eye and hold it there for ~2 seconds. Then remove the

Table 6.2 Examples of recordings from the cover test

Abbreviation	Description
With Rx: NMD @ D or N	No movement detected (hence deviation <2–3Δ) during distance and near viewing wearing appropriate refractive correction.
N without Rx: <3Δ SOP (Phi)	Unaided, at near, a small esophoria (<3Δ) is present but not seen; it is reported subjectively.
D with Rx: ~4Δ XOP	A small exophoria, estimated to be 4Δ, is present during distance viewing with appropriate refractive correction.
8Δ SOP @ N with Rx, slow rec.	An esophoria with slow recovery, measured to be 8Δ, is present on cover/uncover testing, during near viewing with appropriate refractive correction in place.
~4Δ R/L @ D & N, with and without Rx	Right hyperphoria, estimated to be 4Δ, is present during distance and near viewing. The deviation is unchanged by refractive correction.
Int (50%) ~10Δ RSOT @ N without Rx	Intermittent right esotropia is present about 50% of the time during near viewing without refractive correction and estimated to be 10Δ.
8Δ R hyper T @ D & N, with and without Rx	Constant right hypertropia, measured with a prism bar to be 8Δ, is present during distance and near viewing with and with refractive correction.
25Δ Alt XOT c̄ 4 R/L @D without Rx	Constant alternating exotropia of 25Δ with a much smaller vertical component (R hypertropia) during distance viewing without refractive correction.

cover and observe the response of the previously covered eye. If the eye changed its position when covered, the recovery movement of the eye will be opposite to that which took place behind the cover. For example, in EXOphoria the eye moves IN when the cover is removed as it drifted out (away from the nose) behind the cover. To confirm your observations, repeat the cover/uncover test by covering and uncovering the right eye. If there is a phoria, the movements seen on cover-uncover test will generally be very similar in magnitude irrespective of whether the right or left eye is covered.

(b) The alternating cover test: Place the occluder before one eye for 2–3 seconds and then transfer it quickly to the other eye. Again keep the occluder in front of the eye for 2–3 seconds and then repeat the cycle. The patient must not view the target binocularly at any time, and thus rapid movement of the cover between the eyes is required. If there is a deviation of the eyes, it will be seen as a re-fixation eye movement when the cover is transferred from one eye to the other. As with the cover-uncover test you are observing the recovery movements of the eyes and these are the opposite of the eye movements when they are covered so that the eyes will move outwards in esophoria and inwards in exophoria. It is important to stress that, unlike the cover-uncover test, the alternating cover test cannot distinguish between a phoria and a strabismus. Thus the pattern of eye movements on an alternating cover test will not differ between a patient with exophoria compared with a patient with exotropia. The advantage of the alternating cover test is that phoria movements are generally much more obvious compared with those seen during cover-uncover test. For this reason, whereas the cover-uncover test is used in all patients, the alternating cover test is only used in patients without a strabismus.

(c) Estimate or measure the magnitude of the phoria. Deviations can be measured by placing prisms of increasing power in front of one eye until no movement is observed during the alternating cover test. The prism is normally placed in front of one eye only. Base-in prism power is used to measure EXOphorias and base-out to measure ESOphorias. A prism bar is most conveniently used for this purpose, although estimates made by experienced clinicians can be in good agreement with measurements made using prism bars.[10]

(d) During a cover-uncover test in a patient with a phoria, observing the latency, speed, and smoothness of the fusional recovery movement can give clues as to the strength of the fusion reflex.[8] The movement should be smooth and fast. Poor fusion reflexes are slow and hesitant, often with jerky movements. Sometimes, although an eye has deviated behind the cover, there is no recovery when the cover is removed and a strabismus that was not there initially is now present (see Box 6.1). Note that the speed and smoothness of the movements seen during the alternating cover test hold little diagnostic value. This is because binocular vision is suspended during the alternating cover test. Judgements about the speed and smoothness of recovery are more valuable during the cover-uncover test because, unlike in the alternating cover test, the movements are taking place to restore binocular vision following the removal of the cover.

(e) **Subjective cover test and phi movements:** If, using the alternating cover test, you cannot detect any heterophoria and the patient can provide good subjective responses, continue to perform the alternating cover test and ask the patient if the target appears to move when the occluder is switched from one eye to the other. Subjectively reported movements of the target are called 'phi' (pronounced as 'fy' as in 'why') movements. The type of deviation present can be inferred according to whether the target appears to move in the same or opposite direction as the cover. For example, esophoria will cause the target to move 'against' the movement of the occluder and an exophoria will cause the target to move 'with' it. In 'with' movements: for example, when the cover is moved from the left eye to the right eye, the target is also seen to jump to the right. Extracting the direction of movement perceived by the patient can be difficult and it is best not to ask whether the movement was 'with' or 'against or to the left or right, as these are easily confused.' Instead, ask the patient to indicate to you whether the target moves towards you (the clinician) or in the opposite direction as you move the occluder.

6.2.3 Adaptations to the standard procedure

1. **When examining children:** Pictures can be used to retain attention, but they should be of an appropriate size. Pictures (or letters) that are too large do not provide an accurate stimulus for fixation or accommodation, which is important for an accurate cover test. In order to check compliance with your fixation instructions, occasionally it is useful to move the stick a little to one side. If the eyes are seen to follow the target, you can be confident that the patient is looking at the target.

2. **When examining older patients:** In presbyopic patients, cover testing needs to be conducted with their multifocal or varifocal lenses, and the target should be held in the correct location to ensure clear vision. Alternatively the appropriate correction should be provided by the phoropter or trial frame and trial case lenses. During near cover testing, it can sometimes be difficult to see an older patient's eyes because of drooping upper lids and the downward gaze needed to view the fixation target with multifocal spectacles. First, asking the patient to tilt their head back slightly may improve the visibility of their eyes. If the problem is owing to drooping upper lids, they may need to be gently held up. In this case, you should ask the patient to hold the fixation

stick. Finally, if it is otherwise not possible to see the patient's eyes sufficiently well, ask the patient to hold their multifocal spectacles up slightly and to view the fixation target with their head erect and looking straight ahead with their eyes in the primary position of gaze. In this case, you should note that the near cover test has been performed in primary gaze rather than the preferred, slight downward gaze.

3. **If a strabismus is suspected in a patient with equal visual acuity in the right and left eye:** (see online video 6.6). When visual acuity is the same or very similar in the two eyes, investigate the possibility of an alternating strabismus. With an alternating strabismus, the right eye will exhibit the strabismus when the left eye fixates during the cover test and the left eye will exhibit the strabismus when the right eye fixates. The difficulty with diagnosing an alternating strabismus is that the strabismus movement only occurs during the first run of the cover-uncover test. This is because the preciously deviating eye has now become the fixating eye. Thus, when the cover-uncover assessment is repeated a second and third time, the eye being observed does not move. In this scenario, the strabismus will become apparent again during the first cover-uncover assessment of the other eye. When asked to view binocularly after completion of the cover-uncover test, some patients with an alternating strabismus will continue to fixate with the eye that fixated the target during the last iteration of the cover test procedure. In some cases there is no preferred fixating eye, whereas in others, there is a definite preference for fixation with one eye over the other and, although the non-preferred eye might continue to fixate for a short period (e.g., a few seconds) after the cover has been removed, fixation then switches back to the preferred eye. Some patients with alternating strabismus can switch the eye that is fixating if you ask them, and some may even switch fixation as the occluder approaches the fixing eye, so that they can be very confusing to diagnose.

4. **In patients with an abnormal head posture (head turn or tilt):** Ask the patient to straighten their head position before testing commences. If the abnormal head position is a permanent feature for a particular patient, the cover test should be carried out with the head in the habitual (i.e., turned/tilted) position and again when the head is straightened. If the deviation differs markedly with adjustment of the head position, it is likely that the head is being turned/tilted to address an underlying binocular vision issue. This can be further investigated if the head is tilted/turned in the opposite direction to the direction that the patient typically exhibits. If the deviation becomes even more pronounced, an incomitancy is certainly present (section 6.16) and you can conclude that the abnormal

head posture is linked to a binocular vision condition rather than to another, non-visual cause.

6.2.4 Recording

Examples are given in Table 6.2.

1. Write 'cover test' or 'CT' and record separately for distance (D) and near (N).
2. Indicate the Rx, if any, the patient was wearing during testing.
3. Record NMD (no movement detected) if this was the case. NMD is preferred to 'orthophoria' or similar, as even experienced clinicians cannot detect eye movements less than 2–3[Δ,6].
4. Heterophorias found using the subjective cover test, but not seen by you, should be recorded in the usual manner and followed by the term 'phi'.
   If strabismus or phoria is detected, then record:
5. The size of the deviation (if estimated, precede your result with the symbol '~').
6. The laterality of the strabismus (right, left, or alternating recorded as R, L, or 'Alt'; Table 6.1).
7. The direction of the strabismus or phoria (Table 6.2).
8. The type of deviation using P for phoria and T for tropia.
9. If the tropia is intermittent rather than constant (Table 6.1), include an estimate of the percentage of time that the eye deviates.
10. Record phoria recovery movements on the cover-uncover test that were slow, hesitant, and/or jerky. This is of particular relevance when the heterophoria is large (i.e., when there is more chance it may be decompensated). Examples of cover test recordings are given in Table 6.2.

6.2.5 Interpreting the results

Hering's law states that the innervation to synergist muscles of the two eyes is equal. This would imply that the eyes would always move by equal amounts (in the same direction in version movements and in the opposite direction in vergence movements). The common cover test response, in which the fixating eye remains still and the previously covered eye, when the cover is withdrawn, moves to restore fusion thus contravenes Hering's law. Hering's law would predict that when one eye is uncovered, both eyes would make a version movement equal to half the deviation, and then both eyes would make an equal fusional (vergence) movement, to restore bifoveal fixation. This response does occur in some patients and it is important that it is not confused with heterotropic movements (Fig. 6.3). Note that heterotropic cover test movements are in one direction and take place when the cover is *introduced* to

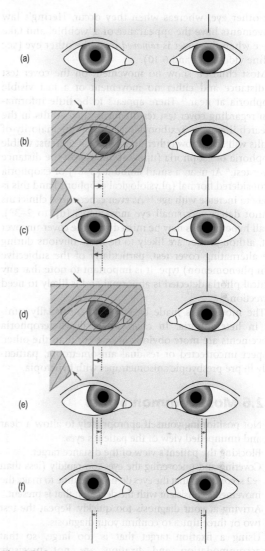

Fig. 6.3 Cover test in a patient with esophoria. (a) to (c) show the simple pattern of movements that are usually seen, and (d) to (f) show the more rare versional pattern of movements that can occur when one eye is dominant. (a) Both eyes look straight ahead. (b) The right eye is covered and the left eye does not move, indicating that there is no strabismus in the left eye. Behind the cover the right eye moves inwards. (c) The right eye is uncovered and the right eye moves out to resume fixation with the other eye. Note that during the movements of the right eye, the left eye has not moved, and disobeys Hering's law to maintain fixation. (d) The right eye is covered as before and it moves inwards behind the cover. (e) The right eye is uncovered and both eyes move to the patient's right by the same amount, obeying Hering's law. (f) Both eyes diverge by the same amount, again obeying Hering's law, and take up fixation. (Reprinted with permission from Pickwell D. *Binocular Vision Anomalies.* Oxford: Butterworth-Heinemann; 1989.)

the other eye, whereas when they occur, Hering's law movements have the appearance of a 'wobble' and take place when the cover is *removed* from the other eye (see online videos 6.7 and 6.10).

Most children show no movement on the cover test at distance and either no movement or a just visible exophoria at near.[11] There appears to be little information regarding cover test results for normal adults in the research literature. Textbooks suggest that the majority of adults will also show either no movement or a just visible exophoria or esophoria (up to about 4^Δ) on the distance cover test.[8] At near, a small amount ($3–6^\Delta$) of exophoria is considered normal (physiological exophoria) and this is likely to increase with age.[12] As even experienced clinicians cannot detect very small eye movements (up to $2–3^\Delta$), small hyperphorias may be missed with the cover-uncover test, although they are likely to be more obvious during the alternating cover test, particularly of the subjective (phi phenomenon) type. It is important to note that any vertical phoria detected is abnormal and is likely to need correction.[6]

The movements made by each eye are usually similar in heterophoria. In cases where the heterophoria movements are more obvious in one eye than the other, suspect uncorrected or residual anisometropia, particularly in pre-presbyopic anisometropes with hyperopia.

6.2.6 Most common errors

1. Not positioning yourself appropriately to allow a clear and unimpeded view of the patient's eyes.
2. Blocking the patient's view of the distance target.
3. Covering and uncovering the eyes too rapidly (less than ~2 seconds) so that the eyes do not have time to make the movements consistent with the deviation that is present.
4. Arriving at your diagnosis too quickly. Repeat the test two or three times to confirm your diagnosis.
5. Using a fixation target that is too large, so that accommodation and fixation are not precisely controlled.
6. Not moving the occluder in an appropriate fashion. For example, not swiftly transferring the cover from one eye to the other during an alternating cover test with the result that binocular vision is not fully suspended.
7. Mistaking a Hering's law movement for a strabismus (Fig. 6.3e and f).
8. Failing to record information about the speed and/or smoothness of recovery in patients with a heterophoria during cover-uncover test. Conversely, recording information about recovery in patients with strabismus.
9. Not realising that the cover test results can change dramatically when the viewing distance is altered (e.g., from distance to near) or whether or not glasses are worn.

6.3 Other tests for the detection and measurement of strabismus

6.3.1 The evidence base: when and how alternative tests for strabismus should be used

In very young children, who may be unable to maintain fixation for long enough to allow the cover test to be performed, other tests to detect and strabismus can be used. The Hirschberg test compares the position of the corneal reflexes of the two eyes. It is quick and easy to perform, and requires little co-operation on the part of the patient, but it can really only be performed at near and intermediate distances. The penlight target provides a poor stimulus to accommodation and the test is more useful for detecting the presence of strabismus than for measuring its size, with even experienced clinicians obtaining results that differ by up to 10 prism dioptres.[13] The Krimsky test extends the Hirschberg test by using prisms to equalise the apparent positions of the corneal reflexes in the two eyes, but is similarly inaccurate for measuring strabismus size.[13] The Bruckner test relies on a comparison of the brightness of the retinal reflex in the two eyes. In the presence of a strabismus the reflex can be brighter and whiter in the deviating eye compared with the reflex from the darkly pigmented macular area of a normally fixating eye (see online video 6.13). The test can be useful in identifying which is the strabismic eye but it is prone to false–positive findings,[14] indicating that a strabismus is present when it is not and hence the usefulness of the Bruckner test is controversial.[15,16] Given their limited accuracy, the cover test (section 6.2) should be used in preference to these tests as soon as the child can co-operate with the cover test requirements. The tests described in this section are typically performed without spectacles, although a comparison with and without spectacles can also be made, for example in patients with significant hyperopia.

6.3.2 Procedure: Hirschberg and Krimsky

(See online video 6.14).
1. Keep the room fully illuminated. Additional use of localised lighting is recommended so that the patient's eyes can be easily seen without shadows.
2. Hold a penlight horizontally 40 to 50 cm from the patient with the light directly in front of the patient's face and aimed at the bridge of the patient's nose. The back of the penlight should be very close to the tip of your nose so you are viewing from directly behind it.

3. Ask the patient to look at the light with both eyes open. Young children will automatically tend to look toward the bright light, but may need a little encouragement.
4. Note the location of the corneal reflex in each eye individually. To do this you should briefly cover each eye in turn; you can do this with the palm of your hand. Remember that the reflex is frequently decentred about 0.5 mm nasally with respect to the centre of the pupil because angle kappa is normally positive.[17]
5. Now compare the location of the corneal reflexes in the two eyes as the patient views the light with both eyes open. The eye that has the its corneal reflex in the same position as in the monocular test is the fixing eye. The location of that reflex should be considered the reference position.
6. If a strabismus is present, the corneal reflex of the other eye will have shifted in a direction opposite to the strabismus. For example, in the case of an ESOtropia, the corneal reflex will be displaced temporally on the patient's cornea relative to the position of the reflex in the fellow eye.
7. **Hirschberg:** Estimate the magnitude of the deviation from the displacement of the reflex in millimetres (mm) relative to the reference position using the approximation of 1 mm = $\sim$22$^\Delta$.
8. **Krimsky:** Use a prism bar in front of the fixating eye and vary the prism power to achieve symmetrical positioning of the reflexes in the two eyes.

6.3.3 Procedure: Bruckner test

▶ (See online video 6.13).
1. Turn down the lights so the room is dimly lit.
2. Hold a penlight 1 m from the patient with the light aimed at the bridge of the patient's nose. The back of the penlight should be very close to the tip of your nose.
3. Ask the patient to look at the light with both eyes open. Young children will automatically tend to look toward the bright light but may need a little encouragement.
4. Compare the colour and brightness of the fundus reflexes. Differences in the apparent brightness of the fundal reflexes can signal the presence of a strabismus.

6.3.4 Recording Hirschberg, Krimsky, and Bruckner test results

Note the test used, the eye that deviates, and the direction of the strabismus. For example:

Hirschberg @ 50 cm: No Strab; Hirschberg @ 50 cm §
Rx: $\sim$10$^\Delta$ RSOT; Krimsky @50cms: 15$^\Delta$ L XOT.
Bruckner @1 m: L SOT.

6.3.5 Interpreting Hirschberg, Krimsky, and Bruckner test results

For the Krimsky and Hirschberg tests, the displacement of the reflex indicates the type of strabismus: nasally displaced reflex indicates exotropia; temporally displaced indicates esotropia; superior displacement indicates hypotropia, and inferior displacement indicates hypertropia. In visually normal eyes, both corneal reflections are usually displaced slightly nasally relative to the pupil centres because of the separation between the pupillary and visual axes (quantified by angle kappa). Thus if there is a large angle kappa, it may result in the misdiagnosis of strabismus or failure to detect a strabismus. Interestingly, patients with exotropia appear to have higher angle kappa values when compared with those who are esotropic.[17] All of this raises questions about the reliability of the results of Hirschberg and Krimsky tests. For the Bruckner tests, any brightness difference may indicate the presence of at least a moderate sized strabismus, although the brightness difference gives no indication of its type or size. Also, when interpreting the results of the Bruckner test, remember that there are other causes of interocular brightness differences, including cataract and retinoblastoma.[18]

6.3.6 Most common errors using Hirschberg, Krimsky, and Bruckner tests

1. Hirschberg and Krimsky: Basing your decision on the absolute position of a single reflex relative to the pupil centre rather than on a comparison of the relative locations of the corneal reflexes in the two pupils.
2. Not viewing the patient's eyes from a position that is directly behind the penlight for the Hirschberg and Bruckner tests or from directly in front of the deviating eye in the case of the Krimsky test.
3. Placing too much trust on the sensitivity and accuracy of these tests.
4. For the Bruckner test, not realising that interocular differences in reflex brightness may be caused by factors other than strabismus.

6.4 Motility test: detection and assessment of incomitant strabismus

In a comitant strabismus the angle of deviation is constant in all directions of gaze, although it may differ in size (or in whether it is present at all) depending on whether the patient is viewing a near or distant target. In an incomitant strabismus, the angle of deviation varies with direction of gaze. Longstanding incomitancies tend to become more comitant as time passes owing to the process of contracture.[9]

An incomitancy can result from a paralysis, a paresis, or a mechanical restriction. In paralysis, the action of one muscle, or a group of extra-ocular muscles, is completely abolished, whereas in a paresis, the action of a muscle is impaired but not abolished. An incomitancy caused by mechanical restriction continues to exhibit the same restricted movement when assessed monocularly (i.e., with the fellow eye closed), whereas the movements of a paretic eye are more normal when assessed monocularly. It is on this basis that a paresis can be distinguished from mechanical restriction.

If there is a problem with an extra-ocular muscle, the angle of deviation is largest when the eyes are turned in the direction of maximum action of the affected muscle. For example, it there is a problem with an elevating eye muscle, this will be most apparent during the motility test when the patient is asked to look upwards. The size of the deviation can also vary with respect to the eye that is used to fixate. The primary angle of deviation is observed when the non-affected eye fixates. The secondary angle of deviation is observed when the affected eye fixates. A difference between the primary and secondary angles of deviation distinguishes a paralytic from a non-paralytic strabismus. The secondary angle is usually larger than the primary angle in recently acquired incomitancy.[7]

6.4.1 The evidence base: when and how to assess incomitancy

A test to detect and, where present, classify incomitant strabismus is part of all first eye examinations of a patient. It is typically part of the 'entrance tests' that are performed subsequent to case history and prior to refraction.[1] Congenital incomitant strabismus is caused by a developmental problem in the anatomy or functioning of one or more of the six extra-ocular muscles or their nerve supply. Acquired incomitant strabismus can occur from conditions such as diabetes, hypertension, multiple sclerosis, thyrotoxicosis, temporal arteritis, or tumour and can be the first sign of the underlying disease and it is therefore essential to distinguish recent-onset from long-standing incomitant strabismus.[19] Missing the signs of these conditions represents a significant cause of malpractice claims in the United States.[20] Signs and symptoms that can differentiate between new and old ocular muscle palsies are given in Table 6.3.

The motility test (or broad H test) is currently the simplest method of evaluating a deviation in the six diagnostic positions of gaze.[21] It is relatively quick and easy to perform and requires only a pen torch and an occluder.

Table 6.3 Signs and symptoms that can help to differentiate between an old and new ocular motor palsy

Sign/symptom	Long-standing	Recent-onset
Diplopia	Rare	Almost always present
Onset	Generally unknown	Usually sudden
Amblyopia	Common	Rare
Recent trauma?	Not usual	Common
Symptoms	Not usual	Common and extreme
Comitance	Spread of comitance may obscure original palsy	Always incomitant
Abnormal head posture	If present, well established and difficult to alter	Can be marked but easy to alter. Covering paretic eye eliminates problem
Past-pointing	Absent	Present
General health	Not usually a factor	Current health may be a significant issue

6.4.2 Procedure: motility test

See online videos 6.15–6.17 of the motility test being used to detect incomitant deviations.

1. Be attentive to the possibility of incomitant strabismus (particularly recent-onset) via indicators from the case history (see Table 6.3).

2. Keep the room lights on and illuminate the eyes without shadows. Explain the test to your patient: "This test checks whether all your eye muscles are working well to move your eyes together."

3. Ask the patient to remove their spectacles, if worn. Spectacles can make observation of the eyes more difficult, and the frame may hide the fixation target. In addition, in peripheral gaze, diplopia can be induced by the prismatic effect produced by anisometropic spectacles and the 'jack-in-the-box' effect of myopic spectacles, particularly with small, modern frames. Sit directly in front of the patient so that both eyes can be clearly viewed.

4. The target used is not critical as long as the patient can easily see it, although a penlight is particularly useful because it allows you to observe the corneal reflexes

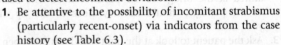

and it will indicate when the light has moved from the binocular field into the monocular field, when one of the corneal reflexes will disappear. A small picture on a fixation stick may be used when examining children.

5. Instruct your patient: "Please watch the light/picture and follow it with your eyes. Keep your head still. Tell me if the light/picture appears doubled at any time or if your eyes feel particularly uncomfortable or painful in any of the positions. Don't worry if the light/picture appears blurred." Patients sometimes mistake diplopia for blur so this can be a very important distinction to make in your instructions.

6. Shine the penlight at eye level towards the patient from a distance of approximately 40 cm. First ask the patient if the light appears single in the straight-ahead position. If it appears single, start to move it in an arc with the bridge of the patient's nose at the centre, so that as the light is moved, it continues to be aimed at the bridge of the nose. For each gaze direction, move the penlight to the edge of the binocular field. The loss of the corneal reflex will indicate to you that you have moved into the monocular field. Note that at the limits of movement, even those with normal ocular motility can feel uncomfortable and end-point nystagmus may be visible.

7. If a strabismus is present in the straight-ahead position, no diplopia may be reported in that gaze direction owing to strabismic suppression. This may mean that the patient will not report diplopia in any direction of gaze, even if there is marked incomitancy. In such situations, objective judgements about relative eye positioning are more important than the subjective responses from the patient.

8. Move the penlight into the six diagnostic positions of gaze by moving the target in a cross or broad H formation. Either type of movement is acceptable.[21] During downgaze, you may need to ask the patient to open their eyes widely or to hold up the patient's eyelids to gain a view of the eyes and corneal reflexes. Transfer the target/penlight from your left to your right hand when switching between the patient's right and left visual fields.

9. Carefully look for any misalignment of the eyes in all positions of gaze (the corneal reflexes can help you in this). Also determine whether the movements of the eyes are smooth and accurate (see pursuit eye movements, section 6.17).

10. If the eye movements were smooth and accurate with no reported diplopia, and both eyes appeared to the practitioner to track the moving target, the test is complete and the results can be recorded.

11. If, in one or more gaze directions, the two eyes appear not to be looking at the pen torch from your position directly in front of the patient, a useful tip is to switch

your viewing position to directly behind the pen torch as the patient looks in this gaze direction. This will enable you to ascertain whether both eyes are in fact looking at the light, and if not, which eye is not adopting the appropriate position.

12. Note and record the position of the eyes when any of the following occur:
    (a) The patient reports any diplopia.
    (b) The patient reports pain or discomfort in one or more positions of gaze that exceeded that experienced in other gaze directions.
    (c) Any underaction or overaction in one eye.
    (d) Jerky or inaccurate pursuit eye movements.
    (e) The size of the palpebral apertures differs between the right and left eyes and/or varies as a function of the direction of gaze.

13. Locate the gaze direction that yields the greatest diplopia because this indicates the field of action of the affected muscle(s). This can be difficult for some patients as similar separations of the doubled images may be reported in two or more directions of gaze.

14. Establish whether the doubled images are horizontally or diagonally separated. Pure horizontal diplopia does arise (e.g., along the horizontal meridian), but purely vertical diplopia does not arise because of the secondary actions of the elevating and depressing extra-ocular muscles.[7] Thus diagonal separation is found most commonly in cases where one (or more) of the oblique or vertical recti muscles is affected.

15. When diplopia is reported, briefly cover each eye in turn to identify which eye is seeing which image. When the eyes are elevated, the eye that sees the higher image is seen by the eye which is physically lower than in its fellow; if there is an underaction this is the eye with the underacting muscle. Alternatively, it could be that there is an overaction in which case the fellow eye has risen too high. Similarly, when the eyes are looking down, the eye seeing the lower image is seen by the eye with the underacting muscle if there is an underaction present; if not, the other eye has an overacting muscle and it has descended too far. Similarly, when the eyes are looking right or left, the eye that sees the image that is further to the right or left, respectively, represents the eye that has moved less from the primary position. A cover test (section 6.2) performed in this direction of gaze can be used to confirm the diagnosis.

16. If an incomitancy is observed, repeat the testing monocularly (assessment of ductions) to help discriminate between paretic and mechanical incomitancy.

6.4.3 Recording motility findings

If the ocular movements appear full and no diplopia is reported in any position, a normal result has been

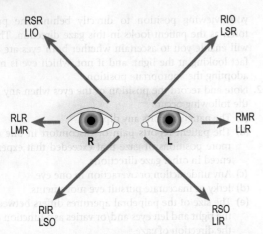

RSR
LIO

RIO
LSR

RLR
LMR

R

L

RMR
LLR

RIR
LSO

RSO
LIR

Fig. 6.4 The six cardinal diagnostic positions of gaze, showing the Yoke muscles that principally maintain the eyes in these positions. Assessment of motility in the vertical midline is necessary for the diagnosis of conditions such as A and V patterns. The three diagnostic positions on the midline supplement the six positions of fixation demonstrated in the figure. R = right eye, L = left eye; LR = lateral rectus, MR = medial rectus, IR = inferior rectus, SR = superior rectus, SO = superior oblique and IO = inferior oblique.

obtained and may be recorded using the acronym SAFE (or FESA). This indicates that the ocular motility movements were (S) Smooth, (A) Accurate, (F) Full, and (E) Extensive. For a patient with strabismus, normal motility can be recorded as 'no incomitancy detected' if the size of the strabismus did not change objectively in different directions of gaze.

In cases where you detect an incomitancy or where diplopia is reported by the patient in some directions of gaze, but not others (or more in some than in others), record a cross/H-pattern to clearly indicate where diplopia was indicated by the patient and where it was maximal. Fig. 6.4 shows the six cardinal diagnostic positions of gaze, showing the Yoke muscles that principally maintain the eyes in these positions. Record any apparent underactions or overactions, clearly stating which eye and in which gaze direction this was observed. Increasingly, incomitancies are recorded using a 9-point scale.[22] Using this system, overactions and underactions are recorded on a basic template in the primary field of action of each muscle. Underactions are recorded as negative numbers on a scale from −1 to −4, where −4 represents the greatest underaction. Similarly, overactions are recorded using positive numbers on a scale from +1 to +4, where +4 represents greatest overaction. For example, underactions that are scored as −4 indicate that the eye is unable to move at all into the primary position into the field of action of that muscle. Overaction of a horizontal rectus muscle is graded

according to the amount of cornea covered by the canthus; in extreme overaction (+4), half of the cornea is concealed. This diagrammatic representation also provides a useful way of signalling the presence of an A or V pattern, restrictions of movements as well as other ocular movement abnormalities (e.g., up- and down-drifts, up- and down-shoots).[22]

If a head tilt/turn is present, it should be noted and you may find it useful to perform the motility in the head-straight and head-tilted/turned conditions so that the results can be compared. The movements observed during a motility test may conform to one of the so-called alphabet patterns.[7] For example, if the deviation is significantly (>15Δ) more convergent (i.e., more eso or less exo) in upgaze than in downgaze, this is referred to as an A-pattern. Similarly, the term V-pattern describes a situation where the deviation is significantly more divergent (i.e., more exo or less eso) in upgaze than in downgaze. Note that incomitancies of this nature do not always conform strictly to the A and V patterns. For example, some patterns may be more correctly described as Y- or inverted Y-patterns.

6.4.4 Interpreting motility results

The results of motility testing are relatively straightforward to interpret if there is a problem with the lateral or medial rectus muscles. A movement to the patient's right along the horizontal meridian will examine the right lateral rectus and left medial rectus. Eye movements to the patient's left will assess their left lateral rectus and right medial rectus.

The clinical interpretation of motility test results is more complicated when diplopia is experienced on upwards or downwards gaze, because there are four extraocular muscles that help to elevate (the right superior rectus, RSR; left superior rectus, LSR; right inferior oblique, RIO; and left inferior oblique, LIO) and four that depress the eyes (the right inferior rectus, RIR; left inferior rectus, LIR; right superior oblique, RSO; and left superior oblique, LSO). By having the patient look in the various directions of gaze, a clinical determination of affected muscle(s) can be made because the eyes will appear most misaligned (and the diplopia noticed by the patient will be maximal) when the eyes move into the field of action of the affected muscle. Diplopia experienced in peripheral gaze can be caused by an underaction or overaction of one or more muscles. An underaction could be caused by a mechanical restriction or a muscle palsy/paralysis. An overaction will occur in the non-paretic eye if the paretic eye is fixating the target.

Duction (monocular) testing (step 16) helps to differentiate between an incomitant deviation owing to paresis/paralysis (underactions are less obvious monocularly) and one caused by mechanical restriction (underactions are similar monocularly and binocularly). To aid or confirm a diagnosis of an underaction/overaction, or to measure the extent of the deviation and to assess the degree of incomitancy, further tests such as the 9-point cover test are required (section 6.16).

6.4.5 Most common errors with motility testing

1. Allowing the patient to turn their head towards the target. The head should remain in the straight-ahead position so as to fully test the ocular motility.
2. Not using a penlight. This makes it difficult to determine when the target is entering the monocular field.
3. Relying too much on the patient to report doubling and not paying enough attention to symmetry of corneal reflexes and the appearance of the relative positioning of the eyes.
4. Moving the target too quickly or too slowly.
5. Moving the target in a straight line rather than an arc, so that increasing unequal angular demands are made of the two eyes as the target is moved into a peripheral position of gaze.
6. Not elevating the top eyelid when viewing the eye movements in downgaze.

6.5 Convergence assessment: near point of convergence

The near point of convergence (NPC) is the point where the visual axes intersect under the maximum effort of convergence, whilst still maintaining binocular single vision.

6.5.1 The evidence base: when and how to measure NPC

NPC is often included in the 'entrance tests' of a typical eye examination[1] as part of the assessment of the binocular vision system. The test determines convergence ability in the patient's habitual state (i.e., with their glasses if worn). It is used with cover test results to screen for convergence insufficiency, which has a relatively high prevalence,[23] and is a treatable condition.[23–25] Note that a lack of symptoms does not in itself indicate good convergence because a remote NPC can be associated with suppression or with the avoidance of near work.

The NPC is a quick and easy test to perform. It requires no special equipment and it provides a very repeatable result.[26] It is the standard test for convergence ability and it provides both subjective and objective information. In patients who are presbyopic the choice of target does not seem important, but in those who are pre-presbyopic there may be a difference in NPCs measured with accommodative and non-accommodative targets.[27–29] Although such differences may not be clinically significant in patients with normal vision, Scheiman et al. suggest that individuals with convergence insufficiency show more remote break and recovery NPCs with a penlight compared with when an accommodative target is used.[27] The NPC can be measured without glasses or with the distance or near correction, depending on when symptoms occur.

6.5.2 Procedure: NPC

(See online video 6.18).

1. Seat the patient comfortably with their head erect and eyes in a slightly downward gaze. Sit directly in front of the patient so that you have a clear view of the two eyes.
2. Keep the room lights on. If necessary, position additional lighting to illuminate the patient's eyes and/or the target without causing glare.
3. Explain the measurement to the patient: "This test determines how well your eyes can turn in to follow a close object."
4. Position the target at a distance of ~50 cm directly in front of the patient slightly below the midline. A target with fine detail should be avoided because otherwise patients (particularly presbyopes) often confuse blur with diplopia. In adults, the tip of a pen can be used. A medium sized, coloured picture on a fixation stick can be used with children.
5. Instruct your patient: "Please keep looking at the pen/picture as I move it towards your eyes. Let me know as soon as it becomes doubled—not blurred but doubled. Try really hard to keep it single. Don't worry if you feel your eyes pulling."
6. Make sure that the patient is looking at the target with both eyes. It can be useful to move the target to the side slightly to check that the patient is maintaining fixation.
7. Slowly but steadily move the target towards the bridge of the patient's nose. The speed should be such that it takes 5–10 seconds to move the target from 50 cm to the bridge of the patient's nose.
8. Observe the patient's eyes for loss of convergence. Measure the distance the target is from the eyes when one of the eyes loses fixation by flicking outwards (objective NPC) and/or the patient reports diplopia (subjective NPC).
9. If the target becomes doubled (subjective NPC) more than 10 cm from the bridge of the nose, encourage the patient to make an extra effort to make the target single again. Moving it away slightly will help this before the target is again moved towards the patient.

When single binocular vision is re-established, advance the target again towards the patient.

10. If a patient reports diplopia at 7 cm or above[30] yet both eyes appear to be converging to the target, the patient may be confusing diplopia with blur. Check this by covering one eye and asking the patient if the target is still double. Continue to move the target in until the objective NPC is found.

11. Once the NPC has been reached, slowly move the target away from the patient's eyes and ask when the target becomes single again. Measure this point and record it as the recovery NPC point. Repeat the test. If the patient can keep the target single to their nose, this is recorded as 'to nose' and thus a recovery point is not measured.

12. If the history indicates that the patient requires prolonged and/or excessive convergence in a specific position of gaze, repeat the procedure under those circumstances.

6.5.3 Recording NPC

NPC: Record the break and recovery NPC points in centimetres from the bridge of the nose. Record the break point first, followed by the recovery point. Distinguish between objective and subjective NPC measures. Examples are given in Table 6.4. If the subjective NPC is much larger than the objective NPC, it is likely that the patient has confused blurring with diplopia and the objective NPC should be recorded. If the patient reports that the target is still seen singly when the eyes are seen to be misaligned, suspect suppression and investigate further.

6.5.4 Interpreting NPC results

Normative NPC values show considerable variation between studies. One source of variation arises from the fact that, although some patients *can* converge, they may not do so on clinical testing.[3] This makes it important not to overinterpret one abnormal test result and to consider results in combination (section 6.18). Scheiman et al. suggest a clinical cut-off value of 5 cm for the NPC break and 7 cm for the NPC recovery with either an accommodative target or a penlight in children and adults.[27] Children and adults should be able to converge to within about 7.5 cm and recovery should return within 10.5 cm.[31] A recent study in children by Menjivar et al. recommends an NPC-break cut-off of 7 cm or above as potentially problematic.[30] Thus NPC values 7 cm or above suggest possible convergence insufficiency and should be investigated further. This investigation should include jump convergence[8,9], distance and near heterophoria (sections 6.2 and 6.11), near fusional reserves (section 6.12), and near fixation disparity (section 6.13). Given the reported high prevalence of accommodative insufficiency in children with convergence insufficiency, tests of accommodation should also be conducted in these patients.[31] The effect of correcting refractive error on convergence ability should be assessed.

Instead of a failure of the eyes to converge, it is possible that diplopia will be reported because of overconvergence. This is rarely encountered, but when it does arise it suggests that the patient may have an abnormally high accommodative convergence to accommodation (AC/A) ratio (section 6.14) or significant uncorrected hyperopia. This should be recorded, and additional investigations should be carried out.

6.5.5 Most common errors (NPC)

1. Relying on *subjective* NPC measures. Objective estimates should also be gained from careful observation of the eyes as they converge.
2. Carrying out the test once only; the test should be carried out at least twice to gain an impression of sustained and repeated convergence ability.
3. Moving the target too rapidly can lead to overestimation of convergence ability. Moving the target too slowly could cause the patient to lose interest. This is particularly true in children, especially if the target does not capture the child's attention.
4. Not encouraging the patient enough to keep the NPC target single (particularly in children).
5. Testing the eyes in primary gaze instead of slight downward gaze.
6. Testing individuals who have a strabismus at near.

Table 6.4 Examples of recordings of the near point of convergence (NPC)

Abbreviation	Description
NPC: 6 cm/9 cm	A break point of 6 cm and recovery point of 9 cm (normal convergence).
(Obj.) NPC: 5 cm/8 cm	Objective NPC recording of a 5 cm break point and 8 cm recovery point.
NPC: to nose	Normal convergence to the nose.
NPC: 12 cm/ 16 cm, RE diverges	Abnormal convergence, with 12 cm break and 16 cm recovery points. The right eye moves out at the break point.
NPC: 14 cm/ 18 cm, LE diverges, no diplopia, suppression	Abnormal convergence with likely suppression. The break point is 14 cm and the recovery point is 18 cm. The left eye moves out at the break point, but no diplopia is reported.

6.6 Suppression testing: worth 4-Dot and mallett test

Suppression testing provides an indication of whether the patient is capable of fusing the images from the right and left eyes, thus meeting the conditions necessary for stereopsis, the highest level of binocularity (section 6.7). Suppression takes place to avoid diplopia and is associated with a variety of conditions including aniseikonia, anisometropia, amblyopia, strabismus, and unilateral eye disease.

6.6.1 The evidence base: when and how to measure suppression

The Worth 4-dot test, which is often included in the 'entrance tests' of a typical eye examination[1] as part of the assessment of the binocular vision system, determines the presence of suppression in the patient's habitual state (i.e., with their glasses if worn).

The Worth 4-dot test is widely available and relatively cheap; it easy to use and can be used to assess fusion or reveal suppression at distance and near. It provides a rather imprecise indication of whether or not suppression is present, because a patient with unstable but functionally useful binocular vision may exhibit a suppression response on the test.[7] Similarly, Worth 4-dot testing at near may incorrectly suggest that no suppression is present because of the large angular size of the lights when viewed at near.[9] A major disadvantage of the test is that luminance of the red and green targets can vary widely between tests, as can the transmission characteristics of the red and green goggles, with the result that the test outcome can vary depending on whether the goggles are used in the standard format (red goggle in front of the right eye) or reversed.[32] Another disadvantage of the test is that a patient with constant strabismus and abnormal retinal correspondence might achieve a normal result. For these reasons, a positive test result does not guarantee normal binocular vision. Because of this, the test result is only useful when considered alongside cover test results (section 6.2).[7] Another test of suppression is provided by the Mallett unit which uses Polaroid filters to provide different information to the two eyes, although this equipment is primarily used to assess fixation disparity at distance and near (section 6.13).

6.6.2 Preparation for suppression test

1. Prior to performing a suppression test, be aware of possible suppression associated with conditions such as anisometropia, amblyopia, strabismus, unilateral eye disease, reduced visual acuity in one eye, no diplopia reported during NPC testing despite an objective failure to converge, and so on.

2. Explain the test to your patient: "This test checks whether you are using both eyes at the same time to see."

6.6.3 Worth 4-dot procedure

3. Do not allow the patient to see the 4-dot stimulus before putting on the red–green spectacles. Place the red–green spectacles on the patient (over their spectacles if worn for that particular test distance). Except in cases where the test is presented on a computer screen, the eye with the red filter in front of it (usually the right eye) will see the red dots and the eye with the green filter in front of it (usually the left eye) will see the green dots. When presented on a computer screen, the eye wearing the red filter will see the green dots, and vice versa. You need to be aware of which eye is seeing which dots in order to be able to interpret an abnormal test result (Fig. 6.5).
   (a) For testing at 6 m: Ensure that the patient is wearing their distance refractive correction.
   (b) For testing at 40 cm, hold the Worth 4-dot torch/flashlight at the patient's reading position, so that the patient looks slightly downward at it. In the case of patients who are presbyopic, ensure that the patient wears appropriate refractive correction for the near test distance. The torch is usually held with the red light at the top and white light at the bottom (see Fig. 6.5).
4. Keeping the room lights on, turn on the Worth 4-dot instrument.
5. Ask the patient: "How many dots do you see?"

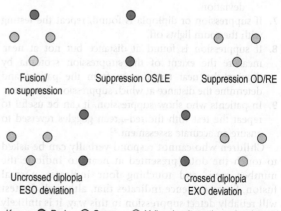

Fusion/ no suppression   Suppression OS/LE   Suppression OD/RE

Uncrossed diplopia ESO deviation   Crossed diplopia EXO deviation

Key: ● Red ○ Green ○ Yellow (or alternating red and green)

Fig. 6.5 Possible patient responses to the Worth 4-dot test.

6. There are four possible responses (see Fig. 6.5).

   (a) '4 dots seen.' This generally indicates that the patient has normal fusion and no suppression. The response can be checked by asking "How many red dots do you see?" "How many green ones?" Normally, patients will see one red, two green, and one white/yellow dot. The white dot may appear yellow, or alternate between red and green owing to retinal rivalry.

   (b) '2 dots seen.' These will be the red and white dots, seen by the patient as two red dots. This indicates suppression of the eye with the green filter in front of it (usually the left eye). To detect alternating and/or intermittent suppression ask: "Is the number of dots changing as you look at them?" If the number of dots seen is constant, check to see if fusion can be achieved by briefly occluding the non-suppressed eye.

   (c) '3 dots seen.' These will be the two green dots and the white dot, seen by the patient as three green dots. This indicates suppression of the eye with the red filter in front of it (usually the right eye). Again, to detect alternating and/or intermittent suppression ask: "Is the number of dots changing as you look at them?" If the number of dots seen is constant, check to see if fusion can be achieved by briefly occluding the non-suppressed eye.

   (d) '5 dots seen.' This indicates diplopia. The right eye (usually with the red filter) will see two red dots. The left eye (with the green filter) will see three green dots. Ask the patient to indicate where the red dots are in relation to the green ones. If the red dots (usually seen by the right eye) are to the right of the green dots, this indicates uncrossed diplopia and an eso deviation. If the red dots are to the left of the green dots, this indicates crossed diplopia and an exo deviation. If the red dots are above or below the green dots, this signals the presence of a vertical deviation.

7. If suppression or diplopia is found, repeat the testing with the room lights off.

8. If suppression is found at distance but not at near, measure the extent of the suppression scotoma by moving the near target away from the patient and determine the distance at which suppression first occurs.

9. In patients who show suppression, it can be useful to repeat the test with the red–green goggles reversed to ensure an accurate assessment.[32]

   Children who cannot respond verbally can be asked to touch the dots (presented at near) to indicate the number seen, and touching four indicates normal fusion. Some evidence indicates that, although the test will reliably detect suppression in this way, it is unlikely to differentiate between normal fusion and alternating fixation.[33]

6.6.4 Procedure: Mallett unit suppression testing

3. Do not allow the patient to see the Mallett unit until the Polaroid filters are worn over the eyes. The filters should be placed over any spectacles worn for that particular test distance.

4. For distance testing, suppression is present if the two monocular markers are not simultaneously visible to the patient. Cover each eye in turn and ask the patient to confirm seeing one of the markers (the red lines that are above and below the X of the OXO, section 6.13; Fig. 6.6). Then, with the eyes uncovered, ask the patient how many lines they can see. If two lines are not seen, it can be helpful to occlude the non-suppressed eye briefly. Occasionally, the patient will perceive two lines following this brief occlusion.

5. For near viewing, the same procedure is used. The patient should wear near correction, if appropriate. Now the monocular markers are green. In addition to the markers, one of the displays on the wheel of the near unit contains letters of different sizes. Whilst viewing through the polaroid filters, some letters are seen only by the right eye, some are seen only by the left eye, and the remainder are visible to both eyes. Thus if the patient reads all of the letters there is no suppression. The small letters provide a more detailed check on suppression than that offered by the markers. If one eye is suppressed the letters presented only to that eye will be omitted from the patient's verbal reading of the letters. The clinician needs to be familiar with the letters that are presented to each eye and to both eyes. The letters on the left side of each line are presented to the left eye, those near the end of the line are visible only to the right eye, and those in the middle

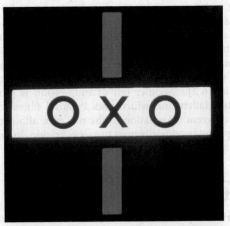

Fig. 6.6 A distance Mallett fixation disparity target.

are presented to both eyes. In cases of mild suppression, the patient may read the larger letters but begin to omit letters on the smaller lines.

6.6.5 Recording suppression results

For the Worth 4-dot test, record the normal perception of four dots at 6 m and 40 cm as: 'W 4-dot: 4-dots seen, DV and NV' or similar. If suppression is found, indicate which eye was being suppressed and whether the suppression is continuous or intermittent. Indicate whether suppression was found at both distance and/or near, in both light and dark room conditions. Indicate whether the evidence of suppression was intermittent or constant. If diplopia is found, indicate the direction of deviation suggested.

For the Mallett-unit suppression test with the monocular markers, it is only necessary to record the presence of suppression when it interferes with fixation disparity assessment (section 6.13).

For the letter suppression test on the near Mallett unit, record 'no suppression' if all letters were read. If letters were suppressed, record for example 'suppression of RE on lowest two lines' or, for example, 'all RE letters suppressed.'

6.6.6 Interpreting the results of suppression tests

If a patient without strabismus sees all four dots on the Worth dot test, this is a normal test result. Note that absence of suppression does not mean that binocularity is necessarily normal. If a patient with strabismus sees four dots with the test, then this indicates that they have abnormal retinal correspondence (ARC). If the response is suppression of the right eye (i.e., the response is 'three green dots') or suppression of the left eye (i.e., the response is 'two red dots') (see Fig. 6.5), then there is a suppression scotoma larger than the angular subtense of one of the four dots. Because the dots on the distance target have a smaller angular subtense than those on the near target, suppression is found more frequently for distance viewing than for near. If the patient achieves fusion in the dark but not in the light, this indicates a shallower level of suppression as compared with the situation where suppression is present in both the dark- and light-room conditions.

The monocular markers on the Mallett unit provide a fairly gross test of suppression, meaning that if both markers cannot be perceived simultaneously, there is marked suppression. The letters on the near unit offer a more fine-grained check of suppression, although a disadvantage is that there is no quantitative scale to record the depth of suppression. One possible outcome is for larger letters to be perceived by both eyes but for the smaller letters to be suppressed by one eye. However, this is a fairly unusual result as suppression tends to be either present or absent.

6.6.7 Most common errors with suppression tests

1. Not performing the tests with the patient's optimal refractive correction in place.
2. Asking the patient the leading question "Can you see four dots?" (Worth 4-dot test) or "Can you see the two lines?" (Mallett unit).

6.7 Stereopsis

The fundamental characteristic of binocular vision in humans is stereoscopic vision. The two eyes receive slightly disparate views of objects owing to being separated horizontally by around 6 cm and this disparity can be used to signal the relative depth of objects. Any obstacle to normal visual development early in life will have consequences for the level of stereoacuity attained, so that stereopsis is typically not measurable in patients with strabismus and is either extremely poor or absent in patients with amblyopia. Other vision disorders (e.g., significant refractive error) are also associated with significantly worse stereoacuity in preschool children and the more severe the disorder, the greater the impact on stereopsis.[34]

6.7.1 The evidence base: when and how to measure stereopsis

Stereopsis is often included in the 'entrance tests' of a typical eye examination[1] in children because the presence of stereopsis strongly suggests roughly equal and good visual acuity at near in the two eyes and the absence of strabismus and/or amblyopia.[34,35] However, stereopsis testing has an important role to play in the visual assessment of all age groups (section 3.11). There is growing evidence, for example, that stereoacuity levels are linked to the level of fine motor skills.[36]

Distant stereoacuity tests, such as the Frisby-Davis Distance test and Distant Randot test,[37] are not in common clinical use and are not discussed here. The TNO, Fly, Randot graded-circles, and Randot Pre-school tests may be difficult to use with young children because they may not be happy to wear goggles, although children from the age of about 3 years can usually be tested.[34,38] For younger children (6 months to 4 years) it is best to use tests that do not require goggles to be worn, such as the Frisby test, or if this test cannot be used, the Lang test.[39] The Frisby test has the advantage that it provides the only test of real depth; all of the others create depth effects by artificial means; for this reason the Frisby is popular amongst many clinicians. Its drawback (monocular clues to depth) can be minimised with careful administration of the test.

The main advantage of the TNO test is that monocular cues are completely eliminated. The patient is required to describe the shape of the raised figure and because this shape is only seen if stereopsis is present there is no possibility of 'cheating' so you can be certain that stereopsis is present if the correct answers are given. The same is not necessarily true for the other tests because of monocular cues (e.g., Titmus Fly, Randot Circles test) and/or because head tilts or viewing from an oblique angle (e.g., Frisby) can help the patient to achieve a result that is not reflective of the genuine presence of stereopsis. However, by carefully following the correct procedures, this drawback should not be critical for the non-TNO stereotests. A disadvantage of the TNO is that the transmission characteristics of the red and green lenses may lead to different contrast levels being experienced by the patient.[32] In some patients this can lead to a different test result depending on which way the goggles are worn (i.e., red before right eye or green before right eye).[32] The Stereo Fly test is popular with children, although the Fly can frighten nervous or timid youngsters. The Randot graded-circles and Randot Pre-school tests operate on the same principle as the Fly test in that they use Polaroid spectacles to provide the disparate stimuli. Even when the polaroid spectacles are worn, a monocular, alert patient could identify which is the 'odd one out' by observing which of the circles is slightly displaced from the centre see (Fig. 6.7).[40] This disadvantage can be overcome to some extent by asking the patient, carefully and without leading them, what is odd about the target they selected, or whether the target seen in depth lies in front of or behind the other animals/circles. The target seen in depth is usually seen in front of the others, but by turning the book

upside-down the target in depth is seen behind the other animals/circles. Other more recent versions of polaroid-based stereo tests include the Randot graded-circles and the Randot Pre-school tests.[41] These tests have the advantage that they feature at least some material which, like the TNO, is constructed on a random dot principle, and thus which requires stereopsis in order to be able to detect the depth effects. The newer Randot Pre-school test has the added advantage that it has been validated on large sample sizes.[41]

6.7.2 Procedure: TNO stereo test

This test works using a random-dot principle and red-green goggles.

1. Explain the test to your patient: "I am now going to test your 3-D vision." Place the red-green goggles over the patient's habitual correction. For patients who are presbyopic, appropriate near correction should be worn.
2. Hold the booklet at about 40 cm, angled to be parallel to the plane of the patient's face.
3. Keep the room lights on. Additional lighting over the patient's shoulder can be used to illuminate the booklet if required.
4. For a general screening test, the first four plates are useful because the disparity is large and provides a qualitative assessment of stereopsis. If the patient has a short attention span, it is advisable to present Plate III alone because this gives a good early qualitative indication if stereopsis is present. Find out if the following images can be seen:

   Plate I: In this plate there are two butterflies, one can be seen monocularly, whereas the other can be

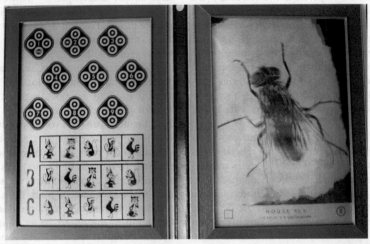

Fig. 6.7 The Titmus stereopsis test. Notice that monocular cues provide the correct answers for some of the tests (compare this with other stereotests in Figures 6.8–6.11).

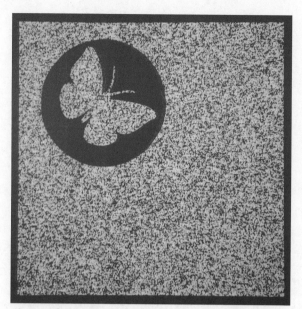

Fig. 6.8 The butterfly plate from the TNO stereo test. One butterfly is shown in the figure and is seen monocularly. There is another butterfly that can only be seen with stereopsis through the red and green goggles.

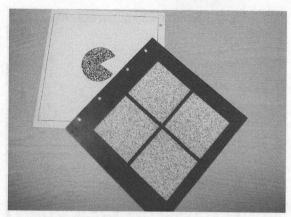

Fig. 6.9 TNO stereo plates in which the patient has to indicate whether the 'missing pizza slice,' 'missing cake slice,' or 'Pac-man mouth' is pointing up, down, or to the right or left. The disparities range from 15" to 480".

seen only if stereopsis is present (Fig. 6.8). Ask the patient: "How many butterflies can you find on this page?" and "Can you point to them?"

Plate II: There are four discs and two can be seen without stereopsis. Ask the patient: "How many circles do you see?" and then "Which is the biggest?"

Plate III: Four 'hidden' shapes (circle, square, triangle, and diamond) are arranged around a central cross that is visible without stereopsis. Ask the patient: "Can you find a cross/square/triangle/circle/diamond? Can you point to it?" This plate is very useful with children, because they like to find and name shapes. You will need to remember the correct locations of the shapes in order to verify the accuracy of their responses because they are only visible with the goggles.

Plate IV: This is a suppression test and consists of three discs. When viewed through the goggles, one disc is seen only with the right eye, one is seen only by the left eye, and one is seen binocularly. Ask the patient: "How many circles can you see on this page?"

Plates V to VII: These plates present disparities from 480 to 15 seconds of arc. At each disparity level, two discs with a sector missing are presented in different orientations (Fig. 6.9). Using the demonstration on the left of the display, ask the patient: "In each of these squares there is a cake

with a piece missing. Can you find the cake and point to the piece that is missing?"

5. If the patient is hesitant about an answer, allow them plenty of time to view the test plate. If only one of the two tests for each stereo level is called correctly, allow them a second attempt at the incorrect one, but if called incorrectly again, or if the patient does not volunteer an answer, record the result as the previous correctly identified stereo level.

6. Record the test (TNO) and the patient's stereoacuity in seconds of arc.

7. In patients achieving a poor test result, it can be useful to repeat the test with the red-green goggles reversed to ensure that stereoacuity is not underestimated.

6.7.3 Procedure: the Frisby test

The Frisby test is a test of sensitivity to real depth using perspex sheets containing contoured figures (Fig. 6.10). One element of the contour that is the shape of a circle is printed on one side of the sheet, whereas the remainder are printed on the opposite side. The thickness of the plate thus generates the real depth effect. No goggles are needed and the patient has to select the square that contains the circle in depth.

1. Explain the test to your patient: "I am now going to test your 3-D vision." In the case of younger children you could say "We are going to play a game where you have to find the ball."

2. In patients who are presbyopic, the test should be properly positioned for near-point viewing and appropriate near correction should be worn.

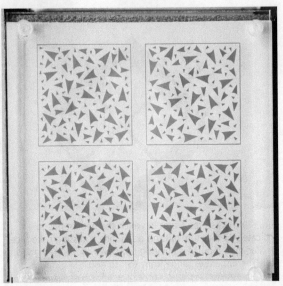

Fig. 6.10 One of the Frisby plates. The faint dark areas in the background are shadows produced by the photographic flash.

3. Keep the room lights on. Additional lighting over the patient's shoulder can be used to illuminate the test, if required, but make sure there are no reflections from overhead or any additional light sources from the perspex plates because these could interfere with the visibility of the target.

4. Hold the thickest of the three perspex plates (6 mm) a distance of 40 cm from the patient and angled so that it is parallel to the plane of the patient's face. The sheet should be held against the white background card that is part of the box provided with the test. Because monocular cues can be provided with movement of the plate or of the patient's head it is very important that the plate is displayed squarely and the patient's head kept still to minimise parallax effects.

5. Ask the patient to point to the square that is the 'odd one out' (older children and adults) or 'to point to the square that contains the ball'. If the patient answers correctly, you should ask why it's the odd one out; the patient may volunteer at this point, that they can see a 'shape' or a 'ball' or a 'circle'. To establish that they are seeing in depth, you should ask if the ball is in front or behind the rest of the 'pattern' or 'background' or 'picture'. All of this additional information, if provided, is very positive and strongly suggests that the patient is seeing real depth.

6. You can tell which is the correct plate by using your sense of touch. One of the buttons at the four corners has a flat top and this signals the location of the circle, and the side (front/back) of the Perspex on which the

circle is printed.[42] This avoids having to look at the sheet to tell if the response was correct. Encouraging the patient (especially children) is a useful way to ensure continued co-operation and thus to gain a reliable measure of the stereoacuity.

7. Repeat step 5 whether or not the response was correct. With the thickest plate, next turn and flip the plate so that the target circle now occupies a new position. Sometimes patients will get the answer correct the second time because they are more sensitive to crossed versus uncrossed disparities, or vice versa. This would manifest itself when the patient shows that they can detect the location of the circle more easily when it is, for example, in front rather than behind the surrounding contours.

8. If the patient is correct on two successive occasions, move to the intermediate plate (3 mm) and repeat steps 5 to 7.

9. If, using the intermediate plate, the patient is correct on two successive occasions, move to the thinnest plate (1.5 mm) and again repeat steps 5 to 7.

10. From 40 cm, the best level of stereoacuity that can be assessed for using the Frisby test is 85 seconds of arc. If you wish to measure the stereopsis (as opposed to just establishing that it is 85" or better), a longer viewing distance is used in combination with the thinnest plate. The lid of the box presents a table which can be used to determine the stereoacuity for different test distances.

6.7.4 Procedure: Stereo Fly test/ Stereo Butterfly test/Randot graded-circles test/Randot Pre-school test/ Random dot 'E' test

These tests operate on similar principles to one another in that they use crossed polaroid filters to present slightly different aspects of the same object to each eye. The vectograph consists of two superimposed, similar patterns that are polarised at right angles to each other. Some aspects of each pattern are identical, whilst for others, small crossed and uncrossed disparities are introduced.[38] When the patterns are viewed with Polaroid goggles, the patterns are seen in depth if stereopsis is present. Although these tests all differ from one another, they contain many similar aspects and are run procedurally in a very similar fashion. The following is a description for the Stero Fly test. After this some additional points relating to the other tests are listed.

1. Explain the test to your patient: "I am now going to test your 3-D vision."

2. Ask the patient to hold the booklet at about 40 cm angled so that it is parallel to the plane of the patient's face.

3. Keep the room lights on. Additional lighting over the patient's shoulder can be used to illuminate the booklet if necessary.

4. If you are measuring stereopsis in children, first show them the fly (see Fig. 6.7). Ask the patient to wear the polaroid goggles (you could refer to these as 'magic glasses' to younger children to make the test more of a game). Note the patient's reaction and ask them to pinch the wings of the fly. A positive test result is indicated if in attempting to touch the wings, the child pinches the air a few centimetres above the chart.

5. Cartoon animals: Ask the patient to look at the top row of animals (see Fig. 6.7) and to tell you which is the odd one out. Then ask the patient why this one appears to differ from the others. If the patient volunteers that it is different because it is closer to them (or because it stands out) this is a strong indication that stereopsis is present. If there is any doubt that the patient may know the answer that was expected (e.g., sibling tested previously when the child was present), turn the test upside down and the figure that appeared in front should now appear behind. Repeat this for the two lower rows of animals.

6. Circle patterns (also known as the Wirt test, see Fig. 6.7): Starting at the top array of circles, ask the patient which one of the four circles (top, bottom, left, or right) is the odd one out. Check the test card to ensure that the patient gave the correct answer and, as with the cartoon figures, ask why it appears different. Continue with this process until the patient cannot tell which is the unique circle ('odd one out') or until they give a wrong answer. The stereo level measured with the test is the smallest disparity that could be correctly detected.

7. Record the result in seconds of arc.

8. For the Randot graded-circles test, the graded circles element works in a similar fashion to the Wirt circle test described above in step 6, except that there are 10 versions of a 3-circles test and one of the three contains depth. This test features disparities from 400″ to 20.″ The cartoon figures are identical to those in the Stereo Fly test (400″ to 100″). This test differs from the Stereo Fly test mainly in that it offers six geometric forms created using the random dot principle (500″ to 20″). This element of the test can be administered by asking the patient to name the shapes that they see or, in the case of younger children, to perform a matching task where the same shapes are made available on a separate, printed sheet.

9. For the Stereo Butterfly test, the same Wirt circle and animal cartoon tests as in the Fly test are presented. The only difference is that the butterfly is created using random dots and offers a test of gross stereopsis (2500″ to 1200″).

10. The Randot Pre-school test is designed for children from the age of two. All of the figures in depth are generated using the random dot principle and the test takes the form of a matching test in which the child matches the 2-D pictures on the left side of the booklet with the 3-D/random-dot figures on the right hand side. The disparity range is 800″ to 40″.

11. The Random dot 'E' test. In this test, which is suitable for children aged 3 years and above, the patient is asked to distinguish between a raised E and a non-stereo target.

6.7.5 Procedure: Lang stereotest

This test was designed to enable stereopsis screening to take place in very young children (e.g., around 18 months to 2 years). The test is a single card that should be held by the practitioner or, if not, by the parent/guardian. It only assesses gross stereopsis and provides targets of a moon arc (200″), star (200″), car (400″), and an elephant (600″) (Fig. 6.11).

1. Hold the card at a distance of 40 cm from the child who sits on the parent/carer's lap.

2. The star can be seen monocularly to help attract the attention of young children.

3. Ask the child what they can see.

4. Pre-verbal children should be encouraged to respond by reaching for the images and this action can be used to indicate that some stereopsis is present. The test can become a matching game; if the child cannot name the targets they see but can match them with the same targets shown on paper, this is a good indication that stereopsis is present.

5. A preferential-looking procedure can also be adopted in pre-verbal children: this involves comparing the child's

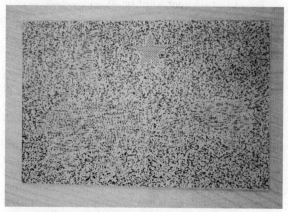

Fig. 6.11 The Lang stereotest II showing the monocularly visible star. Other figures (elephant, car, and moon) can only be seen binocularly with stereopsis.

fixation when the card is held in the normal fashion as compared with when it is rotated by 90 degrees. This is a useful test to have available because it is easy to use, does not require goggles, provides valuable information, and is relatively inexpensive.[43]

6.7.6 Recording stereopsis results

1. Always record the test used to measure the stereopsis.
2. TNO: If the stereo shapes are identified in Plates I–III but not V–VII, record 'Gross Stereopsis; TNO Plates I–III correct.' If the response to Plate IV is incorrect, record which eye is being suppressed. For Plates V–VII, record the stereoacuity as the smallest disparity where both responses were correct. If the patient responds correctly to the lowest disparity presented (Plate VIII), record the stereoacuity as 'TNO ≤15″, because it is possible that stereoacuity may have been even better if lower disparites were shown.
3. Fly-Test: If the patient's reaction and pinching of the fly's wings indicates they could see the fly in depth, record 'Gross Stereopsis (Titmus Fly).' The disparities of the animals range from 400″ to 100″ and the disparities of the circles range from 800″ to 40″. Record the smallest disparity that was correctly identified for this and the other tests, and indicate which element of the test this result is based on (e.g., graded-circles 50″, cartoon 200″, etc). If all of the answers are correct, record the result as 'Titmus Fly ≤40′ because it is possible that stereoacuity may have been even better if lower disparites were shown.
4. Frisby: Again record the stereoacuity as 'at least' the highest level if testing was at 40 cm and the responses were all correct (e.g., Frisby ≤85″).
5. For the Lang test, record as positive or negative the responses to the shapes. For example, if the elephant (600″) was seen/pointed to, but not the car (400″), record as: Lang 400″–600″ (Elephant +ve, car –ve).

6.7.7 Interpreting the results of stereopsis tests

Stereoacuity of around 60″ can be normal, but most adults and very many young (e.g., 5-year-old) children will achieve better (i.e., lower) thresholds.[38,41] In young children, an abnormal test result should prompt you to repeat the test on another occasion because there is a strong likelihood that children exhibiting an abnormal result on the first occasion of testing will achieve a normal test result when the test is repeated.[44] Constant strabismus, amblyopia, or other causes of visual loss (in particular monocular visual loss) usually leads to a seriously degraded or complete loss of stereoacuity.[45] In addition, small amounts of blur (binocular or monocular) and/or aniseikonia can reduce stereoacuity so that a patient's optimal stereo

threshold is only obtained with their optimal refractive correction; for example, reduced stereopsis when viewing with the patient's existing spectacles could be caused by refractive blur if the correction is not optimal.[46,47] In addition, fixation disparity may lead to reductions in stereopsis.[48] If performance is poor on one stereotest, you should try another because some patients perform quite differently on different tests, often for unknown reasons. For example, some patients may not respond well to red/green rivalry of the TNO test but achieve a normal result on tests using Polaroid spectacles to create depth effects or on tests of real depth perception (Frisby).

6.7.8 Most common errors when testing stereopsis

1. Not having appropriate lighting. Lighting should good and without glare sources.
2. Instructing the patient in a manner that leads the patient to the answers. For example, asking "Can you see the two butterflies?" (Plate I, TNO) or "Can you see that the wings of the fly are nearer to you?" (Stereo Fly test).
3. Allowing head tilting by the patient or viewing from oblique angles in an effort to see the depth. This applies mainly to the Lang and Frisby tests and does not affect the TNO or other random-dot tests.
4. Not using the appropriate test distance. Most of the tests are calibrated for 40 cm and the clinician should hold the test to ensure this viewing distance is maintained.
5. Not allowing sufficient time for the patient to view the stereo figures.
6. Using inappropriate refractive correction. For example, using the patient's own spectacles, which may not be optimal or using a distance correction in presbyopes.
7. Not repeating the test in cases where an abnormal result is obtained.[44]
8. Polaroid-based tests: Allowing the child to view the stimuli before the polaroid goggles are worn.

6.8 Accommodation assessment

Accommodation is the focusing ability of the eye that allows targets to be kept clear over a range of distances. There are a variety of tests of accommodation. Two of these are described here in the 'entrance' tests section of the chapter, namely the amplitude of accommodation (AoA) and dynamic retinoscopy. Other tests of accommodation (e.g., accommodation facility) are problem-oriented, supplementary tests that are much less commonly used and are described in section 6.15.

The AoA measures the full range of accommodation, from the far point, where accommodation is fully relaxed, to the near point, with maximum accommodation exerted. If the far point is at infinity (as in the case of emmetropes and those wearing optimal refractive correction for distance vision), then measurement of the near point allows the AoA to be calculated by taking the inverse of the near point in metres. For example, if the far point is at infinity and the near point is at 10 cm, the AoA is 1 ÷ 0.10 = 10.00 D. The AoA gradually falls with age, and causes patients over the age of around 45 years to have difficulty with near work and require reading glasses (i.e., presbyopia). Dynamic retinoscopy provides a measure of accommodation accuracy as it measures how closely the accommodative response matches the accommodative demand.

6.8.1 The evidence base: when and how to measure accommodation

The AoA is often included in the 'entrance tests' of a typical eye examination[1] of patients who are pre-presbyopic to determine accommodative ability in the patient's habitual state (i.e., with their glasses, if worn). Accommodation accuracy is increasingly advocated in the examination of children with hyperopia.[49] Measurement of AoA in early presbyopes is usually measured after the distance refraction and used to estimate a tentative reading addition (section 4.13). The objective AoA becomes zero at age 55 to 60[50] so that subjective measurements are not typically measured in those of this age or older as they reflect only assessments of the depth of field. All tests of accommodation can be conducted monocularly or binocularly, with binocular measures generally being slightly higher than monocular ones. There are a variety of ways in which the AoA can be measured.[51,52] One is to bring a target closer and closer to the patient's eyes until it first blurs; this is called the push-up amplitude. Another is to start with the target right in front of the eyes and move it away until it first becomes clear; this is the pull-away method. Some clinicians take an average of the push-up and pull-away values as the AoA because it provides a useful compromise between the slight overestimate of the push-up technique and the slight underestimate of the pull-away technique.[52,53] The technique advocated here is the pull-away method. The advantage of this method is that the patient responds by naming the letter/target as soon as they can identify it rather than when they first notice the subjective impression of blur (as in the push-up method). In the pull-away method, you should hold the fixation stick and place your thumb beneath an isolated 20/30 letter (or use an RAF rule, Fig. 6.12; or an appropriately sized picture target in the case of young children). The patient should not know the identity of the target/letter before the test starts. A very different method for AoA measurement involves using increasing amounts of minus

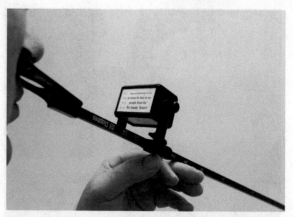

Fig. 6.12 A Royal Air Force (RAF) rule being used to measure amplitude of accommodation. It can also be used to measure the near point of convergence.

spherical lens power until distance vision blurs ('Sheard's technique'). This method typically provides lower estimates of AoA than those provided by the push-up method and it can only be satisfactorily measured using a phoropter.[54] In addition, the minus lens method provides a less clinically relevant measure than the push-up or pull-away techniques, which provide more direct measurements of the near point of clear vision.[53]

Accommodation accuracy measurements are useful because they indicate the behaviour of the patient's accommodation system when a near task is actually being carried out. Accommodative lag and lead indicate whether a patient's accommodation level to a target is less (lag) or more (lead) than expected. Measurements of accommodation accuracy are useful in helping to decide whether or not to prescribe low-to-moderate plus corrections in young hyperopes.[49,55] The clinical significance of increased accommodative lag in patients who go on to develop myopia is controversial.[56–58] Accommodative lag and lead can be measured objectively using various dynamic retinoscopy techniques or subjectively using relative accommodation measurements or the binocular crossed-cylinder method. Dynamic retinoscopy requires minimal extra equipment and provides accommodative accuracy measurements that are quicker and more repeatable, yet as valid as the crossed-cylinder or near duochrome techniques.[59,60] As with most clinical techniques, practice is required in order to develop proficiency in carrying out the tests, especially in relation to the short time in which the retinoscopy judgements need to be made. One study has suggested that the Nott technique provides more accurate estimates of the accommodative response because it does not require the introduction of supplementary lenses.[59] To help to measure the two distances in Nott

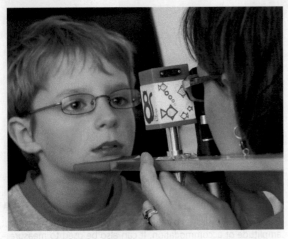

Fig. 6.13 The Ulster-Cardiff Accommodation Cube enables distances to be measured accurately during dynamic retinoscopy. (Photograph courtesy of Prof Kathryn Saunders, Ulster University.)

dynamic retinoscopy, a convenient measurement scale and target has been developed and validated (Fig. 6.13).[59,61] In the monocular estimate method (MEM) of dynamic retinoscopy, the lenses should only be introduced as briefly as possible to try to ensure that the accommodative system does not change in response to any added lenses.

6.8.2 Procedure: pull-away AoA

1. Explain the test to your patient: "I am going to measure the focusing power of your eyes."
2. The test is ideally performed with the patient wearing their optimal distance correction, but is frequently performed with the patient's spectacles provided the optimal and current refractive errors are not substantially different (e.g., > 1.00 D different in spherical equivalent refractive error in either eye). If the test is to be performed on older presbyopes, they should wear a partial addition (~+1.00 for 45–55 years) to facilitate measurement. In young children likely to have high amplitudes, slight linear differences of the near point produce large dioptric differences (e.g., the small difference between 7 cm and 10 cm is > 4.00 D), and it is useful to add a −4.00 D lens to place the near point further from the spectacle plane. This also ensures that depth-of-focus errors are minimised.[53]
3. You should sit directly in front of the patient to allow an unobstructed view of the two eyes. Direct additional lighting over the patient's shoulder to illuminate the reading card without shadows.

4. The test is usually performed monocularly (right then left) followed by a binocular measure of accommodation amplitude. The procedure is common for monocular and binocular testing. For monocular measures occlude one eye.
5. Instruct your patient: "In a moment I am going to ask you to close your eyes. When you open them there will be a letter/target right just above my finger. At the start it will be too close for you to see but I will start to move it away from your eye. Please tell me what the letter/target is as soon as you can see it."
6. With the patient's eyes closed, place the fixation stick so that it is almost touching the eyelid (monocular measures) or tip of the nose (binocular measures) and place your finger just below an appropriately sized letter/target. When you instruct your patient to open their eyes, begin to move the target slowly away from the patient. Remind the patient to tell you as soon as they know what the letter/target is. In the case of children this can take the form of a game to try to optimise compliance and engagement. Small text stimulates accommodation to a greater extent than less demanding targets (e.g., cartoon characters) and hence, even in children, the use of letter/word targets will help to ensure that accommodation is not underestimated.[62]
7. When the patient correctly identifies the target/letter, stop the movement and measure the distance to the spectacle plane and convert this distance to dioptres by taking the inverse of the distance (in metres). For example, if the target was first identified correctly at 10 cm, the AoA as assessed using this method is 10 D (i.e., $1 \div 0.1$ m).
8. Add the effect of any additional lenses to the measured dioptric near point to obtain the true amplitude. For example, if a +1.00 DS lens was provided and the measured amplitude was 4.50 D, the actual AoA is 3.50 D. If a −4.00 DS lens was added and the measured amplitude was 7.00 D, the actual amplitude is 11.00 D.
9. Repeat at least once or twice if the values obtained from the first and second tests are significantly different from each other (e.g., ≥1.5 D difference) or from what would be expected on the basis of the patient's age. In young adults, differences of less than 1.50 D between recorded and age-matched values, or between recordings on two separate occasions, are not usually clinically significant.[51] To avoid memorisation, choose a different letter/target for repeat testing.
10. Repeat for the left eye, again choosing a different letter/target.
11. Repeat binocularly.

6.8.3 Procedure: Nott dynamic retinoscopy for accommodation accuracy measurement

1. To get an impression of the habitual accommodation accuracy, the patient should wear their existing spectacles

if worn. If there is a significant refractive correction, or a significant difference between current and optimal prescription, the test can be repeated with the optimal refractive correction in place.

2. The phoropter should not be used for this test because of the risk of inducing proximal accommodation.
3. Explain the test to your patient: "I am going to check the focusing ability of your eyes using this torch that will shine a light into your eye."
4. The test should be carried out in conditions that approximate, in so far as possible, normal reading conditions and the card to be viewed by the patient needs to be located close to the patient's typical reading distance. The card should contain letters (or pictures for young children) in a position that permits you to perform retinoscopy close to the patient's visual axis (see Fig. 6.13). A near chart with a central aperture works well. If letters are being used they should be bigger (by one line) than the binocular near visual acuity (typically N6, 0.5 M, 20/30).
5. The room lights can be left on and use additional lighting if necessary to ensure that the near chart is well illuminated.
6. Ask the patient to focus on the letters/targets.
7. Perform retinoscopy along the horizontal meridian (with the streak vertical) on the right eye from 40 cm (typically 10 cm behind the near point card). Perform retinoscopy as quickly as possible as the retinoscope light will interfere with binocularity.
8. If neutrality is not observed at 40 cm, change the working distance (move further away if 'with' movements are seen, and closer if 'against' movements are seen) until the neutral point is seen. Note the distance of your retinoscope when the neutral point is obtained. To establish the result you need to know the distance at which the target was presented and the distance from the patient's eyes at which the retinoscope was positioned when reversal was observed.
9. If the neutrality point is behind the near chart position, then there is a lag of accommodation. If the neutrality point is in front of the near chart position, then there is accommodative lead. For example, if the near chart is at 40 cm and neutrality is observed at 57 cm, then the accommodative lag is +2.50 D − 1.75 D = +0.75 D. It is useful to learn corresponding distances and dioptric values, such as 80 cm (1.25 D), 67 cm (1.50 D), 57 cm (1.75 D), 50 cm (2.00 D), 44 cm (2.25 D), and 40 cm (2.50 D).
10. Repeat the procedure on the left eye.

6.8.4 Procedure: MEM dynamic retinoscopy for accommodation accuracy measurement

1. Attach a MEM card or hold a fixation stick to the front of your retinoscope. The card should contain letters

or pictures around a central aperture, through which retinoscopy is performed.
2. The room lights can be left on and use additional lighting if necessary to ensure that the near chart is well illuminated.
3. Ask the patient to focus on the letters/targets. To maintain appropriate fixation and accommodation, you may need to ask children to read some of the letters out aloud or to name details in the picture.
4. Perform retinoscopy along the horizontal meridian (with the streak vertical) on the right eye from the patient's typical working distance. Retinoscopy should be performed in the usual manner, but the lenses should only be placed in front of the patient's eyes for the least amount of time possible (e.g. ~ 0.5 seconds).
5. Record the dioptric power of the lens that provides neutrality.
6. Repeat the procedure on the left eye.

6.8.5 Recording

For AoA, record the number of dioptres of accommodation for each eye. Examples:

AoA (pull-away) R(OD) 8.50 D, L(OS) 8.50 D, BE(OU) 10.00 D

For accommodation accuracy, positive lenses indicate a lag of accommodation and negative lenses indicate a lead of accommodation. Record the technique and the dioptric value of the accommodative lead or lag. For example, Nott: +0.75 lag R & L; MEM: R +1.00 lag, L +1.25 lag.

6.8.6 Interpreting the results: AoA and accommodative accuracy

Pull-away values tend to be lower than push-up values for the AoA. Normal values of monocular spectacle accommodation are shown in Table 6.5. If the measured amplitude is significantly (>1.50 D) lower than the age-matched normal values, the patient may have accommodative insufficiency.[51] Binocular values of AoA are usually a little higher (1.00 to 2.00 D) than the monocular values as the convergence response helps to induce additional accommodation (convergence accommodation).[63] Presbyopia is diagnosed if the patient (aged 40 or above) has an AoA of 5D or below and has difficulties seeing clearly at near whilst wearing an appropriate distance correction. In children aged 4 to 11 years, Adler et al. found large intra-individual variation in measures of AoA and suggested that, in this age group, the test may prove useful mainly as a pass/fail check as to whether accommodative amplitude is more or less than 8.00 D.[63] Evidence indicates that accommodation measures in children are highly dependent on the target being viewed and that using N5 (0.4 M)

Table 6.5 Expected values (mean ± SD). The 95% confidence limits of normal could be calculated as mean ± 2 SD

Test	Jimenez et al. (children aged 6–12)[64]	Morgan[65]	Scheiman and Wick[66]
Horizontal phoria (distance)	0.6Δ±1.7Δ	−1Δ±2 Δ	−1Δ±2 Δ
Horizontal phoria (near)	−0.4Δ±3.1Δ	−3Δ±3 Δ	−3Δ±3 Δ
Vertical phoria (distance)	0.0±0.2Δ		
Vertical phoria (near)	0.0±0.3Δ		
Negative fusional reserve blur/break/recovery (distance)	−/6±2Δ/4±2Δ	−/7±3Δ /4±2Δ	Smooth −/7±3Δ /4±2Δ Step (children aged 7–12 yrs) Step (adults) −/7±3Δ/4±2Δ
Positive fusional reserve blur/break/recovery (distance)	−/17±7Δ/11±6Δ	9±4Δ / 19±8Δ /10±4Δ	9±4Δ /19±8Δ /10±4Δ Step (adults) −/11±7Δ/7±2Δ
Negative fusional reserve blur/break/recovery (near)	−/11±3Δ/7±3Δ	13±4Δ /21±4Δ /13±5Δ	Smooth 13±4Δ /21±4Δ /13±5Δ Step (children 7–12 yrs) −/12±5Δ/7±4Δ Step (adults) −/13±6Δ/10±5Δ
Positive fusional reserve blur/break/recovery (near)	−/18±8Δ/13±6Δ	17±5Δ /21±6Δ /11±7Δ	Smooth 17±5Δ /21±6Δ /11±7Δ Step (children 7–12 yrs) −/23±8Δ/16±6Δ Step (adults) −/19±9Δ/14±7Δ
Vergence facility (cpm)	3.2±1.7 (6–8 yrs) 8 BO/8 BI 4.5±2.3 (9–12 yrs)) 8 BO/8 BI		15±3 (12 BO/3 BI)
Near point of convergence break/recovery (cm)	5.2±4.4/11.4±7.2 [penlight push-up] 6.5±5.7/14.3±11.2 [red lens push-up]		2.5±4/4.5±5 [penlight and red/green glasses] 2.5±2.5/4.5±3 [accommodative target]
AC/A ratio [gradient method] [calculated method]	[2.2±0.8Δ/D] [5.0±0.9Δ/D]	[4.0±2.0Δ/D]	[4.0±2.0Δ/D]
Amplitude of accommodation (D) (push-up) (minus lens method)		18-1/3xage ±2D	18-1/3xage ±2 D 2D less than push-up
Negative relative accommodation (D)		+2.00±0.50D	+2.00±0.50 D
Positive relative accommodation (D)		−2.37±1.00D	−2.37±1.00 D
Monocular accommodation facility (cpm)			5.5±2.5 cpm (6 year olds) 6.5±2.0 cpm (7 year olds) 7±2.5 cpm (8–12 year olds) 11±5 cpm (13–30 year olds)

Table 6.5 Expected values (mean ± SD). The 95% confidence limits of normal could be calculated as mean ± 2 SD—cont'd

Test	Jimenez et al. (children aged 6–12)[64]	Morgan[65]	Scheiman and Wick[66]
Binocular accommodation facility (cpm)			3±2.5 cpm (6 year olds) 3.5±2.5 cpm (7 year olds) 5±2.5 cpm (8–12 year olds) 10±5cpm (adults*)
Accommodative accuracy (D) (monocular estimate method)			+0.50±0.25D
Stereoacuity (Randot) (secs arc)	25±10		

*Using lens power range scaled to 30% of the amplitude of accommodation (e.g., if the amplitude is 10.00 D, lens flippers of ±1.50 D are used). All other accommodation facility estimates refer to testing with flippers of ±20.00 D. cpm: cycles per minute; D: Dioptre

text will reveal higher accommodation compared with using, for example, a cartoon character.[62] However, there is variability in accommodation between participants even when N5 text is used. Another source of variation stems from the fact that, although some patients who *can* accommodate, do not do so on clinical testing.[3] This makes it important not to over-interpret one abnormal test result and to consider results in combination (section 6.18).

Anomalies of accommodation may be associated with a wide variety of conditions including various systemic and ocular medications (probably the most common cause), trauma, inflammatory disease, metabolic disorders such as diabetes, and other systemic diseases.[52] Reduced amplitudes of accommodation have also been reported in children with Down syndrome and cerebral palsy.[67,68] Wick and Hall found that a battery of tests (amplitude, lead/lag of accommodation, accommodative facility, and a cycloplegic refraction) was required to completely rule out accommodative dysfunction, and that just because a patient had an adequate AoA did not mean that accommodative function was normal.[69]

Most young patients have a small accommodative lag, meaning that the accommodative response to a target is slightly less than the accommodative stimulus. For example, a target positioned at 40 cm provides an accommodative stimulus of 2.50 D. If the accommodative response is only 2.00 D, there is an accommodative lag of 0.5 D. The size of the lag depends on the accommodative demand. When the demand is 4.00 D, the mean (± SD) lag in children aged 4 to 15 years has been estimated at 0.30 D (± 0.39) using the Nott method.[61] When the demand is higher, the lag is also higher, 0.74±0.58 D for a 6.00 D demand, and 2.50 ± 1.27 D when the demand is 10.00 D. The lack of an accommodative lag or an accommodative lead can indicate pseudomyopia or accommodative spasm. It has been claimed that the MEM technique provides lags which are around twice those found using the Nott method,[70] but most studies find results that are similar.[52,71] In children with low to moderate hyperopia for whom it is not clear whether they would benefit from refractive correction, there is a growing belief that assessment of accommodative accuracy using dynamic retinoscopy offers a means of identifying those who are likely to benefit from spectacle correction.[72] It is difficult to pinpoint a threshold value of lag that is clinically significant because the exact value depends on the demand, but a lag of 2.00 D or above is very likely to be significant.[49] Hyperopes with a larger lag of accommodation (e.g., > 1.00 D) may benefit more from spectacle correction than those with smaller lags (≤ 0.5 DD).

6.8.7 Most common errors with accommodation testing

AoA

1. Not stressing to the patient to report the letter/target as soon as it is seen.
2. Carrying out the test without the patient's glasses, where glasses are habitually worn. This overestimates the amplitude in myopes and underestimates it in hyperopes.
3. Moving the fixation stick too quickly from the patient, which leads to an underestimation of the accommodative amplitude.
4. Using an inappropriate target (i.e., one that does not require precise accommodation).

Accommodation Accuracy

1. Not realising that a small lag of accommodation is normal.
2. Taking too long to make a judgement as to whether the reflex is moving 'with' or 'against.'

3. Nott method: inaccurate measurement of the distance of the target to the patient and the retinoscope distance from the patient that gives reversal.
4. MEM method: leaving the lens in place for too long. The lens can alter the accommodation of the eye.

6.9 Further assessment of binocular vision and accommodation ('functional tests')

Once case history, initial screening of binocular vision, and accommodation using the entrance tests described, and refraction has occurred, the results up to that point need to be considered to determine whether further testing of binocular vision and accommodation is necessary; if so, what tests may be appropriate? These additional tests are often called 'functional tests.'[1] Further testing may be appropriate in patients whose symptoms are not explained by the clinical data currently gathered, such as a patient with symptoms at near but no significant refractive error. Further testing is also indicated where one or more core/entrance test result(s) (e.g., NPC) is abnormal. The nature of the further testing is governed by a number of factors.

First, it is governed by the overall framework that the clinician uses to evaluate the binocular vision and accommodation system. A clinician may adopt the graphical analysis approach (particularly popular in the United States), in which the clinical measures needed to determine the zone of clear and single binocular vision (section 6.18), such as the positive and negative fusional reserve measures to blur at both near and distance (section 6.12), would be used.

Second, the nature of the symptoms and any previous abnormal test result will direct subsequent testing. For example, if the patient reports difficulties switching between distance and near viewing, tests of accommodative/vergence interaction are called for; if the NPC (section 6.5) has been found to be abnormal, other tests of vergence (in particular, positive fusional reserves at near) and of accommodation/convergence interaction (in particular, the AC/A ratio, section 6.14) are required.

6.10 Further assessment of binocular status in strabismus

6.10.1 The evidence base: when and how to further assess patients with strabismus

The Worth 4-dot test (section 6.6) or stereopsis testing (section 6.7) may indicate that there is residual binocularity in patients with strabismus. In such patients, the majority of whom will have small angle strabismus and mild amblyopia, further testing may be indicated. The 4^Δ base-out test is often used as an indirect test of suppression in the specific case of a suspected microtropia, which typically shows screening test results indicating anisometropia, a 1- to 2-line reduction in visual acuity in one eye and no movement detected on the cover test.[8] The 4^Δ base-out is used in combination with tests of eccentric fixation, abnormal retinal correspondence, and stereopsis to confirm a diagnosis of microtropia. It differs from the Worth 4-dot test of suppression in that it is entirely objective; the result does not rely on a verbal response from the patient but rather is determined by a comparison of the pattern of eye movements that result when the 4^Δ (base-out) is introduced in front of one eye and then the other. Thus this test requires little additional equipment and is quick and straightforward to perform. However, its repeatability is relatively poor and visually normal children can show atypical responses.[73]

6.10.2 Procedure: 4^Δ base-out test

1. Seat the patient comfortably. Keep the room lights on and, if necessary, use additional lighting so that the patient's eyes can be easily seen without shadows. The test cannot be performed using a phoropter; a trial frame with the optimal distance refractive correction (or the patient's spectacles) should be used.
2. Explain the measurement to the patient: "I am going to perform a test to see if and how your eyes move when I introduce this lens."
3. Provide a single letter on a featureless background for the patient to view. The letter should be one line larger than the distance visual acuity of the weaker eye.
4. Ask the patient to keep looking at the letter, even if it appears to move.
5. Place the 4^Δ base-out prism over the eye with the better visual acuity (Fig. 6.14). The eye should make a swift movement inwards due to the prism. The fellow eye, which is likely to have slightly reduced visual acuity (caused by amblyopia and/or eccentric fixation if the patient has microtropia), should initially make a conjugate, versional movement (i.e., in the same direction as the sound eye) before returning to its original position. This wobble of the fellow eye (eye not receiving the base-out prism) is due to Hering's law. You should repeat this several times to confirm your result.
6. Now place the 4^Δ base-out prism over the eye with reduced visual acuity (see Fig. 6.14). In a microtropia (which is generally of the esotropic type) the 4^Δ base-out prism will merely shift the retinal image within the suppression scotoma of the amblyopic eye. In such cases, neither eye will move. Again, you should repeat

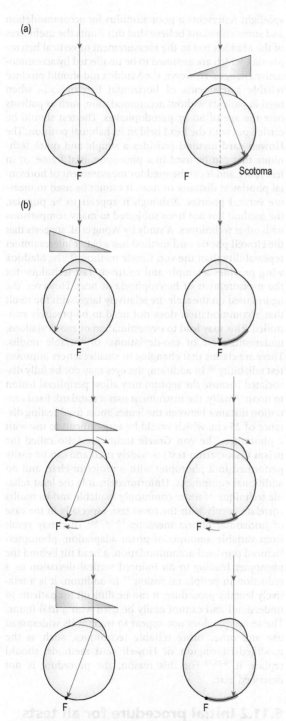

Fig. 6.14 Diagram illustrating the eye movements that should occur during a 4-prism dioptre test when the prism is placed in front of (a) a microtropic eye (there are no eye movements) and (b) the fellow normal eye.

this several times to confirm your result. Obtaining the expected pattern of eye movements when the fellow eye views through the prism but the absence of eye movements when the prism is placed in front of the eye with poorer visual acuity is confirmation of an abnormal ('fail') result.

6.10.3 Recording of the 4^Δ base-out prism test

Record 'fail' if there is no movement of the weaker eye when the 4^Δ base-out prism is placed before the weaker eye (note that in this case, the fellow eye will also not move, as described above). This indicates suppression. For example, 4^Δ base-out test: fail LE (OS). Record 'normal' if the expected pattern of eye movements was seen when the 4^Δ base-out prism was introduced before each eye in turn.

6.10.4 Interpreting the results of the 4^Δ base-out prism test

If neither eye moves when the 4^Δ base-out prism is introduced before the eye with reduced visual acuity but the expected pattern of movement is observed when the prism is placed before the fellow eye, this confirms the presence of suppression in the weaker eye. Along with reduced visual acuity, anisometropia, the presence of eccentric fixation, and degraded but measurable stereopsis, this result on the 4^Δ base-out test strongly suggests a diagnosis of microtropia.[8] The test does have drawbacks. Many normal and microtropic patients exhibit atypical test results, and there are questions about the test-retest reliability of the test.[73] More direct evidence of suppression can be gained with Bagolini lenses,[7] although this test is not discussed further here because the test is seldom conducted in primary care optometry.

6.11 Further assessment of heterophoria

Further assessment of heterophoria may be required post-refraction.

6.11.1 The evidence base: when and how to measure post-refraction heterophoria

In cases where there has been little change to the refractive error, there may be no need to re-measure the heterophoria with the new refractive correction in place. However, when the refractive correction has changed significantly or when signs or symptoms call for it (section 6.9), the clinician will want to assess the heterophoria with the new refractive correction. Because a phoropter/trial frame can limit the

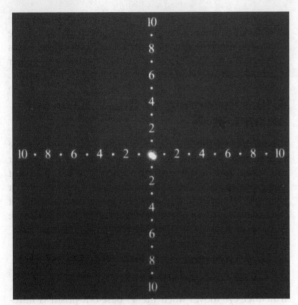

Fig. 6.15 A Thorington card.

visibility of the patient's eyes, the cover test is seldom used to assess the phoria after refraction. Heterophoria tests are more repeatable with a trial frame than with a phoropter.[74]

There are a variety of post-refraction phoria tests. The **modified Thorington** technique is a very simple and quick technique that can be used in a phoropter, trial frame, or in free space. It produces the most repeatable results of the most commonly used subjective techniques[74-76] and is similar to a cover test in terms of its repeatability.[14,77] The modified Thorington overcomes the Maddox rod's problem of lacking an accommodative target by using a target that consists of small letters or numbers (Fig. 6.15). It is principally used at near, but Thorington cards are available for both distance and near. In view of its many advantages it is somewhat surprising that it is not more widely used at present. Normative data from large study populations of children have been published.[78] The **Maddox rod** test can be easily performed with a phoropter (video 6.19), trial frame, or the patient's own spectacles and with modest additional equipment requirements; typically the test is performed with the Maddox rod and a spotlight. Some versions of the Maddox rod test do not employ a spotlight, but present a line stimulus so that the patient sees two lines, one clear and one blurred. These are not discussed further here because the test was designed for use with a spotlight and because the alternative line stimulus is only advised when a suitable spotlight is not available. The Maddox rod is widely used, easy for patients to understand, and can be performed relatively quickly. One drawback is that a

spotlight represents a poor stimulus for accommodation and some clinicians believe that this limits the usefulness of the Maddox rod to the measurement of vertical heterophorias, which are assumed to be unaffected by accommodative changes. However, the Maddox rod should produce reliable assessments of horizontal heterophoria when used in patients without accommodation, such as patients over the age of 60 or pseudophakes. The test should be carried out with the head held in its habitual position. The **Howell card** method provides a simple and quick technique that can be used in a phoropter, trial frame, or in free space and it can be used for measurement of horizontal phorias at distance or near. It cannot be used to measure vertical phorias. Although it appears to be popular, the method has not been subjected to many comparisons with other techniques. A study by Wong et al. suggests that the Howell phoria card method has a better interexaminer repeatability than the von Graefe method.[79] The **Maddox wing** provides a simple and relatively fast technique for the measurement of heterophoria at near. However, the figures used on the scale are relatively large, with the result that accommodation does not need to be precisely controlled. This may lead to overestimation of exo-deviations, underestimation of eso-deviations, or variable results. There are claims that changing to smaller letters improves test reliability.[80] In addition, the eyes may not be fully dissociated because the septum may allow peripheral fusion to occur. Finally, the instrument uses a standard, fixed centration distance between the lenses and a fixed testing distance of 25 cm, which would be very difficult to use with a phoropter. The **von Graefe** technique (also called the **prism dissociation test**) is widely used and can be easily performed in a phoropter with a projector chart and no additional equipment. Unfortunately, it is the least reliable technique of those commonly available and its results correlate poorly with the cover test, especially in the case of horizontal phoria measures.[74-76,79,81] This may result from variable amounts of prism adaptation, phoropter-induced proximal accommodation, a head tilt behind the phoropter leading to an induced vertical deviation or a reduction in peripheral fusion.[74] In addition, it is a relatively lengthy procedure; it can be difficult for patients to understand and cannot easily be used with a trial frame. The technique does not appear to warrant its widespread use and other more reliable techniques, such as the modified-Thorington or Howell card methods, should replace it.[74-76,79] For this reason, the procedure is not described here.

6.11.2 Initial procedure for all tests

1. Inform the patient about the test: "This test is to check how your eye muscles work together with today's prescription."

2. Measure near phorias immediately after the distance heterophoria measurements in patients who are pre-presbyopic and after inclusion of the required reading in addition in those who are presbyopic.
3. For near phoria measurement, adjust the trial frame/phoropter to the near centration distance.

6.11.3 Procedure: modified Thorington test

This test is similar for distance and near, except for the fact that the card is held at 6 m (20 feet) or at 40 cm or 16 inches. Because the cards feature a tangent scale it is vital that the viewing distance is correct. Different cards use numbers only or numbers with letters.

Horizontal phoria

1. Place the Maddox rod in front of the right eye, making sure that the 'grooves' are horizontal. Dim the room lights.
2. Hold the Thorington near card at the appropriate distance and shine the light from a penlight through the central aperture of the card.
3. Direct the patient to look at the letters and keep them clear. Ask the patient to then look at the spotlight, and tell you whether the vertical red line is seen to the right, left, or straight through the spotlight.
4. Some patients have difficulty seeing the red line initially. If they cannot see the red line, cover each eye in turn to demonstrate that one eye sees the spotlight, letters, and numbers and the other sees the red line. Once patients are aware of the test format they are often able to see the red line and spotlight, letters, and numbers simultaneously. Placing a green filter before the eye viewing the spotlight can also help the patient to perform the test. If difficulty is still experienced, place the Maddox rod in front of the left eye and try again. If the spotlight and red line cannot be seen together, then suppression may be present and follow-up tests should be performed (section 6.6).
5. With the Maddox rod in front of the right eye the following responses may be given:
   (a) If the line is seen to pass through the spot, the patient has no horizontal phoria.
   (b) If the line is to the left of the spotlight (crossed images), the patient has an exophoria. If the line is to the right of the spotlight (uncrossed images), the patient has an esophoria.
   (c) Determine the size of the deviation by asking the patient which number (number or letter on some cards) the line passes through. This is the number of prism dioptres of horizontal heterophoria.

Vertical phoria

1. Rotate the Maddox rod so that the 'grooves' are vertical.
2. Ask the patient if the red line is seen above, below, or straight through the spot.
3. With the Maddox rod in front of the right eye the following responses may occur:
   (a) If the line is seen to pass through the spotlight, the patient has no vertical phoria.
   (b) If the line is below the spotlight, the patient has a right hyperphoria; if above, the patient has a left hyperphoria. The size of the deviation is determined by asking the patient which number (number or letter on some cards) the line passes through.

6.11.4 Procedure: Howell cards

This test is similar for distance and near, except that for distance the card is held at 3 m (10 feet) and at 33 cm or 13 inches during near testing (Fig. 6.16). Because the cards feature a tangent scale it is vital that the viewing distance is correct. A piece of string of the appropriate length is provided with the near card.

Horizontal heterophoria

1. Place the 6^Δ stick-mounted or loose vertical prism in front of the right eye to generate vertical diplopia so the patient should see two scales and two arrows.
2. Ask the patient "Do you see two arrows and two sets of numbers?"
3. After a positive response, instruct your patient: "Please look at the top arrow and you will see it points downwards from the '0' on the top set of numbers. Please follow it down with your eyes, and tell me which number on the lower set of numbers it points to. If it points between two numbers, please tell me between which two numbers it seems to point."

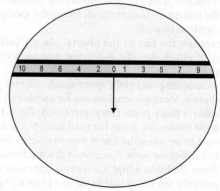

Fig. 6.16 A representation of a typical Howell card.

4. Because the scale is a tangent scale, the number corresponds to the magnitude of the phoria.
5. Assuming the prism is placed base-up in front of the right eye, if the arrow points down towards an odd number, the patient is EXOphoric. If it points to an even number the patient is ESOphoric. Because the patient may extrapolate between two numbers, you should ask if the numbers appear on the yellow or blue part of the scale. Numbers on yellow are odd and those on the blue part of the scale are even.

6.11.5 Procedure: Maddox rod

This test is similar for distance and near (video 6.19), except in one the spotlight is at 6 m (20 feet) and in the other it is a hand-held pen torch at 40 cm (16 inches) or the patient's near working distance.

Horizontal heterophoria

1. Place the Maddox rod in front of the right eye making sure that the 'grooves' are horizontal.
2. Provide a spotlight target at distance using the chart (or hold the penlight at the near working distance) and then dim the room lights.
3. Ask the patient to look at the spotlight, and to indicate if the vertical (red) line is seen to the right or left of the spotlight, or whether it runs straight through the spotlight.
4. Some patients have difficulty seeing the red line initially. If this occurs, use the techniques described in section 6.11.3, step 4)
5. With the Maddox rod in front of the right eye the following responses can occur:
   (a) If the line is seen to pass through the spot, the patient has no horizontal phoria.
   (b) If the line is seen to the left of the spot (crossed images), the patient has an exophoria. If it is to the right of the spot (uncrossed images), the patient has an esophoria.
   (c) If the line is seen to be continuously in motion, ask the patient to concentrate on seeing the spotlight as clearly as possible.
6. To measure the size of the phoria, place a prism in front of either eye. The following approach can be adopted:
   (a) Increase the power of the appropriately oriented prism (base-in for exophoria, base-out for esophoria) using either a Risley prism (Phoropter-based; Fig. 6.17) or loose prisms or a prism bar (trial frame). Ask the patient to say when the line is seen to overlap the spot and record the prism power when this is achieved.
   (b) Some clinicians adopt a screening approach when using the test with a trial frame and place a 2^Δ prism with appropriately oriented base-in front of one eye.

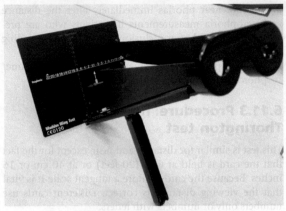

Fig. 6.17 A Maddox wing

If the line moves to the opposite side, the horizontal heterophoria can be recorded as $<2^\Delta$.

Vertical distance heterophoria

1. Rotate the Maddox rod so that the 'grooves' are vertical.
2. Ask the patient if the red line is seen above, below, or straight through the spot.
3. With the Maddox rod in front of the right eye the following responses can occur:
   (a) If the line is seen to pass through the spotlight, the patient has no vertical phoria.
   (b) If the line is above the spotlight, the patient has a left hyperphoria. Use base-down prism power before the left eye (or base-up prism power before the right eye) until the line and spot overlap.
   (c) If the line is below the spotlight, the patient has a right hyperphoria. Use base-up prisms (or base-down prism power before the right eye) before the left eye until the line and spot are coincident.

6.11.6 Procedure: Maddox wing

1. This test is carried out with the room lights on. Ensure there is sufficient lighting to allow the scale on the Maddox wing to be seen with ease (Fig. 6.18). The wing has the facility to insert trial case lenses.
2. Direct the patient to look through the horizontal slits to view the chart, which comprises horizontal and vertical scales, and horizontal and vertical arrows. The right eye sees only the arrows, whilst the left eye sees only the scales. The arrows are positioned at zero on the scales but through the dissociation, any departure from orthophoria will be indicated by an apparent movement of the arrow along the scale.

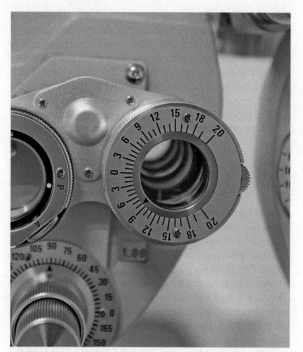

Fig. 6.18 A Risley prism in position to provide prism base-up or base-down (8$^\Delta$ base-down here).

3. Some patients have difficulty seeing the arrows and the scales simultaneously and require help to position the instrument correctly. If necessary, demonstrate to the patient, by covering the aperture in front of each eye in turn, that one eye views the arrows and the other eye views the scales. If the arrows and scales cannot be seen together, then suppression may be present and follow-up tests should be performed (section 6.6).

4. Ask the patient to say whether the white arrow is to the right or left of the zero on the scale. This will inform you whether exophoria or esophoria is present. Allow the patient plenty of time before asking "Which white number does the white arrow point to?" The number on the scale indicates the magnitude of the deviation in prism dioptres and the direction (even numbers correspond to exophoria, odd numbers to esophoria). If, over time, the arrow moves to higher and higher numbers on the scale, wait until the arrow has stopped moving before taking the reading. If the arrow is varying between a maximum and a minimum value, record the value of the midpoint between the extremes. The arrow position will be more stable if you remind the patient to focus on the tip of the arrow and ensure that it is kept as clear as possible. Often the white arrow is seen

to move immediately after a blink. The measurement should thus be taken between blinks.

5. To measure a vertical heterophoria, ask the patient "Which red number does the red arrow point to?" The number on the scale indicates the magnitude of the deviation and the direction.

6.11.7 Recording subjective heterophoria tests

1. The technique, which is used to measure heterophoria, should be included.

2. Record 'ortho H and V' (i.e., orthophoria) if there is no horizontal or vertical phoria. Another way to record orthophoria is to use the symbol ϕ to record that there is no horizontal phoria, $\ominus$ to record that there is no vertical phoria, or $\oplus$ to signal that there is no horizontal or vertical phoria (i.e., similar to the orthophoric patient's perception when using the Maddox rod).

3. Record the amount of deviation in prism dioptres ($^\Delta$) and the direction of the phoria (e.g., 3$^\Delta$ SOP, 5$^\Delta$ XOP). Vertical phorias can be recorded in a variety of ways. For example 2 prism dioptres of R hyperphoria can be recorded as 2$^{\Delta\ R}/_L$ or '2 R hyper'. Record the test distance corresponding to each heterophoria measurement.

4. Note if any suppression took place during the test; for example, if the patient could not simultaneously perceive the line (streak) and spot during Maddox rod or modified-Thorington methods.

5. Also record if the result was variable; for example, if the arrow in the Maddox wing or Howell card methods is not stable on the tangent scale.

6.11.8 Interpreting the results of subjective heterophoria tests

Most people with normal binocular vision have some slight degree of heterophoria. Lyon et al. reported 25th to 75th percentiles for phorias of 0 to 1$^\Delta$ esophoria (distance) and 2$^\Delta$ exophoria to 1$^\Delta$ esophoria (near) in a large sample of first-grade children (aged ~5 years).[75] In older children (aged ~8 years), distance and near phorias measured with the modified Thorington method were 0 to 1$^\Delta$ esophoria (distance), and 2$^\Delta$ exophoria to 2$^\Delta$ esophoria (near). Mean distance heterophoria in children and young adults is 1$^\Delta$ exophoria ± 1$^\Delta$ and mean near heterophoria is 3$^\Delta$ exophoria ± 3$^\Delta$.[19] In older adults, there is a tendency towards greater amounts of exophoria (physiological exophoria) and up to 6$^\Delta$ of exophoria is not uncommon.[8] In adults and children, only about 0.5$^\Delta$ of vertical phoria may be considered normal; in some patients even this amount can give rise to symptoms. Vertical phorias should be checked to make sure they are not caused by a head tilt (unseen behind a phoropter) or abnormal head posture or a non-level trial frame or phoropter.

The heterophoria determined using the subjective tests and measured with optimal refractive correction should be compared with the corresponding cover test result measured using the patient's spectacles, if worn. If there is no significant change in refractive error, the horizontal heterophoria measurements post-refraction should be similar to those found with the cover test. Vertical heterophorias should not differ pre- versus post-refraction, even if there is a substantial change in refractive correction. If a change in refractive correction has occurred, this should lead to a predictable change in the horizontal heterophoria so that if the optimal correction shows an increase in plus (or a decrease in minus) power from the patient's spectacles, then an increase in exophoria or a decrease in esophoria should be expected. Similarly, an increase in minus/decrease in plus power could lead to a decrease in exophoria or increase in esophoria. Patients with unexplained symptoms or signs (e.g., poor recovery on the cover/uncover test) may need further testing that could include fusional reserves (section 6.12), fixation disparity (section 6.13), and the AC/A ratio (section 6.14).

6.11.9 Most common errors with subjective heterophoria tests

1. Attempting to determine the presence of heterophoria in a patient with strabismus.
2. Failing to distinguish between lens-induced deviations and true heterophorias, particularly with vertical phorias, commonly caused by a head tilt behind the phoropter or the phoropter or trial frame not being level.
3. Believing that the results from different heterophoria tests are interchangeable when research evidence shows that this is often not the case.[76]

Modified-Thorington

Not attempting the various procedures that may be necessary to enable the patient to simultaneously perceive the red line and spot. This also applies to the Maddox rod technique.

Maddox wing

1. Not allowing the patient sufficient time for the arrow to stop moving with horizontal phoria measurement. Also, not encouraging the patient to keep the arrowhead in sharp focus to help reduce its apparent movement on the scale.
2. Mistaking the direction of horizontal heterophoria present because the patient has interpolated between the numbers on the scale. For example, if the arrow

is seen to be between the 11 and 13 scale positions (esophoria), the patient may state that 'the arrow is pointing to 12.' You may mistakenly record this result as 12^Δ of exophoria because even numbers are employed on the test for exo-deviations. The way to avoid this problem is initially to ask whether the line is seen to the left or right of the zero position or to introduce a pen and to ask if the tip of the pen is near the arrow. This is also a potential issue with the Howell card method.

6.12 Fusional reserves

Several names are attached to tests that involve determining the prism power that leads to a breakdown in fusion and the perception of diplopia.[8] The names in common use include Fusional Reserves, Fusional Amplitudes, Fusional Vergences, Prism Fusion Range, Vergence Amplitudes, and Prism Vergences! The term 'fusional reserves' will be used here as it provides a clear indication of the clinical information provided by the measurement. Fusional reserves are measured when the clinician wishes to know how much stress the heterophoria is placing on the binocular vision system.[82] It is thought that between one-third and two-thirds of the fusional reserves may be used to overcome the heterophoria without placing the binocular system under undue stress. Positive and negative fusional reserves can be measured at distance and nearby placing appropriate prisms before the eyes. Increasing prism power is introduced before the eyes until fusion breaks down and diplopia results.[83] Placing base-out prism before the eyes forces the eyes to converge and the amount required to produce diplopia is called the positive fusional reserve (PFR). Because the eyes are forced to converge, accommodation is stimulated (convergence accommodation), but often it cannot be maintained at an appropriate level for the target distance. This usually leads to the patient noticing that the target blurs before diplopia occurs.[84] Placing a base-in prism before the eyes forces the eyes to diverge and the amount required to produce diplopia is called the negative fusional reserve (NFR). When measuring NFR at near distance, a blur point is usually reported prior to diplopia as accommodation relaxes when the eyes are forced to diverge. However, it is unusual to obtain a blur point when measuring NFR at distance, as accommodation is already at a minimum (provided the eyes are emmetropic or appropriate distance correction is worn) and cannot relax beyond this point.

6.12.1 The evidence base: when and how to measure fusional reserves

Fusional reserves should be measured to help decide if a heterophoria is compensated or decompensated. Large heterophorias are often found in patients who are symptom free as they can be compensated by large fusional reserves, whereas small heterophorias can occasionally be associated with symptoms because of greatly reduced fusional reserves. The fusional reserves that oppose the phoria should be measured first. Thus if the patient has exophoria, measure the positive fusional reserves first. This is to ensure that an accurate measurement of the key reserve is obtained, because fusional reserves that are measured subsequently may be modified by vergence adaptation and by fatigue.[85] Risley or rotary prisms are an ideal method of changing the amount of prism before the eyes in a smooth manner (video 6.20) and they provide repeatable results in young adults, although results are less repeatable in children.[26,83] Although phoropters typically feature rotary prisms, they have the disadvantage that they greatly limit the view of the patient's eyes (video 6.20). This is important because clinicians can often identify the break and recovery points by observing the eye movements.[8] Fusional reserve tests in free space, typically using prism bars, more closely mimic natural viewing conditions and are particularly useful because the eyes can be viewed more easily and thus allow an objective assessment of the fusional reserves to be obtained.[86]

6.12.2 Procedure for fusional reserves

See online videos 6.20 for fusional reserves measurement in a phoropter and videos 6.21–6.22 for measurement in free space.

The following description is for the measurement at 6 m. The technique at near is the same, except that the trial frame/phoropter should be adjusted to the near centration distance with the fixation target positioned at the appropriate distance.

1. Explain the test to your patient: "This test measures the range over which your eye muscles can keep objects clear and single." The patient should wear their distance refractive correction. Keep the room lights on.
2. Position yourself in front of the patient so that you can view the patient's eyes easily without obstructing their view of the target.
3. To ensure accurate fixation and accommodation, isolate a single letter of a size that is slightly larger than the patient's visual acuity of the poorer eye (alternatively, a vertical line of letters can be used). For young children, a small, isolated picture may be better for holding their attention.
4. Instruct your patient: "I would like you to look at the letter/target at the other end of the room. I am going to make the picture want to go double and I would like you to try as hard as you can to keep it both clear and single. Please tell me as soon as the letter/target

becomes blurred or doubled, but do remember to try to keep it clear and single for as long as you can even it takes a big effort to achieve this."

Horizontal fusional reserves

5. If you are using a phoropter, ask the patient to close their eyes and introduce the Risley prisms (set at zero) in front of both eyes. If you are using a prism bar, position it so that the horizontal prism will be introduced from a zero starting point over one eye.
6. Let us take the example of measuring PFR (measured with base-out prism): Slowly increase the amount of base-out prism at a rate of around 1Δ to 2Δ per second.[8] If you are using a phoropter, increase the prism in both eyes at an equal rate, remembering that the amount of prism present is the sum of the prism powers before each eye.
7. Instruct your patient to report the first perceptible blur. As soon as the blur is reported, stop increasing the base-out prism and instruct your patient to attempt to make the letter/target clear again. If the letter can be cleared, continue to slowly increase the base-out prism power until the patient reports the first sustained blur. This is the *blur point* and it indicates that the prism power has caused the patient's accommodation response to be over-exerted (base-out prism) or under-exerted (base-in prism) for the viewing distance in question. In other words, the error in accommodation response just exceeds the depth-of-focus at the blur point. Make a mental note of the amount of prism at this point. If the patient does not report blur but instead reports diplopia first, then there is no blur point.
8. Ask the patient to report when the letter now doubles. Further increase the amount of prism until the patient reports sustained double vision. This is the *break point* and it corresponds to the situation where the eyes can no longer make the motor response that is needed to overcome the prism power. Make a mental note of the prism power at this point.
9. Throughout the procedure, watch the patient's eyes carefully. Convergence is difficult to observe initially when small amounts of base-out prism power are introduced; however, when prism power is 6Δ and above, the eye (s) receiving the prism should be seen to converge and increasingly converge with further additional prism. Watch carefully for the objective break point. When the break point is reached, the eye receiving the base-out prism will be seen to make a swift, large outwards movement (so as to make the visual axes parallel again) or the eye not receiving the base-out prism will make a swift and large outwards movement that leaves the visual axes more parallel.

10. It is important to note that in some cases the patient will not report diplopia even though the break point has been passed. When questioned, such patients will usually notice that there is another target 'away to the side' and because the two images are widely separated the second image can be ignored, or is not noticed, by the patient. Careful observation of the patient's eyes will alert you to the possibility that this may have happened.

11. Once the break point has been reached, slowly reduce the amount of prism until the patient reports that the two images have moved together again to form a clear and single image. This is the *recovery point*. Make a mental note of the amount of prism in front of the patient's eye(s) and remove all prism power. If you are using a phoropter, ask the patient to close their eyes and return the Risley prism power to zero.

12. Record the results before you forget them.

13. Repeat the measurement for the other horizontal fusional reserve (steps 6–12). For example, if PFR was measured first, now measure the NFR. In the example above base-out prisms were used to measure the PFR, so base-in prisms should now be used to measure the NFR. Remember that with NFR measurement at distance there is usually no blur point.

Vertical fusional reserves

14. If you are using a phoropter, ask the patient to close their eyes and introduce a Risley prism in front of one eye only (e.g., base-up before RE). If you are using a prism bar, position it so that vertical prism will be introduced from a zero starting point over one eye.

15. To measure vertical fusional reserves, slowly increase the amount of prism placed before the eye(s). Note that vertical fusional reserves are much smaller than the horizontal reserves, and thus the rate of increase of prism power should be slower than that used for measuring horizontal vergences (e.g., $0.5–1^\Delta$/second).

16. Measure the break and recovery points for right supravergence (base-up before right eye) and infravergence (base-down before right eye). Vertical fusional reserves do not have a blur point.

6.12.3 Recording of fusional reserves

1. If there is no blur point, record 'X'.

2. Sample recording: NFR @ 6 m: X/14/10 means that there was no blur point, the break point was 14Δ base-in, and the recovery point was 10Δ base-in. Other examples of recordings:
   a. PFR @ 6 m: 12/18/10; R(OD) infra @ 40 cm: 3/1; R(OD) supra @ 40 cm: 3/1

3. A recovery point that requires prism of the opposite base to that initially used to produce the diplopia (e.g.,

a base-in prism being needed for recovery from diplopia when using base-out prisms to produce diplopia and measure PFR) is recorded as a minus value. For example, PFR @ 6 m: 3/5/−1 indicates that 1^Δ base-in was required to achieve recovery from the diplopia that resulted when 5^Δ base-out had produced diplopia and 3^Δ base-out had produced the first sustained blur.

4. If the limit of the prism power is exceeded, record as $>40^\Delta$ (or the maximum prism value) provided you are certain that the break point has not been exceeded and that is not a case where the patient simply failed to report diplopia (see step 9).

6.12.4 Interpreting the results of fusional reserves

Fusional reserves can be compared with normal data (see Table 6.5), and several tables of comparison have been published for adults and children.[64,66,76] It is clear from these comparisons that a wide variety of 'normal' data have been published over the years. Although you should have some awareness of values that can be expected at distance and near for the various measures, it is desirable that each clinician obtain their own impression of the normative values (average and range) that they can expect using their own equipment and their own technique. The value of fusional reserve measures is greatest when considered, not in isolation but when compared with the heterophoria measurements. For example, a patient with an exophoria will use part of their PFR to overcome the deviation. The measured PFR therefore represents the amount of fusional vergence in reserve to maintain single binocular vision. Similarly, a patient with esophoria will use part of their NFR to overcome their deviation. Knowledge of the heterophoria size and of the magnitude of the opposing fusional reserves can be useful in the assessment of a patient's binocular status, specifically in relation to whether the heterophoria is likely to be giving rise to the patient's symptoms. The proportion of the total fusional vergence used to correct the phoria can be determined. For example:

Distance phoria	9^Δ exophoria
Measured positive fusional reserves (PFR)	18^Δ
Total positive fusional reserves	$18^\Delta + 9^\Delta = 27^\Delta$

Therefore, $1/3$ (9^Δ) of the total positive fusional reserves (27^Δ) are used to correct the phoria, which is within normal limits. This approach has been formalised in Sheard's and Percival's rules, which are used to compare the fusional reserves with the heterophoria and to indicate whether the phoria is likely to be decompensated now or to decompensate in the future under conditions of stress (e.g., when tired or around examination time in the case of students). Sheard's rule proposes that the fusional reserve blur point should be at least twice the size of the phoria. Sheard's criterion works best for exophoric cases so that the PFR to blur should be at least twice the size of the exophoria in order for it to be compensated.[87] Sheard's criterion further suggests that the prism required to correct a decompensated exophoria is:

Prism required = $^2/_3$ exophoria – $^1/_3$ PFR. Thus, for example, if the exophoria is 6$^\Delta$ and the PFR is also 6$^\Delta$, Sheard's criterion suggests that a prism of 2$^\Delta$ base-in should be prescribed. Percival's rule suggests that a patient should operate in the middle third of their binocular vergence range. Percival's rule should only be used for near phorias, because PFR and NFR measured in distance viewing are typically very unbalanced and Percival's rule tends to work best for near esophoric cases.[87] Percival's rule suggests that the PFR and NFR should be balanced and that one should not be more than double the other. Percival's criterion suggests:

Prism required for esophoria = $^1/_3$ total range – NFR. For example, if the PFR is 11$^\Delta$ and the NFR is 4$^\Delta$, the prism required is 15/3 – 4 = 1$^\Delta$ base-out.

It is important to stress that even if Sheard's or Percival's criteria are violated, prisms should not be prescribed unless there is good reason to do so. Such reasons may include the presence of symptoms which can be explained by a decompensated phoria, better performance (e.g. better stereopsis, section 6.7) with the prism in place and clinical scenarios where exercises are not appropriate.

6.12.5 Most common errors when measuring fusional reserves

1. Providing an inappropriate stimulus to accommodation through poor choice of target.
2. Not emphasising to the patient that they must make maximal effort to keep the target clear and single for as long as possible, and that in so doing, the eyes may well feel very tired and strained.
3. Not observing the eyes carefully as the prism power is increased so as to gain an objective estimate of the break point.
4. Increasing the prism power too quickly or too slowly.
5. Carrying out the test in patients who have a strabismus at the test distance.

6.12.6 Acceptable alternative: the 20Δ base-out test

(See online video 6.23.)

This technique is suitable for use in those patients who may not be able to co-operate with fusional reserve measurement (e.g., young children). Rather than obtain responses from the patient regarding the blurring or doubling of the target, this test relies on qualitative judgements made by the clinician in response to the

introduction of a high-powered prism. Typically, a 20$^\Delta$ base-out prism is used (although in theory any significant prism power or direction can be employed) and the clinician examines whether the eye behind the prism makes a swift and smooth movement in order to restore the image of the object of regard on the fovea. Also, the clinician will search for a swift recovery movement in the opposite direction when the base-out prism is removed. The test is repeated with the prism in front of the other eye. In principle the test is similar to 4-prism base-out test (section 6.10.2), but it is much easier for the clinician to establish whether the appropriate motor fusion response has taken place following the introduction of this high powered prism. A normal response on this test can allow the clinician to generalise about the effectiveness of the motor fusion system and thus the ability of the visual system to maintain fusion throughout the day. A normal response on this test may be recorded in the following fashion: '20$^\Delta$ base-out overcome with either eye; good recovery.' A positive response on this test (i.e., an appropriate motor fusion response) is a very strong indicator that peripheral fusion exists and thus the 20$^\Delta$ base-out test can prove useful in children who are too young to undergo formal sensory testing.[88] Unfortunately the same is not true in reverse, because a negative result on the 20$^\Delta$ base-out does not guarantee that peripheral fusion is poor or absent.

6.13 Fixation disparity

Fixation disparity describes binocular vision when the two retinal images do not fall on corresponding retinal points, but remain within Panum's area, so that they are still seen singly. Because Panum's areas are small, fixation disparities represent small (typically less than a few minutes of arc) misalignments.[89,90] The advocates of fixation disparity maintain that a fixation disparity arises when the visual system is under stress; indeed the presence of fixation disparity is considered by some to represent that part of the phoria that is decompensated.[91,92] Unlike in phoria assessments (section 6.11), the eyes are only partially dissociated during fixation disparity assessment and most of the target (the binocular lock) is seen by both eyes, whereas a small portion of the target (the monocular locks) is visible to only one eye.

Two approaches can be taken when a fixation disparity is present. One is to have physical control over the monocular markers so that they can be independently moved by the patient to achieve perceptual alignment. The other approach is to have fixed monocular markers in physical alignment and use prisms (or less commonly, spherical lenses) to eliminate the perceptual misalignment. This prism power is called the 'aligning prism', and these measures are sometimes referred to as the 'associated phoria,' although these terms are not universally popular.[8]

6.13.1 The evidence base: when and how to measure fixation disparity

The use of fixation disparity varies widely between countries. In the United Kingdom, fixation disparity has been made popular through the Mallett unit, and clinicians either conduct the test routinely post-refraction as an alternative to post-refraction phoria measurement or they use it when there has been a significant change in the refractive correction, or when signs or symptoms suggest that a binocular vision problem may exist. In other countries, the Mallett unit is less commonly used and tests, such as the Wesson and Saladin cards,[93,94] tend to be used, but as an additional rather than a routine test.

The presence of fixation disparity may indicate that the phoria is decompensated. Jenkins et al. found that 1^Δ and 2^Δ of fixation disparity was associated with symptoms in pre-presbyopes and presbyopes, respectively, and it may be the best indicator that a phoria is decompensated.[91,92] Mallett believed that the aligning prism corresponded to the decompensated portion of the phoria. This is supported by the finding that fixation disparity has been shown to increase under binocular stress, such as working under inadequate illumination or at too close a working distance, and at the end of a working day.[92,95] There are also claims that the magnitude of fixation disparity is linked to the level of stereopsis that can be achieved and that the size of the aligning prism at near is inversely correlated with the fusional reserves, supporting the view that both measures may be indicators of decompensation of heterophoria.[48,96] Near Mallett unit measurements are likely to be changed by previous phoria measurement, particularly if von Graefe's technique was employed. It is recommended, therefore, that the near Mallett unit should be used before the dissociated phoria is measured in patients regarded as having unstable binocular vision, past or present.[97]

The Saladin and Wesson cards provide a means for establishing the shape of the fixation disparity curve, something that was originally possible only with the Sheedy Disparometer, a device that is no longer commercially available.[93,94] As opposed to the aligning prism measure (which corresponds to just one point on the fixation disparity curve) provided by the Mallett unit, the Saladin and Wesson cards provide estimates of fixation disparity when different amounts of prism are introduced and from these measures the key components of fixation disparity curves (e.g., slope in central region, as well as the

x- and y-intercepts) can be deduced.[93,94] The Saladin card is reported to have good test-retest reliability.[98]

The fixation disparity approach has a number of significant disadvantages. One is that fixation disparity measures seem to be critically dependent on the method used to measure them. For example, results obtained with the Wesson and Saladin cards are not comparable, raising the possibility that the measures indicate more about the equipment than about the visual system they are testing.[93] The size and position of the binocular lock and monocular markers appear to exert an influence on the magnitude of the fixation disparity.[99] This is a problem given that computer-based versions of the fixation disparity test employ different test formats. For this and other reasons, many remain unconvinced about the clinical relevance of fixation disparity and view it instead as a physiological phenomenon.[7] For example, if fixation disparity does reflect the decompensated portion of the phoria, the type of fixation disparity present should always match the direction of heterophoric deviation (e.g., an exo fixation disparity should only be present in a patient with exophoria). However, this is not always the case and a small but significant proportion of patients have so-called paradoxical fixation disparity[100,101] where the fixation disparity and/or the associated phoria are in the opposite direction to the phoria.[90] This in itself may be a sign of binocular vision or accommodative disorder.[66]

The distance Mallet unit uses red monocular strips and a central fixation lock (OXO), but does not have a peripheral fusion lock (see Fig. 6.6). The near Mallett unit (Fig. 6.19) uses green monocular strips, as green is usually more sharply focused at near due to a slight lag of accommodation, a central fixation lock (OXO), and a surrounding paragraph of print providing a peripheral fusion lock. The near Mallett unit also contains paragraphs of text of various sizes (typically N5 to N10), a retractable ruler, a near duochrome, and targets that allow investigation of suppression and stereopsis (sections 6.6 and 6.7). Like the Mallett unit, the Wesson Fixation Disparity card and the Saladin Near Point Balance card use a polarisation method to render the monocular markers visible to the right or left eye. In the newer Saladin card, a penlight is held behind the card and is used to illuminate each circle.

6.13.2 Fixation disparity (or aligning prism) procedure

For all tests:
1. Explain the test to your patient: "This is a test that will help to determine how well your eyes are working together."

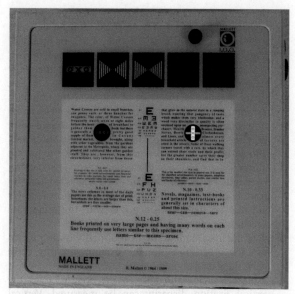

Fig. 6.19 A near Mallett unit.

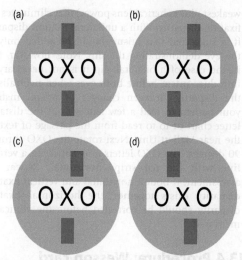

Fig. 6.20 Diagram illustrating the possible patient responses to the Mallett fixation disparity test.

2. Fixation disparity should be assessed when the appropriate refractive correction is in place for the viewing distance (i.e., with reading addition in patients who are presbyopic) and with the appropriate centration distance.

6.13.3 Procedure: Mallett unit

The distance and near assessment procedures are similar, except that a paragraph of small text should be read prior to viewing the near Mallett OXO to ensure accurate accommodation on the target.

3. Orient the OXO in a horizontal position with the red (distance Mallett) or green (near unit) strips vertical. Keep the room lights on to illuminate the unit's surroundings; this provides para-macular and peripheral fusion stimuli.

4. Prior to placing the polaroid visor in front of the patient's eyes, ask the patient to "Look at the X in the middle of the OXO; do you see two red (distance)/ green (near) strips, one above and one below the OXO? Are the two strips exactly in line with each other and in line with the middle of the X?" This ensures that the patient is aware of what alignment looks like (Fig. 6.20a), so that any subsequent misalignment is more easily noticed.

5. Now place the polaroid visor in front of the patient's eyes. Normally the top red strip is seen by the left eye, and the lower strip by the right eye.

6. Next ask the patient "Can you still see the two strips?" If only one strip is seen, show the patient the two individual strips by covering each eye in turn. If only one strip is still seen when both eyes are viewing, central suppression may be present, and no further measurement is possible. Most patients, however, will see both strips without difficulty.

7. Ask the patient "Are the strips in line with each other and the middle of the X?"

8. If both of the strips are reported to be aligned, no fixation disparity is present (see Fig. 6.20a).

9. Several other results could be reported:
   (a) If the lower red strip (usually seen by the RE) is to the left of the X and the upper strip (usually seen by the LE) is to the right, an EXO fixation disparity is present in both eyes (see Fig. 6.20b).
   (b) If the lower strip (RE) remains below the X, but the upper strip (LE) moves to the right, an EXO fixation disparity is present in the left eye only (see Fig. 6.20c). When the disparity is unilateral, there is a view that it is the non-dominant eye that demonstrates the deviation. Unilateral fixation disparity is unusual is most common in vertical imbalance, whereas horizontal fixation disparities are usually bilateral.
   (c) If an ESO fixation disparity is present, the lower strip (RE) will be to the right of the upper strip (LE) (see Fig. 6.20d).

10. The fixation disparity should be neutralised using the lowest prism power (or in rare cases of esophoria, the

weakest plus spherical lens power) that eliminates the fixation disparity. With a unilateral fixation disparity, it is suggested that prism should be added only to the eye demonstrating the slip. Note, however, that in the case of a bilateral slip it is not necessary to introduce prism before both eyes when neutralising the disparity. Between changes of prism, instruct your patient to read a few letters from the distance letter chart or to to read from the passage of text on the near Mallett Unit. Next rotate the OXO through 90 degrees. The OXO letters now appear in a vertical line with the red strips horizontal. Repeat the assessment. If both a horizontal and vertical fixation disparity exists together, the horizontal fixation disparity should be corrected before the vertical is measured.

6.13.4 Procedure: Wesson card

1. The Wesson card can be used at 40 cm or at 25 cm. Appropriate refractive correction and centration distance should be used, and the card should be properly illuminated.
2. Wearing the polarising goggles, the patient reports which line the arrow is pointing towards when no prism is in place and then when 3 base-in (BI), 3 base-out (BO), 6 BI, 6 BO, etc., in 3^Δ increments up to 24 BI and 24 BO or up to the prism power where non-transient diplopia is reported. In so far as possible, the prism should be split evenly between the eyes.
3. Because of the risks of prism adaptation it is recommended that the prism should not be in place for more than 15 seconds and that patients should close their eyes for at least 15 seconds between measurements with successive prism powers.[102,103]
4. Note the magnitude of fixation disparity from the card for each prism and plot the fixation disparity curve using the data gathered.
5. To obtain vertical fixation disparity measures, the card is turned through 90 degrees. Vertical fixation disparity measures are taken only once, without any prism in place.

6.13.5 Procedure: Saladin card

1. The Saladin chart is used at 40 cm and appropriate refractive correction and pupillary distance should be used. The card should be properly illuminated.
2. Wearing the polarising goggles, the patient reports which circle contains the vertically oriented lines that are in alignment. The physical misalignment of the lines in these circles provides the measure of horizontal fixation disparity.

3. The above procedure is carried out when no prism is in place and then when 3 BI, 3 BO, 6 BI, 6 BO, etc., in 3^Δ increments up to 24 BI and 24 BO, or up to the prism power where non-transient diplopia is reported. In so far as possible, the prism should be split equally between the eyes.
4. Again, because of the risks of prism adaptation it is recommended that the prism should not be in place for more than 15 seconds and that patients should close their eyes for at least 15 seconds between measurements with successive prism power.[94] Similarly, if the patient fails to achieve fusion with the new prism power within 5 seconds of its introduction, it is suggested that no fixation disparity be recorded for that prism power and that no higher prism power with the same base direction be offered.[94]
5. Note the magnitude of fixation disparity from the card for each prism and plot the fixation disparity curve using the data gathered.
6. Using the circles with horizontally oriented lines, the vertical fixation disparity can be measured. Vertical fixation disparity measures are taken only once, without any prism in place.

6.13.6 Recording fixation disparity results

If the monocular markers of the Mallett unit are not simultaneously visible to both eyes, record the eye that was being suppressed and whether the suppression was intermittent or constant.

If a fixation disparity was present, record the minimum prism power or spherical lens power required to align the strips. If the fixation disparity was found in one eye only, this should be recorded. For example, 'Mallett: No FD D or N; 'Mallett, Dist: 2^Δ BI; Near: 1^Δ BI LE'.

For the Saladin and Wesson cards, the recording consists of the fixation disparity in minutes of arc corresponding to each prism power introduced. If one of the targets disappears during measurement, this indicates suppression and the eye that is being suppressed should be recorded.

6.13.7 Interpreting the results of fixation disparity

Most patients will be able to simultaneously perceive the monocular markers on the distance and near Mallett unit; usually the markers appear in alignment without the need for any prisms. It is important to remember that the prism power required to align the markers is not predictable from the magnitude of the fixation disparity (e.g., small fixation disparities are not always eliminated by low prism powers) and two patients exhibiting the same amount of fixation disparity may require very different prism powers to perceive the lines as aligned. Due to possible prism adaptation it is advisable to leave the lowest prism power that neutralises the fixation disparity in place for a period of time (several minutes). In patients with normal binocular vision, prism adaptation takes places so that two to three minutes after the introduction of a prism, the slip that was initially corrected by the prism reappears.[8,102] However, it is claimed that if there is a binocular vision problem, no adaptation or only partial adaptation will take place to the prism.[103] The prism power that neutralises any vertical fixation disparities can be used to prescribe vertical prism.

For the Wesson and Saladin card, the horizontal fixation disparity data gathered are used to plot fixation disparity curves and from these curves four key characteristics are identified; they are the type (I, II, III, or IV), the slope, and the x- and y-intercepts. A discussion of fixation disparity curves is beyond the scope of this chapter except to say that most asymptomatic patients have type I curves, featuring shallow slopes in the central region, and most show low numerical values for the x- (aligning prism) and y- (fixation disparity in minutes of arc) intercepts. Scheiman and Wick maintain that the fixation disparity curve method provides the best means for determining the amount of prism to prescribe.[66]

6.13.8 Most common errors when testing fixation disparity

1. Decentration errors due to poorly fitting trial frame/phoropter or badly centred lenses.
2. Mallett:
   (a) Not taking the lowest possible prism as the measure.
   (b) Not checking for potential prism adaptation.
3. Wesson/Saladin card:
   (a) Assuming that the results obtained with these cards are interchangeable.[25]
   (b) Leaving the prism in place for too long before measures are taken.
   (c) Not allowing enough time between the introduction of new prism powers.

6.14 The accommodative convergence to accommodation relationship

The coupling of accommodation and vergence allows clear, stable, single binocular vision across a range of viewing distances. The amount of accommodative convergence in

prism dioptres (Δ) evoked by 1.00 D of accommodation is known as the AC/A ratio.

6.14.1 The evidence base: when and how to measure the AC/A relationship

The AC/A ratio is measured when the patient's signs or symptoms suggest that a binocular vision problem may exist, particularly in patients in whom there is a significant difference between near and distance phoria measures.[66] AC/A ratios that are abnormally high or low can give rise to binocular vision problems.[104] The AC/A relationship remains fairly constant throughout life until the onset of presbyopia, but measurements after the age of 45 years are of little value because of the reduced AoA.[105] The change in vergence obtained with a fixed change in the *stimulus* to accommodation (e.g., a −1.00 DS lens), known as the *stimulus* AC/A ratio, is measured. Due to typical accommodative lag (section 6.8), the accommodative response is less than the stimulus to accommodation. The modified gradient test allows a quick and reliable measure of the AC/A ratio using phoria measurements with and without a negative lens, but the use of only two measures can lead to errors.[106] The full gradient test overcomes this problem by measuring heterophorias with dioptric powers ranging from +3.00 D to −3.00 D in 1.00-D steps and plotting a graph of lens power against induced phoria. The gradient of this line gives the AC/A ratio in Δ/D. The 'calculated' AC/A ratio compares the distance and near heterophoria (see section 6.14 below), but in addition to errors from the use of only two measurements, it also has the disadvantage that proximal accommodation is present in one heterophoria measure (near) but not the other. Irrespective of the method used, the target viewed by the patient should require precise accommodation as the ratio obtained has been shown to depend on the fixation target.[107]

6.14.2 Procedure: gradient AC/A ratio

1. Ensure the patient is wearing an appropriate refractive correction, either their own spectacles or, preferably, the optimal correction determined during the eye examination.
2. Measure the horizontal near heterophoria using the modified Thorington or Howell card method (section 6.11) or some other method that carefully controls accommodation.
3. Add −2.00 DS to the refractive correction in both eyes and measure the new horizontal phoria (any pair of minus lenses can be used but −2.00 DS provides a reasonable accommodative stimulus for most patients).
4. The above procedure is normally carried out at near. However it is just as valid to determine the AC/A ratio

by comparing the horizontal heterophoria at 6 m when viewing with optimal refractive correction with the heterophoria that exists when the patient looks through a pair of −2.00 D lenses.

6.14.3 Recording AC/A ratio results

Use the following formula to calculate the AC/A ratio. Use positive numbers for esophoria and negative numbers for exophoria.

$$AC/A = \frac{\text{Phoria with additional minus lenses} - \text{Baseline phoria}}{\text{Absolute power of additional minus lenses}}$$

The calculation required to determine the AC/A ratio is the same, irrespective of whether the heterophoria measurements were taken during near or distance viewing. For example, if a patient exhibits 6^Δ esophoria during distance viewing when −2.00 D lenses are added to their normal refractive correction but 2^Δ exophoria with the normal refractive correction in place, the AC/A ratio is calculated as:

$$AC/A = 6 - (-2)/2 = 8/2 = 4^\Delta : 1.00 \text{ D}$$

6.14.4 Interpreting the results of AC/A

Normally the AC/A is around 4^Δ/D.[8] A low AC/A ratio may, depending on the distance heterophoria, result in convergence insufficiency. Similarly, a high AC/A ratio may lead to a problem of convergence excess.[66] Knowledge of the AC/A ratio can be useful when determining plus lens power for the correction of decompensated esophoria. As the amount of convergence induced by 1.00 D stimulus to accommodation is known, it is possible to calculate the extra plus lens power required to reduce the esophoria to an acceptable level. Similarly, in young exophoric patients, knowledge of the AC/A ratio is crucial if prescribing minus lens power to reduce the exophoria is being considered.[66] One drawback of the methods described here is that in order to determine the value of the AC/A ratio accurately, we need to take into account the lag or lead of accommodation that the patient exhibits (section 6.8). This relates to the difference between the stimulus and response AC/C ratio discussed earlier (section 6.14).

6.14.5 Most common error when measuring AC/A ratios

1. Attempting to measure the ratio in presbyopic patients who have low or no accommodation remaining.
2. Using an unreliable method of heterophoria assessment to determine the AC/A ratio such as the von Graefe prism dissociation method (section 6.11).

6.14.6 Alternative technique: calculated AC/A

The calculated $AC/A = PD_{cms} + (n - d)/D$, where PD = interpupillary distance measured in cm; n = near phoria; d = distance phoria; D = accommodation. Exophorias are negative and esophorias are positive:

For example: PD = 6 cms and D = 2.5 D (accommodation required at 40 cm), distance phoria is ortho and near phoria is 5 exo, AC/A = $6 + (-5/2.5) = 4^\Delta : 1.00$ D.

Without using the above formula, it is possible to get an impression of whether the AC/A ratio is normal or not by comparing the near and distance heterophorias. For example, an exophoria that is much greater at near than at distance will be found in a patient with a low AC/A ratio. Similarly, esophoria that is greater at near than at distance suggests either a high AC/A ratio or significant uncorrected hyperopia. In cases where the near and distance phorias are the same, the formula above indicates that the AC/A ratio is given by the patient's PD (in cm) and will be approximately $6^\Delta : 1.00$ D.

6.15 Further assessment of the relationship between convergence and accommodation

In a small subset of patients it can be appropriate to consider tests of accommodation and vergence facility and/or positive and negative relative accommodation. A properly functioning visual system allows accommodation to be altered to a small extent without automatically being associated with a change in vergence. If accommodation and convergence are too tightly linked, the patient is vulnerable to symptoms. Accommodation and vergence facility measures reflect the ease (i.e., the speed) with which accommodation can be made independently of vergence, and vice-versa. Positive relative accommodation (PRA) and negative relative accommodation (NRA), on the other hand, represent the full extent to which accommodation can be exerted without vergence. Thus, they are the accommodation equivalents of blur points in the positive and negative fusional reserves (section 6.12), because the latter represent measures of how much vergence can be exerted without accommodation.

6.15.1 The evidence base: when and how to further examine accommodation, vergence, and their relationship

Further tests of accommodation and convergence are appropriate when patients complain of symptoms changing from near to distance viewing, or vice versa, and in the presence of unexplained symptoms that are potentially accommodative or binocular in nature. These investigations are also appropriate when other test results suggest that a binocular vision or accommodation problem exists and warrants further investigation. Measures of accommodation and vergence facility reflect the ability to exercise accommodation without vergence (accommodation facility) or vergence without accommodation (vergence facility) quickly. Unlike vergence facility measures, accommodation facility measurements can be taken under monocular conditions. These tests require additional equipment in the form of prism flippers and lens flippers but they are straightforward to perform.

The results of vergence facility testing may explain symptoms not readily explained by other tests.[108] Gall et al. reported that the combination of 3^Δ base-in and 12^Δ base-out prism flippers provides good repeatability and the best discrimination between symptomatic and non-symptomatic patients.[109] However, normative values have also been published for other powers of prism flippers.[64,109] Accommodative facility should be measured in young patients (i.e., those with appreciable accommodation) with symptoms experienced in near viewing, even when other accommodative measures, such as the AoA, are at normal levels.[69] Growing evidence from clinical studies indicate that the responsiveness of accommodation is amenable to treatment and evidence of objectively measured improvement in accommodation responsiveness following training is emerging from clinical studies.[110-112] Using established pass/fail criteria, a recent study of the prevalence of persistently reduced accommodative facility in 4- to 12-year-old children is 3.6%.[113] The ± 2.00 DS flippers test of accommodative facility can be performed rapidly with minimal additional equipment. Measures of accommodative facility may be useful in diagnosing disorders in symptomatic patients whose phorias and visual acuity are normal.[108] It appears to have diagnostic value in that a reduced facility correlates with near symptoms and facility increases as symptoms are alleviated through treatment. Indeed, flippers can be part of the treatment. There is little justification for the use of the ± 2.00 DS flippers other than they are the powers traditionally used. Indeed, it may be that what is required is a range of flipper powers that relate to the patient's AoA.[114] For example, for a young patient with an amplitude of 12.00 D, ± 2.00 DS flippers cover only 33% (-2.00D to $+2.00$D; i.e., a 4.00 D change) of the amplitude, whereas they cover 67% of the amplitude in an older patient with an amplitude of 6.00 D. Yothers et al. suggest using an amplitude-scaled test for adults, which uses a test distance that requires 45% of the AoA to be exerted and lens flippers that cover 30% of the amplitude.[115] For example, in a patient with 7.00 D of accommodation a

working distance of 32 cm (45% of 7.00 = 3.15 D; 1/3.15 = 0.32 m) and a flipper power of ± 1.00 D (flipper range of 2.10 or 30% of 7.00) is recommended. This is also the approach advocated by Scheiman and Wick in adult patients.[66] Many authors recommend measuring the binocular accommodative facility with a suppression check (typically using polaroid glasses with the Bernell No. 9 vectogram). For appropriate comparison, the monocular measurements should be made with the same set-up except that one eye is now fully occluded.

Both PRA and NRA should be assessed in younger patients with symptoms at near, which could indicate a decompensated phoria and/or an accommodative problem. Because the test results reflect the ability to exert and relax accommodation, it is not appropriate to take relative accommodation measures in patients who are presbyopic. As well as providing a measure of the ability to relax accommodation, the NRA also gives an indirect measure of the positive fusional vergence.[66] This is because, as accommodation is relaxed, there will be less accommodative convergence. The result is that the patient will experience uncrossed diplopia unless the positive fusional vergence takes place to prevent this. Similarly, PRA gives an indirect measure of the negative fusional vergence,[66] because when accommodation is stimulated during PRA, accommodative convergence is increased and this will lead to crossed diplopia unless negative fusional vergence takes place.

6.15.2 Procedure: prism flippers

(See online video 6.24.)

This test can be carried out at any test distance, although it is normally carried out at near. If, however, symptoms are reported at a non-reading test distance, testing should be carried out at that distance. The patient should view a single isolated letter/target or a vertical line of letters; the letter/target should be approximately one line bigger than the smallest letters that can be read at the test distance. The patient should wear the habitual near correction for the test. You should sit down during the test so that you can observe the patient's eyes as the prisms are flipped.[116]

1. Instruct your patient as follows: "I am now going to test how well your eyes can maintain clear and single vision when I introduce some lenses".
2. First demonstrate the task required of the patient by introducing the prisms and asking the patient to appreciate that it can take some time for the letters to become clear and single again after the introduction of the prisms. Remind the patient that they will be required to let you know as soon as the letters are clear and single, and also that they should attempt to make them clear and single as quickly as possible.

3. Once the patient appears to understand the test, start the clock and introduce the 12^Δ base-out prism power. When the patient reports 'clear', flip the handle to introduce the 3^Δ base-in prism power. When the patient again reports 'clear' this represents one cycle, and flip the handle again.

4. Observing the patient's eyes as the prisms are introduced provides very useful objective confirmation that the patient understands what is required in the test, that they are complying with your instructions and therefore that the result is valid. When base-out prism power is introduced, expect to see the eyes converge and when the prisms are flipped to provide base-in power the eyes should be seen to diverge. The ease with which this pattern of eye movements can be seen by the practitioner naturally depends on the prism powers, but except in the case of very low powers (e.g., 2 BI/2 BO), careful observation should reveal the expected pattern if the test is proceeding properly.

5. As the eyes are being observed, count the number of cycles achieved by the patient in a 60-second period.

6.15.3 Procedure: lens flippers

(See online video 6.25.)

1. If testing monocularly, occlude one eye. Keep the room lights on and, if necessary, use localised lighting so that the patient's eyes can be easily seen without shadows.

2. Explain the measurement to your patient: "I am now going to test how quickly your focusing can change."

3. Ask the patient to hold a near chart at 40 cm. Maintaining a stable viewing distance is crucial because viewing distance affects the results obtained and because published normative data are generally based on a 40-cm test distance.[66,117] Ask the patient to look at a letter on a line that is one line larger than the near visual acuity in the circumstances. This would typically be about N6 (0.4 M, 20/30).

4. Explain the test to your patient: "I want you to keep looking at the word/letter. I am going to place a lens in front of your eye that may make the word appear blurred. I want you to focus and make the print clear again as soon as you can. As soon as it becomes clear, say 'clear'. I will then flip another lens in front of the eye that may make the word appear blurred again. As before, I want you to refocus quickly and make the word clear again, and then say 'clear'. We will repeat this for 60 seconds." Demonstrate the procedure to the patient so that they understand what is required before the test is started.

5. Start the clock as soon as you place the $+2.00$ D lens in the lens flippers (twirls) in front of the patient's right eye and ask the patient to tell you as soon as the target becomes clear by saying 'clear'.

6. As soon as the patient reports that the target is clear, quickly flip the lens flippers to the -2.00 lens and ask the patient to again inform you as soon as the letters become clear again.

7. Count the number of times the patient utters 'clear' in 60 seconds. One cycle consists of clearing both the plus and the minus lenses.

8. Repeat for the left eye.

9. Repeat the test binocularly if the patient does not suppress at near. Some clinicians use a polaroid bar reader placed over the near chart while the patient wears polaroid glasses. This provides a check on suppression because the patient will only be able to see half of the text if suppression is present. In binocular testing, the patients is asked to indicate to you as soon as the target becomes both clear and single.

6.15.4 Procedure: positive and negative relative accommodation

1. Adjust the phoropter to the near PD and attach the near-point card. Make sure that the optimal distance refractive correction is in place and that both eyes can view the near-point card. The viewing distance should correspond to the patient's typical working distance for near tasks. If the test is conducted with trial frame and lenses, it is vital to ensure that the viewing distance is held constant as the lenses are changed.

2. Direct the patient's attention to letters one or two lines larger than their best near visual acuity on the near-point card. Both eyes remain open throughout testing. The patient must maintain fixation on the same-sized letters throughout the test and is asked to keep the letters clear and single for as long as possible as increasing positive and negative spherical lens power is added.

3. For NRA, add plus lenses binocularly, $+0.25$ D at a time, until the patient reports the first sustained blur. If the letters become less clear, the patient should be asked to try to make the letters clear again. 'First sustained blur' means that the patient notices that the letters are not as sharp and clear as they were initially, even if the patient can still read them. The total amount of plus power added when then letters exhibit the first sustained blur is the NRA. Note the amount of plus power added and then remove it.

4. For PRA, add minus lenses binocularly, -0.25 D at a time, until the patient reports the first sustained blur. The total amount of minus lens power added is the PRA.

6.15.5 Recording

For vergence facility: Record the number of cycles achieved (e.g., vergence facility at 40 cm: 10 cycles/minute [12 BO/3 BI]).

For accommodation facility: Record the number of cycles/minute for each eye and then for the binocular viewing condition (e.g., 'accomm. facility: 12 cycles /min [RE], 11 cycles/min LE), 10 cycles/min (Binocularly) using (+2 D/–2 D)'. If the patient cannot clear one of the two lenses, the recording should note this.

For NRA and PRA: Record the positive (NRA) and negative (PRA) lens powers which lead to the first sustained blur or first sustained diplopia at near. Sample recording: PRA @ 40 cm: −2.50 DS, NRA @ 40 cm: +2.25 DS.

6.15.6 Interpretation

Vergence and accommodation facility measurements depend on the powers of the prisms and lenses that are presented in the flippers. Normal values for the vergence facility test using 12 BO/3 BI are in the region of 15 cycles/minute (see Table 6.5).[66] Normative data reported for accommodation facility in the literature are variable, possibly because data were gathered across a range of ages but reported as a grand average or because they were collected from unselected samples (e.g., samples may have included patients with symptoms and accommodative or vergence dysfunctions). For these reasons, published normative data cannot be completely relied on and you are encouraged to have an impression of normative data for a range of age groups based on your own measurements.[114] Suggested 'clinical pass' criteria in young adults are 11 cycles/minute (monocular) and 8 cycles/minute binocularly.[114] For children aged between 8 and 12 years, 'clinical pass' criteria are 7 cycles/minute (monocular) and 5 cycles/minute (binocular).[113] There is considerable intra-individual variability in raw accommodation facility measures in children.[118] When considered in terms of pass/fail, children who initially exhibit normal accommodative facility continue to do so on repeat testing. Conversely, however, most children with initially reduced accommodative facility exhibit normal performance on repeat testing. This suggests that a diagnosis of reduced accommodative facility in children should not be based on a single, below-expected measure.

Measures of PRA and NRA are taken binocularly. For this reason, PRA and NRA measures can be affected by fusional vergence or by the ability to relax or engage accommodation. To establish whether NRA primarily represents a failure or accommodation or vergence, there are two options. The first is to repeat the NRA measure under monocular conditions. If the NRA is, for example, +2.00 D monocularly but only +1.00 D binocularly, this suggests that the binocular measure is affected by reduced positive fusional amplitude. If the monocular and binocular NRA measures are similarly low, the problem is one of inability to relax accommodation. The second approach is simply to cover one eye when the target exhibits the first sustained blur. If the target clears when one eye is covered, vergence rather than accommodation is implicated. The second approach is also used for interpreting PRA measures. Comparison of PRA under binocular and monocular conditions is not useful because monocular measures merely reflect the AoA (negative spherical lens power to first sustained blur; see section 6.8).

For a viewing distance of 40 cm, the expected NRA is +2.00 D ± 0.50 D and we expect to see balanced PRA and NRA values (see Table 6.5). Based on the dioptric demand at 40 cm, the maximum expected NRA is +2.50 D. Thus if −2.50 D can be added whilst maintaining clear and single vision, there is no need to offer higher negative power and the PRA can recorded as ≥2.50 D.

6.15.7 Most common errors

Facility testing

1. Not allowing the patient to practice before starting the test or not explaining the test in sufficient detail as to what is expected.
2. Using an inappropriately sized target for the test (e.g., letters that are too large) or using a target that is surrounded by other targets so that appreciation of diplopia or blur is made difficult for the patient.
3. Counting the recovery from each prism/lens introduction as a cycle and thus over-estimating the test performance by a factor of two.
4. Not observing the eyes closely during the vergence facility test and therefore failing to check that the eyes move in the expected fashion when base-in and base-out prism powers are added.
5. Not recording the power of prisms/lenses in the flippers and/or the test distance and/or the reason for any test failure (e.g., not indicating if the patient failed to clear the positive or negative lens power during accommodation facility testing).
6. Not being aware of the normative values for the prism/lens powers used (see Table 6.5).

NRA and PRA

1. Attempting to measure PRA and NRA in patients with no/minimal accommodation.
2. Attempting to measure PRA and NRA under monocular conditions.
3. Not knowing how to distinguish a problem of vergence from one of accommodation when PRA and NRA measures are below expected values (see Table 6.5).

6.16 Further evaluation of incomitant strabismus

Incomitant deviations are screened for using the motility (broad H) test (section 6.4).

6.16.1 The evidence base: when and how to evaluate incomitancy

Evaluation of incomitancy is warranted when the motility test (section 6.4) reveals that an incomitant deviation is present and a variety of tests are available. The cover test or Maddox rod can be used in peripheral directions of gaze.[7] Cover testing in peripheral gaze has an advantage over the Maddox rod test in that it is an objective test and, therefore, it can be used in patients with suppression. Although considerable dexterity is required, an experienced clinician will be able to carry out the procedure swiftly and smoothly. The technique of assessing movements of the eyes as the head is tilted successively toward one shoulder and then toward the other was introduced by Hoffmann and Bielschowsky, but has since come to be known as the Bielschowsky head tilt test.[7] The manner in which this test is normally used in the clinical setting is referred to as the Parks 3-step test. Head tilting is used to reveal the defective vertically acting muscle(s) (it is not needed if a problem with the lateral or medial rectus muscles is suspected). If there is a problem with one of the elevating or depressing muscles, head tilting causes a change in the vertical alignment of the eyes because the muscle which is affected is not able to cancel the vertical action of its ipsilateral antagonist. Cover testing in peripheral gaze and the Parks-3 step test should not be seen as alternative tests but rather as complementary tests. If cover testing in peripheral gaze suggests a particular explanation for the incomitancy (e.g., superior rectus underaction), this can be further subjected to testing via the Park-3 step test. In other words, the latter generally follows cover testing in peripheral gaze and is carried out to explain the results of previous testing. The Parks 3-step test is useful in cases of paresis of any of the cyclovertical muscles, but the results are more dramatic when the oblique muscles are affected compared with when the vertical rectus muscles are involved. No additional equipment is required to perform this test; the added advantage is that the test is objective, thus making it suitable for use in young children. However, the test result can be affected by a number of factors, including the paresis of more than one muscle and mechanical restrictions by previous surgery to the extra-ocular muscles. Furthermore, interpretation of results may be more difficult than in the case of the Hess screen test.

6.16.2 Procedure: 9-point cover test

Perform a near cover test in each of the nine positions of gaze. A cover-uncover test for strabismus (see Box 6.1) in a peripheral gaze direction can help to reveal which eye is not looking at the spotlight. An alternating cover test is often carried out because the direction of movements will be more obvious than in a cover-uncover test. However, a major disadvantage of the alternating cover test is that it will not tell you which eye is the fixating eye. For this reason a cover-uncover test is preferred. Note that in the cover-uncover test, the deviation may differ depending on which eye is fixating (primary versus secondary deviation, see section 6.4). If quantitative measures are required, horizontal and vertical prism bars are needed in order to neutralise the vertical and horizontal deviations.

6.16.3 Procedure: Parks-3-step test

In order to carry out the Parks 3-step test, you should attempt to answer the following three questions:

1. Which is the hyper-deviated eye in the primary position? The answer to this question may be obvious by simply viewing the patient or it may require you to carry out a cover-uncover test in the primary position (section 6.2).
2. Is the hyper-deviation greater in right or left gaze?
3. Is the hyper-deviation greater with head tilted to the right shoulder or to the left shoulder? This portion of the test is the Bielschowsky head tilt test.

6.16.4 Recording incomitancy

The peripheral cover test result is normally recorded in a fashion that identifies the muscle(s) that is/are affected (e.g., 'peripheral cover test: bilateral super rectus underaction'). The Park's 3-step test result also describes the problem muscle identified (e.g., 'Park's 3-step: bilateral inferior-oblique underaction').

6.16.5 Interpreting incomitancy results

9-point cover test: The results of motility testing are relatively straightforward to interpret if there is a problem with a lateral or medial rectus muscle.

The clinical interpretation of motility test results is more complicated when diplopia is experienced on upward or downward gaze, because there are four extra-ocular muscles that help to elevate (the right superior rectus, RSR; left superior rectus, LSR; right inferior oblique, RIO; and left inferior oblique, LIO), and four that depress the eyes (the right inferior rectus, RIR; left inferior rectus, LIR; right superior oblique, RSO; and left superior oblique, LSO). By having the patient look in the various directions of gaze, a clinical determination of affected muscle(s) can be made because the eyes will appear most misaligned (and the diplopia noticed by the patient will be maximal) when the eyes move into the field of action of the affected muscle.[8] Diplopia experienced in peripheral gaze can be caused by an underaction of one or more muscles or by an overaction. An underaction could be caused by a mechanical restriction or a muscle palsy/paralysis. An overaction will occur in the non-paretic eye if the paretic eye is fixating the target. It is important to remember that longstanding incomitancies tend to become more comitant as time passes due to the process of contracture.[9] Other ways that can help to distinguish between long-standing and recent onset strabismus are provided in Table 6.3.

Parks 3-step test: Determine the muscle that the Parks 3-step test suggests is paretic by matching the test result to the information provided in Table 6.6. If, for example, the *right* eye is the hyper-deviated eye in the primary position (Answer to Question 1), the deviation is greater on *leftwards* gaze (Answer to Question 2), and greater when the head is tilted to the *right* (Answer to Question 3), the muscle implicated is the *Right Superior Oblique (RSO)* (see Table 6.6).

It is easier to recall the result patterns associated with the oblique muscles being affected. In the case of superior oblique muscles, the answers to the three questions will be *right-left-right* when the right superior oblique is affected, and *left-right-left* when the left superior oblique is affected. In the case of the inferior oblique muscles, the result will be *right-right-right* in the case of the left inferior oblique, and *left-left-left* for the right inferior oblique. The head tilt test is particularly useful for distinguishing a fourth nerve palsy from a skew deviation, a general term for any vertical deviation caused by a brainstem lesion that is not caused by a third or fourth nerve palsy. In both cases, there is vertical, oblique, and/or torsional diplopia. However, in the case of a fourth nerve palsy, the affected, hypertropic eye is extorted, whereas in a skew deviation there is intorsion of the hypertropic eye.[19]

6.16.6 Most common errors when assessing incomitancy

9-point cover test

1. Not keeping the viewing distance fixed in the various positions of gaze.
2. Failing to ensure occlusion in peripheral gaze directions.
3. Introducing and removing the cover too quickly and thus not allowing the eyes time to take up position when prompted to fixate.

Parks 3-step test

1. If using prism, not holding the prism with its base parallel to the palpebral fissure when the head is in the tilted position, rather than parallel with the floor. This is to ensure that the prism has the same relation to the eye as in the primary position.[7]

6.17 Assessment of eye movements

Saccadic eye movements are used to redirect our eyes quickly so that an object of interest falls on the fovea. They are conjugate eye movements in that the eyes move by the same degree and they are the fastest of all eye movements with velocities as high as 700 degrees per second.[119] Saccades are used continually to scan the environment and are particularly important during reading. They originate in the left and right frontal eye fields (Brodmann's area 8) of the frontal lobes. Pursuit eye movements are those used when following a moving target. Most patients can pursue targets moving at 30 degrees per second. Pursuit movements should be both smooth and accurate. When a foveated target moves, the pursuit response begins after a latency of around 100 to 150 milliseconds and the pursuit movements are at the same

Table 6.6 Parks three-step method for identifying the paretic muscle when the deviation is vertical								
1. Which is the hyper eye?	RE (OD) hyper				LE (OS) hyper			
2. Is the deviation greater on left or right gaze?	Left gaze		Right gaze		Left gaze		Right gaze	
3. Is the deviation greater on head tilt to the right or left?	Right	Left	Right	Left	Right	Left	Right	Left
Likely paretic muscle	RSO	LSR	LIO	RIR	LIR	RIO	RSR	LSO

LE (OS), Left eye; *LIO*, left inferior oblique; *LIR*, left inferior rectus; *LSO*, left superior oblique; *LSR*, left superior rectus; *RE (OD)*, right eye; *RIO*, right inferior oblique; *RIR*, right inferior rectus; *RSO*, right superior oblique; *RSR*, right superior rectus.

velocity as the target.[120] Because of the latency, a small, catch-up saccade is seen initially to allow the moving target to be foveated, but there should be no need for any further catch-up saccades. Assuming the target moves in a predictable fashion (constant speed and direction), it can then be closely followed using pursuit movements.

6.17.1 The evidence base: when and how to assess eye movements

Eye movements should be assessed when symptoms are unexplained. Because saccadic eye movements are the eye movements primarily used in reading, assessing saccades is potentially informative in patients experiencing symptoms during close work (which may include older patients; e.g., Parkinson's disease[121]) and in children who are not doing well with their school work. It is important that both saccades and pursuits are assessed because the relative magnitude of any deficit in pursuits compared with saccades can be characteristic of different brain disorders.[19] In most clinical settings, the equipment required to assess eye movements quantitatively is not available. Hence, clinical assessment of pursuit and saccadic eye movements is usually qualitative. A simple assessment of saccadic eye movements can be made by direct observation of the patient's eyes as they switch fixation from one target to another. Very little additional equipment is required and these eye movements can be assessed in a simple, quick, and reasonably reliable fashion.[122,123] It should be pointed out that a simple and repeatable assessment of pursuit eye movements can be made by direct observation of the patient's eyes as they follow a moving target and, as this task is performed during motility/Broad H testing for incomitancy (section 6.4), the pursuit reflexes can be assessed at the same time.[122] Alternatively, pursuit eye movements can be assessed separately and this is preferred. The tests of pursuits and saccades described here are the NSUCO (Northeastern State University College of Optometry) tests, which are claimed to be both reliable and repeatable.[66,122,123]

6.17.2 Procedure: NSUCO pursuits test

1. Ask the patient to stand directly in front of you.
2. Inform your patient that the test is to "look at how well your eyes can follow a target" and instruct them to "follow the target as closely as possible as it moves around." No instructions are given about head/body movements because you will want to observe whether these spontaneously take place as the target is followed.
3. One target is used (e.g., brightly coloured bead on a stick) and it is held at 40 cm. The target is first positioned directly in front of the patient along

the midline. Then it is moved in, tracing a circle of around 20 cm.
4. Look for jerky pursuit movements, fixation losses, or other eye movements that are not at the same speed or in the same direction as the movement of the target. Also, look for body or head movements that are made.
5. Four rotations are made, two clockwise and two counter-clockwise. A sweep horizontally along the midline may be made when you are switching from clockwise to counter-clockwise movements.

6.17.3 Procedure: NSUCO saccades test

1. The patient should stand directly in front of you.
2. Keep the room lights on. Position additional lighting to illuminate the patient's eyes or the target (whichever is necessary) without shadows.
3. Inform your patient that the test is to "look at how quickly your eyes can switch to a new position."
4. Hold two fixation sticks, one with a red sticker, one with a green sticker, approximately 10 cm either side of the patient's midline and at a distance of approximately 40 cm from a point midway between the patient's eyes.
5. Instruct your patient: "Do not move your eyes until I instruct you. When I say green, please turn to look at the green target as quickly as you can. Keep looking at the green target until I say to look at the red target." Repeat for five cycles. No instructions are given about head/body movements because you will want to observe whether these spontaneously take place.
6. Grade the saccadic movements out of five, giving separate scores for 'ability,' 'accuracy,' 'head movement,' and 'body movement' using Table 6.7.

6.17.4 Recording

The NSUCO method uses a 5-point scale for recording ability, accuracy of movement, and the extent to which head and/or body movements have taken place during the test (see Table 6.7). An example of a record would be: 'pursuits: ability 4, accuracy 3, head movement 4, body movement 5.' Descriptive terms may be also used. For example, if normal pursuit eye movements are seen, record 'smooth and accurate pursuits' or similar. If pursuits are abnormal, record the type of abnormality (e.g., 'jerky eye movements' or 'unable to maintain fixation') and indicate if one eye is more at fault than the other. An equivalent 5-point scale is used to grade saccades (see Table 6.7).

6.17.5 Interpretation of eye movement results

All saccadic eye movements should be fast (completed in much less than 1 second), conjugate and accurate,

Table 6.7 NSUCO oculomotor test: scales for grading pursuits and saccades[123]

Eye movement	Ability	Accuracy	Head movement	Body movement
Pursuits				
	1. Cannot complete ½ rotation in either the clockwise or anti-clockwise direction. 2. Completes ½ rotation in either direction. 3. Completes one rotation in either direction but not two rotations. 4. Completes two rotations in one direction but less than two rotations in the other direction. 5. Completes two rotations in either direction.	1. No attempt to follow the target or requires >10 re-fixations. 2. Re-fixations 5–10 times. 3. Re-fixations 3–4 times. 4. Re-fixations ≤2 times. 5. No re-fixations noted.	1. Large movement of the head at any time. 2. Moderate movement of the head at any time. 3. Slight movement of the head (>50% of the time). 4. Slight movement of the head (<50% of the time). 5. No movement of the head.	1. Large movement of the body at any time. 2. Moderate movement of the body at any time. 3. Slight movement of the body (>50% of the time). 4. Slight movement of the body (<50% of the time). 5. No movement of the body.
Saccades				
	1. Completes less than two round trips. 2. Completes two round trips. 3. Completes three round trips. 4. Completes four round trips. 5. Completes five round trips.	1. Large over- or undershooting is noted one or more times. 2. Moderate over- or undershooting is noted one or more times. 3. Constant slight over- or undershooting noted (>50% of the time). 4. Intermittent slight over- or undershooting noted (<50% of the time). 5. No over- or undershooting noted.	1. Large movement of the head at any time. 2. Moderate movement of the head at any time. 3. Slight movement of the head (>50% of the time). 4. Slight movement of the head (<50% of the time). 5. No movement of the head.	1. Large movement of the body at any time. 2. Moderate movement of the body at any time. 3. Slight movement of the body (>50% of the time). 4. Slight movement of the body (<50% of the time). 5. No movement of the body.

with no overshoots requiring secondary compensatory eye movements. A small undershoot with a compensatory eye movement is normal. Dysmetria denotes inaccurate saccadic eye movements and includes hypometria (undershooting) or hypermetria (overshooting). Abnormal saccadic and/or pursuit eye movements could indicate certain conditions including ocular motor nerve paresis, cerebellar disease, or Parkinson's disease, or could be caused by systemic medications (e.g. particular antidepressants). In cases of abnormal saccadic and/or pursuit eye movements, additional testing is warranted and referral may be necessary. It is worth remembering that disorders of saccadic, pursuit, and fixational eye movements generally occur together.

6.17.6 Most common errors when assessing pursuits and saccades

1. **Pursuits:** Moving the target at an inappropriate speed, or in a non-smooth fashion.
2. **Saccades:** Misinterpreting the results due to lack of experience. For example, not realising that small undershoots are frequently seen.

6.18 Making a final diagnosis and management plan

Although this chapter describes many procedures that test diverse aspects of the accommodation and binocular visual systems, the results from any one test need to be considered alongside the results from other tests in order for you to decide if there is a problem, and if so, to reach a diagnosis and develop a management plan. Clinicians should be aware that a single abnormal test result is unlikely to be significant on its own. Single abnormal test results should be always be rechecked because of a strong likelihood that the result will be (more) normal on repeat testing.[63,113] This is particularly true in the case of children who may perform poorly on initial testing, perhaps due to unfamiliarity with test expectations or instructions. In fact, if there is a problem with the accommodative or binocular vision system it is highly likely that abnormal performance will be evident on a number of tests. This is because most of the tests presented in this chapter simultaneously test both accommodation and vergence, although to a greater or lesser degree. For example, when the AoA is measured binocularly, the eyes need to accommodate appropriately to achieve a clear view of the target, but the vergence system also needs to respond appropriately if diplopia is to be avoided. Thus a vergence problem could 'contaminate' a measure of binocular AoA, although listening closely to what the patient reports (diplopia before blur) could alert you to this fact. Similarly, if there is a primary problem of accommodation, this could produce an abnormal result on a test that is primarily designed to test vergence function (e.g., fusional reserves). From the clinician's perspective the fact that many of the tests described in this chapter assess both accommodation and vergence simultaneously make identification of the presence of an accommodative/vergence problem quite straightforward but definite diagnosis of the primary problem more difficult. For example, an abnormal (i.e., elevated) NPC, exophoria at near greater than at distance, a low AC/A ratio, and a reduced positive (i.e., base-out)

fusional reserve at near strongly suggest a diagnosis of convergence insufficiency; but patients with this condition might, for the same reason, exhibit a reduced AoA when tested binocularly, a reduced binocular accommodative facility, and an increased lag of accommodation.[66] To establish whether the primary problem has its origins in the accommodation or vergence system, it is necessary to resort to less frequently used tests or to versions of tests in which accommodation is tested independently of vergence, or in which vergence is tested without changing the stimulus to accommodation. An example of the former is the monocular AoA test (section 6.8) and an example of the latter is vergence facility (section 6.15).

A number of analytical approaches are available to clinicians to help them to understand the results from tests of binocular vision and accommodation, and which are therefore aimed at providing a framework for diagnosis and management. These include graphical analysis, fixation disparity, Morgan's system of normative analysis, and the Optometric Extension Program's analytical analysis. The advantages and disadvantages of each of these system are described by Scheiman and Wick[66] who also describe what they refer to as an integrative analysis approach. The latter is an approach that attempts to draw on the positive aspects of the other case analysis approaches. It includes the following steps: (1) comparing the individual test results with expected findings; (2) grouping findings that deviate from expected findings; and then (3) identifying the syndrome based on steps 1 and 2.

Once test results have been compared against the expected values (see Table 6.5), it is time to evaluate whether the pattern of results points to a diagnosis. Duane proposed a 4-way classification of convergence excess and insufficiency, and divergence excess and insufficiency[124] for strabismus cases and this was later applied to non-strabismic binocular vision anomalies. Further developing this approach, Scheiman and Wick[66] list 15 common accommodative, ocular motility, and binocular vision problems which include:

Heterophoria with low AC/A ratio: (a) Orthophoria at distance and exophoria at near: *convergence insufficiency;* (b) exophoria at distance, greater exophoria at near: *convergence insufficiency;* (c) esophoria at distance, orthophoria at near: *divergence insufficiency.*

Heterophoria with normal AC/A ratio: (d) Orthophoria at distance, orthophoria at near: *fusional vergence dysfunction;* (e) esophoria at distance, same amount of esophoria a near: *basic esophoria;* (f) exophoria at distance, same amount of exophoria a near: *basic exophoria.*

Heterophoria with high AC/A ratio: (g) orthophoria at distance and esophoria at near: *convergence excess;* (h) esophoria at distance and greater esophoria at near: *convergence excess;* (i) exophoria at distance and less exophoria at near: *divergence excess.*

(j) *Vertical heterophoria*

Accommodative anomalies: (k) accommodative insufficiency; (l) ill-sustained accommodation; (m) accommodative excess; (n) accommodative infacility

(o) *Ocular motor dysfunction*

Each of these conditions is diagnosed when a spectrum of signs is present. For example, in convergence insufficiency, we would expect to see higher exophoria at near than at distance, a low AC/A ratio, a receded NPC, poorer than expected positive fusional reserve measures at near, along with poor performance to base-out prism introduction during vergence facility testing and to positive sphere power introduced during accommodation facility testing. Scheiman and Wick[66] give details of the expected spectrum of test results for each of the conditions listed above.

References

1. Carlson N, Kurtz D. *Clinical Procedures for Ocular Examination*, ed 4. New York: McGraw-Hill; 2016.
2. Horwood AM, Toor S, Riddell PM. Screening for convergence insufficiency using the CISS is not indicated in young adults. *Br J Ophthalmol.* 2014; 98:679–83.
3. Horwood AM. 2016 International Orthoptic Congress Burian Lecture: Folklore or Evidence? *Strabismus.* 2017;25:120–7.
4. Weddell L. Optometric examination of children—child's play. *Optom in Pract.* 2014;15:109–20.
5. Rabbetts RB. *Bennett and Rabbett's Clinical Visual Optics*. Oxford: Butterworth-Heinemann Ltd; 2007.
6. Fogt N, Baughman BJ, Good G. The effect of experience on the detection of small eye movements. *Optom Vis Sci.* 2000;77:670–4.
7. von Noorden GK. *Binocular Vision and Ocular Motility: Theory and Management of Strabismus*. London: CV Mosby; 2002.
8. Evans BJW. *Pickwell's Binocular Vision Anomalies*, ed 5. Oxford: Butterworth-Heinemann; 2007.
9. Eperjesi F, Rundstrom MM. *Practical Binocular Vision Assessment: A Practical Guide*. Oxford: Butterworth-Heinemann; 2003.
10. Rainey BB, Schroeder TL, Goss DA, Grosvenor TP. Reliability of and comparisons among three variations of the alternating cover test. *Ophthalmic Physiol Opt.* 1998;18:430–7.
11. Walline JJ, Mutti DO, Zadnik K, Jones LA. Development of phoria in children. *Optom Vis Sci.* 1998;75:605–10.
12. Freier BE, Pickwell LD. Physiological exophoria. *Ophthalmic Physiol Opt.* 1983;3:267–72.

13. Choi RY, Kushner BJ. The accuracy of experienced strabismologists using the Hirschberg and Krimsky tests. *Ophthalmology.* 1998;105:1301–6.
14. Griffin JR, Cotter SA. The Brückner test: evaluation of clinical usefulness. *Am J Optom Physiol Opt.* 1986;63:957–61.
15. Miller JM, Hall HL, Greivenkamp JE, Guyton DL. Quantification of the Brückner test for strabismus. *Invest Ophthalmol Vis Sci.* 1995;36:897–905.
16. Gräf M, Alhammouri Q, Vieregge C, Lorenz B. The Brückner transillumination test: limited detection of small-angle esotropia. *Ophthalmology.* 2011;118:2504–9.
17. Basmak H, Sahin A, Yildirim N, Saricicek T, Yurdakul S. The angle kappa in strabismic individuals. *Strabismus.* 2007;15:193–6.
18. Kanski J, Bowling B. *Clinical Ophthalmology: A Systematic Approach*, ed 8. Saunders Ltd, Philadelphia; 2015.
19. Pane A, Miller NR, Burdon M. *The Neuro-Ophthalmology Survival Guide*, ed 2. Elsevier, Philadelphia; 2017.
20. Classe JG, Rutstein RP. Binocular vision anomalies: an emerging cause of malpractice claims. *J Am Optom Assoc.* 1995;66:305–09.
21. Clement RA, Boylan C. Current concepts of the actions of the extraocular muscles and the interpretation of oculomotility tests. *Ophthalmic Physiol Opt.* 1987;7:341–4.
22. Vivian AJ, Morris RJ. Diagrammatic representation of strabismus. *Eye (Lond).* 1993;7:565–71.
23. Scheiman M, Gwiazda J, Li T. Non-surgical interventions for convergence insufficiency. *Cochrane Database Syst Rev.* 2011;3:CD006768.
24. Convergence Insufficiency Treatment Trial Group. Long-term effectiveness

of treatments for symptomatic convergence insufficiency in children. *Optom Vis Sci.* 2009;86:1096–103.
25. Scheiman M, Kulp MT, Cotter S, et al. Vision therapy/orthoptics for symptomatic convergence insufficiency in children: treatment kinetics. *Optom Vis Sci.* 2010;87:593–603.
26. Rouse MW, Borsting E, Deland PN. Reliability of binocular vision measurements used in the classification of convergence insufficiency. *Optom Vis Sci.* 2002;79:254–64.
27. Scheiman M, Gallaway M, Frantz KA, et al. Nearpoint of convergence: test procedure, target selection, and normative data. *Optom Vis Sci.* 2003;80:214–25.
28. Siderov J, Chiu SC, Waugh SJ. Differences in the near point of convergence with target type. *Ophthalmic Physiol Opt.* 2001;21: 356–60.
29. Adler PM, Cregg M, Viollier AJ, Woodhouse MJ. Influence of target type and RAF rule on the measurement of near point of convergence. *Ophthalmic Physiol Opt.* 2007;27:22–30.
30. Menjivar AM, Kulp MT, Mitchell GL, Toole AJ, Reuter K. Screening for convergence insufficiency in school-age children. *Clin Exp Optom.* 2018;101:578–84.
31. Rouse MW, Borsting E, Hyman L, et al. Frequency of convergence insufficiency among fifth and sixth graders. The Convergence Insufficiency and Reading Study (CIRS) group. *Optom Vis Sci.* 1999;76:643–9.
32. Simons K, Elhatton K. Artifacts in fusion and stereoscopic testing based on red/green dichoptic image separation. *J Pediatr Ophthalmol Strabismus.* 1994;31:290–7.

33. Lueder GT, Arnoldi K. Does "touching four" on the Worth 4-dot test indicate fusion in young children? A computer simulation. *Ophthalmology.* 1996;103:1237–40.

34. Ciner EB, Ying GS, Kulp MT, et al. Stereoacuity of preschool children with and without vision disorders. *Optom Vis Sci.* 2014;91:351–8.

35. Schmidt P, Maguire M, Kulp MT, Dobson V, Quinn G. Random dot E stereotest: testability and reliability in 3- to 5-year old children. *J APPOS.* 2006;10:507–14.

36. O'Connor AR, Birch EE, Anderson S, Draper H, FSOS Research Group. The functional significance of stereopsis. *Invest Ophthalmol Vis Sci.* 2010;51:2019–23.

37. Chung YW, Park SH, Shin SY. Distant stereoacuity in children with anisometropic amblyopia. *Jpn J Ophthalmol.* 2017;61:402–7.

38. Heron G, Dholakia S, Collins DE, McLaughlan H. Stereoscopic threshold in children and adults. *Am J Optom Physiol Opt.* 1985;62:505–15.

39. Broadbent H, Westall C. An evaluation of techniques for measuring stereopsis in infants and young children. *Ophthalmic Physiol Opt.* 1990;10:3–7.

40. Hall C. The relationship between clinical stereotests. *Ophthalmic Physiol Opt.* 1982;2:133–43.

41. Birch E, Williams C, Drover J, et al. Randot preschool stereoacuity test: normative data and validity. *J AAPOS.* 2008;12:23–6.

42. Saunders KJ, Woodhouse JM, Westall CA. The modified Frisby stereotest. *J Pediatr Ophthalmol Strabismus.* 1996;33:323–7.

43. Manny RE, Martinez AT, Fern KD. Testing stereopsis in the pre-school child: is it clinically useful? *J Pediatr Ophthalmol Strabismus.* 1991;28:223–31.

44. Adler P, Scally AJ, Barrett BT. Test-retest variability of Randot stereoacuity measures gathered in an unselected sample of UK primary school children. *Br J Ophthalmol.* 2012;96:656–61.

45. Friedman JR, Kosmorsky GS, Burde RM. Stereoacuity in patients with optic nerve diseases. *Arch Ophthalmol.* 1985;103:37–8.

46. Menon V, Bansal P, Prakash P. Randot stereoacuity at various binocular combinations of Snellen acuity. *Indian J Ophthalmol.* 1997;45:169–71.

47. Odell NV, Hatt SR, Leske DA, Adams WE, Holmes JM. The effect of induced monocular blur on measures of stereoacuity. *J AAPOS.* 2009;13:136–41.

48. Saladin JJ. Stereopsis from a performance perspective. *Optom Vision Sci.* 2005;82:186–205.

49. Mutti DO. To emmetropize or not to emmetropize? The question for hyperopic development. *Optom Vis Sci.* 2007;84:97–102.

50. Charman WN. The path to presbyopia: straight or crooked? *Ophthalmic Physiol Opt.* 1989;9:126–32.

51. Rosenfield M, Cohen AS. Repeatability of clinical measurements of the amplitude of accommodation. *Ophthalmic Physiol Opt.* 1996;16:247–9.

52. Rosenfield M. Accommodation. In: Zadnik K, ed. *The Ocular Examination: Measurements and Findings.* Philadelphia: WB Saunders; 1997.

53. Atchison DA, Capper EJ, McCabe KL. Critical subjective measurement of amplitude of accommodation. *Optom Vis Sci.* 1994;71:699–706.

54. Kragha IKOK. Amplitude of accommodation: population and methodological differences. *Ophthalmic Physiol Opt.* 1986;6:75–80.

55. Somer D, Karabulut E, Cinar FG, Altiparmak UE, Unlu N. Emmetropization, visual acuity, and strabismus outcomes among hyperopic infants followed with partial hyperopic corrections given in accordance with dynamic retinoscopy. *Eye (Lond).* 2014;28:1165–73.

56. Gwiazda J, Thorn F, Held R. Accommodation, accommodative convergence, and response AC/A ratios before and at the onset of myopia in children. *Optom Vis Sci.* 2005;82:273–8.

57. Mutti DO, Mitchell GL, Hayes JR, et al. Accommodative lag before and after the onset of myopia. *Invest Ophthalmol Vis Sci.* 2006;47:837–46.

58. Koomson NY, Amedo AO, Opoku-Baah C, Ampeh PB, Ankamah E, Bonsu K. Relationship between reduced accommodative lag and myopia progression. *Optom Vis Sci.* 2016;93:683–91.

59. McClelland JF, Saunders KJ. The repeatability and validity of dynamic retinoscopy in assessing the accommodative response. *Ophthalmic Physiol Opt.* 2003;23:243–50.

60. Rosenfield M, Portello JK, Blustein GH, Jang C. Comparison of clinical techniques to assess the near accommodative response. *Optom Vis Sci.* 1996;73:382–8.

61. McClelland JF, Saunders KJ. Accommodative lag using Nott dynamic retinoscopy: age norms for school age children. *Optom Vis Sci.* 2004;81:929–33.

62. Ludden SM, Horwood AM, Riddell PM. Children's accommodation to a variety of targets - a pilot study. *Strabismus.* 2017;25:95–100.

63. Adler P, Scally AJ, Barrett BT. Test-retest reproducibility of accommodation measures gathered in an unselected sample of UK primary school children. *Br J Ophthalmol.* 2013;97:592–7.

64. Jiménez R, Pérez MA, García JA, González MD. Statistical normal values of visual parameters that characterize binocular function in children. *Ophthalmic Physiol Opt.* 2004;24:528–42.

65. Morgan MW. The analysis of clinical data. *Am J Optom.* 1944;21:477–91.

66. Scheiman M, Wick B. *Clinical Management of Binocular Vision: Heterophoric, Accommodative, and Eye Movement Disorders.* Philadeplphia: Wolters Kluwer (Lippincott, Williams and Wilkins); 2013.

67. Woodhouse JM, Meades JS, Leat SJ, Saunders KJ. Reduced accommodation in children with Down's syndrome. *Invest Ophthalmol Vis Sci.* 1993;42:2382–7.

68. Leat SJ. Reduced accommodation in children with cerebral palsy. *Ophthalmic Physiol Opt.* 1996;16:385–90.

69. Wick B, Hall P. Relation among accommodative facility, lag and amplitude in elementary schoolchildren. *Am J Optom Physiol Opt.* 1987;64:593–8.

70. del Pilar Cacho M, Garcia-Muñoz A, García-Bernabeu JR, López A. Comparison between MEM and Nott dynamic retinoscopy. *Optom Vis Sci.* 1999;76:650–5.

71. Locke LC, Somers W. A comparison study of dynamic retinoscopy techniques. *Optom Vis Sci.* 1989;66:540–4.

72. Horwood AM, Riddell PM. Hypo-accommodation responses in hypermetropic infants and children. *Br J Ophthalmol.* 2011;95:231–7.

73. Frantz KA, Cotter SA, Wick B. Re-evaluation of the four prism dioptre base-out test. *Optom Vis Sci.* 1992;69:777–86.

74. Casillas EC, Rosenfield M. Comparison of subjective heterophoria testing with a phoropter and trial frame. *Optom Vis Sci.* 2006;83:237–41.

75. Rainey BB, Schroeder TL, Goss DA, Grosvenor TP. Inter-examiner repeatability of heterophoria tests. *Optom Vis Sci.* 1998;75:719–26.

76. Antona B, Gonzalez E, Barrio A, Barra F, Sanchez I, Cebrian JL. Strabometry precision: intra-examiner repeatability and agreement in measuring the magnitude of the angle of latent binocular ocular deviations (heterophorias or latent strabismus). *Binocul Vis Strabolog Q Simms Romano.* 2011;26:91–104.

77. Cebrian JL, Antona B, Barrio A, Gonzalez E, Gutierrez A, Sanchez I. Repeatability of the modified Thorington card used to measure far heterophoria. *Optom Vis Sci.* 2014;91:786–92.

78. Lyon DW, Goss DA, Horner D, et al. Normative data for modified Thorington phorias and prism bar vergences from the Benton-IU study. *Optometry.* 2005;76:593–9.

79. Wong EP, Fricke TR, Dinardo C. Interexaminer repeatability of a new, modified prentice card compared with established phoria tests. *Optom Vis Sci.* 2002;79:370–5.

80. Pointer JS. An enhancement to the Maddox Wing test for the reliable measurement of horizontal heterophoria. *Ophthalmic Physiol Opt.* 2005;25:446–51.

81. Calvin H, Rupnow P, Grosvenor T. How good is the estimated cover test at predicting the von Graefe phoria measurement? *Optom Vision Sci.* 1996;73:701–6.

82. Sheedy JE, Saladin JJ. Phoria, vergence, and fixation disparity in oculomotor problems. *Am J Optom Physiol Opt.* 1977;52:474–81.

83. Penisten DK, Hofstetter HW, Goss DA. Reliability of rotary prism fusional vergence ranges. *Optometry.* 2001;72:117–22.

84. Schor CM, Narayan V. Graphical analysis of prism adaptation, convergence accommodation, and accommodative convergence. *Am J Optom Physiol Opt.* 1982;59:774–84.

85. Rosenfield M, Ciuffreda KJ, Ong E, Super S. Vergence adaptation and the order of clinical vergence range testing. *Optom Vis Sci.* 1995;72:219–23.

86. Rosner J. A procedure for measuring the near-point fusional vergence reserves of young children. *J Am Optom Assoc.* 1979;50:473–4.

87. Sheedy JE, Saladin JJ. Association of symptoms with measures of oculomotor deficiencies. *Am J Optom Physiol Opt.* 1978;55:670–6.

88. Kaban T, Smith K, Beldavs R, Cadera W, Orton RB. The 20-prism-dioptre base-out test: an indicator of peripheral binocularity. *Can J Ophthalmol.* 1995;30:247–50.

89. Saladin JJ, Sheedy JE. Population study of fixation disparity, heterophoria, and vergence. *Am J Optom Physiol Opt.* 1978;55:744–50.

90. Sheedy JE. Fixation disparity analysis of oculomotor imbalance. *Am J Optom Physiol Opt.* 1980;57:632–9.

91. Jenkins TCA, Pickwell LD, Yekta AA. Criteria for decompensation in binocular vision. *Ophthalmic Physiol Opt.* 1989;9:121–5.

92. Yekta AA, Pickwell LD, Jenkins TCA. Binocular vision, age and symptoms. *Ophthalmic Physiol Opt.* 1989;9:115–20.

93. Ngan J, Goss DA, Despirito J. Comparison of fixation disparity curve parameters obtained with the Wesson and Saladin fixation disparity cards. *Optom Vis Sci.* 2005;82:69–74.

94. Frantz KA, Elston P, Michalik E, Templeman CD, Zoltoski RK. Comparison of fixation disparity measured by Saladin card and disparometer. *Optom Vis Sci.* 2011;88:733–41.

95. Mallett R. Techniques of investigation of binocular vision anomalies. In: Edwards K, Llewellyn R, eds. *Optometry.* London: Butterworths; 1988:238–69.

96. Conway ML, Thomas J, Subramanian A. Is the aligning prism measured with the Mallett unit correlated with fusional vergence reserves? *PLoS One.* 2012;7:e42832.

97. Brautaset RL, Jennings JA. The influence of heterophoria measurements on subsequent associated phoria measurement in a refractive routine. *Ophthalmic Physiol Opt.* 1999;19:347–50.

98. Corbett A, Maples WC. Test-retest reliability of the Saladin card. *Optometry.* 2004;75:629–39.

99. Evans BJW. Optometric prescribing for decompensated heterophoria. *Optom Pract.* 2008;9:63–78.

100. Flom B, Fried A, Jampolsky A. Fixation disparity in relation to heterophoria. *Am J Ophthalmol.* 1957;43:97–106.

101. London R. Fixation disparity and heterophoria in ocular assessment. In: Barresi B, ed. *Ocular Assessment: The Manual of Diagnosis for Office Practice.* Boston: Butterworth-Heinemann; 1984:141–50.

102. Henson DB, North R. Adaptation to prism-induced heterophoria. *Am J Optom Physiol Opt.* 1980;57:129–37.

103. North RV, Henson DB. Adaptation to prism induced heterophoria in subjects with abnormal binocular

vision or asthenopia. *Am J Optom Physiol Opt.* 1981;58:746–52.

104. Schor CM, Horner D. Adaptive disorders of accommodation and vergence in binocular dysfunction. *Ophthalmic Physiol Opt.* 1989;9:264–8.

105. Ciuffreda KJ, Rosenfield M, Chen HW. The AC/A ratio, age and presbyopia. *Ophthalmic Physiol Opt.* 1997;17:307–15.

106. Rosenfield M, Rappon JM, Carrel MF. Vergence adaptation and the clinical AC/A ratio. *Ophthalmic Physiol Opt.* 2000;20:207–11.

107. Le T, Koklanis K, Georgievski Z. The fixation target influences the near deviation and AC/A ratio in intermittent exotropia. *J AAPOS.* 2010;14:25–30.

108. Gall R, Wick B. The symptomatic patient with normal phorias at distance and near: what tests detect a binocular vision problem? *Optometry.* 2003;74:309–22.

109. Gall R, Wick B, Bedell H. Vergence facility: establishing clinical utility. *Optom Vis Sci.* 1998;75:731–42.

110. Rouse MW. Management of binocular anomalies: efficacy of vision therapy in the treatment of accommodative deficiencies. *Am J Optom Physiol Opt.* 1987;64:415–20.

111. Sterner B, Abrahamsson M, Sjostrom A. The effects of accommodative facility training on a group of children with impaired relative accommodation—a comparison between dioptric treatment and sham treatment. *Ophthalmic Physiol Opt.* 2001;21:470–6.

112. Maxwell J, Tong J, Schor CM. Short-term adaptation of accommodation, accommodative vergence and disparity vergence facility. *Vision Res.* 2012;62:93–101.

113. Adler P, Scally AJ, Barrett BT. Test-retest reproducibility of accommodative facility measures in primary school children. *Clin Exp Optom.* 2018;101:764–70.

114. Wick B, Yothers TL, Jiang BC, Morse SE. Clinical testing of accommodative facility: part 1. A critical appraisal of the literature. *Optometry.* 2002;73:11–23.

115. Yothers T, Wick B, Morse SE. Clinical testing of accommodative facility: part II. Development of an amplitude-scaled test. *Optometry.* 2002;73:91–102.

116. Gall R, Wick B, Bedell H. Vergence facility and target type. *Optom Vis Sci.* 1998;75:727–30.

117. Siderov J, Johnston AW. The importance of the test parameters in the clinical

assessment of accommodative facility. *Optom Vis Sci.* 1990;67:551–7.

118. Zellers JA, Alpert TL, Rouse MW. A review of the literature and a normative study of accommodative facility. *J Am Optom Assoc.* 1984;55:31–7.
119. Kowler E. Eye movements: the past 25 years. *Vision Res.* 2011;51:1457–83.
120. Büttner U, Kremmyda O. Smooth pursuit eye movements and optokinetic nystagmus. *Dev Ophthalmol.* 2007; 40:76–89.
121. Jehangir N, Yu CY, Song J, et al. Slower saccadic reading in Parkinson's disease. *PLoS One.* 2018;13:e0191005.
122. Maples WC, Ficklin TW. Interrater and test-retest reliability of pursuits and saccades. *J Am Optom Assoc.* 1988;59:549–52.
123. Maples WC. *NSUCO Oculomotor Test.* Santa Ana: Optometric Extension Program Foundation; 1995.
124. Duane A. A new classification of the motor anomalies of the eye based upon physiological principles, together with the symptoms, diagnosis and treatment. *Ann Ophthalmol Otol.* 1896;5: 969–1008.

Chapter | 7 |

Ocular health assessment

C. Lisa Prokopich, Patricia Hrynchak, John G. Flanagan, Alexander F. Hynes, and Catharine Chisholm

7.1 Examination of the anterior segment and ocular adnexa

This includes the eyelids, eyelashes, conjunctiva, tear layer, cornea, anterior chamber, iris, crystalline lens, and anterior vitreous.

7.1.1 The evidence base: when and how to assess the anterior segment and adnexa

This is typically performed during most full oculo-visual assessments and contact lens assessments and some partial oculo-visual assessments, plus before and after any procedure that touches the eye, such as tonometry and gonioscopy, to determine any iatrogenic damage. Certain symptoms and other case history information would lead to specific procedures being used and specific areas being assessed in more detail. For example, 'acute flashes and floaters' would lead to the assessment of the anterior vitreous for Shafer's sign; 'ocular foreign body' symptoms might lead to ocular surface staining with fluorescein and lissamine green and lid eversion; gradual onset blurred vision plus problems with glare in an older patient suggests a careful assessment of the lens for cataract; a history of previous ocular disease/surgery would suggest searching for keratic precipitates after iritis and posterior capsular remnants after cataract surgery; a history of certain recurring diseases, such as trichiasis, corneal erosion, and blepharitis, suggests you search for these conditions again; some systemic medications can cause anterior segment changes: beta-blockers can cause dry eyes and long-term, high dosage oral corticosteroids can cause posterior subcapsular cataracts, etc.

Slit-lamp biomicroscopy, which is the current standard, offers excellent resolution, depth of field, control of a large range of illumination, and variable and high magnification (~10× to 40×; involuntary eye movements reduce the clarity of highly magnified images and limit the value of increasing the magnification beyond 40×). The quality of the image is better in slit-lamp models that have higher optical quality lenses that use multi-aspheric lens designs and anti-reflection coatings. Patients who are obese or have neck or back problems may find positioning themselves at a table slit-lamp uncomfortable such that a hand-held slit-lamp may be preferred. Anterior segment optical coherence tomography (OCT) is becoming increasingly used to quantify some abnormalities, such as cells and flare in anterior uveitis (section 7.1.3, No. 7)[1] and its use seems certain to increase further. Direct ophthalmoscopy, penlight, and loupe or Burton lamp assessment can be used when slit-lamp assessment cannot be undertaken, but they are very limited in resolution, illumination control, and magnification (~2 to 4×).

7.1.2 Procedure for general slit-lamp examination

▶ See video 7.1 for general slit-lamp examination. Familiarity with the adjustment controls of the slit-lamp is required. The positions of the controls differ for different models, but it should be possible to change the position, width, height, and intensity of the light beam and place filters over it (Table 7.1); change the magnification of the biomicroscope and adjust its position in all directions; change the angle between the illumination and viewing systems and break the linkage between the these systems (decoupling), which allows focus on a point other than that being illuminated. Magnification is provided in one of three ways: a flip magnification system (the most basic with magnification typically provided at 10× and 16×), a rotating barrel, or a zoom continuous magnification (typically from 10× to 40×). Slit-lamps also differ in the degree of convergence of the microscope and clinician preference seems to vary depending on their own convergence stability.

1. Wash your hands thoroughly and clean the slit-lamp contact surfaces with an alcohol wipe in front of the patient.
2. Many clinicians will perform the slit-lamp examination without glasses because the field of view is greater the closer your eyes are to the slit-lamp eyepieces. If you have a high cylinder in your glasses, you may need to wear your correction to obtain adequate resolution.
3. Focus the eyepieces: Place the focusing rod in the appropriate holder, with the flat surface towards the viewing system. Switch on the illumination system to produce a slit-image on the focusing rod. Look through one eyepiece and turn it fully anti-clockwise; then, while viewing the focusing rod, turn the eyepiece clockwise until the slit-image on the rod is first in sharp focus. Repeat the procedure for the other eyepiece. The eyepiece should be set at approximately zero if you are an emmetrope or wearing your correction and set to your mean sphere correction (sphere + half of cylinder) if you are uncorrected. More minus/less plus might be required in younger practitioners due to proximal accommodation. Once you have each eyepiece focused, adjust the distance between the eyepieces so that the image is centred in the field of view of each eye. You should see a single clear image.
4. Seat the patient comfortably on a stable chair without rollers and ask the patient to remove any glasses. Explain the procedure in lay terms: "I am going to use this special microscope to carefully examine the front of your eyes."
5. Adjust the height of the slit-lamp table so that the patient may lean forward comfortably and place their chin in the chin rest and forehead against the forehead rest. Adjust the chin rest so that the patient's eyes are at an appropriate height to provide a large enough vertical range to allow adequate examination of the adnexa. Many slit-lamps have an eye alignment marker on a supporting beam of the headrest that should be level with the patient's outer canthus. If your patient is obese, an exaggerated bend at their waist will often allow satisfactory positioning. Having the patient hold onto the handles (if available) can also be helpful.
6. Dim the room lights and ask the patient to look at your ear (your right ear for the patient's right eye and your left ear for the patient's left eye) or the instrument's fixation device so that the patient's gaze is straight ahead.
7. Use one hand to control the joystick (focusing and lateral/vertical movement) and the other to control the

Table 7.1 Filters available on most slit-lamp biomicroscopes

Filter	Typical symbol	Use
Cobalt blue	Blue filled circle	Enhances the view of fluorescein dye in the tear film of the eye. Typically used for fluorescein staining and Goldmann tonometry.
Red free	Green filled circle	Used to enhance the view of blood vessels and haemorrhages.
Neutral density	Circle with hashed lines	Decreases maximum brightness for photosensitive patients.
Heat absorbing	Built into most slit-lamps	Decreases patient discomfort.
Grey	Circle with thick line	Decreases maximum brightness for photosensitive patients.
Yellow filter	Yellow filled circle Located in the observation system	For good contrast enhancement when using fluorescein and the cobalt blue filter.
Diffuser	May be a flip-up filter placed on the illumination source	Used for general overall observations of the eye and adnexa.

magnification and illumination and to manipulate the patient's eyelids. Use a low rheostat setting for a wide, diffuse beam (for patient comfort) and a high rheostat setting for a narrower beam, or when filters are used, to give sufficient illumination.

8. There are several techniques that, with experience, you will use alternately or in combination to examine the anterior segment and adnexa thoroughly. A general procedure is to use diffuse illumination followed by a parallelepiped, which is described below. This is followed by descriptions of additional techniques with examples of when they might be used.

9. **Diffuse illumination:** Provides an overall assessment under low magnification (~10×). Adjust the illumination to a wide beam and place a diffusing filter in front of it to systematically examine the components of the anterior segment and adnexa as described below.

10. **Direct illumination using a parallelepiped:** Use low to moderate magnification (~10×) because magnification that is too high will result in missing obvious, moderately sized abnormalities. Set the illumination system at approximately 45° from the microscope position on the temporal side and use a beam width of approximately 2 mm. An illuminated block of corneal tissue in the shape of a parallelogram should be visible (Fig. 7.1). A beam that is too narrow will make it difficult to detect abnormalities. Assess each of the structures described below in a systematic manner using the following procedure: Focus on the temporal tissue first with the illumination coming from the temporal side. Move the slit-lamp laterally across the tissue until the centre is reached, maintaining good focus at all times. Then sweep the illumination system across to the nasal side, taking care not to bump into the patient's nose, and examine the nasal tissue. This scanning procedure may be repeated several times to examine all areas of the tissue concerned and may require more than one level of magnification. Being able to keep a parallelepiped sharply in focus as you scan from temporal limbus to central cornea and then nasal limbus to central cornea is the foundation for good slit-lamp technique.

(a) Eyelids and lashes: Examine the superior eyelid and lashes first using the scanning procedure described above. This can be easier with the patient's eyes closed. Examine the inferior lid and lashes in the same manner, but with the patient's eyes open, while also examining lid apposition to the eye and meibomian gland orifice appearance (section 7.2.9). Assess the lid for anomalies, including an abnormal lid position (e.g., ptosis, entropion, ectropion), redness, inflammation, ulcers, and growths. Inspect the lashes for colour (e.g., white), areas where the lashes are missing or misdirected, and the presence of scales.

(b) Direct and indirect illumination: With increasing experience you will be able to look at both the area illuminated (direct illumination; see Fig. 7.1) and the area just outside the area of illumination (indirect illumination, Fig. 7.2 and see Fig. 8.18). Indirect illumination is used to view areas that become bleached with excessive light using direct illumination, such as fine blood vessels at the limbus, fine infiltrates or other opacities, and microcysts.

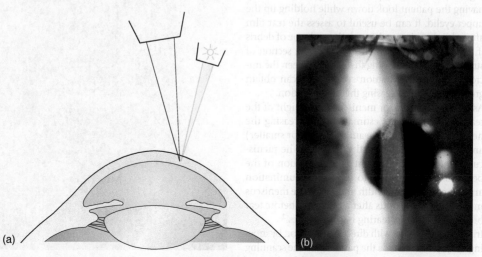

Fig. 7.1 (a) Diagram illustrating the position of the illuminating and viewing systems when using direct illumination. **(b)** A parallelepiped section of the cornea showing an irregularity above the corneal apex.

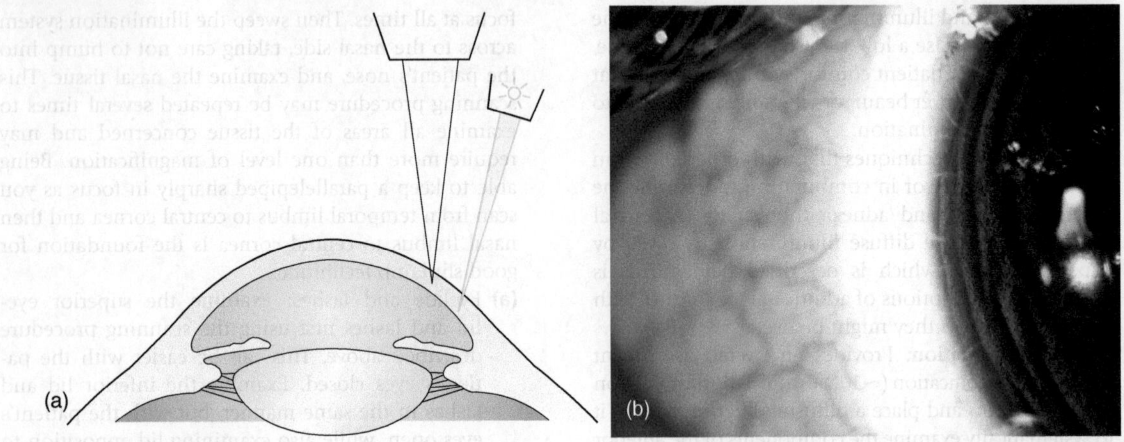

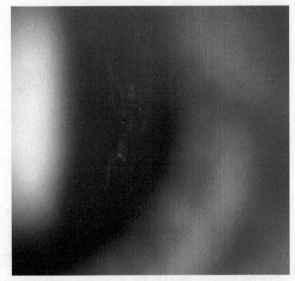

Fig. 7.2 (a) Diagram illustrating the position of the illuminating and viewing systems when using indirect illumination. **(b)** Corneal nerve fibres seen in indirect illumination.

(c) Conjunctiva: Ask the patient to look upwards while you pull the lower eyelid gently downwards to expose the lower fornix for examination. Examine both the bulbar and palpebral conjunctiva using a scanning process. Next ask the patient to look downwards and gently pull up the upper eyelid, thereby exposing the superior bulbar conjunctiva for examination. Finally ask the patient to look in right and then left gaze to allow examination of the entire conjunctiva, plica, and the caruncle.

(d) Cornea and tear film: Use the scanning process to examine the cornea in three sweeps: inferior, central, and superior. Examine the inferior cornea by having the patient look up and the superior cornea by having the patient look down while holding up the upper eyelid. It can be useful to assess the tear film after a blink and note the quantity and type of debris if any. You can increase the width of the section of stroma seen by increasing the angle between the microscope and illumination system. You can obtain greater detail by increasing the magnification.

(e) Assessment of the tear meniscus: The height of the tear meniscus can be estimated by decreasing the height of the slit-lamp beam to 1 mm (or smaller) and then judging the relative height of the meniscus at the lower lid margin as a proportion of the beam height. Use a low to moderate illumination and a medium beam width and assess the meniscus more than two seconds after a blink and before tear break-up and reflex tearing become issues.[2]

(f) Iris: Examine the iris with direct illumination by moving the joystick towards the patient. Use the scanning technique described above. Take note of the depth of the anterior chamber and the shape of the pupil.

(g) Lens: For a non-dilated pupil the illumination angle must be reduced until an optic section of the lens is just seen. This may be as small as 15° for an elderly patient with a small pupil. Further discussion of slit-lamp assessment of cataract with mydriasis is provided in section 8.4.

(h) Anterior vitreous: Moving the joystick further towards the patient allows viewing of the anterior vitreous with a parallelepiped when the pupil is dilated. To look for anterior vitreous floaters (Fig. 7.3), it can be useful to ask the patient to look

Fig. 7.3 Vitreous floaters seen in the anterior vitreous by direct illumination.

up, look down, and then straight ahead, so that the opacities become visible as they float through the field of view (see video 8.1). Assessing the anterior vitreous for 'tobacco dust' (Shafer's sign) is a specialised technique described in section 7.1.3, No 6.

7.1.3 'Specialised' slit-lamp techniques

(See video 7.2.)

If an abnormality/anomaly is suspected from the case history or detected during a routine slit-lamp examination, one or more of the following slit-lamp techniques may be used. With experience many or all techniques are used in quick succession. The slit-lamp magnification can be varied to examine the anomaly more carefully noting its size, shape, appearance, depth, and location.

1. Optic section

The illumination beam is narrowed and viewed at a wide angle to provide a cross-sectional view of the cornea and lens (Fig. 7.4). It can be used to judge the depth of a foreign body in the cornea, whether a cataract is anterior or posterior cortical or subcapsular and is the technique used to grade nuclear cataract (section 8.4; Fig. 7.5).

1. Set the illumination system at approximately 45° from the microscope and use approximately 10× magnification.
2. If the area of the cornea/lens you wish to view is temporal, place the illumination on the temporal side; if it is nasal, place it on the nasal side.

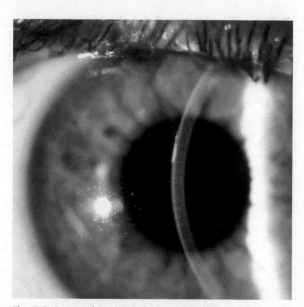

Fig. 7.4 A corneal section indicating that the corneal abrasion shown in Fig. 7.1 is in the corneal epithelium.

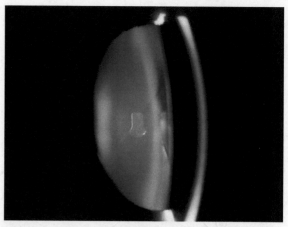

Fig. 7.5 An optical section of the lens showing nuclear cataract (*yellowing and increased light scatter in the lens nucleus or centre*). The blurred arc to the right is the out-of-focus cornea. There is also increased light scattering (seen in direct illumination) indicating anterior cortical cataract (compare with the cortical cataract seen in retro-illumination in Fig. 7.8).

3. Narrow the beam to the narrowest possible width and sharply focus on the cornea/lens using the joystick. As you have greatly narrowed the beam, you need to increase the illumination using the rheostat.
4. A slice of the cornea and lens should now be visible (cornea, see Fig. 7.4; nuclear cataract, see Fig. 7.5). If the illumination system is temporal to the viewing system, the corneal epithelium or anterior lens will be on the temporal side of the image with the corneal endothelium or blurred posterior lens on the nasal side.
5. The section of the cornea can be broadened by increasing the angle between the microscope and illumination system. The focusing should be precise enough to allow the graininess of the stroma to be visualised.
6. To view the posterior lens, the joystick needs to be moved further forward and the angle of the illumination system may need to be reduced, depending on the pupil size.
7. Once the object of interest is identified, increase the magnification to obtain greater detail.

2. Specular reflection

Specular reflection is used to examine the endothelium for polymegathism (cell size variability) and pleomorphism (cell shape variability), the precorneal tear film, and variations in contour of the epithelium. When learning this technique, it is best to start by attempting to obtain an image of the anterior lens surface by specular reflection (Fig. 7.6).

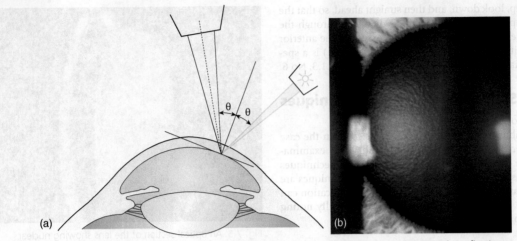

Fig. 7.6 (a) Diagram illustrating the position of the illuminating and viewing systems when using specular reflection to view the corneal endothelium. **(b)** Specular reflection from the anterior surface of the lens showing its orange peel appearance.

1. Set the illumination system at approximately 30° to 45° from the microscope, using a moderately wide 2 to 3 mm parallelepiped. Look through the eyepieces and focus the parallelepiped on the anterior lens.
2. Change the angle of illumination until the reflection of the instrument lamp is seen from the lens surface. This occurs when the angle of incidence equals the angle of reflection from the lens (see Fig. 7.6a).
3. View the orange peel textural appearance of the anterior lens (see Fig. 7.6b) to the side of the bright reflex.
4. To examine the tear film and epithelium, set the illumination system at approximately 45° to 60° from the microscope, using a moderately wide 2 to 3 mm parallelepiped. Look through the eyepieces and focus the parallelepiped on the cornea. Ask the patient to blink and use the particles floating in the tear film to help you focus.
5. Change the angle of illumination until a bright reflection is seen from the pre-corneal tear film. This occurs when the angle of incidence equals the angle of reflection from the cornea. This can also be obtained by moving the illumination/microscope system laterally until the two angles are equal.
6. To examine the endothelium, set the magnification to about 16× with a fairly wide 2 to 3 mm parallelepiped and initially focus on the tear film.
7. Alter the illumination angle and/or lateral position of the slit-lamp until the bright corneal reflexes (Purkinje images) fall on top of the corneal section. There should be two reflexes: on the epithelial side of the corneal section there should be a bright white reflex from the tear film (conjugate with the epithelium) and on the endothelial side a less bright, slightly yellowed reflex

from the endothelium. You may need to alter the angle of illumination very slightly to separate the two reflections.
8. Increase the magnification to about 40× and move the joystick slightly forward to focus on the endothelium. If you then look to the side of the dull endothelial slightly yellowed reflex (nasal or temporal to the reflex, depending on the position of the illumination system), the duller picture of the endothelial hexagonal cells will be in view.

3. Retro-illumination from the iris

Retro-illumination from the iris (Fig. 7.7) is used in the examination of corneal vessels, epithelial oedema, pigment

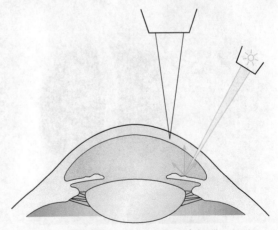

Fig. 7.7 Diagram illustrating the position of the illuminating and viewing systems when using retro-illumination from the iris.

deposits, or keratic precipitate on the endothelium and small scars on the cornea using light reflected from the iris. Opaque features appear dark against a light background.

1. Use a 1 to 2 mm parallelepiped with low magnification and set the illumination system to an angle of about 45°.
2. If it is possible to view the abnormality in direct illumination, bring it into focus and then lock the joystick position.
3. Decouple the illumination and viewing systems by loosening the knob at the back of the illumination system.
4. Direct the light onto the iris and view the structure against the light reflected from the iris. The magnification can be varied, as necessary.

4. Retro-illumination from the fundus

Retro-illumination from the fundus is used to examine cataracts and iris disorders using light reflected from the fundus. Cortical (Fig. 7.8; see Figs. 8.29 and 8.30) and posterior subcapsular cataracts (Fig. 7.9; see Fig. 8.27) are seen as dark opacities against the red background glow from the fundus. Iris abnormalities, such as peripheral iridotomies and loss of pigment, are shown by the red fundal glow being seen through the iris (iris transillumination).

1. Use a 1 to 2 mm parallelepiped with low magnification and set the illumination system to an angle of 0°. Adjust the beam height to the height of the pupil.

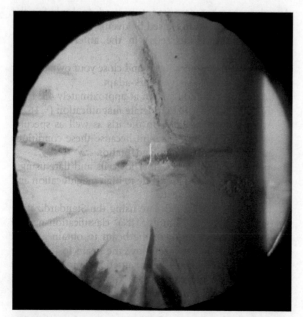

Fig. 7.8 Cortical cataract, seen in retro-illumination from the fundus.

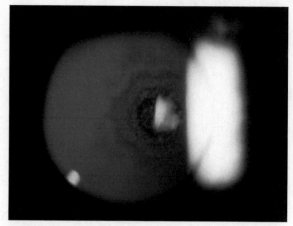

Fig. 7.9 Posterior subcapsular cataract, seen as a dark central opacity in retro-illumination from the fundus.

2. Focus on the iris or lens, as appropriate.
3. You will only be able to focus the anterior or posterior part of the lens at any one time. You can gain an approximate focus on the anterior lens by focusing the iris. To focus the posterior lens, you will need to push the joystick forwards (towards the patient). To gain a retro-illumination image of the lens with an undilated small pupil, you may need to decouple the instrument slightly and alter the angle of illumination by a small amount.
4. Observe any illumination coming through the iris. Although lens opacities are best observed with the pupil dilated, iris transillumination is best observed before dilation.

5. Sclerotic scatter

Sclerotic scatter can be used to view iatrogenic damage due to novice contact tonometry or gonioscopy use, foreign bodies, scars, and central corneal clouding caused by rigid contact lens wear; it involves observing the cornea while the illumination is directed at the limbus. The light is totally internally reflected in a healthy cornea and creates a glowing halo of light where it escapes from the opposite limbus (Fig. 7.10).

1. Turn off the room lights to keep the surrounding light levels as low as possible so you can observe subtle amounts of light scatter.
2. Set the magnification at about 10× and use a 1 to 2 mm slit at about 45°. Focus the central cornea by ensuring the particles in the tear film are focused. Asking the patient to blink will move the tear film debris making them easier to find. Lock the slit-lamp position to ensure the viewing system remains focused on the central cornea.

211

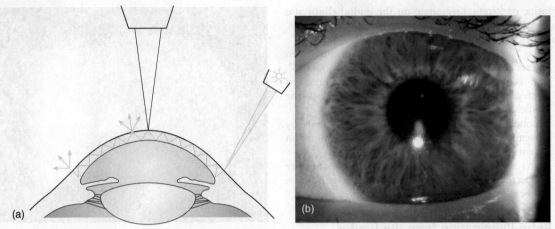

Fig. 7.10 (a) Diagram illustrating the position of the illuminating and viewing systems when using the sclerotic scatter technique. **(b)** Sclerotic scatter showing an S-shape of contact lens deposits.

3. Decouple the illumination and viewing systems by loosening the knob at the back of the illumination system.
4. Move the illumination system onto the temporal limbus. Ideally, shorten the length of the slit because extra slit length can produce light scatter from the sclera that may reduce the visibility of subtle defects.
5. Although you can scan the cornea for areas of light scatter with the naked eye, it is preferable to view it using the decoupled slit-lamp viewing system.

6. Shafer's sign

(See video 7.3.)

Shafer's sign is pathognomonic for a retinal break in phakic eyes, with a sensitivity of 92% to 96%,[3] so that this technique should be used in all patients you suspect might have a retinal tear, such as a patient with symptoms of acute-onset flashes and floaters (section 7.12.1). A standardised patient study in 2009[4] suggested that the use of Shafer's sign by optometrists in the United Kingdom in a patient with acute-onset flashes and floaters was very low (13%) at that time. This should be a routine test in such patients.

1. Set the illumination system at approximately 30° from the microscope using moderate magnification (~16×) and then turn off the room lights.
2. Obtain a thin optical section (increase the rheostat to compensate) of the anterior lens and subsequently the posterior lens. Then push the system forward very slightly from the position when the posterior lens is in focus to view the anterior vitreous.
3. Ask the patient to move their eyes (look up and then down) and then straight ahead, as the particles are easier to detect when moving.

4. Look for red-brown pigmented cells floating in the anterior vitreous (Fig. 7.11, these are retinal pigment epithelium (RPE) pigments and/or blood from vessel injury caused by the retinal break) and not wisps or strands, which are more likely to be vitreous floaters (compare videos 7.3 and 8.1).

7. Anterior chamber assessment for cells and flare

Anterior chamber assessment is used to look for the signs of inflammation caused by uveitis of flare (protein) or cells (white blood cells) in the anterior chamber (Fig. 7.12).

1. Turn off all the room lights and close your own eyes for a few minutes to start to dark-adapt.
2. Set the illumination system at approximately 45° from the microscope using moderate magnification (~16×). Avoid having the light on the iris as well as specular reflection from the tear film because these conditions are likely to decrease dark adaptation.
3. Assess the anterior chamber for cells and flare using a parallelepiped and moderate to high magnification and brightest beam intensity.
4. To grade the cells and flare using the Standardization of Uveitis Nomenclature (SUN)[5] classification narrow the height and width of the beam to obtain a beam 1 mm by 1 mm in size. Move the beam to the centre of the pupil and focus in the anterior chamber midway between the anterior surface of the crystalline lens and the posterior surface of the cornea. Focusing forward and backward within the anterior chamber will facilitate the viewing of cells. Note that the convection currents in the anterior chamber will cause any cells to

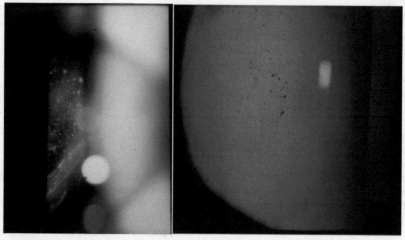

Fig. 7.11 Shafer's sign. Best seen in direct illumination as the particles can be seen as *red-brown* (left image), rather than in *retro-illumination* (right image). (Courtesy of Mr. Paul Sullivan.)

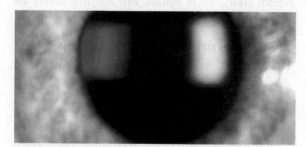

Fig. 7.12 Flare. The image has been enhanced to more easily show the cells in the anterior chamber.

rise where it is warmer (near the iris) and fall where it is cooler (near the cornea).

5. Count cells and grade the degree of obscuration of the iris details (see recording in section 7.1.4).

8. Eyelid eversion

Eyelid eversion is used to examine the superior and inferior palpebral conjunctivae, particularly in contact lens wearers, and when looking for allergic conjunctival changes, papillae, and foreign bodies.

1. Ask the patient to look down and grasp the superior eyelashes and pull them slightly away from the eye. It can be useful to press a cotton bud onto the superior lid to lift it away from the inferior lid, making it easier to grab just the superior lashes.

2. Gently press down on the superior margin of the tarsal plate at the crease using a cotton swab (or the index

finger or thumb of the other hand); at the same time pull the eyelashes up and over the cotton bud. This technique will evert the eyelid to permit viewing of the superior palpebral conjunctiva (Fig. 7.13) using a parallelepiped.

3. To re-evert the eyelid, hold the eyelashes and ask the patient to look up and gently pull the eyelashes away from the eye.

4. To evert the lower eyelid, pull the eyelid down and press under the eyelid margin while moving your finger upwards. The eyelid will evert over your finger.

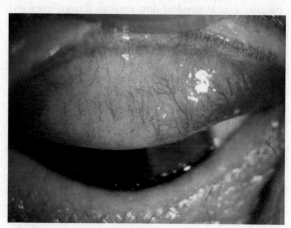

Fig. 7.13 The superior palpebral conjunctiva viewed after lid eversion.

9. Double eyelid eversion

Double eyelid eversion is used to find small foreign bodies in the superior fornix. Care should be taken to minimally irritate the palpebral conjunctiva. The eyelid is not actually everted twice.

1. Wipe a Desmarres lid retractor using an alcohol pad.
2. Instil anaesthetic and fluorescein into the eye.
3. With the patient at the slit-lamp, single-evert the upper eyelid. Use the Desmarres lid retractor to hook under the everted tarsus with the blade placed between tarsus and bulbar conjunctiva.
4. Gently pull up and out to expose the fornix.
5. Observe for any small foreign bodies using fluorescein and the cobalt blue filter on the slit-lamp or irrigate the fornix in free space to try to dislodge any foreign bodies.

7.1.4 Recording of slit-lamp findings

Normal appearance: If no abnormalities are detected, record 'clear' if the tissue is transparent, such as the cornea and lens. Otherwise record 'within normal limits' (WNL) or equivalent.

Specific chief complaints: If the patient has a presenting complaint that could suggest an anterior segment abnormality and no abnormalities are detected, your recording should be more detailed to highlight that your examination was full and appropriate. For example, for a patient complaining of a foreign body (FB) sensation, you might record 'cornea clear, no FB found, no trichiasis, no fl. (fluorescein) staining, no infiltrates, no ulcers, lids everted—all clear, no papillae,' or similar. A patient with acute-onset flashes and floaters should have the results of a Shafer's sign test recorded.

Any normal variation in appearance should be recorded (e.g., melanosis, concretions, corneal arcus, pingueculae, Mittendorf dot, vitreous floater, iris naevi, iris heterochromia, see sections 8.1 and 8.2) and imaged if appropriate.

Anomalies/abnormalities: Take a digital image of any abnormalities/anomalies, if possible, and/or use grading scales[6] to record fluorescein staining, corneal oedema, conjunctival anomalies (papillae, follicles), injection, vascularisation, and forth. Record the size, shape, appearance, and location of other anomalies using a diagram and written description.

Cataracts: Image cortical and subcapsular cataracts using retro-illumination (see Figs. 7.8 and 7.9), otherwise draw them (Fig. 7.14). If there are cortical opacities in both the anterior and posterior cortex, both should be imaged and recorded. Image nuclear cataracts using optical sections (see Fig. 7.5), otherwise nuclear yellowing and opacification can be graded separately using a cataract grading system, such as the LOCS III[7] in which a photograph of the

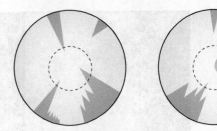

Fig. 7.14 Recording of cataract.

cataract is graded on a decimal scale against standardised colour photographs.

Cells and flare: Cells in the anterior chamber are graded (see Fig. 7.12) according to the number observed with grade 0 = < 1 cell, 0.5+ = 1–5 cells, 1+ = 6–15 cells, 2+ = 16–25 cells, 3+ = 26–50 cells, and 4+ = >50 cells.[5] Aqueous flare is graded from 0–4+ depending on the visibility of the iris detail, with grade 0 = no flare, grade 1+ = faint flare, 2+ = moderate (iris and lens details remain clear), 3+ = marked (iris and lens details are hazy), and 4+ = intense (fibrous or plastic aqueous).

7.1.5 Interpretation of slit-lamp findings

A good understanding of the normal anatomy and physiology of the anterior segment, variations in normal appearance (sections 8.1 and 8.3), the normal changes expected with age (sections 8.2 and 8.4), and anterior segment disease is required. You need to consider whether any significant findings of slit-lamp assessments helped in your differential diagnosis of any pertinent symptoms and signs and whether they lead to a final diagnosis or an indication of the need for further testing.

7.1.6 Most common errors when using a slit-lamp

1. Poor positioning of the patient so that they are not able to maintain their forehead against the headrest, resulting in the image going in and out of focus.
2. Not focusing the eyepieces to compensate for your refractive error.
3. Not increasing the brightness when narrowing the beam or using a filter.
4. Not maintaining a sharp focus as the beam is swept across the eye.
5. Not developing a smooth, logical routine that can be repeated.
6. Using an optic section with high magnification and low illumination during the initial phases of the assessment.

7. Not examining the superior cornea and conjunctiva by having the patient look down and raising the upper eyelid.

7.2 Tear film and ocular surface assessment

7.2.1 The evidence base: when and how to assess the tear film and ocular surface

The tear film, which is assessed during slit-lamp examination, is specifically indicated in patients with any symptoms of an ocular surface condition and particularly dry eye disease (DED). DED is a multifactorial disease diagnosed by characteristic ocular symptoms and a loss of homeostasis of the tear film,[8] and signs and symptoms are more likely when the tear film and ocular surface homeostasis is under stress (section 7.2.2). Specific diagnostic indicators from the Tear Film and Ocular Surface Society (TFOS) dry eye workshop II (DEWS II) are a positive symptom score plus one of the three markers of abnormal homeostasis (tear film instability, ocular surface damage, and osmolarity),[8] In addition, assessments of tear volume and meibomian gland structure and function can identify the aqueous deficiency and evaporative elements of DED, respectively, to help differentiate DED subtypes and determine correct management. Tests are being developed at a rapid rate, and this is an area that particularly requires regular attention to the literature.

Tear film instability is measured by the time taken for the tear film to break up after a blink. It can be measured invasively with fluorescein tear film break-up time (FBUT) or non-invasively (NIBUT) and both are simple, quick measurements. Fluorescein reduces the stability of the tear film and FBUT shows a wide variability in patients with mild and moderate DED, so that its usefulness seems limited.[2] However, it is very widely used and perhaps for that reason, it is included in the DEWS II DED diagnostic test battery. NIBUT has the inherent advantage of not altering the tear film before measurements are taken and is thus preferred by DEWS II.[2,8]

Ocular surface damage is best assessed using a combination of the vital dyes fluorescein and lissamine green. Fluorescein is the standard dye for assessment of corneal surface damage, because it is taken up by damaged cells, adheres to the surface of cells and pools in depressed areas of the ocular surface. Lissamine green stains dead and devitalised cells and mucin, with staining properties that are similar to rose bengal, but with significantly less toxicity and discomfort, so that it has largely replaced rose bengal in clinical use. Both dyes are important for viewing

conjunctival damage, including bulbar, tarsal, and lid margin. Lissamine green is particularly useful in highlighting lid wiper epitheliopathy, which is damage to the lid wiper region (Fig. 7.15) that is responsible for spreading the tear film during blinks.[9]

Increased tear film osmolarity has been shown to have a central role in the pathophysiology of DED.[10] However, measurements of tear film osmolarity have been reported to be highly variable,[11-13] particularly those provided by the iPen system.[11,12] Although the TearLab device has been shown to provide more reliable and accurate measurements,[11] others have reported that 28% of TearLab scores from patients without DED give osmolarity values above the standard cut-off of 308 mOsm/L,[13] which suggests poor validity of results. However, Nolfi and Caffery[11] provide an alternative view that such scores are valid and indicate an unstable ocular surface before traditional clinical signs have revealed DED.

Tear volume helps to determine the relative contribution of *aqueous deficiency DED* and contributes to the diagnosis of Sjögren syndrome.[8] Reduced tear volume increases the osmolarity of the tear film and produces friction between the lid wiper and the ocular surface, both

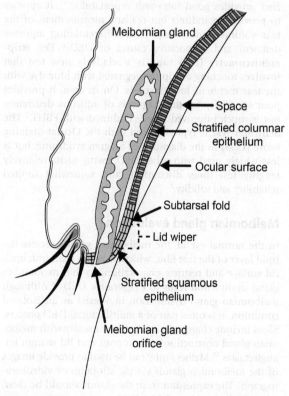

Fig. 7.15 The anatomy of the eyelid. (Courtesy of Samantha Strong.)

Labels in figure:
Meibomian gland
Space
Stratified columnar epithelium
Ocular surface
Subtarsal fold
Lid wiper
Stratified squamous epithelium
Meibomian gland orifice

of which contribute to ocular surface inflammation.[14,15] Although the components of aqueous deficiency and evaporative DED are on a continuum in many patients, the identification of aqueous deficiency can alter management strategies, such as the use of lacrimal occlusion earlier in the treatment paradigm, for example. The clinical assessment of tear volume may be undertaken using meniscometry, phenol red thread test, SM-tube (strip meniscometry tube), and Schirmer test. **Meniscometry** using the slit-lamp shows poor inter-visit repeatability due to poor visualisation of the meniscus (without the introduction of fluorescein), and variables such as time after a blink, location of measurement, environment (e.g., temperature and humidity), and illumination (part of section 7.1.2).[2] Many commercial instruments are introducing imaging software to try to quantify the tear meniscus, but normative values and direct comparisons between instruments are not yet available. Clinicians with access to an OCT with anterior segment functionality can capture a repeatable measure of the tear meniscus height or area using a line scan (section 7.11.1) that has been shown to correlate with Schirmer, FBUT, and symptoms.[16] The **Phenol red thread** test is tolerated well by patients owing to the relative comfort of the test and short duration; it also provides good intra-visit repeatability.[17] It appears to provide an indirect but realistic measurement of the tear volume and is helpful in differentiating aqueous deficient and evaporative causes of DED.[2] The **strip-meniscometry (SM) tube** is a relatively new test that involves touching a strip impregnated with blue dye with the tear meniscus for 5 seconds. On its own, it provides poor specificity for the diagnosis of aqueous deficiency, but is much improved when combined with FBUT.[2] The **Schirmer test** is typically used with the Ocular Staining Score (OSS) in the diagnosis of Sjögren syndrome, but is less widely used with other DED owing to its relatively lengthy test time, discomfort, and somewhat limited reliability and validity.[2]

Meibomian gland evaluation

In the normal eyelid, the meibomian glands secrete the lipid layer of the tear film, which provides a smooth optical surface and restricts evaporation, so that meibomian gland dysfunction leads to evaporative DED.[18] Although meibomian gland dysfunction may exist as an isolated condition, it is often part of a multifactorial DED process. Signs include changes in lid structure usually with meibomian gland obstruction and dropout and lid margin telangiectasias.[19] Meibography can be used to provide images of the meibomian glands via the slit-lamp or videokeratograph. The expression from the glands should be clear, whereas dysfunction yields cloudy to opaque expression or no excretion at all.

Test order and recommended procedures. The order of testing of the tear film and ocular surface is important because some tests may influence the results of others, so that tear film instability measured by a non-invasive method should be undertaken before any invasive measures or any procedures that may stimulate tearing.[20] Similarly, a measure of tear volume or production should precede the instillation of vital dyes. The tests listed below are ordered with this in mind. The procedures described are based on the recommendations of DEWS II.[2]

7.2.2 Symptoms assessment

A three-step process for symptoms assessment is proposed:
1. Any patient reporting symptoms indicative of DED in the chief complaint of the case history should undergo a full DED assessment. Symptoms typically include irritation, dryness, grittiness, foreign body sensation, burning, stinging, pain, tearing, contact lens intolerance, and transient blurred vision; less commonly mentioned symptoms include haloes around lights (especially at night), excessive tearing, stringy mucus discharge, redness, photophobia, itching, and asthenopia.
2. Patients at risk of DED should be identified in the case history. Risk factors include[20]:
   (a) Contact lens wear
   (b) Post refractive or cataract surgery
   (c) Occupations/hobbies that include extended concentrated tasks that reduce the blink rate, such as prolonged reading, viewing screens, or driving
   (d) Occupations/hobbies associated with environmental factors that can exacerbate DED, such as wind, air conditioning, airline travel, low humidity indoors in winter months
   (e) Cigarette smoking
   (f) Systemic medications, including but not limited to beta-blockers, antihistamines, oral contraceptives, and acne medications.
   Patients identified as at risk of DED from the case history or other elements of the eye examination should be asked a four-item set of 'DED screening' questions[20]:
   • "Do your eyes feel uncomfortable?"
   • "Do you have watery eyes?"
   • "Does your vision fluctuate, especially in a dry environment?"
   • "Do you use eye drops?"
   If the patent responds positively to any of the four questions, then ask "Do you have dry mouth?" to screen for Sjögren syndrome.
3. An essential component of DED diagnosis is a symptom assessment questionnaire such as the OSDI (Ocular Surface Disease Index) and the DEQ-5 (Dry Eye Questionnaire-5).[21] Links to both questionnaires, as well as others, and their scoring systems are available online.

7.2.3 Non-invasive tear film (NIBUT) procedures

A video clip of the NIBUT procedure and many other of the diagnostic tests described here are provided on the TFOS DEWS II website (www.tearfilm.org).

NIBUT or tear thinning time measurements involve projecting a pattern on to the tear film and observing the specular image. Keratometer mires may be used in clinical practice, but grids are also available: the tearscope is a commercially available test for measuring NIBUT and many corneal topographers (section 5.4) have a NIBUT module.[2]

1. The illumination of the room should be low to provide the best image contrast.
2. With the patient's head in position on the chin rest, focus the instrument so that a clear view of the pattern is seen. If using a keratometer, the mires should be centrally positioned and sharply in focus.
3. Instruct the patient to blink fully and normally three times, and then to hold their eye wide open and not blink until instructed.
4. Record the time between the last complete blink and the first indication of pattern break-up.
5. Repeat the measurement two more times and take an average.

7.2.4 Procedure for tear film osmolarity testing

A variety of instruments are commercially available and their measurement procedures are well described in the instrument manuals. In addition, a video clip of the Tear-Lab instrument procedure is available on the TFOS DEWS II website (www.tearfilm.org) and is summarised below.

1. Ensure the TearLab is calibrated as directed in the user manual.
2. Explain the purpose of the procedure to the patient: "This test determines how concentrated your tears are and will help us determine whether you have dry eye and how we can best treat it if you do."
3. Remove a TearLab pen from the reader station and insert a single use test card. Remove the protective cover from the test card.
4. With the patient looking up and away, gently touch the tear meniscus above the temporal lower lid next to the lateral canthus area (Fig. 7.16; no significant pressure needs to be applied). After the tear sample has successfully been collected via passive capillary action the pen will beep. **Note**: Do not collect tear fluid within 2 hours of any topical eye drops being applied. It should be performed before any fluorescein is instilled or slit-lamp examination has been conducted.
5. Each test card will have a code number. Enter the code after docking the pen into the reading station. After

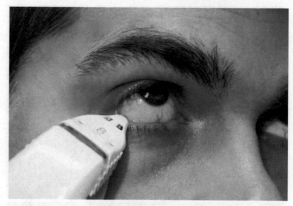

Fig. 7.16 TearLab instrument about to take osmolarity assessment.

following instructions, the osmolarity reading will be displayed.
6. Perform steps 3 through 5 on the other eye with a fresh single-use test card.

7.2.5 Procedure for phenol red thread test

1. The test may stimulate some degree of reflex tearing and should be undertaken prior to manipulation of the eyelids or to instillation of any fluid or dye into the tear film.
2. Lower the room lights. Instruct the patient to look up slightly and blink normally during the test.
3. Remove the threads by gently peeling the plastic film covering from the unsealed end of the aluminium sheet. Make sure that the folded 3 mm end of the thread is bent open at an angle that allows for easy placement onto the palpebral conjunctiva (Fig. 7.17a).
4. Pull the lower eyelid away from the globe slightly and place the folded 3 mm portion of the thread on the palpebral conjunctival junction, approximately one-third of the distance from the lateral canthus of the lower eyelid with the eye in the primary position.
5. Begin timing as soon as the thread touches the tear layer (see Fig. 7.17b).
6. After 15 seconds, gently remove the thread.
7. Measure the length of the red portion of the thread in millimetres from the very tip (ignoring the fold; Fig. 7.18).
8. Because tear volume can vary, reliability can be improved by repeating the test on different days. It may also be helpful to ask the patient if they could feel the thread during testing, because it could be indicative of a reflex tearing component to the measurement. Excessively high measures (approaching 30 mm+) should be repeated.

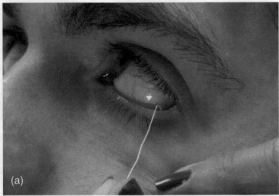

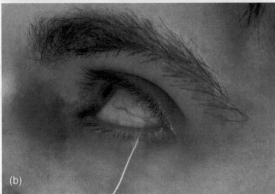

Fig. 7.17 Phenol red thread, with **(a)** the folded end bent open at an angle that allows for easy placement onto the palpebral conjunctiva; **(b)** it is placed approximately one-third of the distance from the lateral canthus of the lower eyelid with the eye in the primary position.

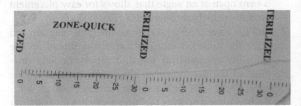

Fig. 7.18 Scoring the Phenol red thread test. It is ~23 mm (measured from the thread end).

7.2.6 Procedure for Schirmer tear test

1. The test may stimulate some degree of reflex tearing and should be undertaken prior to manipulation of the eyelids or to instillation of any fluid or dye into the tear film.
2. Bend the round wick end of the test strips at the notch approximately 120° before opening the sterile

pouch. Peel back the pouch and remove the strips. Only handle the strips by the non-wick ends to avoid contamination.

3. Have the patient look up and gently pull the lower eyelid down temporally. Place the bent hooked end of the strip at the junction of the temporal and central third of the lower eyelid margin (Fig. 7.19a). The strip should not touch the cornea when the eyelid is released (see Fig. 7.19b). Release the eyelid and have the patient continue to look up, blinking normally. The patient can close their eyes if this is more comfortable, but should not squeeze the eyes shut. Both eyes should be measured at the same time.
4. Note the time of insertion. Remove the strip after 5 minutes or when it is completely wet, whichever comes first. Measure the wetted portion of the strip from the notch towards the flat end in millimetres and record this value.

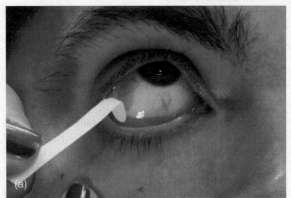

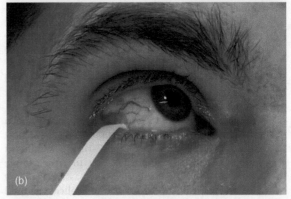

Fig. 7.19 Schirmer test, with **(a)** the bent and hooked end of the strip allows easy placement onto the palpebral conjunctiva; **(b)** it is placed at the junction of the temporal and central third of the lower eyelid margin.

7.2.7 Procedure for fluorescein tear film break-up time

(See video 7.4.)

Topical anaesthetics should not be used prior to the test.

1. Fluorescein instillation: Wet the tip of a fluorescein strip with sterile saline solution. Be careful not to contaminate the saline by touching the strip to the tip of the bottle. Shake excess fluid from the strip over a sink (too much fluid will delay the time to maximum fluorescence and may drip onto and stain the patient's lids and cheeks).
2. Ask the patient to look up and touch the strip to the inferior bulbar or tarsal conjunctiva, being careful not to touch the cornea. Do not use a sweeping movement to 'paint' the conjunctiva because it can provide too much fluorescein and create unnecessary discomfort for the patient. The strip can also be touched to the upper bulbar conjunctiva, but this has the disadvantage that if the patient blinks or attempts to blink, the eye will rotate and the strip may scratch the superior cornea. Ask the patient to blink several times to allow the fluorescein to spread across the cornea. Remove any excess fluorescein using a tissue and be careful not to spill the dye on the patient's face or clothing as a stain will result.
3. Warn the patient that they may note colour if they blow their nose due to drainage through the nasolacrimal system.
4. Soft contact lens wearers can replace their lenses after a biomicroscopic investigation using fluorescein as long as the dye is irrigated out of the eye using saline prior to lens reinsertion. Otherwise irrigation is not necessary.
5. Measure FBUT 1 to 3 minutes after fluorescein instillation.
6. Examine the tear film at the slit-lamp with a wide 2 to 3 mm parallelepiped and low magnification. Switch to the cobalt blue filter so that the tear film should appear as a fine green film due to the fluorescein. The use of the Kodak Wratten yellow filter number 12 held over the observation system is helpful.
7. With the patient positioned at the biomicroscope, ask them to blink three times and then hold their eyes open without blinking until instructed.
8. From the time of the last blink, time how long it takes in seconds before dark spots or streaks appear in the even green tear film after a blink.
9. If the patient blinks before 10 seconds have passed, the measurement cannot be made and the procedure must be re-started.
10. Repeat the measurement two more times and take an average.

11. If the tear film breaks up immediately and consistently in the same location, there may be an epithelial basement membrane defect in that location on the cornea. The test should be repeated, not considering this defect, to get an indication of tear film stability.

7.2.8 Procedure for assessing ocular surface damage

Fluorescein is used to detect any corneal surface damage, and lissamine green is used to detect any interpalpebral bulbar conjunctival and/or lid margin damage. Both fluorescein and lissamine green dyes may be instilled at the same time, or in any order. Generally, clinicians use fluorescein first, then add lissamine, because they are using the fluorescein to also measure FBUT and the additional fluid of the lissamine green could alter FBUT measurements.

Corneal staining

1. If not instilled for FBUT, instil fluorescein as described above (section 7.2.7, steps 1 through 4).
2. Assess the cornea between 1 and 3 minutes after instillation.[2]
3. With the patient at the biomicroscope, observe the cornea with cobalt blue light and medium magnification. When using the cobalt blue light, you will need to increase the illumination. A Kodak Wratten number 12 yellow gelatine filter held in front of the biomicroscope viewing system will facilitate the view by filtering out the reflected blue light. This filter may be built in over the observation system or can be hand-held.
4. It can be useful to examine the eye using both diffuse illumination and then a wide parallelepiped beam, altering the angle of the illumination throughout.
5. Use a grading system to record any staining and ideally photograph or draw the staining distribution, coalescent patches, proximity to both inferior and superior lid, and whether or not there is staining in the pupillary area. Record the number of punctate spots.

Interpalpebral bulbar conjunctival staining and lid margin staining

1. The procedure for lissamine green is performed in a similar way to fluorescein, but make sure the saline drop is retained on the strip for at least 5 seconds and do not shake any excess saline off the strip, so that approximately twice the volume of the dye is used.[2]
2. Assess the interpalpebral bulbar conjunctiva and lid margins between 1 and 3 minutes after instillation.
3. Bulbar staining: Count the number of spots on the interpalpebral bulbar conjunctiva, on both the nasal

and temporal sides, and use a grading scale to record the amount of staining.

4. **Lid margin staining:** Lid wiper epitheliopathy is also evaluated using lissamine green dye. Wet the tip of a lissamine green strip with sterile saline solution. With the patient looking up gently tap the palpebral conjunctiva of the lower lid beneath the lid wiper region or the inferior bulbar conjunctiva. Ensure a generous amount of dye is instilled without sweeping the conjunctival surface.

5. With the patient behind the slit-lamp, examine the lower lid wiper region for staining by gently everting the lower lid. It is imperative not to mistake lid wiper epitheliopathy with the line of Marx which stains naturally in a normal eyelid.

6. Evert the upper lid with a sterile cotton swab (or other preferred method) and inspect for lid wiper epitheliopathy.

7. Estimate the extent of the staining in millimetres and the percent width of staining relative to the lid margin width (excluding Marx's line).

7.2.9 Meibomian gland evaluation

1. With the patient at the biomicroscope, use white light and medium magnification to inspect the lower eyelid margins.

2. Look for stenosis and closure of the meibomian gland orifices, thickened (inspissated) secretions, blocked glands, tear frothing on the eyelid margins, telangiectasias ('spider veins' because of their fine, web-like appearance) of lid margin vessels, notching of the Meibomian gland openings, and migration of these openings towards the posterior surface of the lids; all indicative of chronic disease.

3. Pull the lower eyelid down and look for concretions (section 8.2.7) in the palpebral conjunctiva, as well as any inflamed, blocked, or missing glands.

4. Another method of assessing the meibomian gland function is to determine the position of the line of Marx, which is a clear line running along the lower lid margin, after fluorescein or lissamine green is instilled into the eye. In normal eyes this line is located on the conjunctival side of the meibomian gland orifices, and in meibomian gland dysfunction it is located on the cutaneous side of the orifices.[22]

5. Slit-lamp examination only allows assessment of the meibomian gland orifices, but images of the glands can be taken using infrared light and several meibography imaging devices are available. The procedures of the various instruments are provided by the instrument manuals and are not provided here. The images provide clear evidence of meibomian gland changes (Fig. 7.20).

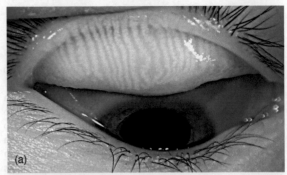

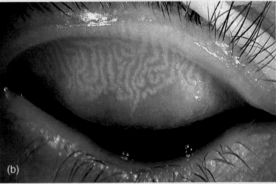

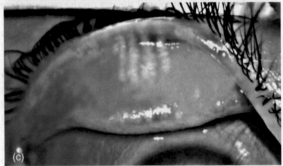

Fig. 7.20 Infra-red meibomography images of **(a)** healthy meibomian glands (grade 0) and two levels of meibomian gland drop-out: **(b)** level 2 and **(c)** level 4.

Meibomian gland expression

1. Assessment should be done after other tests used in the diagnosis of ocular surface disease so that, for example, tear film assessment, including tear break-up time, is not affected by meibomian gland diagnostic expression.

2. Inform the patient that you are going to press on their eyelid and that they will feel some pressure. With the patient looking up, apply moderate pressure on the lower eyelid margins near the eyelashes, while observing the meibomian gland orifices and assess the expressibility and secretion quality. Clear fluid should be expressed. If this is not the case apply pressure

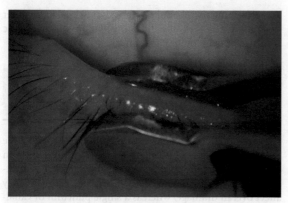

Fig. 7.21 Meibomian gland expression using Collins expressor forceps.

over the central third of the upper and particularly the lower lids[23] to determine the extent and severity of the dysfunction. Meibomian gland pressure devices (Fig. 7.21) can be used instead of digital pressure.

7.2.10 Recording

Symptoms. Record the patient's symptoms if part of their chief complaint as normal and indicate whether these symptoms only occur/are exacerbated under certain conditions (e.g., prolonged reading, airline travel, wind, contact lens wear). If the 4/5-item set of 'DED screening' questions[20] were used, record both negative and positive responses. If a standardised questionnaire, such as OSDI, DEQ-5, was used, record as described within the instructions provided with each test.

Tear instability. The FBUT or NIBUT value should be recorded in seconds for each eye individually. Indicate the method that was used to determine this value. For example, NIBUT with grid pattern, RE: 10 s, LE: 12 s.

Ocular surface damage. A large number of grading and scoring systems exist for the documentation of ocular surface damage, with a variety of pros and cons.[24] The grading scales used most commonly by optometrists are the CCLRU-Brien Holden Institute, original Efron, Johnson & Johnson (modified Efron), and Alcon scales.[6] The scores of these scales should be accompanied by photographs and descriptions and drawings of any corneal and conjunctival staining patterns. Lid wiper epitheliopathy can be graded by the extent of staining as described in Table 7.2.

Osmolarity. Record the instrument used and the osmolarity in mOsm/L (milliosmoles/litre).

Tear volume. Record the distance in millimetres that the thread is red (phenol red test) or that the strip is wet (Schirmer test) for each eye. For example:

Schirmer: RE 8 mm; LE 5 mm in 5 minutes
Phenol red thread: OD 12 mm; OS 15 mm in 15 seconds

Table 7.2 Grading scale for lid wiper epitheliopathy

Length of staining (horizontal)	Grade	Width of wiper staining (sagittal)
<2 mm	0	<25% of width of wiper
2–4 mm	1	25% to 50% width
5–9 mm	2	50% to 75% width
>10 mm	3	≥75% of wiper

Meibomian gland evaluation. Record any meibomian gland obstruction and dropout, lid margin telangiectasias, and expressibility of the glands. A 'Meiboscore' can also be used to grade meibomian gland dysfunction[18] and the expressibility can be graded by the amount of pressure required to express the glands (1: light pressure, 2: moderate pressure, and 3: heavy pressure) and the quality of the expressed meibum (0: clear, 1: cloudy, 2: granular, and 3: toothpaste).[25]

7.2.11 Interpretation

Symptoms. A score of 13 or more on the OSDI and 6 or more (and 12 or more for Sjögren syndrome) on the DEQ-5 are considered significant for DED. A detailed review of available questionnaires and their value is provided by Guillemin et al.[21]

Tear instability. Normal NIBUT (keratometer or topographer) is between 28 and 60 seconds and a normal FBUT is between 15 and 45 seconds. NIBUTs and FBUTs of less than 10 seconds are indicative of an unstable tear film.[2] Although FBUT measurements are significantly lower than NIBUT values, the disparity is smaller for short break-up times associated with poor tear quality.[26] Normal FBUT and NIBUT measurements are sometimes limited by the patient's ability to keep their eyes open and not blink.

Ocular surface damage. Surface damage on both the cornea (fluorescein) and conjunctiva (lissamine green) generally shows a characteristic distribution confined to the interpalpebral area of the ocular surface. Lissamine green staining is dose-dependent; therefore, if a very small amount is used the staining will be very minimal.[27] Temporal and nasal interpalpebral bulbar conjunctival lissamine green staining is predictive of dry eye. More than five punctate fluorescein spots on the cornea is diagnostic of DED and more than nine punctate lissamine green spots on the conjunctiva is diagnostic of DED.[2] Lid wiper epitheliopathy is diagnosed by staining greater than 2 mm and/or greater than 25% of the lid margin width (excluding Marx's line).

Osmolarity. 308 mOsm/L is widely accepted as a cut-off value to help diagnose mild-moderate DED and an

8 mOsm/L difference between the eyes is indicative of a loss of homeostasis due to DED in the eye with the higher osmolarity.[2] Further, this inter-eye variability has been shown to reduce with successful treatment of DED, making osmolarity measures important for monitoring treatment as well as diagnosis.[28]

Tear volume. For the phenol red thread test, a measurement of <less than 10 mm wetting represents true dryness, whereas 10 to 20 mm wetting is considered borderline, and more than 20 mm is generally considered normal (see Fig. 7.18). Measurements in the high 20s or 30s are most likely caused by reflex tearing. For the Schirmer test, a measurement of 10 to 15 mm or more without anaesthesia is regarded as normal tear production. A value of less than 5 mm represents a significant aqueous dry eye. Several measurements should be made on repeated visits and averaged to obtain as accurate a result as possible.

Meibomian gland evaluation. The importance of evaluation of the meibomian glands cannot be overemphasised given that obstructive meibomian gland dysfunction is significantly more common than previously understood (see Fig. 7.21).[20] Digital (or other forms) expression should be utilised on evaluation of all lids (see Fig. 7.19). Poor expression may be due to gland atrophy or meibomian gland obstruction.

7.2.12 Most common errors

1. Touching the cornea with a fluorescein strip or wiping the fluoret against the conjunctiva, causing discomfort and reflex tearing.
2. Not obtaining a sharply focused image of the grid or mires before measuring NIBUT.

3. Performing the Phenol red thread or Schirmer test after manipulation of the lids, instillation of diagnostic drugs or dyes, or applanation tonometry.

7.3 Assessment of the lacrimal drainage system

Lacrimal drainage system obstruction can occur at the punctum, vertical or horizontal canaliculus, common canaliculus, and the nasolacrimal duct (Fig. 7.22). The latter two are more likely to cause significant tearing as they affect overall drainage, whereas a single punctum or canaliculus will reduce outflow through one of the two channels, but will not impede it completely.

7.3.1 The evidence base: when and how to assess the lacrimal drainage system

Patients who complain of excessive eye watering (epiphora) need assessing to determine whether this is caused by true nasolacrimal system obstruction or eyelid abnormality, such as ectropion (lower eyelid droops away from the eye) and eNtropion (eyelid turns iNward), or is caused by paradoxical reflex tearing associated with DED or other ocular surface problem. If nasolacrimal system obstruction is suspected, an assessment of the lacrimal drainage system is required. The dye disappearance test and/or the Jones 1 test helps to determine whether there is a stenosis (abnormal narrowing) or blockage of the nasolacrimal system. If the tests results suggest a stenosis or blockage, then dilation and irrigation of the system is indicated.

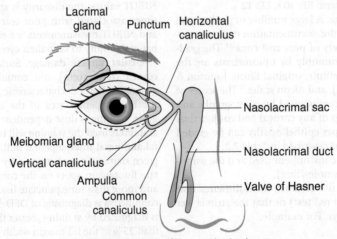

Fig. 7.22 The anatomy of the nasolacrimal system.

Contraindications for dilation and irrigation include symptoms and signs of canaliculitis and dacryocystitis (including regurgitation of discharge from the punctum). Lacrimal sac palpation may help to determine if dilation and irrigation of the system are contraindicated. Dilation and irrigation itself may dislodge a concretion or mucous plug that has blocked the canaliculus. In this respect it is a therapeutic procedure. However, it is also a diagnostic procedure in that it helps to determine if the system is patent (open and unobstructed). Jones 2 testing, which attempts to determine the site of any blockage, is rarely used in primary eye care because if dilation and irrigation were unsuccessful the patient would likely be referred.

7.3.2 Procedure for fluorescein dye disappearance test

1. Explain the procedure and obtain informed consent. Encourage the patient to blink normally and not to squeeze the eyes during the procedure(s).
2. Ask the patient to blow their nose and clean it thoroughly with tissues.
3. Instil equal amounts of fluorescein in each eye and observe the patient for 5 minutes.
4. Compare the relative heights of the tear meniscus at the inferior margin of each eye and the degree of fluorescein spilling over the patient's eyelids.
5. Do not allow the patient to blot the fluorescein because this might draw an excessive amount of fluorescein and tears out of the conjunctival sac. Wipe away any excess fluorescein dye that has spilled onto the patient's cheek to avoid unnecessarily staining the skin.

7.3.3 Procedure for Jones 1 or primary dye test

1. Moisten two to four fluorescein strips with sterile saline and touch to the inferior nasal palpebral conjunctiva, introducing a large amount of dye and fluid into the conjunctival sac. False test results are more likely if insufficient dye is applied.[29]
2. Allow the patient to blink normally for 5 minutes. Ensure that fluorescein dye does not remain in contact with the facial skin long enough to dry.
3. Note that the dye disappearance test may be undertaken simultaneously with the Jones 1 test by observing the dye distribution and disappearance characteristics.
4. Instruct the patient to occlude the nostril on the unaffected side (if tearing problem is unilateral) or one nostril at a time (if tearing problem is bilateral) and blow into a white tissue.
5. Inspect the tissue for fluorescein using a Burton lamp or the cobalt blue light on the slit-lamp biomicroscope.

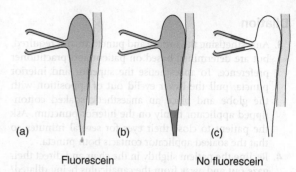

(a) (b) (c)

Fluorescein   No fluorescein

Fig. 7.23 Jones I test. **(a)** Fluorescein is recovered, indicating that the system is patent. **(b)** and **(c)** The absence of fluorescein indicates a blockage or stenosis in the system and the need for dilation and irrigation; **(b)** shows a lower system blockage and **(c)** an upper system blockage.

6. If no fluorescein is detected and especially if the dye was noted to have cleared from the eye other than over the lids onto the face, a false result may have been noted. Consider repeating the test or ask the patient to roll a sterile swab about 1 cm into the nose against the inferior turbinate. Check the swab for fluorescein with the cobalt blue light.
7. If *fluorescein is recovered* (Fig. 7.23a), no further tests are required as the nasolacrimal system is patent. Reflex tearing from DED and other causes should be reconsidered. Dilation and irrigation may still be considered if it is thought that there may be a partial blockage that might be relieved with irrigation.
8. If *no fluorescein is recovered* (see Fig. 7.23b and c), there is either some degree of blockage of the drainage, there is a failure of the lacrimal pump mechanism, or a false test result was obtained, likely due to insufficient fluorescein being used.
9. Consider dilating the punctum on the affected side and repeating steps 1 to 5. If fluorescein is now recovered, the source of the poor drainage was likely stenosis of the punctum.

7.3.4 Procedure for dilation and irrigation

Dilation and irrigation are generally undertaken if no fluorescein is recovered with the Jones 1 test.
1. Prepare the instruments with appropriate disinfection of internal and external surfaces. Attach a reinforced 23-gauge cannula to a 3, 5, or 10 mL syringe.
2. Fill the syringe with 3 to 5 mL sterile saline. Push most of the saline through the cannula to thoroughly rinse the disinfectant, reserving approximately 1 mL for irrigation.

Dilation

3. Anaesthetising the surface and puncta are not required, but are determined based on patient and practitioner preference. To anaesthetise the superior and inferior puncta, pull the lower eyelid out of apposition with the globe and place an anaesthetic soaked cotton-tipped applicator firmly on the inferior punctum. Ask the patient to close their eyes for several minutes so that the soaked applicator contacts both puncta.
4. Recline the patient slightly in the chair and direct their gaze out and away from the canaliculus being dilated/irrigated. For example, have the patient look superior temporally to irrigate the inferior system.
5. Pull the inferior eyelid away from the globe and place a long-tapered dilator vertically into the inferior punctal opening (<2 mm).
6. If the punctum is tight around the dilator, gently roll the dilator back and forth between your fingers to begin to dilate the punctum.
7. Once the dilator is inserted 1 to 2 mm, advance the dilator a little further while pulling laterally on the eyelid to straighten out the canaliculus. Continue to roll the dilator back and forth while directing the tip of the dilator nasally towards the location of the opening into the common canaliculus (i.e., orientation of the dilator is now horizontal). Whitening of the punctal ring indicates expansion of the opening. Do not force the dilator too deeply into the canaliculus and retract it if resistance is encountered or the patient experiences significant discomfort or a sharp pain.
8. If the punctum is not sufficiently enlarged or closes down before the cannula can be inserted, dilate again with the long-tapered dilator and gently advance it further, again respecting the anatomy and the patient's comfort.
9. The primary dye test (Jones 1) may be repeated after only punctal dilation; however, generally you will proceed to irrigation.

Irrigation

10. Insert the cannula immediately after dilating the punctum. If the punctum cannot be opened sufficiently to insert the cannula, consider a smaller gauge cannula or a wider dilation of the punctum.
11. Pull the eyelid away from the globe slightly and insert the cannula 1 to 2 mm vertically then pull the eyelid taut laterally to continue 1 to 4 mm into the horizontal canaliculus, as with the dilator. If the cannula meets with gentle resistance, this is termed 'soft stop,' and the cannula should not be advanced further as an obstruction exists in the canaliculus. The 'hard stop' position indicates that the cannula has come into contact with the nasal bone. This can only be achieved with a sufficiently long cannula to transverse the vertical, horizontal, and common canaliculi and the lacrimal sac (>10 mm advancement).

12. Reach up with the thumb of the hand *not* holding the cannula/syringe. While watching carefully that the position of the cannula is maintained (i.e., that it is not inadvertently advanced further into the canaliculus), apply pressure to the plunger to introduce a small amount of saline (<0.5 m) into the system. Never force the fluid if resistance is encountered. If resistance is encountered, first withdraw the cannula and test that the cannula/syringe combination itself is not obstructed by pushing fluid through the syringe and cannula. Reintroduce the cannula.
13. Once a small amount of saline is introduced, ask the patient to report when it is detected in the throat, at which time pressure on the plunger of the syringe is stopped and the cannula carefully withdrawn (go to step 15). Keep talking to the patient throughout the procedure to ensure that they remain still until the cannula is withdrawn safely.
14. If saline regurgitates from the canaliculus being irrigated, it is likely that this canaliculus is obstructed or stenosed.
15. If saline regurgitates from the contravertical punctum, a common canaliculus blockage should be suspected. Hold a sterile cotton-tipped applicator firmly on that punctum and try to irrigate again. Carefully withdraw the cannula.
16. Offer the patient a mint or lozenge because the saline can have an unpleasant taste for some patients.

7.3.5 Recording of lacrimal drainage tests

Fluorescein dye disappearance: Record if the meniscus height is equal in each eye and if dye runs down over the patient's cheek or disappears into the nasolacrimal drainage system. Relative speed of disappearance between the eyes is also relevant. Take note of the completeness of the blink, including apposition of the puncta, and the lid position.

Jones 1: Record whether or not dye was recovered on each side. Note that some sources label the presence or recovery of dye as 'positive' and absence of dye as 'negative,' so that a 'positive Jones 1 test' means that the system is patent. This is opposite to the usual convention of a positive test result being one that indicates a problem, so it is best to record whether or not dye is recovered in each test in order to avoid confusion (e.g., dye recovered in left nostril [left nasolacrimal system patent]).

Dilation and irrigation: Record whether or not the patient tasted salt or felt the solution in the throat. Also note if saline was regurgitated from the same canaliculus or from the contravertical canaliculus.

7.3.6 Interpretation of lacrimal drainage test results

Fluorescein dye disappearance: If the heights of the tear meniscus are unequal, it implies that the eye with the larger meniscus may have impaired tear drainage. It is less likely that there is a unilateral poor meniscus due to dry eye or unilateral pseudoepiphora from reflex tearing from the dry eye.

Jones 1: If fluorescein is recovered, no further tests are required as the nasolacrimal system is patent. However, some clinicians may consider dilation/irrigating if they feel there is a chance to dislodge a partial obstruction. If no dye is recovered, this indicates either a partial or full blockage in the system, a failure of the lacrimal pump mechanism, or it could be a false positive (likely due to insufficient fluorescein).[29] If mucopurulent effluent is recovered, irrigation should *not* be attempted because there is an active infection/inflammation.

Dilation and irrigation: Normally fluid should exit from the system and be noted by the patient in the throat. A blocked system will offer resistance to fluid injection or cause regurgitation from the contravertical punctum. No fluid flow in the throat indicates a complete obstruction. Fluid subsequently noted in the throat indicates that the obstruction was relieved or there had been a partial obstruction or a stenosis.

7.3.7 Most common errors when using lacrimal drainage tests

1. Instilling insufficient fluorescein or making inadequate attempts to recover fluorescein for the Jones 1 test.[29]
2. Not introducing the cannula quickly enough such that the punctum closes down after dilation, making it difficult to insert the cannula.
3. Failing to respect the anatomy of the canaliculi with the dilator/cannula during dilation/irrigation, leading to patient discomfort.

7.4 Anterior chamber angle depth estimation

The anterior chamber angle is important because it is the drainage location for the circulating aqueous humour (Fig. 7.24), and blockage of the angle can lead to a spike in intraocular pressure (IOP) and potentially damage to the optic nerve. The risk of blockage is highest in patients with narrow angles (female, increasing age, hyperopes,

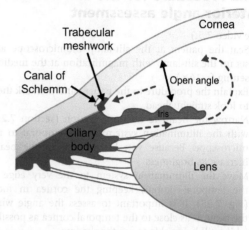

Fig. 7.24 A van Herick grade III anterior angle. (Courtesy of Samantha Strong.)

Inuit or East Asian ethnicity) and when the angle is narrowed because of pupillary dilation (in winter months, at night, with mydriatics). Elderly patients are much more likely to have narrow angles because of the growth of the lens throughout life and children typically have large angles, especially young myopes.

7.4.1 The evidence base: when and how to assess the anterior chamber angle

The most common reason for estimating the anterior angle is as a safety precaution prior to dilating a patient's pupils. The risk of inducing angle closure with a mydriatic is minimal, providing appropriate precautions are used.[30] An estimation of the anterior chamber angle depth may also be used in patients who are taking a systemic medication known to cause pupil dilation and possibly angle closure. It is also used to screen patients with risk factors for angle closure glaucoma.

In most cases the relatively quick and simple van Herick angle assessment is sufficient to indicate whether there is a danger of angle closure although the van Herick angle assessment is unable to assess the narrowest and most-likely-to-close superior angle.[31] If the angle appears narrow using this assessment, gonioscopy is required to determine whether dilation is safe. The van Herick assessment is a conservative one in that many patients with a narrow angle as determined by the test can be safely dilated.[30] Anterior segment OCT can also be used to measure angles, and it gives results similar to van Herick (section 7.11.1).[32]

7.4.2 Procedure for the van Herick anterior angle assessment

(See video 7.5.)

1. Seat the patient at the slit-lamp biomicroscope and set up the slit-lamp with magnification at the medium setting (~16×).
2. Explain the procedure to the patient and then ask them to look straight ahead.
3. Narrow the beam to an optic section (section 7.2.3) with the illumination system at 60° temporal to the microscope. Because you have narrowed the beam, increase its brightness.
4. Move the illumination system to the very edge of the temporal limbus, keeping the cornea in focus (Fig. 7.25). It is important to assess the angle when the beam is as close to the temporal cornea as possible while still being able to see the shadow.
5. Judge the depth of the anterior chamber by the width of the optically clear space between the cornea and the iris. Compare this width to the width of the cornea (Fig. 7.26) as a percentage (so that an angle half as wide as the cornea is 50%).[32]
6. Repeat the measurement on the nasal anterior chamber angle. You may have to rotate both the illumination and viewing systems (keeping them 60° apart) to ensure the illumination system avoids the patient's nose.
7. Repeat for the other eye.

7.4.3 Recording anterior angle size

The original van Herick 4-point grading system is limited, and a 7-point percentage system is preferred.[31,33] Further,

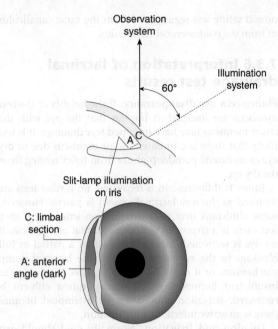

Fig. 7.26 Diagrammatic representation of van Herick's technique for anterior angle estimation.

given the limitations of grading with a small number of step sizes,[34] a full percentage system is recommended.

van Herick: Record the angle as a percentage of the width of the cornea. If only one measurement is recorded, it can be assumed to be temporal. Examples:

van Herick. RE. 100%, LE. 125%
van Herick. OD. 50%, OS. 40%

7.4.4 Interpretation of anterior angle results

The angle should normally be 50% or wider (see Fig. 7.25). If the angle is 25% or narrower, gonioscopy should be performed to determine if it is safe to dilate. Van Herick angle assessment has relatively good specificity, but poor sensitivity in detecting narrow angles as compared with gonioscopy.[35] A large anterior chamber angle (e.g., 300%) can be a sign of pigment dispersion syndrome/glaucoma. In patients with exceptionally wide angles, tests for iris transillumination and pigment in the anterior chamber should be performed.

7.4.5 Most common errors when measuring the anterior angle

1. Failure to position the optical system as close to the limbus as possible. The measured angle will increase in size as you move away from the limbus.

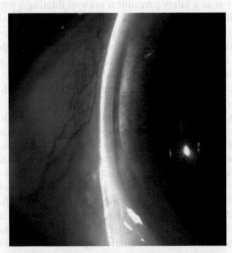

Fig. 7.25 Anatomy of the anterior angle showing the circulation of aqueous humour.

2. Having the angle between the illumination system and the microscope less than 60°.

7.5 Examination of the anterior chamber angle by gonioscopy

7.5.1 The evidence base: when and how to examine the anterior chamber

Specific indications for assessment of the anterior chamber angle include:

1. Narrow anterior chamber angles suggested by van Herick to assess the relative risks for pupillary dilation.
2. Narrow (or closed) angle glaucoma, including evaluation and documentation of peripheral anterior synechiae if present.[36]
3. Primary open-angle glaucoma (POAG) and risk factors for POAG (e.g., elevated IOP) to confirm 'primary' diagnosis.
4. Secondary open-angle glaucoma and risk factors (e.g., pseudoexfoliation, pigment dispersion, chronic uveitis) to contribute the determination of disease severity.
5. Risk of angle neovascularisation (e.g., confirmed rubeosis iridis and ischaemic posterior segment conditions, including vein or artery occlusions and diabetic retinopathy).[37]
6. Risk of angle recession post blunt trauma.
7. Risk of intraocular foreign body.
8. Congenital or acquired structural irregularities of the iris and anomalies of the anterior chamber (e.g., iris cysts or tumours, ectopic pupil).
9. Post laser peripheral iridotomy to assess effect on angle depth.

   Gonioscopy is contraindicated in patients who have experienced:
10. Recent ocular trauma, especially in the presence of hyphaema or microhyphaema.
11. Recent intraocular surgery, including cataract surgery.

Gonioscopy is the standard procedure for examination of the anterior chamber angle and the gold standard technique against which screening tests for narrow angles are compared.[33,35] Light from the anterior chamber angle is totally internally reflected by the cornea, so that the angle cannot be viewed directly. Gonioscope lenses are high minus contact lenses that neutralise the power of the cornea and include appropriately angled mirrors to allow examination of the anterior chamber angle. There is significant physiological variation between normal eyes with regard to the prominence of the various angle structures, including pigmentation. Therefore, gonioscopy should be performed frequently to be able to distinguish between normal and abnormal angle structures.

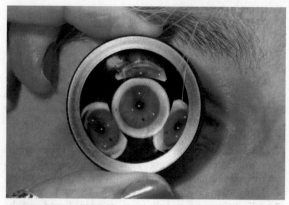

Fig. 7.27 A Goldmann 3-mirror Universal lens on the eye.

Scleral-type lenses, such as the Goldmann 3-mirror lens (Fig. 7.27), provide excellent optics and mirror placement allowing for the detection of subtle angle findings (e.g., early angle neovascularisation), which can be more difficult with the poorer image quality of corneal-type lenses. Scleral-type lenses also provide excellent lens stability on the eye once inserted and good eyelid control even with a patient with blepharospasm. This allows a better view in patients with significant loss of corneal transparency. The image may be more transient with corneal-type lenses as the tear film seal is disrupted easily if the lens is not maintained on the central cornea. The Universal lens also contains two additional mirrors angled for evaluation of the peripheral and midperipheral fundus as well as a central lens for evaluation of the vitreous and posterior pole (section 7.12).

All *corneal-type* lenses have a smaller (9 mm) and flatter area of contact on the cornea compared with the scleral-type lenses and have four or six mirrors, all of which are angled to allow examination of the anterior chamber angle. The smaller, less concave surface enables gonioscopy without the need for a viscous coupling solution and essentially no lens rotation (particularly for the 6-mirror) is required because all the mirrors are angled for gonioscopic assessment. The lens is easily inserted onto the cornea of a cooperative patient, thus facilitating a relatively quick assessment, unlike the more challenging lens insertion and required coupling solution with scleral-type lenses. Corneal compressions can only be undertaken with corneal-type lenses and allows differentiation between appositional and synechial angle closure. Disadvantages of corneal-type lenses include the identification of an artificially wider angle if too much pressure on the cornea causes the angle to appear to widen. Corneal epithelial disruption may also occur if significant lens movement occurs on the corneal surface.

7.5.2 Gonioscopy procedure

1. Describe the specific indications for gonioscopic assessment to the patient and outline the procedure: "I would like to use a contact lens on the front of your eye to examine the hidden part of the front of your eye. I will be putting a drop in your eyes to numb the cornea, so do not rub your eyes for at least half an hour or you could scratch your eye without feeling it." Obtain informed consent.
2. Anaesthetise both eyes. Gonioscopy can be performed immediately following applanation tonometry so that additional anaesthetic is not necessarily required. Fluorescein does not interfere with the examination.
3. Adjust the room and slit-lamp, as needed, and seat the patient comfortably (section 7.1.2, steps 1 through 6). Consider using the lens case under your elbow or hook your little finger over the headrest bar of the biomicroscope to promote stability of the lens.
4. Align the illumination system to be co-axial with the viewing system, set the magnification to a low power (e.g., 10×), and the rheostat to low or medium intensity.

Goldmann 3-mirror (Universal) gonioscopy procedure

▶ (See video 7.6 and summary in Box 7.1).
5. **Lens preparation:** Clean and disinfect the gonioscopy lens. Fill approximately two-thirds of the concave lens surface with a viscous coupling solution, ensuring no bubbles remain to interfere with the view.

Box 7.1 **Summary of gonioscopy procedure**
1. Disinfect the lens and fill the lens surface with viscous coupling solution.
2. Anaesthetise both eyes
3. Align the biomicroscope illumination and observation systems. Set the magnification and the rheostat to low settings.
4. Insert the lens and (for Goldmann 3-mirror) wipe away excess solution.
5. Rotate the Goldmann 3-mirror lens through 360° to establish a good seal.
6. Place the thumbnail mirror at 12 o'clock on the cornea to view the inferior angle first.
7. Identify the *most posterior structure* observable.
8. Position the slit beam horizontally to view the nasal and temporal sides.
9. Examine all quadrants (through 360°) in a systematic manner.
10. Remove the lens by introducing air under the lens and releasing from contact with the cornea.

---

6. **Lens insertion:** Move the microscope off to the side or reach around the microscope to insert the lens. Advise the patient that pressure and a turning feeling may be detected with the lens in place, but that there will be no discomfort. Instruct the patient to look up. Hold the eyelashes of the upper eyelids tightly against the orbital rim with the thumb, then pull the lower eyelid down and away from the globe and introduce the rim of the lens over the lower eyelid margin. Use the lens edge to pull down the lower eyelid further, while quickly rotating the lens upwards onto the eye (video 7.6). Once the lens is on the eye, ask the patient to *slowly* look straight ahead. Keep the flat front surface perpendicular to the line of sight. If air bubbles are present, apply a little pressure and gently rock the lens to see if they can be removed. The angle can often be viewed around air bubbles, but if they remain a significant problem with the view, remove and re-insert the lens. Consider manipulating the lens through a couple of rotations with both hands to establish the lens seal and enable smooth rotation of the lens while observing the various angle quadrants. Wipe excess solution that may have dripped onto the patient's cheek.
7. **Examination/observation procedure:** For examination, it is preferable to hold the lens with the left hand when examining the right eye and vice versa for the left eye. Either two hands can be used to rotate the lens to view all four quadrants, or one hand can be used with stabilisation of the lens between rotations with the middle finger.
8. Start with a vertical parallelepiped beam 1 to 3 mm wide. Keep the illumination moderate to reduce pupillary constriction that may decrease the perceived width of the angle and prevent patient discomfort.
9. Start with the thumbnail mirror placed in the 12 o'clock position to enable a view of the inferior angle first. The inferior quadrant is usually the widest and most pigmented, making it easier to identify the various structures.
10. In normal angles, look for the prominently discernible pigmented posterior structure, the ciliary body band, and identify the adjacent angle structures from posterior through to anterior (Figs. 7.28 and 7.29). Identify the most posterior structure observable and note any abnormal findings.
11. When the ciliary body band is less visible or is not visible at all, such as with a narrow angle, with unusual pigment patterns, or when peripheral anterior synechiae or neovascularisation obscure or distort the angle, use the *focal line technique* to identify Schwalbe's line, which is the last (most anterior) structure visible in a progressively narrow angle. Use a very bright optic section at a 20° angle with the mirror in the 12 o'clock

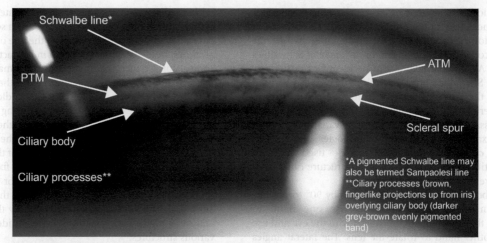

Fig. 7.28 A wide-open angle of a brown iris (Asian). There is pigment on Schwalbe's line (Sampaolesi's line); iris processes overlying the ciliary body, mild pigment in the posterior trabecular meshwork; the *reddish tinge* is blood reflux through Schlemm's canal.

*A pigmented Schwalbe line may also be termed Sampaolesi line
**Ciliary processes (brown, fingerlike projections up from iris) overlying ciliary body (darker grey-brown evenly pigmented band)

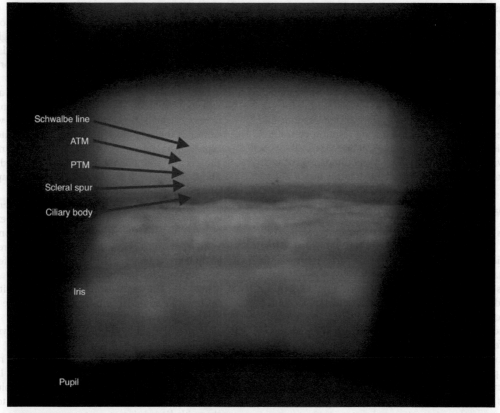

Fig. 7.29 Inferior angle (superiorly placed mirror) with a light blue iris. Note that the structures are more challenging to visualise owing to a paucity of pigmentation. The angle structures in this view are also much deeper, with wide PTM (posterior trabecular meshwork) and ATM (anterior trabecular meshwork) bands, and a challenge to view Schwalbe line. Focal line technique is used to identify Schwalbe line so that errors are not made in interpretation of the angle structures.

position. Two separate beams representing the anterior and posterior surfaces of the cornea will be observed in the domed cornea above the angle. These two beams will collapse into one beam in the angle at Schwalbe's line. All other structures can be identified posteriorly from Schwalbe's line. This technique can also be used with the thumbnail mirror in the 6 o'clock position (superior angle examination), but it is usually not necessary if you follow the structural variations through the examination of all 360° of the angle.

12. The *convex iris technique* can be used to help identify the most posterior angle structure observable before the iris inserts into the angle.

13. Use both hands and rotate the lens by 90° to observe the nasal or temporal angle. Use one hand to hold the lens to maintain contact with the eye and use the other hand to rotate the lens. The lateral angles may be more easily viewed when the slit beam is rotated horizontally.

14. Examine all quadrants (through 360°) in a systematic manner.

15. Lens removal (video 7.6): Instruct the patient to look toward the nose and blink forcefully (the strongest eyelid force is nasally), while applying digital pressure through the inferior eyelid on the temporal side of the globe to introduce air beneath the lens. A popping sound may be heard as the lens releases from the eye. Repeat with more pressure temporally if the first attempt fails to release the lens. Do not use a pulling force to remove the lens. Consider lavage of the superior and inferior cul-de-sacs with irrigating solution (or saline) if viscous, preserved coupling solution was used.

16. Always examine both eyes as relative comparison of angle structures between eyes and quadrants is important.

Corneal-type gonioscopy procedure

1. **Lens preparation:** Clean and disinfect the gonioscopy lens. Solution is not required, but a drop of saline, artificial tear, or viscous solution may improve the contact and therefore the view.

2. **Lens insertion.** Generally, the lens is applied with the handle superior or inferior temporally in a 'square' pattern, although a 'diamond' pattern is preferred by some clinicians. Advise the patient that the lens will be felt if the lids touch it, but otherwise will not be uncomfortable.

3. It is preferable to hold the lens with the left hand when examining the right eye and vice versa for the left eye. Lens stability is critical, so it is important to have good arm support.

4. Instruct the patient to hold their eyes widely and to look straight ahead (a specific target to fixate on is helpful). Pull the microscope back and bring the lens

in from the patient's temporal side. Rotate the lens quickly and directly onto the central cornea so that the flat front surface is perpendicular to the line of sight. At all times, hold the lens just barely in contact with the corneal surface such that the tear prism is maintained. Do not apply excessive pressure with the lens. A wrinkled appearance through the lens indicates that folds in Descemet's membrane are occurring owing to too much pressure on the lens. Maintain the flat lens perpendicular to the cornea to maintain the tear film seal and reposition the lens on the centre of the cornea if sliding is noted or if the patient changes fixation.

5. Position the vertical slit beam in the mirror placed in the 12 o'clock position to enable a view of the inferior angle first. The inferior quadrant is usually the widest and most pigmented, making it easier to identify the various structures.

6. In normal angles, look for the prominently discernible pigmented posterior structure, the ciliary body band, and identify the adjacent angle structures from posterior through to anterior. Identify the most posterior structure observable and note any abnormal findings.

7. When the ciliary body band is less visible or is not visible at all, such as with a narrow angle, with unusual pigment patterns, or when peripheral anterior synechiae or neovascularisation obscure or distort the angle, use the focal line technique to identify Schwalbe's line, which is the last (most anterior) structure visible in a progressively narrow angle. Use a very bright optic section at a 20° angle with the mirror in the 12 o'clock position. Two separate beams representing the anterior and posterior surfaces of the cornea will be observed in the domed cornea above the angle. These two beams will collapse into one beam in the angle at Schwalbe's line.

8. The convex iris technique can be used to identify the most posterior angle structure observable before the iris inserts into the angle and pressure gonioscopy can be used in narrow angles to ensure there are no peripheral anterior synechiae, and to differentiate appositional and synechial angle closure.

9. Rotate the slit beam horizontally and position the beam in the appropriate mirror to observe the nasal or temporal angle.

10. Examine all quadrants (through 360°) in a systematic manner.

11. Lens removal: Remove the lens by simply releasing it from contact with the cornea. No ocular lavage is required because no preserved coupling solution is used. Examine the cornea after the procedure to ensure the epithelium is intact.

12. Always examine both eyes as relative comparison of angle structures between eyes and quadrants is important.

7.5.3 Additional examination technique: the corneal compression technique

The corneal compression technique is also termed compression, pressure, or indentation gonioscopy. This technique can be used to differentiate if an observed angle closure is appositional (i.e., iris is in contact with the angle structures, but is not adherent) or synechial (i.e., the iris is physically and irreversibly adherent to the angle). Pressure is applied with the four-mirror gonioscopic lens directly on the centre of the cornea forcing aqueous into the peripheral chamber and forcing the iris posteriorly. Pressure on an eye with an appositionally closed angle will cause the iris to pull away from the angle to reveal some angle structures, whereas a synechial angle closure will remain closed.

7.5.4 Recording gonioscopy findings

Although there are several published grading systems, the suggested method is to use an anatomically descriptive recording system, thus eliminating the discrepancies and controversies that exist between grading systems. The anterior chamber angle is widest inferiorly and is most narrow superiorly, with the nasal and temporal quadrants in between. All quadrants should be inspected and graded independently. Recording of observations should include the following:

- Most posterior angle structure observed (e.g., posterior trabecular meshwork).
- Angular approach at the recess (approximation, in degrees).
- Iris contour (e.g., 'flat,' 'steep,' or 'convex' in midperipheral iris as in narrow angles; 'convex at iris root' as in plateau iris; 'convex over entire iris' as in pupillary block; or 'concave' or 'posteriorly bowed' as in pigment dispersion).

Other characteristics and pertinent negatives include:

- Amount of pigment.
- Presence of iris processes, angle recession, peripheral anterior synechiae, and normal and abnormal vasculature.
- Other findings: lens cortex material, naevi and surgical alterations such as sclerectomy and peripheral iridotomy.
- Whether or not lens tilt (convex iris technique) was required to observe the angle properly.
- To what degree the angle opens with indentation (if relevant).

Common alternate grading systems include that of Shaffer, which grades the angle by the estimate of the geometrical angle between the iris and angle wall at the recess. This system most closely correlates with the

Table 7.3 Equivalent values with the original van Herick anterior angle recording grades

van Herick grade	van Herick grade (%)
Grade 0 (closed)	Closed
Grade I (<1: ¼)	5–20
Grade II (1: ¼)	25
Grade III (1: ¼–½)	30–50
-	55–95
Grade IV (1: 1+)	100+

van Herick angle estimation method. The original van Herick grades III to IV (Table 7.3; angles 30% to over 100% of the corneal thickness) are widely open angles of 30° to 40°. In both the van Herick and Shaffer systems, angles designated grade II or 25% of the corneal thickness (20°) or less are considered capable of closure. Grade 0 angles are considered closed. The Spaeth grading system uses three criteria to describe the angle. The angle is initially described in a similar way to the Shaffer system but in degrees. The peripheral iris contour is then described as being either regular (r), steep (s), or concave (q for queer). Finally, the site of iris insertion is described anatomically (see further reading for details).

In addition to grading and describing the angle, the trabecular meshwork can be graded with respect to the degree of pigmentation. The scale is somewhat arbitrary, but convention describes 0 as no pigment, 1 as trace, 2 as mild, 3 as moderate, and 4 as dense pigment deposition. The absence of pigment (grade 0) makes the angle assessment difficult as the various structures are highlighted with pigment. The focal line technique helps to delineate the faint Schwalbe's line and therefore to help determine the most posterior structure.

7.5.5 Interpretation of gonioscopy results

It is useful to approach the angle evaluation from an anterior to posterior direction because all structures are not always present (see Figs. 7.28 and 7.29).

Schwalbe's line

Schwalbe's line is the most anterior structure of the angle and is a demarcation line marking the termination of the transparent cornea at Descemet's membrane. It is a very narrow, usually white or translucent line and is not always prominent. Sampaolesi's line is the term applied to a pigmented Schwalbe's line. It appears as pigment deposited in a wavy discontinuous fashion anterior to Schwalbe's line and is a feature of pseudoexfoliation and pigment dispersion syndromes.

Trabecular meshwork

The trabecular meshwork or trabeculum has a translucent appearance and is frequently dull grey or brown in appearance. The anterior portion of the trabecular meshwork is usually less pigmented and is considered the non-filtering portion of the meshwork. The more posterior portion of the trabecular meshwork overlies the Schlemm's canal and is more active in the drainage process. The posterior trabecular meshwork is pigmented and may accumulate pigment with age and in specific eye disease, such as pigment dispersion and pseudoexfoliation syndromes. Trauma, uveitis, and surgery are also causes of pigment deposition in the angle. It is advisable to grade the level of pigmentation in the angle, and it is usually noted that pigment deposits most heavily in the inferior quadrant. Schlemm's canal can be seen through the translucent meshwork only if blood is refluxed back into it from the venous system (see Fig. 7.29). This occurs if excess pressure is applied with the gonioscope (usually a scleral-type lens), such that the pressure in the draining veins exceeds the IOP.

Scleral spur

The scleral spur is a slight protrusion of the white sclera into the anterior chamber. The trabecular meshwork attaches anteriorly and the longitudinal muscle of the ciliary body posteriorly. The scleral spur becomes more visible when the ciliary body and trabeculum are pigmented. If the scleral spur appears unusually wide, angle recession may be present.

Ciliary body

The visible band of ciliary body, which represents the longitudinal muscle, may appear black, brown, grey, or have a mottled appearance. If visible, the angle is widely open. In lightly pigmented eyes, blood vessels can occasionally be observed running circumferentially in the ciliary body. The presence of a very wide ciliary body band along with a history of trauma may indicate angle recession. Iris processes are strands of the iris that are seen to project anteriorly onto the ciliary body or scleral spur and occasionally even more anteriorly on to the trabecular meshwork. These are found in approximately one-third of normal eyes.

Iris root

The iris root runs from the most posterior section of the iris and inserts onto the ciliary body. It can occasionally obscure the view of the ciliary body.

7.5.6 Other gonioscopic findings

Peripheral anterior synechiae are adhesions formed between the iris tissue and the trabecular meshwork or even Schwalbe's line. Their appearance is dependent on the aetiology of the adhesion, so that in angle closure it is usually found where the angle is narrowest, whereas inflammatory peripheral anterior synechiae are often located inferiorly owing to the settling of inflammatory debris. It may also be seen adjacent to surgical incisions, such as for cataract or glaucoma surgery, or in association with posteriorly located laser burns following laser trabeculoplasty.

Neovascular growth may be preceded by rubeosis iridis at the pupillary ruff; however, neovascularisation of the angle may occur without neovascularisation of the iris. Early neovascular bridging vessels across the angle can be very difficult to detect. The risk of missing neovascularisation by not performing gonioscopy in patients with central retinal vein occlusion is about 10%.[37]

7.5.7 Most common errors when using gonioscopy

1. Misinterpreting angle structures. A narrow angle is the most difficult to interpret.
2. Using the wrong amount of solution with scleral-type lenses: too little solution can cause bubbles behind the lens limiting the view of the angle, whereas too much can cause the excess solution to run onto the patient's cheek.
3. Using too much pressure with a *corneal* type lens, which indents the cornea, causing folds in Descemet's membrane as well as falsely widening the angle.

7.6 Pachymetry

Pachymetry is the measurement of the thickness of the central cornea. It has become increasingly used by optometrists in primary eye care,[38] because it allows a more accurate interpretation of IOP measurements (section 7.7.1) and is an important risk factor for which patients with ocular hypertension will develop POAG.[39]

7.6.1 The evidence base: when and how to assess central corneal thickness

Central corneal thickness (CCT) should be measured:
1. In all patients with ocular hypertension
2. When IOP is measured
3. Prior to referral for refractive surgery
4. Screening and/or monitoring corneal oedema
5. Screening and monitoring keratoconus and corneal dystrophies

Despite being the current 'gold standard' measurement of IOP, it is well known that Goldmann applanation tonometry (GAT) only provides valid measurements for corneas with near average thickness (~520 μm) and measured IOPs can be artificially high in patients with thick corneas,[40,41] and artificially low in patients with thin corneas, such as those post refractive surgery.[41] Therefore pachymetry is particularly important in patients with ocular hypertension,[40–42] and normal tension glaucoma.[43] Unfortunately, there is no simple equation between corneal thickness and GAT to provide a validated correction factor,[44,45] perhaps partly because the issue is clouded by changes in corneal rigidity, so that corneal oedema increases corneal thickness but reduces rigidity and leads to a reduced IOP measurement, whereas scarring can increase rigidity and measured IOP.[45] Whether corneal thickness is an independent risk factor for glaucoma is uncertain[46,47] and it seems likely that corneal biomechanical properties may be more associated with POAG than corneal thickness.[47] This is another area that requires careful monitoring of the literature.

Although ultrasound pachymetry is typically considered the gold standard for CCT measurement and is widely used,[45] this seems to be owing to tradition because it requires anaesthetic, is operator-dependent, and is less repeatable than several other techniques, including the Pentacam, Orbscan, and anterior segment OCT devices.[48] Many pachymetry measurements are 'point-and-shoot' type of instruments so that a description of the procedure is not provided.

7.6.2 Recording of Pachymetry results

CCT should be recorded in micrometres to the nearest 1 μm for both eyes. Given that corneal thickness measurements differ depending on the instrument used[48] and the time of day,[49] these should both be recorded. Record all measurements taken if greater than 1.

For example,

Pentacam CCT, 11.30 am, RE: 553 μm; LE: 558 μm

7.6.3 Interpretation of Pachymetry results

Central corneal thicknesses are typically similar in the two eyes, with an average of approximately 550 μm for normal, healthy eyes of most races, with averages quoted in the literature from 520 to 580 μm.[50] Average thicknesses are lower for African American and Japanese patients, and corneas are generally thinner in patients with glaucoma, but thicker in patients with ocular hypertension.[45,50] Patients with ocular hypertension and lower than average corneal thickness (<555 μm) are three times more likely to develop POAG than those with thick corneas of more than 588 μm.[39] Corneal thickness also varies depending on the instrument used,[48] and it is better to collect your own normal data or use normative data provided for your particular instrument.

7.7 Tonometry

Tonometry involves the measurement of IOP.

7.7.1 The evidence base: when and how to measure IOP

Tonometry must be performed in any patient with glaucoma or 'at risk' for glaucoma (e.g., suspicious discs, family history of glaucoma, central visual field defect, and narrow anterior angles). Although tonometry is now known to be a poor screening test for glaucoma compared with optic nerve head and visual field assessment, it identifies ocular hypertensive patients who should subsequently be monitored more closely[51] and is critical in monitoring glaucoma treatment because reducing IOP is currently the only effective approach to slowing glaucoma progression.[52]

Any patient with glaucoma or any risk factors for glaucoma should have pressures measured by Goldmann applanation tonometry, which has long been the gold standard for IOP measurements. GAT measured IOPs are only strictly valid for corneas of near average thickness of approximately 520 μm. For example, in 1978 Johnson et al reported details of a 17-year-old patient with GAT readings between 30 and 40 mmHg owing to extremely thick corneas of 900 μm whose 'real' IOP was 11 mmHg.[40] This long-known inaccuracy of GAT has come to the fore since the findings of significant IOP reductions owing to the corneal thinning induced for refractive surgery.[41] The influence of CCT on applanation IOP may lead to the classification of some normal subjects with thick corneas as ocular hypertensives (section 7.6.1). In addition, this effect could also mean that some patients diagnosed as having normal tension glaucoma using GAT may actually be patients with high IOP but a thin cornea.[43] In this regard, a clinical note reports two cases of post-LASIK patients with steroid response progressing to end-stage glaucoma, and that the late detection may have been partly caused by unreliably low IOP after surgery.[53] Attempts have been made to determine the relationship between corneal thickness and GAT to provide a validated correction factor, but there is wide disagreement among investigators.[44,45] Some reports have suggested that non-contact tonometry provides even higher IOP values than GAT in patients with thick corneas.[54,55] Most non-contact tonometers (NCTs) are now highly automated and simply involve lining up the instrument in the correct position when it will automatically take measurements. They are easier to perform than GAT, do not require corneal anaesthesia, and can be performed by trained clinical assistants. NCT results are typically less reliable than GAT, with slight differences that are model dependent.[56] You should check the literature for information regarding the model type you have. At least three readings are required to average the effects of the arterial pulse, which varies IOP by over 4 mmHg, although averaging four measurements is often recommended in professional guidelines, if not used.[57] If an NCT is used, a useful protocol can be to screen patients who do not have risk factors for glaucoma using NCT measurements taken by a clinical assistant and to repeat any measurements that are high, unequal, or increased from previous visits using GAT or Perkins. The Perkins tonometer is a portable, low magnification, hand-held version of GAT that does not require a slit-lamp and can be used on domiciliary (home) visits (Fig. 7.30).

Given GAT's inherent variability with corneal thickness, new tonometers are being developed that attempt to be less affected by corneal properties. These include rebound tonometry (which offers the possibility of home monitoring),[58] dynamic contour tonometry (which has shown much better repeatability than GAT),[59] and the ocular response analyzer. The gold standard crown of GAT may be slipping further with the finding that corneal compensated IOP measured by the ocular response analyzer, which attempts to correct IOP for the individual differences in corneal biomechanics, has been shown to better predict visual field progression than GAT.[60] This NCT also measures corneal hysteresis, the compliance of the cornea, which has been proposed as an independent risk factor for glaucoma and its progression,.[61] Once again, this is a quickly evolving area of research that needs to be monitored.

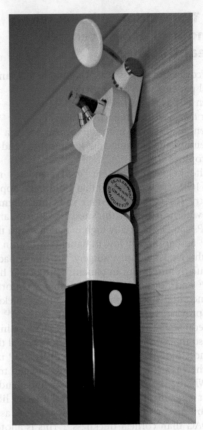

Fig. 7.30 A Perkins tonometer.

7.7.2 Procedure for GAT

(See video 7.7.)

1. Make certain that the tonometer probe tip has been appropriately disinfected. Check the integrity of the cornea for any contraindications to performing the technique.
2. Explain the test to the patient and obtain informed consent. Ask about any sensitivity to the anaesthetic. For example: "I am now going to measure the pressure in your eye, which is one of the tests for glaucoma. This involves putting a drop in your eye. Have you ever reacted badly to drops or an anaesthetic before at an optometrist's or dentist's office?"
3. Inform the patient that the drops will sting at first, but that the stinging will disappear very quickly. Instil one drop of anaesthetic or anaesthetic/fluorescein solution in both of the patient's eyes (section 7.8). You may suggest that the patient closes their eyes because this can be more comfortable. Keep a tissue handy to dab

the patient's tears subsequently. Allow approximately 30 seconds for the anaesthetic to take effect.

4. If required, add a small amount of fluorescein to both conjunctivae. Fluorets can be wet with preserved saline or another drop of the anaesthetic, although the pH of the anaesthetic will reduce the fluorescence of fluorescein. Insufficient fluorescein will result in poorly visible mires.

5. Position the patient comfortably at the slit-lamp (section 7.1.2).

6. With the fluorescein in place, check for corneal staining prior to performing tonometry. Ensure there are no conditions that would contraindicate applanation tonometry, such as a serious corneal injury (this is likely to have been identified in the case history).

7. Insert the tonometer probe into the Goldmann tonometer and align the white line on the carrier with the 0/180° degree line on the probe. Astigmatic corneas produce an error of 1 mmHg for every 4 D of corneal cylinder. To reduce this error, adjust the tonometer head to 43° from the flattest corneal meridian if the corneal cylinder is greater than 3 D. If astigmatism is with-the-rule or against-the-rule, the probe can be aligned with the red line on the probe carrier (at 43°).

8. With older instruments, GAT is a monocular technique. Position the GAT probe in front of the slit-lamp eyepiece that corresponds to your dominant eye. For example, if you are right eye dominant, insert the tonometer body into the right-hand hole on the slit-lamp tonometer plate, so that you will view the probe image through the right eyepiece.

9. Set the tonometer scale to an average setting of about 16 mmHg (1.6 g on the GAT scale), so that minimal movement of the tonometer scale is subsequently required. Use low (~10×) to moderate (~16×) magnification, turn the illumination system to 45° to 60° to the temporal side of patient, and adjust the system to the widest beam and the cobalt blue filter. You may need to increase the slit-lamp illumination.

10. Adjust the biomicroscope to align the probe with the centre of the patient's cornea.

11. Encourage the patient to blink a few times, then to stare straight ahead.

12. Bring the probe towards the cornea. Corneal contact is signalled by either a green glow on the peripheral cornea when you are looking outside the instrument or by the appearance of two green arcs when you are looking into the eyepiece.

13. At first contact, two green hemispherical pools of fluorescein may be seen. These are caused by the tears filling in the gap between the cornea and the tonometer probe. If these are seen, move the probe very slightly

further forward to applanate the cornea. The probe and its arm will then be seen to move backwards.

14. Determine whether you have the correct amount of fluorescein by assessing the diameter of the green arcs. Their thickness should be about one-tenth the size of the diameter of the arcs (Fig. 7.31). If the arcs are too thin, there is insufficient fluorescein and more should be instilled. If the arcs are too thick, a tear meniscus has formed around the outside of the probe and you should attempt to remove excess tears from the eye and probe using a tissue. This is a common problem in patients with a large tear volume.

15. If both the arcs can be seen, but are not correctly positioned (see Fig. 7.31), move the probe while still in contact with the cornea until the two green arcs are of equal size above and below the horizontal line of the probe beam splitter and are centred in your view (see Fig. 7.31). Always move the probe towards the larger ring. If only one (or neither) arc can be seen, remove the tonometer tip from corneal contact to make small adjustments to the position of the tonometer probe until both arcs can be seen.

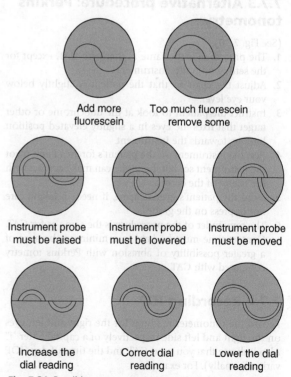

Fig. 7.31 Possible appearances seen with Goldmann applanation tonometry.

16. Some clinicians gently hold the superior eyelid with the forefinger and lower lid with the thumb to ensure the eyelids do not touch the probe. Do not put pressure on the patient's globe as this will artificially increase the IOP.
17. Adjust the tonometer scale until the inner edges of the green arcs are just touching, then remove the probe from the patient's eye. If a pulsation is perceived, adjust the scale such that the pulse centres on the correct alignment pattern.
18. Take the tonometry reading. The dial is calibrated in grams, with each gram being equivalent to 10 mmHg, so that a reading of 1.6 g indicates an IOP of 16 mmHg.
19. Examine the cornea for unintentional damage. Examine the depth of any abrasion using an optical section technique. Deep and/or extensive abrasions made by novices may need analgesic or other treatment and should be monitored.
20. Inform the patient not to rub their eyes and to avoid dusty or windy environments for at least half an hour because of the anaesthetised cornea. Contact lens wearers must be warned not to wear their contact lenses for at least the same time period.
21. Disinfect the probe.

7.7.3 Alternative procedure: Perkins tonometry

(See Fig. 7.30)
1. The procedure is the same as that with GAT, except for the setting up of the instrument
2. Adjust the chair so that the patient is slightly below your eye level.
3. Instruct the patient to look at the duochrome or other target that fixes the eyes in a slightly elevated position looking towards the instrument.
4. Rest the instrument on the patient's forehead and pivot the instrument so that the probe can make contact with the centre of the cornea.
5. Hold the patient's eyelids apart, if needed, taking care not to press on the globe.
6. The remainder of the procedure is the same as for GAT. Contact time must be kept to a minimum because of a greater possibility of abrasion with Perkins tometry compared with GAT.

7.7.4 Recording IOP

Record the tonometer readings for the right and left eyes on the right and left side respectively of a capital letter 'T'. Also indicate that you used GAT and the time of day (IOP varies diurnally). For example:

$_{15}T_{16}$ – GAT – 11:30 am.; $_{18}T_{16}$ – Perkins – 2:30 pm

With NCTs and rebound tonometry, it is best to record all 3 to 4 tonometer readings. For example:

$_{15,16,17,15}T_{16,14,17,\ 18}$ – NCT – 11.: am

Corneal compensated IOP is recorded as: IOP_{cc} – $_{15,16,17,15}T_{16,14,17,\ 18}$

7.7.5 Interpretation of IOP results

The range of normal GAT IOPs is from 10 to 21 mmHg (mean of ~ 15.5 mmHg). However, note that GAT readings are influenced by CCT[41,44] and provide a significant underestimation with corneal epithelial oedema.[41] Various systemic drugs can alter IOP, including systemic and topical steroid use that can significantly raise IOP in steroid 'responders' and beta-adrenergic blockers that can lower IOP. IOPs below 7 mmHg may suggest conditions such as retinal detachment, uveitis, or wound leak. IOPs above 20 mmHg indicate ocular hypertension and may suggest glaucoma. However, note that patients can have POAG and have a normal IOP below 21 mmHg. The difference in IOP between the two eyes should not exceed 4 mmHg. IOPs vary diurnally, with the highest IOP generally measured in the mornings. If a patient suspected of having glaucoma has a normal IOP in the afternoon, ask the patient to return on another day in the early morning, so that IOPs can be remeasured at that time.

7.7.6 Most common errors when measuring IOP

1. Obtaining high IOPs because of patient apprehension. Describing the procedure to the patient in non-threatening terms can help.
2. Taking a reading when a tear meniscus has formed around the GAT probe leading to tonometer arcs that are too thick and an invalid, high-pressure measurement.
3. Not explaining the NCT procedure and demonstrating it to the patient, so that he or she is unnecessarily startled.
4. Not repeating NCT measurements four times on each eye.[57]

7.8 Instillation of diagnostic drugs

The three major types of diagnostic drugs available to many optometrists are anaesthetics, cycloplegics, and mydriatics. Staining agents are discussed in section 7.2.

7.8.1 The evidence base: when and how to instil diagnostic drugs

The advantages to be gained by using anaesthetics, cycloplegics, and mydriatic outweigh the possible adverse ocular and systemic effects that rarely occur if appropriate drug choices are made and recommended precautions taken. For example, in a systematic review of published research between 1933 and1999, Pandit and Taylor concluded that the risk of inducing acute glaucoma following mydriasis with tropicamide alone is close to zero, and the risk with long-acting or combined agents is between 1 in 3380 and 1 in 20,000.[30] Mydriasis with tropicamide alone is safe in patients with POAG and the risk is low (0.6%) even in suspected acute angle closure.[62]

Adverse reactions to two drops of cyclopentolate 1% are common, particularly in younger children (<6 years) and those with a low body mass index; they include drowsiness, excitation, and hyperactivity and behavioural changes.[63] One drop of 1% cyclopentolate is much preferred because it leads to less adverse reactions.[63] Adverse reactions to tropicamide are rare.[63]

7.8.2 Procedure for obtaining informed consent

1. Using lay terms, inform the patient about the technique you wish to use and the rationale for doing so.
2. Inform the patient whether the drops will sting, how long any side effects (e.g., near blur and photosensitivity with mydriatics) will last, and the chances of an adverse reaction.
3. If you wish to use a mydriatic or cycloplegic, ask the patient whether they are going to operate heavy machinery, drive, or perform a similar activity requiring good vision following the eye examination. Ideally patients should be informed not to drive after the examination if possible. If pupillary dilation is likely, it is good practice to advise patients to bring a driver with them or use alternative transport to the practice. Indeed, if pupillary dilation is routine, this advice can be provided to patients when they make the appointment and printed on their appointment card. If driving is their only option for transport home, allow sufficient time for them to adapt to a dilated pupillary state and recommend that they drive only on familiar roads. Commercially available paper sunglasses or attachments could be provided if it is sunny. If the patient has to operate heavy machinery or perform a similar possibly dangerous task, make another appointment for them when they can have their pupils dilated.

7.8.3 Safety checks

1. Case history/case history notes. If the following information is not included in your initial case history notes, make sure you ask about them prior to instillation of the drops.
   (a) Does the patient report symptoms suggestive of angle closure?
   (b) Does the patient have any systemic or ocular disease that could be aggravated by the use of a diagnostic drug? For example, patients with angle closure glaucoma, with or without surgical or laser treatment, should have their pupils dilated with caution.
   (c) Does the patient have a systemic condition that could be aggravated by the instillation of a diagnostic drug? For example, one case highlighted the need to avoid hyperextending the neck of a child with Down syndrome when instilling drops to prevent spinal cord injury.[64]
   (d) Has the patient been given similar drops before and did they have a reaction to them?
2. Visual acuity. Make sure that you record distance visual acuity before any procedure is carried out on the patient. If you have not already measured visual acuity, make sure that it is measured prior to instillation of the drops.
3. Anterior angle assessment. You should estimate the size of the anterior chamber angle before using any drug that has mydriatic effects (section 7.5). Do not use miotics after mydriasis because it is generally unnecessary and pilocarpine can even cause angle closure by producing a mid-dilated pupil. As indicated previously, the risk of inducing acute angle glaucoma using a mydriatic is very low. Indeed, some clinicians take the view that it is better for patients to have a mydriatic-induced angle closure in their office/practice, where appropriate treatment can be provided, than in the patient's home. In situations where you dilate a pupil of a patient 'at risk' of angle closure, make sure that you obtain informed consent, and be prepared to manage any subsequent angle closure. Angle closure is even less likely to occur with mydriasis owing to a cycloplegic, because cycloplegia is generally used on a much younger population than mydriatics.
4. Slit-lamp examination. Prior to mydriatic instillation, check for contraindications, such as synechiae, subluxated crystalline lens, dislocated intraocular lens implant, exfoliation, or pigmentary glaucoma. If any of these conditions are found, avoid mydriasis if possible or proceed with great caution. Determine the integrity of the cornea before any drops are instilled and after any procedure involving the cornea, such as contact tonometry or gonioscopy.

5. Tonometry. Assess IOP prior to the instillation of mydriatics/cycloplegics. Some exceptions include when instilling a cycloplegic in infants and very young children for refractive error assessment.

7.8.4 Choosing the appropriate drug and dosage

1. Case history/case history notes. If the following information is not included in your initial case history notes, make sure you ask about them to help you choose the appropriate drug and dosage.
   (a) Does the patient have any systemic or ocular disease that could be aggravated by the use of a diagnostic drug? For example, phenylephrine 10% should not be used in those patients with severe cardiac disease, systemic hypertension and hypotension, insulin-dependent diabetes, aneurysms, or advanced arteriosclerosis. Phenylephrine 2.5% should only be used with great caution in these patients. There have also been reports of similar problems after the use of hydroxyamphetamine hydrochloride 0.25% used in combination with tropicamide 0.25%.[65]
   (b) Does the patient have any systemic or ocular disease that could have an influence on the choice of a diagnostic drug? For example, it is often difficult to obtain satisfactory mydriasis in patients with diabetes and they may require additional mydriatic drops and/or a combination of mydriatic drops (tropicamide 0.5% or 1% plus phenylephrine 2.5%). Patients with kidney disease can have unusually slow detoxification and elimination of ocular diagnostic drugs systemically absorbed, and care should be given to use the lowest necessary dosage of the drug. Conversely, note that patients with a compromised corneal epithelium can have enhanced penetration of a diagnostic drug.
   (c) Is the patient taking systemic medication that could interact with a diagnostic drug? For example, phenylephrine should not be used if the patient is taking monoamine oxidase inhibitors or tricyclic antidepressants.
   (d) There is a general lack of information on the use of specific drugs in women who are pregnant or breastfeeding. However, diagnostic drugs, including topical ophthalmic dyes, anaesthetics, and mydriatics, are generally considered safe as long as standard cautions, warnings, and contraindications are considered.
   (e) Has the patient had an allergic reaction to eye drops previously?
2. Iris colour. In general, patients with lighter irides will respond quicker and to a greater degree than those patients with dark irides. Therefore, give a higher drug dosage to a patient with dark irides and/or use a combination drug approach.
3. The drug(s) and dosage (concentration and number of drops) will depend on the procedure you are going to perform. Some clinicians choose to use a combination drug routinely and other clinicians use this approach when greater dilation is required, such as when using head-band binocular indirect ophthalmoscopy (BIO). This is achieved either with a drop of two drugs, such as one drop of phenylephrine and one drop of tropicamide, or the use of a combination drop that contains both of these agents (the availability of different concentrations varies).
4. Instilling a topical ocular anaesthetic prior to the use of a mydriatic or cycloplegic agent (one may have been used for contact tonometry) results in an enhanced mydriatic/cycloplegic effect. The anaesthetic, as well as reducing possible discomfort, can reduce lacrimation and thus reduce drug washout for subsequently instilled drugs. It has also been suggested that the mildly toxic effects of a topical anaesthetic on the cornea opens up the intracellular spaces and aids penetration of other drugs.
5. When using cycloplegics in young children, be particularly careful if the child is small and/or thin for their age (section 4.12.1).[63]
6. In all cases, choose the drug with the least possible adverse effects and the lowest concentration that will allow you to efficiently attain the cycloplegia (section 4.12.1) or mydriasis that you require.

7.8.5 Checks prior to instillation

1. Ensure that you have performed all the procedures prior to instillation of the diagnostic drug that would not be possible after it has been instilled. For example, make sure that you assess pupil reflexes, near muscle balance, and accommodation prior to using a cycloplegic and tonometry prior to a mydriatic.
2. Carefully identify any drops before instillation by checking the brand name, ingredients, and expiry date (Fig. 7.32) and check for discoloration and precipitates. If the expiry date has passed, or if there are precipitates, discoloration, or other signs of contamination, the suspect container should be discarded and a new one obtained.
3. Before the installation, record the drug type (preferably by its brand name) and dosage (concentration and number of drops used in each eye), the batch number, and expiry date. The use of the brand name is useful because it uniquely identifies the particular preparation that has been used (see Fig. 7.32). Different brands may well have different preservatives or other non-active ingredients.

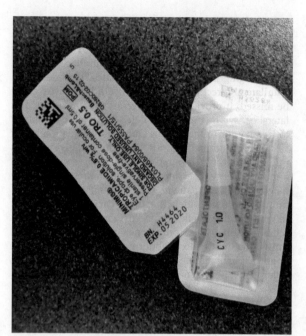

Fig. 7.32 Minims of cyclopentolate 1% and tropicamide 0.5%; note the expiry date and batch number.

4. Recheck the container of the diagnostic drug for its identity and remove the cap in preparation for drug instillation. If a dropper bottle is being used, do not place the dropper cap on any surface in such a way as to risk contaminating the inside of the bottle cap. It is best if you hold it in your hand.

7.8.6 Drug instillation procedure

▶ (See video 7.8.)

1. The patient should be seated in a fixed chair with a proper back support and arm rests. There is a chance that on installation, the patient (especially a child) will abruptly move. Therefore, do not use a stool or a chair on casters.
2. Ask the patient to tilt their head backwards with the chin raised slightly.
3. Gently pull down the lower eyelid or pull it forwards slightly to form a pouch.
4. Instil a drop or drops into the temporal side of the pouch. Avoid touching the eyelashes, eyelids, or conjunctiva with the dropper tip. Gently release the lower eyelid.
5. In the case of ointment, gently squeeze a 1.5 cm ribbon of ointment inside the lower fornix.
6. Ask the patient to look downwards and gently release the upper eyelid over the eye.

7. Press firmly over the lacrimal sac (just medial to the inner canthus) for at least 10 seconds. Nasolacrimal occlusion prevents any excess drug entering the nasolacrimal duct, keeping systemic absorption to a minimum. Nasolacrimal occlusion is not required when an ointment is used. Make sure that you wipe any excess drops/ointment away from the eye with a tissue.
8. If two drops are to be used, wait at least 3 minutes between drops. Instilling two drops consecutively without this wait overfills the lacrimal lake and negates the theoretical effect of applying more drug.

7.8.7 Post drug instillation procedure

1. Return the cap to the bottle (and screw it on securely) or dispose of single dose products such as Minims.
2. Anaesthetics: Inform the patient not to rub their eyes and avoid dusty or windy environments for at least half an hour after use of an anaesthetic. Contact lens wearers must be warned not to wear their contact lenses for at least the same time period.
3. Mydriasis: Measure IOP post mydriasis for patients at risk of angle closure. A rise of more than 5 mmHg should be monitored until it returns to normal levels.
4. Provide commercially available paper sunglasses or attachments after mydriasis, when necessary, to avoid photophobia.
5. Use appropriate follow-up procedures and/or emergency care should any untoward reactions or sequelae occur. All these drugs (with the exception of tropicamide, for which no serious adverse effects have been recorded) can give rise to systemic effects, such as altered mental states and increased heart rates.[63] Patients may also faint. Note that an unwanted reaction, such as a rise in IOP owing to pupil block post mydriasis, can develop some hours later, and 'at risk' patients should be told who to contact in case of an emergency.

7.8.8 Recording drug instillation

Record the drug used, the number of drops and the dosage, the drug batch number (BN) and expiry date, and the time of instillation.

For example:

> 9.30 am: 2 drops 0.5% tropicamide, BN 54321, expiry 11/2023

7.8.9 Most common errors when instilling drugs

1. Instilling two drops consecutively without waiting for 3 minutes after the first drop.

2. Not checking drops carefully enough before instillation by forgetting to check the brand name, ingredients, and/or expiry date and/or not checking for discoloration and precipitates.

7.9 Pupil light reflexes

7.9.1 The evidence base: when and how to assess pupillary function

Evaluation of pupillary function provides valuable information about the integrity and function of the iris, optic nerve, posterior visual pathways, and the third and sympathetic nerves to the eye; some of the conditions that cause pupil reflex abnormalities are life threatening. For these reasons, the assessment of pupil reflexes is a standard part of a primary eye care examination. Afferent pupillary defects are caused by lesions in the 'front end' of the pupillary light reflex pathway and most commonly by lesions in the retina and optic nerve. The afferent pupillary pathways leave the visual pathways in the last third of the optic tracts to reach the pretectal nuclei (Fig. 7.33). Afferent pupillary defects do not cause anisocoria (different pupil sizes), but may produce abnormal pupillary light reflexes. Efferent pupillary defects produce anisocoria, which are caused by lesions to the motor neurone system, which carries signals from the central nervous system to the iris via the 3rd cranial nerve.

Pupil size should be assessed in both bright and dim illumination to investigate any anisocoria. Observing the

pupil reflexes as a light is shone into an eye (the direct reflex) and the fellow eye (consensual reflex) can indicate abnormalities affecting the afferent or efferent neurological pathways responsible for pupillary function. The swinging flashlight test accentuates small defects in a unilateral direct pupil reflex that could otherwise easily be missed. It provides a sensitive assessment of any unilateral or asymmetric afferent defects, and has been shown to be superior to the Marcus Gunn test (redilation under sustained illumination) for detecting relative afferent pupillary defects.[66] Infrared video pupillography provides a more accurate assessment of relative afferent pupillary defect (RAPD) in patients with asymmetric glaucoma,[67] but it is not used widely in clinics. There is no condition in which the near reflex is defective or lost when the light reflex is normal. Therefore, the near reflex need be checked only if the light reflex is abnormal. Patients can show an abnormal light and near pupil reflex or an abnormal light reflex with a normal near reflex (light-near dissociation).

7.9.2 Procedure for pupil assessment

(See video 7.9.)
1. Ask the patient to take off their glasses and look at a letter on the distance visual acuity chart that both eyes can see easily. If the worst monocular visual acuity is less than about 6/18 (20/60), ask the patient to look at a spot of light on the distance chart.
2. Sit in front and to the side of the patient, so that you can easily observe the patient's pupils, but you are not obscuring fixation of the target.
3. Keep the room lights on and check the size, shape, and location of both pupils. Compare the size of both pupils carefully. You can estimate the size of the pupil using the iris as an approximate 12 mm reference scale (Fig. 7.34).
4. If the pupil sizes are unequal in bright light conditions, measure the pupil sizes with a millimetre ruler or a hemisphere scale. In addition, dim the room lights but keep the light levels high enough so that you can clearly see the patient's pupils, and measure the size of the patient's pupils again. An ultraviolet lamp can be used with patients with dark irides as the lens fluoresces to allow pupil sizes to be measured.
5. Direct and consensual light reflexes:
   (a) Ask the patient to remain fixating a letter or spotlight on the distance chart.
   (b) Shine a penlight or transilluminator into the right pupil from the inferior temporal side from a distance of 5 to 10 cm. Observe the extent and speed of constriction of the right pupil (direct light reflex) and left pupil (consensual reflex). Remove the light and observe the direct and consensual dilation. Check this several times because dramatic fatigue

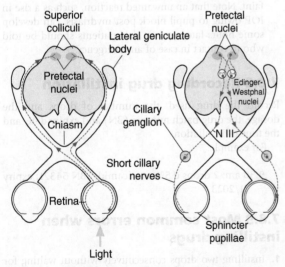

Fig. 7.33 The pupillary reflex pathway.

Labels: Superior colliculi, Lateral geniculate body, Pretectal nuclei, Pretectal nuclei, Edinger-Westphal nuclei, Chiasm, Cillary ganglion, N III, Short cillary nerves, Retina, Sphincter pupillae, Light

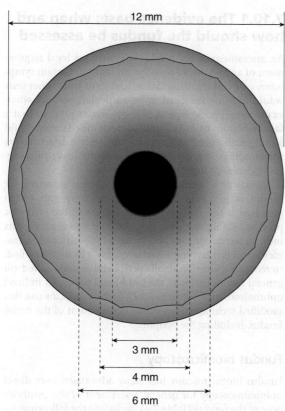

12 mm

3 mm

4 mm

6 mm

Fig. 7.34 The size of the pupil can be estimated using the iris as a 12 mm reference scale.

can occur in an abnormal eye that at first shows a normal response.

(c) Shine the light into the left pupil from the inferior temporal side from a distance of 5 to 10 cm. Observe the extent and speed of constriction of the left pupil (direct light reflex) and right pupil (consensual reflex). Remove the light and observe the direct and consensual dilation. Check this several times.

6. Swinging flashlight test:
   (a) Ask the patient to remain fixating a letter or spotlight on the distance chart.
   (b) Shine a penlight or direct ophthalmoscope into the right eye from below the patient's eyes from a distance of 5 to 10 cm. Pause for 2 to 3 seconds and then quickly switch the light to shine into the left eye.
   (c) Repeatedly alternate between the two eyes, pausing for 2 to 3 seconds on each eye, and look for any change in pupil size as the light is alternated.
   (d) A normal response is that both pupils will constrict as the penlight is shone in one eye. Moving to the other eye will maintain the constriction. A slight hippus or bilateral dilation is normal.

(e) An eye with an RAPD will dilate as the light is turned upon it from the good eye. The direct response is less than the consensual response so both eyes will dilate. This takes a few seconds to observe.
(f) The RAPD can be quantified by adding successively increasing neutral density filters to the 'good' eye, until a normal swinging flashlight response is seen.

7. Near reflex: This need be measured only if the light responses are abnormal or sluggish.
   (a) Ask the patient to remain fixating a letter or spotlight on the distance chart.
   (b) Ask the patient to then look at a target, such as the patient's own thumb, about 15 cm from his or her eyes.
   (c) Observe the extent and speed of pupillary constriction as the patient changes fixation from distance to near.
   (d) Ask the patient to look back at the distance target and observe the dilation as this occurs.

7.9.3 Recording of pupil size and reflexes

Pupil shape and size: Record any irregularity in pupil shape and any anisocoria.

Pupil reflexes: A 0 to 4+ grading system can be used for direct (D) and consensual (C) reflexes where 0 indicates no pupil response, 1+ (or +) indicates a very small, just visible response, 2+ (++) indicates a small, slow response, 3+ (+++) indicates a moderate response, and 4+ (++++) indicates a brisk, large response typical of a healthy young patient. An alternative is to use the acronym PERRL (Pupils Equal Round and Respond to Light), but this does not differentiate between a just visible response and a large, brisk one. If the light reflex is abnormal, the near reflex must be checked. Some disorders produce an absent light reflex with a normal near reflex (light-near dissociation).

Also record the result of the swinging flashlight test as +ve RAPD (if a RAPD is indicated) or –ve RAPD (this indicates that there is no problem). If +ve RAPD is found, record which side was defective. If the defect is quantified using a neutral density filter, indicate the filter density in log units.

Examples:

RE 6, LE 6. D and C 4+ R and L, –ve RAPD
OD 4, OS 4. D and C 3+ OD and OS, –ve RAPD
RE 5, LE 5. PERRL, –ve RAPD
OD 4, OS 4. PERRL, +ve RAPD OS, 0.3 ND filter

7.9.4 Interpretation of pupil size and reflexes

Pupils are normally equal in size and typically vary from 3 to 6 mm in diameter in bright light to about 4 to 8 mm in dim light and show slight physiological fluctuations in size or hippus. The pupil gets smaller with age. Physiological anisocoria is seen in about 20% of normal patients and is generally the same in dim and bright illumination, usually small (<1 mm), shows normal pupil reflexes, and has been present for years. If the diagnosis is in any doubt, this can be checked by asking the patient to bring in some old close-up photographs of themselves looking straight ahead. Pathological anisocoria is caused by an abnormality in the efferent or motor pupil pathway. Anisocoria that is greatest in bright light will generally show an abnormal direct and consensual light reflex. This indicates a problem in the motor leg of the light reflex pathway, such as in the third nerve, ciliary ganglion (including Adie's tonic pupil), or iris, or could be drug induced.

An abnormal direct light response in a pupil capable of a normal consensual response indicates an afferent (visual pathway) defect. There is generally no anisocoria. The swinging flashlight provides a more sensitive assessment of any unilateral or asymmetric afferent defects. It compares each eye's direct response (reflecting the normality of its visual pathway) with its consensual response (reflecting the normality of the other eye's visual pathway). Symmetrical afferent defects do not show a positive RAPD. Some normal subjects may show a persistent but small RAPD in the absence of detectable pathologic disease. Therefore, an isolated RAPD in the range of 0.3 log unit that is not associated with any other significant historical or clinical finding should probably be considered benign.[68] Similarly, patients with unilateral cataract may show a RAPD in the non-cataractous eye that is not reflective of visual pathway disease.[69]

7.9.5 Most common errors when assessing pupils

1. Using too slow a swing in the swinging flashlight test.
2. Using too low a light level to observe the contralateral eye, especially with a darkly pigmented iris.
3. Blocking the patient's view of the visual acuity chart and stimulating accommodation and subsequent pupil constriction.
4. Forgetting to check pupil reflexes prior to instilling a mydriatic or cycloplegic.

7.10 Fundus examination, particularly the posterior pole

Ophthalmoscopy revolutionised eye examinations by allowing observation of the ocular fundus and replacing the diagnosis of 'amaurosis' (an outwardly healthy eye with poor vision) with a multitude of others for which an aetiology and treatment could be sought.

7.10.1 The evidence base: when and how should the fundus be assessed

An assessment of the fundus is typically a legal requirement of any primary eye care examination. Certain symptoms, case history information, and signs from other tests would indicate the need to be particularly careful when examining specific aspects of the posterior pole, so that a family history of POAG and/or other risk factors would highlight the need to assess the optic nerve head and its surroundings in great detail, visual acuity loss could suggest macular changes/disease, and so on.

Stereoscopic techniques are the clinical standard for fundus examination. Fundus biomicroscopy with a high plus lens is the standard for assessment of the posterior pole, including the disc, macula, and vasculature. This indirect technique may also be used for peripheral assessment, and is often employed to enable a more magnified, stereoscopic view of small, peripheral lesions noted on general assessment with the head-band binocular indirect ophthalmoscope (section 7.12). Some clinicians use this modified technique for routine examination of the entire fundus, including the periphery.

Fundus biomicroscopy

Fundus biomicroscopy has many advantages over direct ophthalmoscopy for general assessment of the posterior pole of the fundus (Table 7.4), including the following:

- Stereoscopic viewing is possible through dilated and undilated pupils. The neuroretinal rim (NRR) tissue and the cup-to-disc ratio cannot be evaluated properly without stereoscopic observation of the depression of the cup in relation to the disc structure. Often the depression of the cup extends beyond the area of pallor, which is very difficult to detect without observing the disc stereoscopically.[70] In addition, non-stereoscopic assessment cannot consistently or accurately determine the presence of more subtle elevations, such as oedema of the retina or macula.[71]
- A larger field of view is available compared with direct ophthalmoscopy, even through an undilated pupil.
- The technique is dynamic and all parts of the fundus can be viewed with only minor cooperation from the patient.
- A superior view is obtained through media opacities as compared with direct ophthalmoscopy and this is particularly useful to assess the fundi behind cataract.
- Varied lens diameters and powers are available (see Table 7.4). The SuperField lens is probably the lens of first choice. The Super66 stereo, the older +78 D, and other lower-powered lenses allow more

Table 7.4 Optical and observational characteristics of various fundus examination techniques

Method	Image	Stereopsis?	Diameter (approx.) (mm)	Image mag.[a]	Mag. in slit-lamp (16 ×)	Static field of view[a]	Extent of fundus visible[c]
Direct ophthalmoscope	Erect	No	N/A	15×[‡]		~5°[‡]	To equator
Monocular indirect	Erect	No	N/A	5×		~12°	Beyond equator
SuperPupil™	Reversed and inverted	Yes. Detail in stereopsis improves with lower power (higher magnification); best with 'Super' series	15	0.45×	7×	Variable (generally higher with higher powered lenses)	Beyond equator (generally facilitated with higher powered lenses)
Super VitreoFundus™			25	0.57×	9×		
SuperField™			30.2	0.76×	12×		
Super66 Stereo Fundus Lens™			35	1.0×	15×		
+90 D			19	0.76×	12×		
+78 D			29	0.93×	14×		
+60 D			30	1.15×	18×		
BIO, +20 D	Reversed and inverted	Yes	48	3×	–	~45°	Entire retinal surface
Fundus contact lens	Reversed	Yes	–	Variable	Variable	–	Entire retinal surface

[a]Various manufacturers' claims.
[b]Through a dilated pupil, with direction of patient fixation to regions to be viewed and with manipulation of the slit-lamp.
[c]Varies with refractive error.
BIO, Binocular indirect ophthalmoscopy.

magnification and better stereopsis for viewing details of the optic nerve, macula, and specific lesions. They can all be used with an undilated pupil with practice. The SuperPupil, the older +90 D, and other smaller, higher-powered lenses can facilitate examination when the pupil is undilated or otherwise small. The SuperPupil XL provides a wider field of view for examination of the peripheral retina.

- Variable magnification settings on the slit-lamp allow for varied viewing conditions with the same lens, and a very wide range of magnification options when various lenses are employed.
- The view is relatively independent of ametropia. This is particularly useful in moderate to high myopia, where the high magnification when using direct ophthalmoscopy can limit the field of view substantially. A better estimate of optic disc size can also be obtained. The slit-lamp beam height can be used to increase the accuracy of disc size estimates when used with appropriate magnification factors.[72]

- A red-free filter and various magnification settings facilitate the assessment of the retinal nerve fibre layer (RNFL).[72]
- A yellow filter attachment facilitates examination of individuals who are photosensitive. Clinicians have varied opinions on whether or not to use a yellow filter as some find the colour rendering properties of the filtered lenses unacceptable and question the necessity in a routine, quick assessment. Students first learning the technique, however, should use a yellow filter to reduce the discomfort and exposure of their subjects.[73]

These advantages outweigh the mild inconvenience of the aerial inverted and reversed image, the interpretation of which is soon learned.

Digital fundus cameras

Digital imaging allows immediate viewing (meaning that a repeat photograph can be taken if necessary) and the

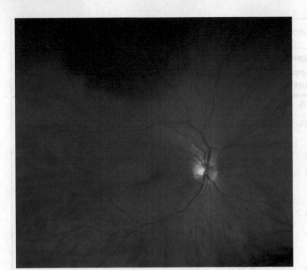

Fig. 7.35 An optomap image of a choroidal naevus; the image can be shown to the patient and an explanation of what it is ('an eye freckle') and the need to monitor it (the very rare chance it may become malignant) can be provided.

ability to analyse, archive, and longitudinally compare images. The images can be shown to patients to provide enhanced patient counselling (section 2.4; Fig. 7.35). Computer manipulation allows for the easy enhancement of images and automated measurements of diagnostic features within images. Some devices allow a colour fundus image to be captured concurrently with an OCT image of the fundus, allowing easy comparison (section 7.11). Finally, transmission of digital images through computer networks introduces the possibility of 'teleophthalmology' referrals from primary eye care, where the secondary eye care clinician is remote from the patient.[74] Over-reliance on imaging must be avoided as the consequences of the Honey Rose case tragically illustrates (section 1.6)

Direct ophthalmoscopy

Direct ophthalmoscopy has the advantages of being a simple technique to perform, providing an erect view of the fundus with moderate to high magnification ($15\times$ with an emmetrope) and can easily be performed with the patient sitting upright. It uses a hand-held instrument that is easily portable. It can be useful for domiciliary (home) visits and when it is not possible to use a table or hand-held slit-lamp. Several disadvantages are described in the previous 'Fundus biomicroscopy' section and it also requires a very close working distance, which some patients find unsettling (students need to learn to overcome the natural avoidance of invading a patient's 'personal space') and if the examiner or patient is ill it may be necessary for the examiner

to wear a surgical mask to prevent the spread of infection. Finally, the bending required can lead to strain injury to the back of the examiner over the long term.[75]

Monocular indirect ophthalmoscopy

Monocular indirect ophthalmoscopy is typically used to provide an assessment of the retina without the necessity of pupil dilation, so that its use was higher in the past when fewer countries allowed optometrists to use mydriatic drugs. It is still used in patients where pupil dilation is not possible or advisable, patients who are not tolerant of the brighter light of a binocular technique, young children and special populations (because of the farther proximity from the patient), and basic screenings. It has also been used, instead of direct ophthalmoscopy, by clinicians who are essentially monocular and cannot use their weaker eye with the direct ophthalmoscope. In reality they are monocular indirect ophthalmoscopes (MIO) that provide an erect view of the fundus. The field of view is close to 25° versus the typical direct ophthalmoscope field of view of 5° and the magnification is similar to that of a direct ophthalmoscope at $15\times$. Although the MIO provides a good view of the majority of the posterior pole, the view of the peripheral fundus and macula is limited.

7.10.2 Fundus biomicroscopy procedure

(See summary in Box 7.2 and video 7.10.)

Box 7.2 **Summary of fundus biomicroscopy procedure**

1. Dilate the patient's pupils (if required and unless contraindicated).
2. Prepare the slit-lamp biomicroscope and clean your lens.
3. Place the illumination system in line with the eyepieces, use a parallelepiped and set the magnification low (~$10\times$). Direct patient fixation.
4. Introduce the lens, ensuring that the light enters the pupil through the lens.
5. Look through the biomicroscope and pull the joystick straight back, first noticing the lens itself in focus, then the red reflex of the retina also coming into focus.
6. Increase the magnification and broaden the illumination, as required.
7. Evaluate the optic nerve head and its immediate surroundings.
8. Systematically examine the rest of the posterior pole while maintaining lens stability.
9. Examine the light-sensitive macula last.
10. Examine the posterior vitreous by pulling even farther back on the joystick.

The fundus biomicroscopy procedure is the same in undilated or dilated pupils. Maintaining a stable, binocular image is easier when the pupil is larger, but with practice, the ability to maintain excellent views through a small pupil improves.

1. Explain the test to the patient: "I am going to examine the health of the inside of your eyes with a microscope and a lens held close to your eye. The light will be bright, so please let me know if you would like a break." If dilation of the patient's pupils is required, obtain informed consent and use an appropriate mydriatic (section 7.8).

2. Set the slit-lamp biomicroscope up for yourself and your patient if this has not already been done and ask them to remove any glasses. Choose an appropriately powered lens for the type of examination required and make sure that it is clean.

3. Place the illumination system in line with the eyepieces of the biomicroscope (0° displacement). Use a parallelepiped of moderate width, moderate height, and low to medium intensity. Set the magnification to low (~ 10×), and dim or turn off the room lights. If you are examining the patient's right eye, ask the patient to look at your right ear (left ear when examining the left eye) or look in a general straight-ahead direction if the patient is visually impaired.

4. Look through the biomicroscope and reduce the height of the slit to the size of the pupil.

5. Either rest your elbow on the slit-lamp table (or on the lens holder placed on the table) or hook your little finger over the forehead rest of the biomicroscope to take the strain off your arm. Holding the lens manually offers more flexibility in manipulation of the lens, and therefore the view, than using one of the available lens mounts.

6. Hold the lens with your thumb and first or second finger. Generally, use your left hand for examination of the patient's right eye and vice versa. The lens should be oriented with the back of the lens facing the patient (i.e., the V of 'Volk' points towards the patient).

7. Introduce the lens into the light path, within 5 mm of the patient's cornea. The optimum lens-to-cornea distance is greater for lower plus lenses (range 5 to 11 mm); however, being closer and pulling away slightly from the patient is preferred to being too far from the eye where the pupil stop prevents a stereoscopic view and reduces the field of view. Make sure that the light enters the pupil through the lens. Rest your other fingers on the patient's cheek and/or bridge of the nose and brow to help stabilise the lens.

8. Once you see the light enter the pupil and the lens is stable, look again through the biomicroscope and pull the biomicroscope joystick straight back. As the slit-lamp is being pulled back, the surface of the lens itself will first come into focus, then the blurred red reflex of the retina should be seen. While maintaining lens stability, continue to pull back until the fundus structures come into focus. The extent of this movement varies with the power of the condensing lens. The lower dioptric powered lenses will create an image farther from the patient's face so the biomicroscope must be pulled back more than with higher powered lenses. Novices must learn *not* to move the lens back at the same time as the slit-lamp is pulled back.

9. Increase the magnification and broaden the illumination, as required. Reflections can be reduced by tilting the lens and/or tilting the illumination system.

10. Encourage the patient to blink normally throughout the procedure, but to hold their eyes open wide between blinks. Make sure the eye not being examined has a clearly visible fixation target because this assists the patient in holding the eyes open. If the patient's eyelids are blepharospastic or ptotic, hold the upper eyelid with the fourth finger of the hand that is holding the lens. You can facilitate examination of the patient who is photophobic by reducing the illumination intensity, beam width, and beam height, and by using a yellow filter.

11. Evaluate the optic nerve head and its immediate surroundings (Fig. 7.36). Note whether the disc is particularly large or small and note its shape

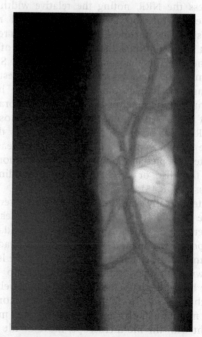

Fig. 7.36 A right optic disc seen with fundus biomicroscopy.

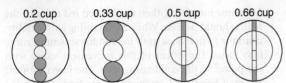

0.2 cup   0.33 cup   0.5 cup   0.66 cup

Fig. 7.37 In general, when the cup is smaller than one-third of the overall optic nerve head, the cup can be visually superimposed on the rims to determine the ratio, and certain mathematical relationships hold. For a 0.20 cup, four more of the same sized cups should be able to fit into the available rim tissue, although not necessarily symmetrically. For a 0.25 cup, three more should be able to be superimposed on the rims. For a 0.33 cup, the cup would be the same size as equally sized rims and a 0.30 cup is slightly smaller than one-third of the optic disc and a 0.35 cup is slightly larger than one-third. In larger cups, the rims can be superimposed on the cup to help to determine the ratio. With a 0.50 cup, both of the rims can be superimposed onto the cup and add up perfectly to the cup size. For a 0.65 cup, both rims superimposed within the cup add up to half of the total cup.

and colour and the clarity of the disc margins. Make sure you are viewing the cup stereoscopically and estimate the cup-to-disc ratio along the vertical meridian (Fig. 7.37) and note the location, slope, and depth of the cup.

12. Assess the NRR, noting the relative width of the superior, inferior, nasal, and temporal rims, if possible. The mnemonic **'ISNT'** is used as a reminder that in most normal discs the thickest part of the rim is the **Inferior** (temporal), followed by the **Superior** (temporal), then **Nasal**, and the thinnest is the **Temporal**. In glaucoma, the NRR often becomes thinner at the superior and inferior (temporal) poles first and a 'notch' indicates the localised loss of the NRR. If this occurs, the NRR will not obey the ISNT rule and the vertical C-to-D ratio will increase.[76]

13. Note the presence of any anomalies/abnormalities of the disc or its immediate surroundings (see Figs. 8.33–8.45).

14. Systematically examine the rest of the posterior pole (see Figs. 8.46–8.52). Follow the arcades (either inferiorly or superiorly) around the macula, to the opposite arcades and back to the nerve head. As the illumination system of the biomicroscope is moved down with the joystick of the slit-lamp through the high plus lens, the light will go up behind the high plus lens to illuminate the superior retina. To maintain the image stability, as you move the light with the biomicroscope, move or tilt the lens

slightly in the same direction as the light source in order that the cone of light from the lens continues to go straight through the pupil. Because the image is inverted and laterally reversed, what appears to be the inferior fundus in the view is actually the superior fundus and vice versa.

15. Note the colour and tortuosity (see Fig. 8.46), and any general or focal narrowing or dilation of the blood vessels. Also carefully examine the arteriovenous (AV) crossings and look for abnormalities, such as venous nipping or right-angle crossings (venule deviations owing to an overlying hardened arteriole; see Fig. 8.54). Estimate the relative width of the arteries and veins between one and three disc diameters from the disc (the AV ratio); it is typically 2:3 or 3:4 when healthy and can be 1:2 or less with hypertension.[77] At the same time, examine the surrounding fundus and look for any abnormalities.

16. Some practitioners recommend that the light-sensitive macula should be examined last. Note that the after-image produced can make patient fixation of the second eye examined difficult.

17. Examine the posterior vitreous by pulling even farther back on the joystick with the patient's gaze in primary position. The most common and prominent finding is the Weiss ring representing the posterior vitreous that has pulled away from the optic disc (Figs. 7.38 and 8.32).

18. If a binocular or adequate view of any part of the fundus, and particularly the optic nerve and macula, is not obtained, or any lesions are noted or a condition, such as glaucoma, is suspected, the patient's pupils should be dilated. If a patient refuses mydriasis, counselling on the relative risks should be undertaken and carefully documented.

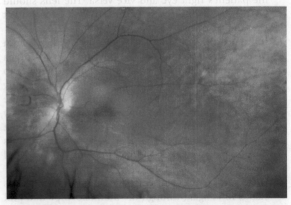

Fig. 7.38 Weiss ring to the left of the optic nerve head.

7.10.3 Peripheral fundus and nerve fibre layer assessment with fundus biomicroscopy

Peripheral views are improved with pupillary dilation. As with headband BIO with a +20 D lens, the patient's gaze is directed towards the sector that the examiner wishes to view. All eight sectors of the fundus are examined in a systematic order (e.g., view the superior fundus first, then the superior-nasal, nasal, inferior-nasal, inferior, inferior-temporal, temporal, and finally the superior-temporal fundus). To view the superior periphery, ask the patient to look up; centre the lens and light to enter the patient's pupil and pull the slit-lamp back, as per instructions for the posterior pole assessment. To view farther into the periphery, move the biomicroscope down (the light will be directed up behind the lens) and tilt the lens slightly to maintain coaxial illumination (Fig. 7.39). Although the view of the superior retina will be inverted and reversed, it is helpful to remember that, if you are directing the light towards the superior retina with the patient looking upwards, you will be looking at the superior retina.

Examination of the RNFL (Figs. 8.33–8.35) with the red-free filter is useful and is especially important in patients in whom you suspect optic neuropathies including glaucoma.[72] As the filter decreases the brightness of the image, the slit-lamp illumination should be increased. A 'bright-dark-bright' pattern is noted in normal individuals, as noted by the light band of white, striated nerve fibres inserting into the superior-temporal and inferior-temporal poles of the disc, and a darker pattern through the macular area. 'Slit' defects appear as slightly darker bands in the striated nerve fibre layer (NFL) band and are approximately one blood vessel width across. These defects can be normal in some individuals. 'Wedge' defects appear as a darker band that widens as it extends away from the optic disc into the NFL. These can be accompanied by a focal loss in the NRR tissue. Diffuse loss of the striations of the NFL can also be noted.[72] Note that the fine tertiary retinal vessels can be seen more prominently in regions of NFL loss and are less visible within the healthy NFL. Nerve fibre loss with age decreases the robustness of the 'bright-dark-bright' pattern as does media opacity and observation with a lens with a yellow filter.

7.10.4 Direct ophthalmoscopy procedure

(See video 7.11.)

Familiarise yourself with the controls of the direct ophthalmoscope. Learn how to vary the intensity of the light beam, its size, shape, and colour. A green ('red-free') filter increases the contrast of blood vessels and vascular lesions (they appear dark against the light background of the fundus) and therefore can be useful when assessing

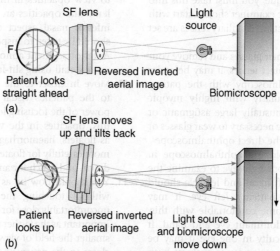

Fig. 7.39 (a) Optics of fundus biomicroscopy with a high-plus lens. The real image is reversed and inverted and lies between the hand-held lens and the observer at the slit-lamp. The image is therefore in focus when the slit-lamp biomicroscope is pulled back towards the observer. (b) Observation of the superior fundus is facilitated by having the patient look up.

patients with diabetes or other vascular disease. Some instruments also have settings that will project a target with the light beam, such as an eccentric fixation target. A slit aperture is sometimes provided to determine the elevation or depression of a lesion using the monocular cue of the beam bending. A polarising filter and a half circle aperture are often available to help decrease annoying reflections from the corneal surface, although the image with the polarising filter is limited in that the luminance across the image becomes variable (in a 'Maltese cross' pattern owing to corneal birefringence). Direct ophthalmoscopes include focusing lenses with ranges that differ depending on the instrument used, but the range is typically from about +30 to –30 D. The power of the lens being used is displayed, with the red numbers indicating minus lenses and the black numbers indicating plus lenses. Some instruments have a second wheel of lenses or a setting for additional lenses that, when used in combination with the first wheel of lenses, allow for higher total dioptric range.

1. Raise the chair to such a position that you can comfortably look into the patient's eye (from the patient's temporal side) by bending over only slightly. This is important to avoid a long-term strain injury to your back.[75]
2. Inform the patient that you are going to examine the health of their eyes.
3. Use the largest aperture beam for patients with large pupils because it provides the largest field of view. For patients with smaller pupils, typically the elderly, the intermediate size aperture is preferred because the field of view is limited by the pupil and the larger aperture creates a larger corneal reflex.
4. Set the lens wheel to about +10 D (if you remove your glasses for this technique, you must take this into account, i.e., a –6 D myopic examiner should start with a +4 D lens). Make sure that any auxiliary lenses are set at zero.
5. Ask the patient to remove their glasses and remove your own. If a patient wears contact lenses, it may be easier to perform direct ophthalmoscopy with the patient wearing the lenses, particularly with highly myopic patients. If you have an unusually large astigmatic or myopic correction, it may be necessary to wear glasses or contact lenses while using the direct ophthalmoscope.
6. Dim the room lights. Hold the ophthalmoscope in your right hand and use your right eye to examine the patient's right eye. Your left hand and left eye should be used to examine the patient's left eye. It may take some practice to become comfortable with this, especially with your non-dominant eye and hand. If you have reduced visual acuity in one eye it may be necessary to use your better seeing eye to evaluate both the patient's eyes. This will take some practice to avoid bumping the patient's nose and to obtain an adequate view of the fundus on your affected side.

7. Instruct the patient to look up and temporally (usually at the corner of the room). Some practitioners find this positioning places less strain on the examiner's back than if the patient looks straight ahead at a target.
8. Place the top of the ophthalmoscope against your brow. You should now be able to view through the aperture. Rotate the ophthalmoscope handle approximately 10° to 20° from the vertical to avoid the patient's nose. Position the ophthalmoscope about 15° temporal to the patient's line of sight. Both of your eyes should be kept open to relax your accommodation. It will take some practice to suppress the other image, especially when you are using your non-dominant eye.
9. Place the hand not holding the ophthalmoscope on the back of the examination chair for stability. With the total dioptric power set at about +10 D (step 2) move closer to the patient until the anterior segment of the eye is in focus (at ~ 10 cm). Now observe the clarity of the media. Opacities will appear as dark areas against a bright red background (the red reflex; Figs. 7.8 and 7.9). You can estimate the location of the opacity by using the principle of parallax motion. Choose a point of focus (e.g., the iris). If the opacity is **Anterior** to the iris, **'Against'** motion will be observed when you move the beam. If the opacity is posterior to the iris, 'with' motion will be observed when you move the beam. If you note that the opacity is anterior (e.g., on the cornea), ask the patient to blink. If the opacity moves, it is floating in the tears (e.g., mucus or debris). If it does not move, it is a true corneal opacity. Instruct the patient to look up, then left, then down, and then right while directing your view in the same direction to view opacities in the lens behind the iris. Cortical lenticular opacities are most commonly found in the inferior nasal aspect of the crystalline lens so care should be taken to inspect this quadrant (section 8.4.3). Anterior segment abnormalities should be assessed in more detail using slit-lamp biomicroscopy.
10. Move in closer to the patient on a line 15° temporal to the patient's visual axis and decrease the dioptric power of the focusing lens as you move closer. By doing this, opacities in the vitreous may be observed, such as floaters, haemorrhage, and asteroid bodies. To look more carefully for floaters, ask the patient to look up and down, and watch for any floaters moving in your view.
11. You should now be as close as possible to the patient without touching the patient's eye. This may feel uncomfortably close for both you and the patient, but it is important as the farther away you are from the patient, the smaller the field of view you will obtain. Also, if you are closer to the patient the corneal reflex will move farther from the viewing axis, making the view less obstructed. If you are viewing 15° temporally from the patient's line of sight, the disc or retinal vessels should now be in view.

12. If both you and the patient are emmetropic and your accommodation is relaxed, the dioptric value of the lens wheel should be close to zero. If you and/or the patient are uncorrected and ametropic, the lens power necessary to focus on the fundus (i.e., the power in the lens wheel) will be the sum of the refractive errors and your accommodative state. Some practitioners use this as an approximate estimation of the patient's spherical refractive state. For example, if you are a -3 myope and your patient is a -5 myope and neither is wearing glasses or contact lenses during the assessment, you will likely need a -8 lens to focus on the fundus.

13. If you do not see the disc straight away but can focus on the vessels, follow the vessels backwards towards the disc. The bifurcation of the vessels forms a 'V' and this will point in the direction you should move to get to the disc.

14. Once you see the disc, focus it clearly using the lens wheel. Bracketing several lens positions may be required before deciding on the optimal focus.

15. Estimate the size of the disc using the middle aperture of the typical 3-aperture system. This is ~ 5° and about the size of an medium-sized disc.[72]

16. Determine whether the NRR follows the ISNT rule and estimate the vertical C-to-D ratio (Fig. 7.37; examples 8.33–8.39; online quiz 8.3). The cup margins should be determined by kinking of the vessels as they pass over the margin. Do not assess the cup as the area of pallor, because the cup can extend beyond this area. This is difficult as you are trying to make judgments about a 3D structure with a 2D image. In deep cupping, the bottom of the cup will focus with less plus than the NRR tissue and it can appear grey with central mottling (the lamina cribrosa; section 8.5.4). Slight parallax movements may help in determining the cup. Note the relative position of the vessels to the cup.

17. Evaluate the optic nerve head and its immediate surroundings. Note its shape and colour and the clarity of the disc margins. Observe the veins as they leave the optic cup and look for venous pulsation. Note the presence of any anomalies/abnormalities of the disc or its immediate surroundings.

18. Systematically examine the vascular arcades and rest of the posterior pole. Follow the arcades (either inferiorly or superiorly) around the macula, to the opposite arcades and back to the nerve head. Carefully note any tortuosity and/or focal narrowing of the arterioles. Also examine the AV crossings and look for abnormalities, such as venous nipping or right-angle crossings. Estimate the relative width of the arteries and veins between one and three disc diameters from the disc (the AV ratio); it is typically 2:3 or 3:4 when healthy and can be 1:2 or less with hypertension.[77] At the same time, examine the surrounding fundus and look for any abnormalities.

19. Examine the retina more peripherally. Ask the patient to look into various positions of gaze (up, up and right, right, down and right, down, down and left, left and up, and left) and systematically examine the retina with a moderately wide beam of light. You must look in the same direction as the patient. For example, when the patient looks up, you must position the ophthalmoscope slightly below the pupil and aim the ophthalmoscope beam upwards, towards the superior retina. It is important to be careful, as moderately large abnormalities can be missed easily owing to the direct ophthalmoscope's high magnification and narrow field of view. When the patient is looking down, it will be necessary to gently hold up the upper eyelid to view the inferior retina.

20. Finally, evaluate the macula using the smallest aperture. This observation is performed at the end so that the patient has a chance to adapt to the light; however, many patients still find the light uncomfortably bright, therefore dimming the illumination may be required to get an adequate view of the macula. The macula is located slightly below centre and approximately 2 DD temporal to the disc. You can either move the light in this direction or ask the patient to look directly into the light. You will often note a bright reflection from the cornea that obscures the view of the macula. This is minimised by using the smallest aperture beam and/or changing the shape of the light beam (a half circle shape is available with some ophthalmoscopes), changing your angle of observation, and/or getting as close to the eye as possible.

7.10.5 PanOptic procedure

1. Seat the patient comfortably in the examination chair with their head held upright and not back against the headrest. The chair should be raised to such a position that you can comfortably look into the patient's eye (from the patient's temporal side) by bending over only slightly. This is important to avoid a long-term strain injury to your back.[75]

2. Inform the patient that you are going to examine the health of their eyes.

3. Ask the patient to remove their glasses. You should be able to continue to wear your own glasses for this technique, but it is recommended that you remove them. Now dim the room lights.

4. Look through the PanOptic with your thumb on the dynamic focusing wheel and focus on an object in the room that is at least 3 to 4 m away so that it is clear and sharp.

5. Make sure that the aperture dial is set to the small aperture position. This setting is marked with a green indicator line on the dial. It is the ideal setting for a typical non-dilated pupil.

6. Turn the PanOptic on and adjust the light intensity rheostat to its maximum position.
7. Explain to your patient that the eyecup will touch their brow. Instruct them to try not to move their head and to look straight ahead.
8. Position yourself about 15 cm away at a 15° to 20° angle on the temple side of the patient. To keep your patient's head steady, you may want to rest your left hand on the patient's forehead.
9. Shine the light at the patient's eye and look for the red retinal reflex. Slowly follow the red reflex towards the patient and into the pupil.
10. The eyecup should be compressed about half its length to maximise the view. At this point, a large view of the entire optic disc and surrounding vessels should be visible.
11. After examining the right eye, repeat the procedure for the left eye.

7.10.6 Keeler wide-angle twin mag procedure

Familiarise yourself with the controls of the ophthalmoscope. The apertures and filters available are a wide angle beam that illuminates a large area of the fundus and is most useful with a dilated pupil, an intermediate beam that is useful for use with an undilated pupil, and in the paediatric examination, a macular beam for use in viewing the macula, a slit, a cup disc graticule, a semi-circle, and red-free and cobalt blue filters.

1. Position the spectacle rest, which is located at the user end of the instrument. When it is in position there will be a click. Pull out the spectacle rest if you are not wearing glasses.
2. Remove the dust cover and store in dust cover holder.
3. Position the brow rest into place.
4. Set the magnification lever to LO and select the small or intermediate aperture by rotating the graticule/aperture/filter selector. Look through the eyepiece and focus the instrument on an object by sliding the focus adjuster up or down.
5. Turn on the lamp by rotating the light intensity adjuster anti-clockwise until the desired intensity is achieved.
6. Position yourself at approximately 60 cm from the patient and view the eye to be examined along the visual axis to observe the red reflex. Move towards the patient and refocus the instrument on a fundus feature. The posterior pole will be in view. The field of view will increase as you move closer to a maximum when you are 15 mm from the patient's cornea. Position your hand on the patient's forehead to steady the instrument.
7. If you are using the brow rest, move the instrument towards the patient until the brow rests on the patient's forehead.

8. The large beam produces a 25° field of view and is used for general examinations. It provides 15× magnification. By flipping the magnification lever to HI, the field of view decreases to 17.5° and provides 22.5× magnification.
9. Corneal examination procedure: administer fluorescein dye to the patient's eye and attach the corneal lens at the front of the instrument. It attaches magnetically. Select the blue filter from the graticule/aperture/filter selection wheel. View the cornea from a distance of 1.5 cm from the front of the instrument.

7.10.7 Recording of fundus examinations

Obtain images of any abnormalities, if possible, and store the image for future comparisons. If the patient has a presenting complaint that could suggest a fundus abnormality and no abnormalities are detected, your recording should be more detailed to highlight that your examination was full and appropriate.

Lens (with direct ophthalmoscopy): If there are no opacities record 'clear.' Sketch any cataracts as shown (Fig. 7.14). The undilated pupil can be recorded as a dashed line on this diagram.

Vitreous: If no abnormalities are detected, record 'clear.' Note that only the posterior vitreous is examined with fundus biomicroscopy and the anterior vitreous is examined with the slit-lamp without an auxiliary lens.

Fundus biomicroscopy: Keep in mind that the image is real, inverted, and aerial, so vertical and lateral directions must be reversed for recording. Two methods may be employed for documentation of the findings with indirect fundus biomicroscopy with a high plus lens. The first involves mentally reversing and inverting the image before drawing the findings. This requires a significant amount of practice and is susceptible to errors in interpretation. The second and often more accurate method if paper records are used: place the form upside down to compensate for the reversed inverted image, and draw exactly what is seen in the lens.

Optic nerve head

(See online quiz 8.3.)
Record the following:

1. Distinctness of the optic disc margins.
2. Optic nerve head size and shape. Indicate whether the optic disc size is small, average, or large.
3. The size, configuration, and location of any peripapillary chorioretinal atrophy, both zone alpha and zone beta.
4. The health of the NRR tissue by its colour, thickness, and uniformity. Whether or not the 'ISNT' rule is followed should be documented.

5. The optic cup size. Draw the shape, size, and location of the physiological cupping on a diagram of the disc (Fig. 7.40). Include a horizontal cross section of the cupping showing the depth and shape and a vertical one, if necessary. Record the size of the optic cup as a decimal fraction of the optic nerve in the vertical dimension (see Fig. 7.37). Note the presence of the lamina cribrosa (section 8.5.4) and spontaneous venous pulsation (video 8.2).

6. In the same diagram include all anomalies/abnormalities of the disc, such as coloboma, crescents, drusen, disc swelling, haemorrhages, myelinated nerve fibres, pallor, pits, and disc tilting. The differential diagnosis of drusen in the disc can be helped by using cobalt blue light and a yellow filter because they autofluoresce.

Example 1: The recording of a normal optic nerve head could include the following: 'Large disc, distinct margins, healthy NRR (follows ISNT rule), C:D 0.40 V, 3D cup, lamina visible, venous puls'n sup. Temp.' Your recording could also include a plan and cross-sectional diagram of the disc.

Example 2: If the patient reported a family history of POAG or other risk factors, your recording should be more detailed to highlight that your examination was full and appropriate for the patient, so that you could

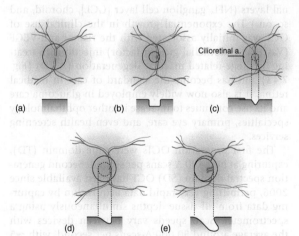

Fig. 7.40 Diagrams of different sizes and types of optic nerve cupping. **(a)** No cup. **(b)** 0.4 cup-to-disc ratio (C:D) in both the horizontal and vertical meridians. Deep, with clearly demarcated edges. **(c)** Shallow cup with gently sloping edges and a C:D of 0.30 H and 0.25 V. **(d)** C:D of 0.60 H and 0.50 V, with nasal displacement of the vessels and a gentle slope temporally. **(e)** Advanced glaucomatous cupping with a C:D of 0.90 and a deep bean pot shape. There is no healthy rim of tissue temporally.

additionally record 'Normal RNFL, no PPA, no haemorrhage' or similar.[72]

Nerve fibre layer: Record the relative brightness and width of the pattern in the superior-temporal and inferior-temporal NFL. Note any diffuse loss, as well as any slit- or wedge-type defects.[72] Patients with a more darkly pigmented retinal pigment epithelial layer often have a more prominent appearance of the RNFL than those with less pigment.

Blood vessels: If no abnormalities are detected, record 'normal for age' or 'negative,' or equivalent and record the AV ratio. Record any abnormality of the blood vessels (e.g., attenuation or dilation, emboli, broadened reflex or copper/silver wiring or vascular sheathing), the artery-vein crossings (90° degree crossings, venule nipping), and any tortuosity of the arterioles (often congenital) and venules (often acquired). Indicate the location of all findings in a diagram.

Fundus (posterior pole, equator, and periphery): If no abnormalities are detected, record 'Normal for age,' 'Negative,' or equivalent. Record this separately for the posterior pole and the periphery/mid-periphery. Note the size, shape, location, colour, elevation, and depth of any abnormality. Specify the size of a lesion and its location with respect to the disc in terms of disc diameters (DD). For example, the lesion may be 2 DD × 1 DD wide and located 4 DD at 4 o'clock from the disc (Figs. 7.41 and 7.42). Determining the appropriate anterior-to-posterior location in the peripheral fundus can be facilitated by certain normal landmarks.

Macula: If no abnormalities are detected, record 'Normal for age,' 'Negative,' or equivalent. Pertinent negative findings should be recorded in certain situations (e.g., 'No clinically significant macular oedema' in those patients who are diabetic). Record any findings or abnormalities noted at the macula, such as drusen, pigmentation changes, haemorrhages, exudates, cotton wool spots, subfoveal neovascular membranes, and thickening (oedema).

7.10.8 Interpretation of fundus examinations

A good understanding of the normal anatomy and physiology of the retina, choroid, and optic nerve variations in normal appearance (sections 8.5 and 8.6), the normal changes expected with age (section 8.7), and posterior segment eye disease is required. You need to consider whether any significant findings of fundus biomicroscopy helped in your differential diagnosis of any pertinent symptoms and signs and whether they lead to a final diagnosis or an indication of the need for further testing.

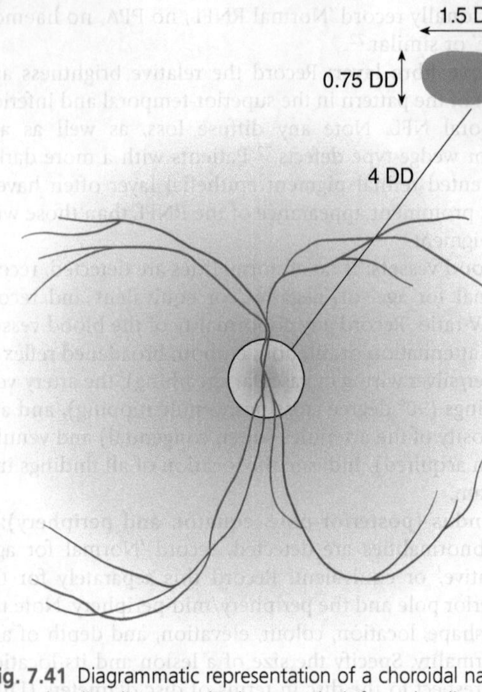

1.5 DD

0.75 DD

4 DD

Fig. 7.41 Diagrammatic representation of a choroidal naevus located 4 disc diameters (DD) at 1 o'clock from the disc. Its size is 1.5 DD by 0.75 DD.

7.10.9 Most common errors when assessing the fundus

Fundus biomicroscopy

1. Misaligning the indirect optical system, causing a poor view and a view with only one eye (no stereopsis). Stability of the lens is critical.
2. Holding the lens too far from the cornea, causing the pupil stop to limit the view and/or a view with only one eye (no stereopsis). You need to learn *not* to move the lens back from the eye when the slit-lamp is pulled back from the eye.
3. Holding the lens too close such that the patient's lashes touch the lens. Patients may be concerned about the lens touching their eye so may either blink frequently or may pull back from the headrest. You may also get condensation on the lens surface, which will obscure your view.

Direct ophthalmoscopy

1. Not getting close enough to an older patient (with a small pupil) when performing the technique, particularly when attempting to view the macula.

2. Using the cup pallor instead of the deflection of the blood vessels to determine the edge of the cup.

Monocular indirect ophthalmoscopy

1. Not getting close enough to optimise the view.
2. Not matching the aperture stop to the pupil diameter. It is best to have the aperture stop less than wide open to avoid reflection from the edge of the pupil.

7.11 Optical coherence tomography

OCT is the most common technology used for routine, high-resolution, digital imaging of the retina and optic nerve (Fig. 7.42). For a review of the optical principles and their application to the eye, see Fujimoto and Huang.[78] OCT enables non-invasive, cross-sectional imaging of the retina by measuring the reflectance (backscatter) and relative delay of light as it journeys through the ocular tissues, comparing it with a known reference path. Line scans (B-scans) are composed of many A-scans captured along a line. The fast scan speeds of modern devices allow multiple cross-sectional B-scans to be captured over an area, creating dense 3D volume scans. Automated segmentation of these data cubes provides thickness data of the retinal layers (NFL, ganglion cell layer [GCL], choroid, and so on.) The exponential growth in the clinical use of OCT was initially associated with the rise of anti-VEGF (Vascular endothelial growth factor) injections in treating 'wet' age-related macular degeneration (AMD) (Fig. 7.43) and has become the standard of care in medical retina. It is also now widely employed in glaucoma care and its use continues to increase in other ophthalmology specialties, primary eye care, and even health screening services.

The first generation OCTs were time domain (TD), capturing at best 400 A-scans per second. Second generation spectral domain (SD) OCT has been available since 2006, permitting very rapid data acquisition by capturing data from all tissue depths simultaneously using a spectrometer. Scan speeds vary between devices with the average around 50,000 A-scans per second, with ~5 microns of axial and ~14 μm of lateral resolution. Both TD and SD OCT use a light source with a peak around 830 nm. Third generation swept source (SS) OCT has been available since 2012 with scan speeds of 100,000 A-scans per second. SS technology provides a high signal-to-noise ratio and longer source wavelength (1050 nm). SD and SS OCTs represent the bulk of OCT devices in use today.

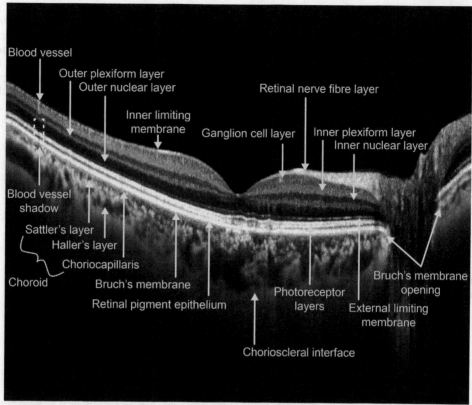

Fig. 7.42 The layers of the retina and choroid provided by optical coherence tomography (OCT) images.

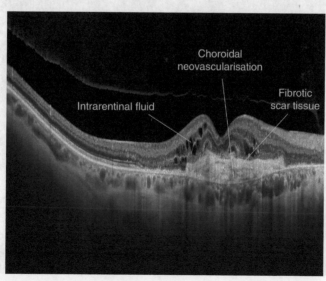

Fig. 7.43 Swept Source Optical Coherence Tomography (OCT) of a case of wet age-related macular degeneration showing macular oedema, intraretinal fluid, exudates, and an area of fibrosis containing a choroidal neovascular membrane. (Courtesy of Dr. Carl Glittenberg.)

7.11.1 The evidence base: when and how should OCT be used

OCT is capable of documenting subtle lesions of the retina and choroid, with high levels of repeatability. In primary eyecare, OCT should be considered in all suspected maculopathies, including AMD (Figs. 7.43 and 7.44), central serous chorioretinopathy (Fig. 7.45), and diabetic eye disease (Fig. 7.46).[79] It is also capable of monitoring macular oedema, aided by thickness and differential maps. It is a useful tool for problem solving when visual acuity is not as expected, and it provides valuable information in cases of vitreomacular adhesion/traction (see Fig. 7.47) and suspected ocular tumour. The ability to measure choroidal thickness is useful, especially in central serous chorioretinopathy and posterior uveitis (Fig. 7.48).[80]

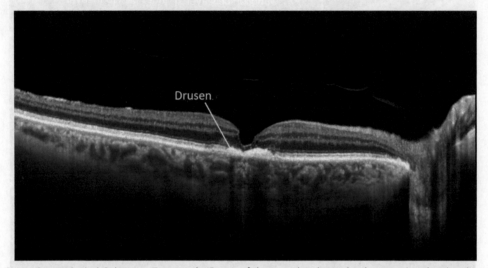

Fig. 7.44 Swept Source Optical Coherence Tomography B-scan of dry age-related macular degeneration showing drusen at the level of the retinal pigment epithelium.

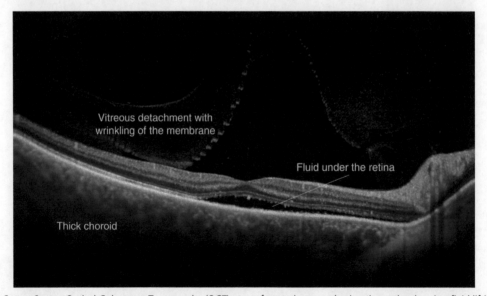

Fig. 7.45 Swept Source Optical Coherence Tomography (OCT) scan of central serous chorioretinopathy showing fluid lifting the retina away from the retinal pigment epithelium (RPE) and swollen photoreceptor outer segments. There is also an unrelated partial vitreous detachment. (Courtesy of Professor P.E. Stanga.)

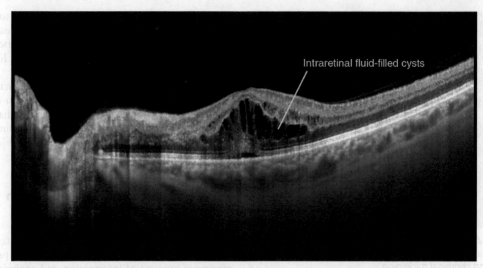

Intraretinal fluid-filled cysts

Fig. 7.46 Diabetic macular oedema showing fluid-filled intraretinal cysts and thickening of the macular region.

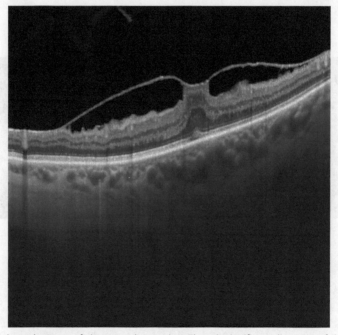

Fig. 7.47 Averaged B-scan through a case of vitreomacular traction. There is significant distortion of the inner retinal layers, but the outer retinal layers remain intact so there will be limited effect on visual acuity

OCT should be considered for all patients with glaucoma or at risk of glaucoma, where it can evaluate the NFL and/or ganglion cell complex (GCC) with respect to a reference database or previous measurements, as well as providing detailed, repeatable optic nerve head metrics (Fig. 7.49).

Other neurodegenerative diseases have also been shown to cause a reduction in NFL and GCC over time,[81] and OCT imaging of the optic nerve head provides additional information when trying to differentiate papilloedema from more benign causes of optic disc swelling (online figures).

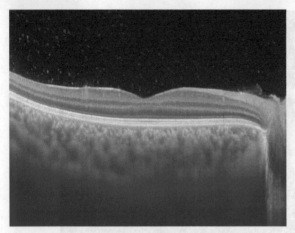

Fig. 7.48 Averaged SS optical coherence tomography (OCT) B-scan of an eye with posterior uveitis, showing cells in the vitreous and choroidal thickening.

Anterior segment OCT (AS-OCT) is used to evaluate the cornea, iris, and anterior chamber angle measurement (Fig. 7.50), with additional use in tear meniscus measurements (section 7.3.1)[82] and scleral contact lens fitting (section 5.12).[83]

A large number of OCT devices are commercially available; they share basic functionality, but vary in a number of other ways (Table 7.5). It is worth noting that because segmentation algorithms differ between manufacturers, layer thickness measurements are not comparable between devices.[84]

7.11.2 Selecting a scan pattern

Retinal imaging

Three-dimensional volume scans or dense raster patterns are standard for macular imaging because they provide the maximum amount of information and analysis options.

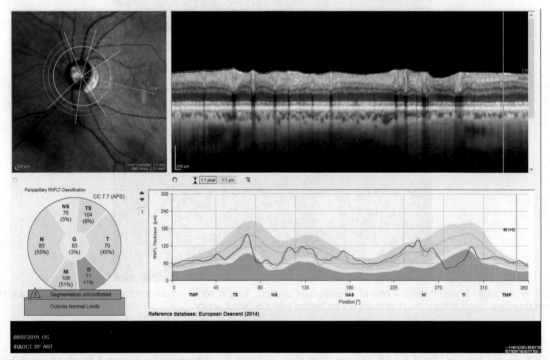

Fig. 7.49 Circumpapillary SD-OCT image of the left eye of a 67-year-old woman with primary open-angle glaucoma. Analysis of RNFL thickness shows significant thinning of the inferior temporal region, as well as possible thinning of the superior nasal region. The accompanying SITA Std 24-2 visual field shows a superior arcuate defect corresponding to the inferior temporal RNFL thinning, and an early inferior defect corresponding to the less marked superior nasal RNFL thinning. (Courtesy Mrs. Habiba Bham and Dr. Jonathan Denniss. © 2014 Carl Zeiss Meditec.).

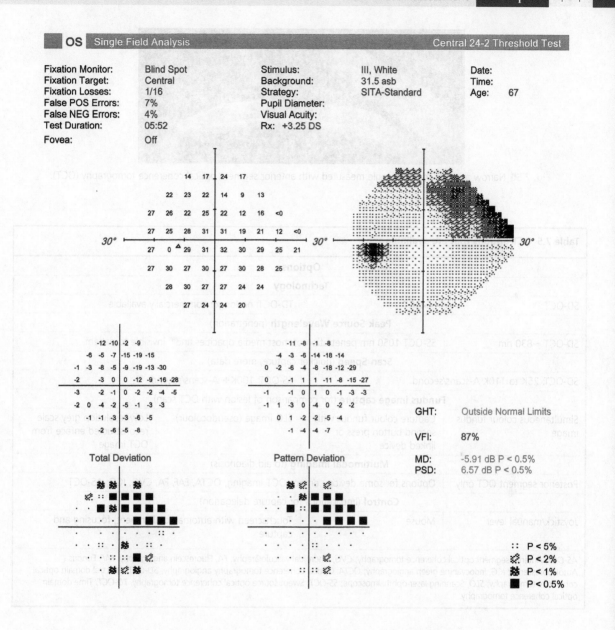

Comments

Fig. 7.49, cont'd

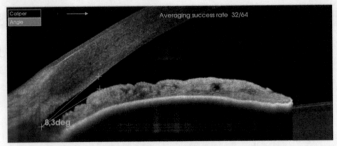

Fig. 7.50 Narrow anterior chamber angle measured with anterior segment optical coherence tomography (OCT).

Table 7.5 OCT options that are available			
Options			
Technology			
SD-OCT	SS-OCT	TD-OCT: no longer commercially available	
Peak Source Wavelength (penetration)			
SD-OCT ~830 nm	SS-OCT 1050 nm penetration of most media opacities and[85] invisible to patient		
Scan Speed (quicker capture, more data)			
SD-OCT: 25K to 110K A-scans/second	SS-OCT: 100K+ A-scans/second		
Fundus image capture (for comparison of lesion with OCT scan)			
Simultaneous colour fundus image	Capture colour fundus with second button press or linked device	SLO image (pseudocolour)	Low resolution grey scale reconstructed enface from OCT image
Multimodal imaging (to aid diagnosis)			
Posterior segment OCT only	Options for some devices: enface OCT imaging, OCTA, FAF, FA, CVG, ICG, AS-OCT		
Control (implications for capture delegation)			
Joystick/manual lever	Mouse	Touchscreen with automated alignment, focusing and capture	
AS-OCT, Anterior segment optical coherence tomography; *CVG*, Choroidal vasculoGraphy; *FA*, Fluorescein angiography; *FAF*, Fundus AutoFluorescence; *ICG*, Indocyanine green angiography; *OCTA*, Optical coherence tomography angiography; *SD-OCT*, Spectral domain optical coherence tomography; *SLO*, Scanning laser ophthalmoscope; *SS-OCT*, Swept source optical coherence tomography, *TD-OCT*, Time domain optical coherence tomography.			

For raster patterns, the line scans should be close together to avoid missing small lesions owing to interpolation between scans.

There may be retinal lesions for which a line scan pattern is preferred; line scans generally provide the highest quality images because they can be averaged (more than one image combined). Common line scan patterns include 5- or 7-line cross patterns, radial (or star) patterns, and single lines. Averaged line scans can be useful when imaging through media opacities with SD-OCT. For steep myopic retinas (Fig. 7.51), the vertical scans within cross patterns are useful where the limited scan depth of SD-OCT makes it difficult to focus both the centre and periphery of the OCT image. The vertical meridian of the myopic retina tends to be less steep than the horizontal, making it easier to capture an in-focus SD-OCT image. This is less problematic for SS-OCT owing to the greater scan depth.

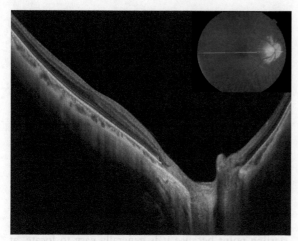

Fig. 7.51 Swept source optical coherence tomography (OCT) image of a highly myopic retina showing the steep retinal profile.

Recognition software available on most devices allows the same location to be scanned at each follow-up visit. This will influence the scan type you select to allow direct comparison. Before selecting a scan, check that the analysis options you require are available for that scan type, for example the ability to compare retinal layer thickness with a reference database.

Glaucoma imaging

Circumpapillary NFL thickness is most commonly based on 3D disc scans or radial disc scans, which also capture useful disc metrics. 3D macula scans to examine the GCC are also informative. Clinic efficiency can be improved by using a single widefield (12 × 9 mm) 3D scan, which captures the disc and macula in one go, and is associated with glaucoma-orientated analysis. A widefield scan is also useful for general screening purposes.

7.11.3 Procedure for OCT

When performing OCT imaging, pupils should be 2.5 mm or greater, whenever possible. Low room lighting and the small pupil function are useful in patients with particularly small pupils. A mydriatic may be necessary in a few patients.

1. Explain the test and the reasons for performing the assessment to the patient.
2. Turn on the instrument, clean the chin and forehead rest and, if necessary, the camera lens using the method recommended by the manufacturer.
3. Seat the patient at the instrument and make any gross adjustments to the height of the instrument.

4. Enter the patient's name using the surname first, date of birth (often formatted as month-day-year), and patient file number, if appropriate. There is usually an option to enter additional data, such as ethnicity and refractive error.
5. Select the eye to be tested.
6. Select the scan type (3D cube size) and location, or line scans (raster, 5-line cross, radial, single line, and so on), and any additional settings offered, such as the type of tracking, spacing, or length of scan lines or number of averages (line scans).
7. With the instrument head pulled back from the headrest, ask the patient to position their head on the chinrest and forehead against the brow bar.
8. Alter the chinrest height to position the eye within the horizontal bands shown on the device screen.
9. Choose a fixation target that the patient can see (larger for poor visual acuity, VA). The fixation location is determined automatically by the scan location, but some devices allow refinement.
10. For fully automated devices, touch the centre of the patient's pupil on the screen to align and focus the device automatically. For joystick-controlled devices, adjust the focus and position of the camera to ensure even illumination, a focused image, and an OCT scan that is oriented correctly (erect) with minimum tilt and within the necessary acquisition window.
11. Instruction the patient: "Take a few blinks and stare wide, while looking carefully at the fixation target."
12. Press the button to acquire the images. Some devices optimise the scan quality and then provide a countdown. This can help improve patient cooperation, allowing better timing of their final blink. Monitor the OCT scan progression and encourage the patient to keep fixating and try not to blink or move. For SD-OCT devices with a visible scan line, the patient should be reminded not to follow the moving scan lines. Tell them as soon as the scan is complete so they can blink. For an OCT device that captures simultaneous colour fundus images, the camera flash signals the end of the process.
13. Select the next scan type and repeat, or select the other eye.
14. Save all scans if not stored automatically.
15. Inspect all scans and ensure that the scan quality is good (quality scores vary between manufacturers), scan patterns are centred appropriately and are without artefact (blink, movement, vertical clipping).
16. Repeat scans, if necessary.

7.11.4 Reviewing and recording OCT

Select a scan in the review software. Ensure that automated segmentation is successful and accurate and, if not, adjust and re-save. For 3D scans, scroll through the B-scans using the slider below the scan view or move the scan line on the fundus image (devices with simultaneous pinpoint registered colour fundus image only) (see video 7.12). Click on any anomalies noted in the scan to show their location on the fundus image, or vice versa. Numerous software options are generally available, providing metrics, overlays, and views of individual layers. Consult your device manual for the options available.

Select the report type (varies with scan type and device) and whether to show results for a single eye or both eyes side by side. Print the results or save/export them to an electronic medical records system. For monitoring changes in layer thickness over time, most devices have the option of selecting scans taken at different points in time and plotting the change in different layer thickness over time.

7.11.5 Interpretation of OCT images

A detailed discussion of OCT interpretation falls outside the scope of this book, but some basic pointers are provided.

Retina

Familiarity with the normal appearance of the retinal and choroidal layers (see Fig. 7.42) can be aided by reviewing the Staurenghi et al. 2014 paper.[86] Assessment

of the retina is somewhat more qualitative than the assessment for glaucoma, and it can take time to gain confidence in your ability to interpret the layers of the retina and common abnormalities. White corresponds to high reflectivity and horizontal structures, such as the NFL, plexiform (connecting) layers, and RPE. Dark colours indicate minimal reflectance and are associated with the cell bodies in the inner and outer nuclear layers, but dark voids may be fluid within the retina. The vitreous is often seen as black, although the vitreous anatomy can often be visualised with SS-OCT (Fig. 7.52).[87] If there is vitreoretinal separation, the posterior hyaloid face may be visible as a reflective line (Fig. 7.53). It is advisable to develop a routine for examining OCT scans–there is no right or wrong technique, but the RPE, a bright white double line, is a good starting point because it is generally easy to locate, at least somewhere within the scan. Work up through the outer then inner retina to the vitreous from the RPE, then down from the RPE through the choroid to the chorioscleral interface. Drusen are seen below the RPE and above Bruch's membrane as reflective 'bumps' (see Fig. 7.44); fluid can be subretinal (above the RPE, but below the retina) or intra-retinal and pigment epithelial detachments (PEDs) are dome-shaped serous fluid elevations of the RPE; hyper-reflective areas above the RPE

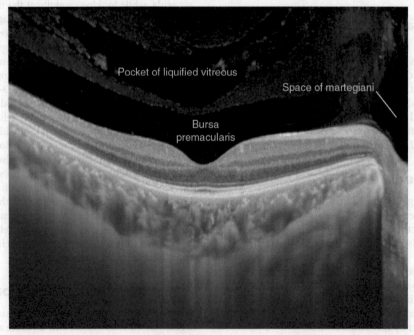

Fig. 7.52 Swept source image of a normal eye, showing features of the vitreous in addition to the retina, choroid, and sclera. (Courtesy of Professor P. E. Stanga.)

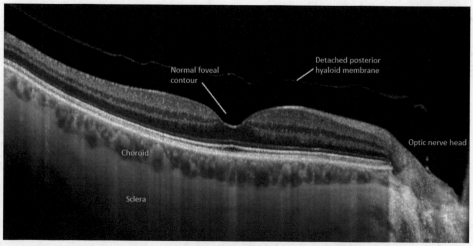

Fig. 7.53 Optical coherence tomography (OCT) scans showing complete detachment of the posterior vitreous membrane. A normal foveal contour confirms that the detachment has not damaged the macular region.

but below the retina are called subretinal hyper-reflective material (SHRM) and can include neovascularisation, fibrosis, exudation, vitelliform material, and haemorrhage. The variety of causes of SHRM highlights that interpretation of OCT images requires information from other assessments, such as fundus assessment/imaging and OCT angiography (section 7.11.6).

Three-dimensional volume scans and radial scans provide retinal thickness maps for comparison with a reference database. Some devices offer choroidal thickness maps. There are specific analysis tools to enable mapping of retinal atrophy and the size or height of lesions.

Glaucoma

Volume disc scans provide the NFL thickness around the optic nerve for comparison with a reference database, generally shown for hemifields, quadrants, and sectors (Fig. 7.54). This comparison should always be interpreted in the context of other clinical findings; a thickness measurement that dips into the red is not a guaranteed abnormality, it is just indicating a relatively high chance of it not being normal, but there may be a good clinical reason for this, such as particularly oblique retinal arcades. Highly repeatable disc metrics are also extracted from these data, allowing easy comparison between the two eyes, or over time.

Three-dimensional macular scans are generally segmented to give full retinal thickness, NFL thickness, ganglion cell layer (GCL+) thickness and, in some cases, the full ganglion cell complex (GCL++) consisting of the

NFL, GCL, and inner plexiform layer. There are differing views on whether macular analysis is more sensitive than circumpapillary NFL for the early detection of glaucoma,[88] and therefore it is advisable to study both. This can be done easily with a single widefield report, available on some devices[89] (see Fig. 7.11e). More informative than an isolated measure of the retinal layers at a point in time is examination of the reduction in thickness over time using the progression tool. A normal age-related decline in NFL of between 0.2 and 0.3 μm per year is expected.[90]

7.11.6 OCT angiograph

The OCT angiography (OCTA) is a relatively new technology that is set to revolutionise retinal imaging to the extent that OCT did when first available. A detailed discussion of OCTA falls outside the scope of this book, and the reader is advised to consult Kashani et al.[91]

The OCTA effectively creates 3D images of the retinal vasculature by taking between two and four B-scans at the same location in very quick succession and comparing the images. Because the tissue itself does not move, any difference in reflectivity between images is associated with red blood cells moving in the vessels, and hence the location of the vessels is identified. The results are similar to fluorescein angiography (FA), but have the advantage of being non-invasive, volume rendered (3D) to show deeper vessels and reveal the tiny capillary networks (Fig. 7.55). Leakage of fluid is not associated with red blood cells, and therefore is not visualised by OCTA. Experts are still learning how to interpret the findings, but the information provided by OCTA, although

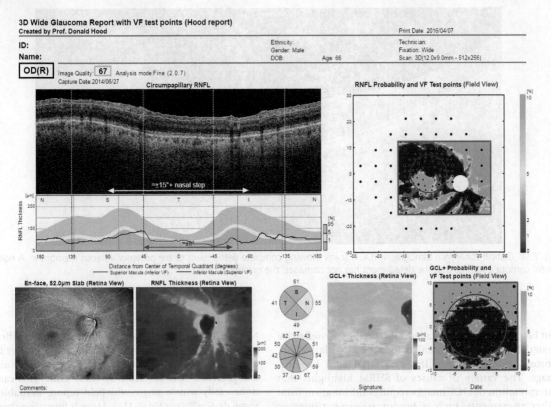

3D Wide Glaucoma Report with VF test points (Hood report)
Created by Prof. Donald Hood

Fig. 7.54 Widefield Glaucoma report based on a 12 × 9 mm scan of the disc and macula in an eye with primary open angle glaucoma. The segmented circumpapillary data are compared with a retinal nerve fibre layer (RNFL) normative database, displayed as NSTIN (nasal, superior, temporal, inferior, nasal) to place the most vulnerable region centrally. The RNFL thickness falls in the thinnest 1% of the reference population at many locations around the disc, but particularly around the inferior temporal region. Arcuate RNFL lesions can be seen on both the enface and RNFL thickness maps (*bottom left*) and the probability of these measurements being normal is shown in the *top right* RNFL probability map, which is displayed in relation to the locations of the visual field test points. The lower right plots show the ganglion cell thickness over the macular region in relation to the visual field test points. (Courtesy of Topcon Healthcare.)

differing from FA, is proving very informative. OCTA can reveal many abnormalities, including neovascularisation owing to wet macular degeneration, new vessels, and retinal ischaemia associated with retinal vascular diseases and glaucoma. A growing number of quantification tools are available, providing metrics, such as vessel density.

7.11.7 Most common errors with OCT

1. Not optimally focusing and aligning the image (joystick devices).
2. Not properly instructing the patient prior to and during capture.
3. Trying to scan a patient with a poor quality tear film without optimising the tear film (ocular lubricants and clear blinking instructions).

4. Not checking scan quality before dismissing the patient.
5. Accepting poor centration, particularly for disc scans and OCTA scans.
6. Analysing thickness measurements of poor quality images.
7. Interpreting OCT or OCTA findings in isolation without considering the full clinical picture.

7.12 Fundus examination of the peripheral retina

The peripheral fundus is the area of the retina that includes the equator, where the retina is at its largest circumference to the anterior limit of the retina at the ora

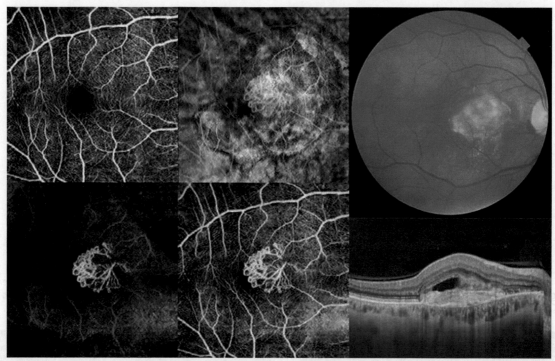

Fig. 7.55 Optical coherence tomography angiography (OCTA) showing choroidal neovascularisation (CNV; four images on the *left*); fundus photograph shows geographic atrophy and OCT shows SHRM (subretinal hyperreflective material) that includes the atrophy and the CNV, which is adjacent to subretinal fluid (Figure courtesy of Dr Carl Glittenberg and Karl Landsteiner Institute, Vienna).

serrata (Fig. 7.56). The equator is located by finding the vortex vein ampullae (Fig. 7.57), which are the dilated sacs of the vortex veins (these drain the choroid) and are typically one per quadrant, although there may be more. The peripheral retina is divided into superior and inferior halves by the long posterior ciliary nerves (Fig. 7.58) found at 3 and 9 o'clock between the equator and ora serrata. Peripheral retinal degenerations are common with increasing age and high myopia and include cystoid, lattice, paving-stone and snail-track degeneration plus white-with or -without pressure. (The Optos images have all been provided courtesy of Dr. Kelly Gibbons, Wodonga Eye Care, Australia.)

7.12.1 The evidence base: when and how to assess the peripheral retina

Minimal evidence exists to support *routine* dilated fundus examinations or any form of routine screening of the peripheral retina (section 1.5). Signs and/or symptoms that would prompt a dilated fundus examination to assess the peripheral retina include symptoms of acute-onset flashes and floaters, myopia, cataract surgery (particularly for high myopes and those with a history of eye trauma),[92] a family history of retinal detachment, monitoring previously recorded anomalies including naevi (see Fig. 7.35 and 8.47), increased likelihood of peripheral diabetic retinopathy,[93] and a small undilated pupil that would restrict the stereoscopic view of the central retina. There is increased risk of retinal detachment (Figs. 7.59 and 7.60) for both low (over 4× for –1 to –3) and moderate-high myopia (10× for –3 to –8),[94] with even higher risks for high myopia,[95] and this risk is increased in patients who are myopic with white-without-pressure (Fig. 7.61) and lattice degeneration (Fig. 7.62) and posterior vitreous detachments (PVDs).[96] Given the similar increased risk of myopic choroidal neovascularisation with the degree of myopia,[97] the importance in attempting to reduce myopia progression given the current pandemic of myopia is clear (section 4.14).

Acute-onset flashes and floaters are a particular concern for optometrists,[98] and a standardised patient study has shown that primary care clinicians use large variations in approaches when examining such patients.[4] The prevalence of retinal breaks (Figs. 7.60 and 7.63) in patients

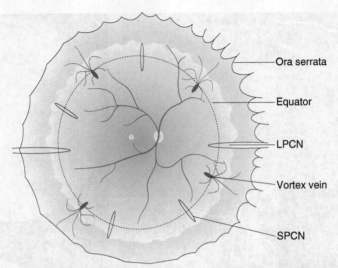

Ora serrata

Equator

LPCN

Vortex vein

SPCN

Fig. 7.56 Peripheral retina landmarks. The ora serrata marks the termination of the retina (and the beginning of the pars plana); the equator is the widest part of the eye (represented here with a *dotted circle*) and is represented by the vortex vein ampullae; the long posterior ciliary nerves (LPCN) and arteries are at the 3- and 9-o'clock positions of the fundus; the short posterior ciliary nerves (SPCN) are located approximately at the equator and may, like the vortex vein ampullae, be asymmetrical in each hemisphere.

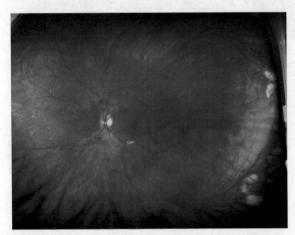

Fig. 7.57 Optomap showing vortex vein ampullae in the superior and inferior peripheral temporal thin retina of a myopic patient, showing chorioretinal atrophy and a highly visible long posterior ciliary nerve.

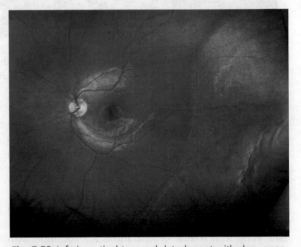

Fig. 7.59 Inferior retinal tear and detachment with slow creep.

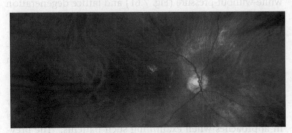

Fig. 7.58 Optomap showing a highly visible long posterior ciliary nerve in a patient with circinate retinopathy.

Fig. 7.60 Horseshoe tear with associated retinal detachment.

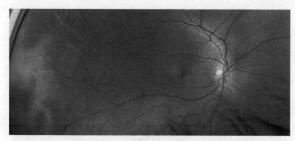

Fig. 7.61 White without pressure.

with symptoms of acute flashes and floaters self-referring or referred to secondary eye care is approximately 14%[3] so that the great majority of such patients have a PVD and not a retinal break. A detailed case history of the flashes and floaters plus determination of other risk factors for retinal detachment, slit-lamp examination of the anterior vitreous for Shafer's sign (section 7.1.3, No. 6), and a dilated peripheral retina examination should be performed.[4]

Many fundus abnormalities in the peripheral retina are missed with direct or monocular indirect ophthalmoscopy through an undilated or dilated pupil, including but not limited to retinal holes/tears (see Figs. 7.60 and 7.63), retinal detachments (see Fig. 7.59 and 7.60), retinoschisis (Fig. 7.64), intraretinal haemorrhages, exudates, and infarcts, neovascularisation, lattice degeneration (see Fig 7.62), white without pressure (see Fig. 7.61), naevi (see Fig. 7.35, 8.47), and tumours (Fig. 7.65) (section 1.5). Dilated fundus biomicroscopy provides a superior assessment of the peripheral retina than direct or monocular indirect ophthalmoscopy (section 7.10.1), but head-band BIO provides the gold standard assessment of the peripheral retina. It provides simultaneous viewing of approximately eight disc diameters (about 35°) of the fundus compared with less than two disc diameters with the direct ophthalmoscope. Other advantages include a quick assessment of the entire fundus periphery and vitreous (see Table 7.4), with subsequent easy localisation of most lesions owing to the very large field of view. This can be especially useful when examining the fundus in children who have been cyclopleged and special populations. Different lenses can be used to create different magnifications. The +20 D or +22 D aspheric lenses are recommended for routine use. Lower-powered lenses (+14 D or +15 D) provide higher magnification and may be used if the patient is bedridden or in a reclined wheelchair such that fundus biomicroscopy is not an option.

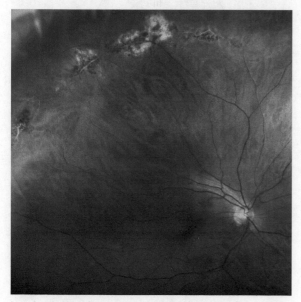

Fig. 7.62 Extensive lattice degeneration.

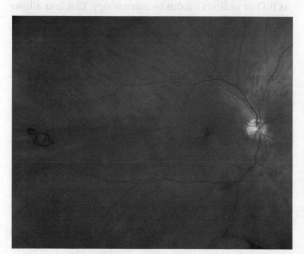

Fig. 7.63 Retinal hole with operculum.

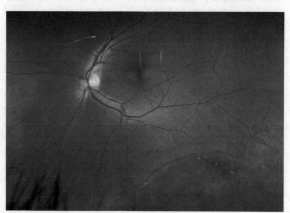

Fig. 7.64 Retinoschisis.

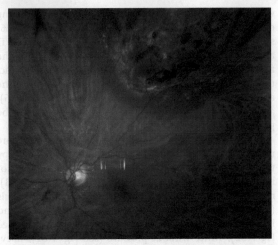

Fig. 7.65 Optomap showing melanoma.

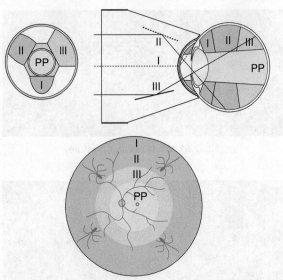

Fig. 7.66 Diagrammatical representation of the Goldmann 3-mirror contact lens demonstrating the central lens for examining the posterior pole (PP); the thumbnail-shaped mirror angled at 60° and used for gonioscopic assessment of the anterior chamber angle as well as examination of the far-peripheral fundus in a dilated eye **(I)**; the rectangular-shaped mirror angled at 66° and used to assess the peripheral fundus (II) and the trapezoidal-shaped mirror angled at 76° and used for examination of the equatorial fundus (III).

They are somewhat more difficult to manipulate because they must be raised farther from the patient's eye to get an image and of course have a smaller field of view. Smaller, higher-powered lenses (+28 D or +30 D) provide a larger field of view, but are rarely used because of their low magnification. They may be considered by a clinician who has small hands and difficulty manipulating the larger +20 D lenses, during scleral indentation owing to easier lens manipulation around the scleral indentor, and when the patient has small pupils. Scleral indentation can be used in conjunction with BIO to further evaluate peripheral areas of the fundus, such as the ora serrata, in a dynamic manner. The main disadvantages of BIO are the reversed and inverted image (making interpretation and recording a challenge to learn initially), the need for a chair that will recline, need for mydriasis, and the lower magnification provided (~3× compared with 9 to 18× with fundus biomicroscopy and 16× slit-lamp magnification, and 15× with direct ophthalmoscopy). Finally, the potential exists for light toxicity with prolonged exposure.[73] Yellow condensing lenses or yellow filters attached to clear lenses may be used and are recommended for students. They can also reduce patient glare and discomfort.

The 3-mirror Universal lens allows the patient to remain at the biomicroscope and does not need to be placed into a supine position; with established slit-lamp skills, the technique is easier to learn than scleral indentation. The 'thumbnail' mirror (angled 59° to 64° from the horizontal plane) is used for gonioscopy (section 7.5), but it can also be used to view the far peripheral fundus through a well-dilated pupil. The rectangular mirror (angled at ~ 66°) is used to examine more posteriorly to the thumbnail, but still in the fundus periphery. The third

mirror is trapezoidal in shape (angled at ~76°) and is used to examine the equatorial fundus (Figs. 7.27 and 7.66). Because of the limited field of view, the 3-mirror lens is not used for general assessment. Instead, it is employed when lesions are detected with other techniques, such as BIO or indirect fundus biomicroscopy. This lens allows a stereoscopic view that is different from the indirect techniques. Note also that the central lens is an excellent tool for assessment of the macula (and disc), especially when fine stereopsis detail is critical (e.g., macula oedema). Other disadvantages of the 3-mirror lens include the need for corneal anaesthesia and the lack of a dynamic view so that layer separation is not possible and there is greater difficulty in lesion localisation.

Ultra-wide imaging uses a scanning laser retinal imaging system to provide a 200° image or 'optomap' of the retina using red and green lasers (Fig. 7.67). It provides all the advantages of other fundus imaging systems (archiving for accurate recording and monitoring; can be shown to patients to provide enhanced patient counselling and allows computer enhancement of images and transmission of digital images through computer networks). The images can be seen in red-free or green-free formats, which allows differentiation between retinal (seen in green-free)

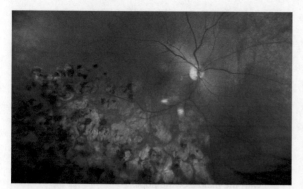

Fig. 7.67 Sectoral pan retinal photocoagulation (PRP) scarring.

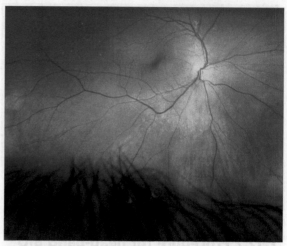

Fig. 7.69 Eyelashes are common on optomap images and can obscure lesions, such as this partly obscured large Congenital hypetrophy of the retinal pigment epithelium (CHRPE).

and choroidal (seen in red-free) abnormalities and the instrument shows excellent resistance to the effects of cataract (although central cataracts can show up as artefacts, even Mittendorf dots, Fig. 7.68, which may appear as a small dark 'retinal' lesion).[99] Eyelashes are very commonly seen (Fig. 7.69). However, although optomaps provide good specificity, they miss treatable conditions in both the mid-peripheral (moderate sensitivity) and particularly the far-peripheral retina (low sensitivity) when compared with a dilated fundus examination.[100-102] Other disadvantages are the need for some manipulation of the patient's position to get their eye in a correct position, the loss of part of the image owing to the patient's eyelashes (Fig. 7.69; this can be improved using eyelid retraction with a cotton bud or tape), and the image colour, in that the fundus does not look the same as it does in the white light of ophthalmoscopy.[101] There are conditions present in the peripheral

retina that do not typically need referral, such as CHRPE (Congenital hypertrophy of the retinal pigment epithelium), bear tracks, naevi, and window defects (sections 8.6–8.9), and these peripheral retina conditions need to be fully understood if ultra-wide image screening is to be conducted because it will otherwise lead to false–positive referrals,[103] which are not in the best interests of patients or the referral system (section 1.5). Fundus autofluorescence assessments have recently been added to the system, which allow useful assessments of conditions that include fluorophores, such as optic nerve and retinal drusen (Figs. 7.70 and 7.71) and retinitis pigmentosa .

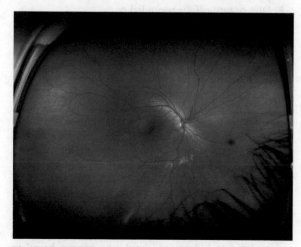

Fig. 7.68 An optomap artefact: the dark 'lesion' is a shadow caused by a Mittendorf dot.

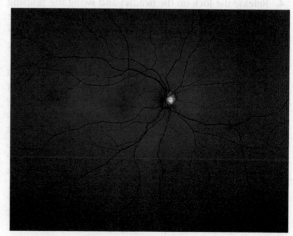

Fig. 7.70 Optomap autofluorescent image of optic nerve drusen.

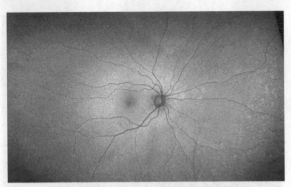

Fig. 7.71 Optomap autofluorescent image of peripheral drusen.

7.12.2 Procedure for head-band BIO

(Summary in Box 7.3)

(See video 7.13.)

1. Wear your glasses if you use them. You will be viewing the areal image between the condensing lens and the instrument. Presbyopic examiners will need to use +2D lenses in the eyepieces of the BIO. Younger examiners sometimes find that removing the +2D lenses allows them to converge on the image more easily.

2. Explain the test to the patient: "I am going to examine the health of the inside of your eyes with light from the head unit and a lens held close to your eye." Obtain informed consent and instil an appropriate mydriatic (section 7.8).

3. Adjust the back and top of the headband of the instrument to allow for a comfortable fit. The fit may need to be readjusted as the eyepieces are adjusted.

4. Release the lock on the headset and swing the housing unit down in front of your eyes until the eyepieces are as close as possible and approximately perpendicular to your line of sight. The closer the eyepieces are to the eyes, the larger the field of view.

5. Direct the ophthalmoscope light at your thumb or at a wall at arm's length and adjust the eyepieces for your interpupillary distance so that the spot of light is exactly centred in the field of view for each eye. Adjust the mirror vertically until the spot of light is situated in the upper half of the field of view (± 4° adjustment arm). This allows the illumination beam to pass above the observation beam to minimise reflections during patient examination. Most instruments possess this adjustment.

6. Adjust the illumination intensity to low to medium-low and the illumination beam to the largest spot size that can be used for the patient's pupil size. For a dilated pupil, use the largest spot size. A smaller spot size may be considered if the pupils are not fully dilated.

Box 7.3 Summary of head-band binocular indirect ophthalmoscopy (BIO) procedure

1. Dilate the patient's eyes.
2. Recline the patient to approximately hip level.
3. Adjust the headband.
4. Adjust the eyepieces and mirror vertically so the spot of light is in the upper half of the field of view.
5. Adjust the illumination intensity.
6. Dim or turn off the room lights.
7. Ask the patient to look straight up to the ceiling.
8. Align the two reflections from the condensing lens with the middle of the pupil.
9. Gradually pull the lens directly towards you until the fundus detail fills the entire lens.
10. Examine the fundus in a systematic, predetermined order (usually clockwise), filling the condensing lens as much as possible.

---

7. Ask the patient to remove any glasses and explain that you are going to recline the chair as at a visit to the dentist. Adjust the chair to the reclining position, so that the patient is at approximately hip level. The supine position allows you to stand approximately opposite the area of the fundus being viewed, optimising stereopsis and the extent of viewing area while minimising back strain.[75] Examination with the patient seated upright can also be performed if reclining is not possible. The inferior and superior fundi are more difficult to examine with a seated patient because the light source must be well above the patient's head to view the inferior peripheral fundus and towards the patient's lap to see the superior peripheral fundus.

8. Dim or turn off the room lights.

9. Pick up the aspheric condensing lens with the white or silver edge of the lens casing towards the patient to minimise reflections and optical aberrations. Hold the lens between the index finger and the thumb. The little (or the third) finger can be used to retract the upper eyelid and allow for stable extension of the lens away from the patient's eye, while acting as a pivot, enabling the observer to tilt the lens in all planes merely by rocking the lens system. The other eyelid may be retracted with the thumb of the opposite hand. Alternatively, the little (or the third) finger of the opposite hand may be employed so that this second index finger can also be used to help stabilise the lens. The lens can be moved with critical control closer or further from the eye by increasing or decreasing the extension of the little finger stabilising on the patient's eyelids. Ambidexterity should be practised and is required for scleral indentation.

10. Novices will want to view the recognisable posterior pole first, so should ask the patient to look straight up to the ceiling if in supine position or over your shoulder if seated upright.

11. Direct the BIO light source so that it is centred on the patient's pupil. Introduce the condensing lens close to the patient's eye (2 to 4 cm) such that the external eye can be seen through the lens and with slight magnification. Centre the pupil in the condensing lens (observe the red reflex) and align the two reflections from the +20 D lens surfaces with each other and in the middle of the pupil. Gradually move the lens away from the patient's eye (towards you), and fundus detail will become progressively magnified until the red reflex fills the entire area of the lens.

12. Keep the pupil centred in the lens at all times or the fundus view will be lost. Only slight misalignment of any part of the optical system will cause shadows, distortion, or complete loss of the view. Stabilisation of the lens with a finger from the second hand helps to minimise this fluctuation. When loss of the image occurs, move the lens towards the eye again, until the pupil can be recognised and centred, and pull the lens back towards you again to maximise the image in the lens.

13. Keep the headband unit at arm's length to the lens. When the examiner moves closer to the lens, difficulties with accommodation, convergence, and loss of binocularity may occur, as will a smaller field of view.

14. If reflections from the condensing lens block visualisation of the fundus, displace the reflections by tilting the lens slightly. Excessive tilting, however, induces astigmatism and will distort the fundus image.

15. To view the different regions of the fundus, change position around the patient and tilt the lens so that the optical system formed by the patient's pupil and fundus, the condensing lens, and your pupils remain aligned along the widest part of the patient's pupil. To examine the superior fundus, for example, ask the patient to look upwards while you direct the illuminating beam towards the superior fundus. A 'full' lens image in this position will show approximately 8 DD of the fundus near the superior equator. Examine farther into the peripheral fundus by moving the light source anteriorly (towards the ora serrata), making sure the elements of the optical system remain in alignment so that the image continues to fill the lens as much as possible. To do this, you must bend along the line of sight, but in the opposite direction (i.e., towards the patient's feet). Because the image is reversed and inverted, attempting to shift the field of view in one direction will cause the image to move in the opposite direction. It helps to remember here that only the lens view is reversed and inverted; that is, if you wish to see more temporally, direct the light in that direction; more superiorly, direct the light towards the superior fundus, and so on.

16. Stereopsis is achieved by imaging both of the examiner's pupils within the patient's pupil. This is facilitated by a large patient pupil with maximum dilation. During the examination of the patient's periphery, the patient's fixation is directed towards the sector that is to be examined. The pupil relative to the examiner's perspective is oval, with the long axis of this pupil perpendicular to the patient's line of sight. To maximise stereopsis in these situations, keep your two pupils aligned with this long axis. If the patient's pupil is very large or they are not looking too far off axis, stereopsis is still possible without this alignment with the long axis, but it is less likely and less consistently achieved.

17. It is advised that you examine the fundus in a systematic, predetermined order. Some clinicians elect to examine the regions of the equatorial and peripheral fundus before the posterior pole to allow the light-sensitive patient time to adapt (unless the posterior pole has just been examined with fundus biomicroscopy anyway). Direct the patient gaze towards each individual sector until all eight sectors of the fundus have been examined (plus the posterior pole). Moving clockwise for the right eye and anti-clockwise for the left eye is a good initial method.

7.12.3 Additional techniques: Scleral indentation, Goldmann 3-mirror, and ultra-wide field retinal imaging

Scleral indentation with BIO provides a dynamic assessment of the peripheral fundus, allowing tissue separation and facilitating the detection of previously undetected retinal tears. The technique also allows further examination of lesions detected with other methods (e.g., retinal breaks for the presence of fluid cuffs; lattice degeneration for the presence of breaks; vitreoretinal traction). Rarely, the clinician may elect to perform scleral indentation in all sectors if risk factors warrant a closer look when first examination with BIO noted no breaks. Generally, however, indentation is targeted to a previously identified lesion.

Procedure for scleral indentation with BIO

1. Perform BIO or dynamic fundus biomicroscopy of all sectors and determine the area(s) of the periphery requiring indentation. Note both the clock position and the anterior-to-posterior position (relative to the equator and ora serrata).

2. Explain the specific reasons for scleral indentation to the patient. For example: "I am now going to apply a slight pressure to the outside of the eye to better view

a region of the inside of the eye. You may note mild discomfort or a pressure-like sensation during the procedure.". Topical anaesthetic may be considered.

3. Recline the patient. Seated examination is not recommended.

4. Ask the patient to look in the opposite direction to the area to be viewed. Place the indentor tip on the fold of the eyelid (just beyond the tarsal plate) at the clock position on the globe where the lesion was localised. The indentor may be placed with the curve following or opposite the globe, depending on patient anatomy.

5. Direct the patient fixation back towards the indentor and, as the patient moves their eye, have the indentor follow the globe back into the orbit. The indentor should be placed approximately 7 mm posterior to the limbus to indent the ora serrata, and 13 to 14 mm to indent the equator. If the orbital anatomy is obstructing the placement of the indentor, tilt the patient's head slightly to facilitate manipulation of the instrument. For example, if the brow is prominent and in the way, tilt the head back somewhat. Maintain indentor position without pressure on the globe. Tangential pressure only is required.

6. Introduce the BIO light source. Note that 'on axis' indentor positioning can be determined in advance of introducing the condensing lens by noting a shadow in the red reflex in the pupil. When the lens is introduced, the optical system formed by the indented region of the fundus, the patient's pupil, the condensing lens, and your pupils must be perfectly on axis to observe the indented retina. Do not apply pressure, but gently roll the indentor laterally and forward and backward. If the indentor is not seen, move the lens away in order to re-orient your view. You may need to alter the orientation so that the light is aimed directly at the indentor tip. Also check the anterior-to-posterior positioning of the indentor. If the elevated area is seen but not in the proper position, move the indentor in the opposite direction expected (away from the centre of the lens) as the view is reversed and inverted. Another way to obtain gross orientation is to remember that when the patient is looking into an extreme position of gaze and you direct your light source directly into their pupil, the equator should be in view. To extend the final four to five disc diameters between the equator and the ora serrata, you must bend away from the area being examined and direct the light up under the iris.

7. Observe all areas in question. For the more difficult temporal and nasal areas, the superior eyelid may be drawn downwards or the inferior eyelid drawn upwards with the indentor. If this is unsuccessful, the indentor may be disinfected and placed directly on the anaesthetised conjunctiva.

Procedure for Goldmann 3-mirror examination

1. Explain the specific reasons for using the lens. Inform the patient that it is a contact lens used with local anaesthetic and a cushioning fluid between the lens and the eye. Explain that they may feel some pressure from the lens and will likely feel the lens on the eyelids, but will feel no discomfort with the instillation of anaesthetic. Obtain informed consent and dilate the patient's pupils (section 7.8).

2. Having determined the anterior-to-posterior positioning of the lesion to be evaluated, choose the mirror most likely to detect the lesion; that is, for a lesion at the ora serrata, use the thumbnail mirror; for a lesion in the peripheral retina, use the rectangular mirror; and for the midperiphery or equatorial fundus, use the trapezoidal mirror.

3. Prepare the patient at the slit-lamp and prepare the lens for insertion. Apply the lens to the eye. Usually, the patient can maintain a primary gaze position for the examination of most areas of the fundus.

4. Rotate the lens such that the chosen mirror is positioned 180° from the lesion. To examine the posterior pole, use the central contact lens.

5. With the biomicroscope in a 'full-back' position, direct the slit-lamp light into the mirror of choice. Move the slit-lamp forwards until the fundus is in focus, then rotate and tilt the lens to locate the lesion. If the lesion is more posterior to that portion of the fundus which is being viewed, tilt the lens away from the mirror; if more anterior (i.e., more peripheral), tilt the lens towards the mirror.

6. Once the lesion has been fully examined, remove the lens.

Procedure for ultra-wide field retinal imaging

A full description of the imaging capture procedure is not provided because it is relatively straightforward, although experience in positioning the patient is needed. Although images can be obtained undilated, dilation is strongly recommended for some patients, including those with diabetes, high myopia (Fig. 7.72), symptoms of acute-onset flashes and floaters, and when monitoring conditions. Keep tape next to the instrument because lid taping is required for patients with ptosis, naturally narrow palpebral fissures, some patients with deep-set eyes, and when attempting to image the inferior retina. In addition, regular cleaning is required to avoid dust artefacts.

7.12.4 Recording of the peripheral retina

If possible, all peripheral retina findings are best recorded as an image and this is where ultra-wide field

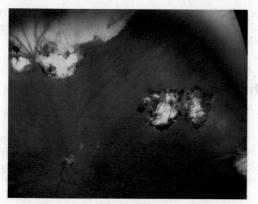

Fig. 7.72 Peripheral myopic chorioretinal atrophy.

imaging is particularly useful (see Figs. 7.59 to 7.72). Otherwise fundus findings should be recorded with a sketch accompanied by brief explanatory notes. By convention, fundus details are recorded with two circles, one within the other. The inner circle represents the equator and

the larger one surrounding it represents the ora serrata (Fig. 7.73). Note that, although the outside circle is larger, the circumference of the ora serrata is actually less than the equator, the widest part of the globe. Determining the appropriate anterior-to-posterior location in the fundus can be facilitated by certain normal landmarks in the fundus (see Fig. 7.56).

Specific chief complaints: If the patient has a presenting complaint that could suggest a peripheral retina abnormality and no abnormalities are detected, your recording should be more detailed to highlight that your examination was full and appropriate. For example, you should record that no retinal breaks or PVDs were seen in a patient with acute-onset flashes and floaters; if there were myopia, it would be appropriate to indicate that there were no lattice degeneration or white without pressure or other myopic peripheral degenerations. The results of a Shafer's sign test should also be recorded (section 7.1.3, No. 6)

Any normal variation in appearance should be recorded (e.g., reticular peripheral degeneration, CHRPE, window defects, naevi; sections 8.8, 8.9, and 8.10) and imaged if appropriate.

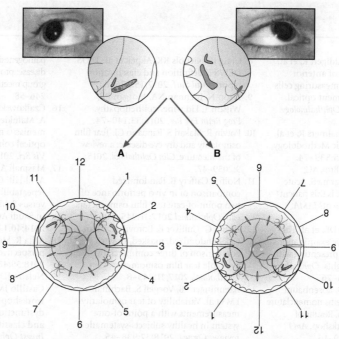

Fig. 7.73 Demonstration of recording methods for binocular indirect ophthalmoscopy (BIO) and other indirect techniques. The top portion of the figure demonstrates the patient's position of gaze and diagrammatic representation of the view in the binocular indirect lens (+20 D). Option A represents mentally reversing and inverting the image seen and recording on the patient's chart. Asymmetric and complicated lesions are more difficult to interpret and document properly in this manner. Option B demonstrates how the examiner may draw the lesion exactly as it was seen and in the proper clock position, but with the recording paper turned upside down.

7.12.5 Interpretation of peripheral retina findings

Many changes can be noted in the peripheral retina, some of which are benign and others that have quite a significant risk to vision if left undetected. Benign ocular findings include peripheral cystoid degeneration, which is present in essentially all patients over the age of 8 years. Disorders, such as posterior vitreous detachment, white without pressure, lattice degeneration, vitreoretinal traction tufts, commotio retinae, pars planitis, retinal breaks, retinal detachment, and others, may be sight threatening and may go undetected without a dilated examination with BIO and possibly scleral indentation. Findings, such as malignant melanoma, can be life threatening. Retinal degenerations, breaks, and shallow detachments are much more obvious with indentation. The contrast of a break is enhanced as the edge of the torn retina appears more whitened, whereas the tear itself appears to open and becomes more red. Subtle breaks and traction may be missed without this technique. Fluid cuffs surrounding breaks are representative of subclinical or progressive retinal detachment and observation is facilitated with scleral indentation.

7.12.6 Most common errors using the head-band BIO

1. Not adjusting the instrument properly, leading to diplopia, eyestrain, or compromised stereopsis.
2. Not reducing the intensity of the light source or using a yellow filtered lens to minimise patient photosensitivity.
3. Starting the examination of a sector while already in the bent position. This not only limits the view of the periphery, but will cause you to miss sections of the equatorial fundus.
4. Getting confused regarding where a lesion is. Understanding and drawing the inverted and reversed image seen with BIO must be practised.
5. Moving the indentor in the opposite direction to that which is needed to facilitate the view owing to the reversed and inverted image orientation.

References

1. Invernizzi A, Marchi S, Aldigeri R, et al. Objective quantification of anterior chamber inflammation: measuring cells and flare by anterior segment optical coherence tomography. *Ophthalmology*. 2017;124:1670
2. Wolffsohn JS, Arita R, Chalmers R, et al. TFOS DEWS II Diagnostic Methodology report. *Ocul Surf*. 2017;15:539–74.
3. Hollands H, Johnson D, Brox AC, Almeida D, Simel DL, Sharma S. Acute-onset floaters and flashes: is this patient at risk for retinal detachment? *JAMA*. 2009;302:2243–9.
4. Shah R, Edgar DF, Harle DE, et al. The content of optometric eye examinations for a presbyopic patient presenting with symptoms of flashing lights. *Ophthalmic Physiol Opt*. 2009;29:105–26.
5. Jabs DA, Nussenblatt RB, Rosenbaum JT. Standardization of uveitis nomenclature for reporting clinical data. Results of the first international workshop. *Am J Ophthalmol*. 2005;140:509–16.
6. Wolffsohn JS, Naroo SA, Christie C et al. Anterior eye health recording. *Cont Lens Anterior Eye*. 2015 ;38:266–71.
7. Chylack LT, Wolfe J, Singer D, et al. The Lens Opacities Classification System III. *Arch Ophthalmol*. 1993;111:831–6.
8. Craig JP, Nichols KK, Akpek et al. TFOS DEWS II definition and classification report. *Ocul Surf*. 2017;15:276–83.
9. Efron N, Brennan NA, Morgan PB, Wilson T. Lid wiper epitheliopathy. *Prog Retin Eye Res*. 2016;53:140–74.
10. Potvin R, Makari S, Rapuano CJ. Tear film osmolarity and dry eye disease: a review of the literature. *Clin Ophthalmol*. 2015; 9:2039–47.
11. Nolfi J, Caffery B. Randomized comparison of in vivo performance of two point-of-care tear film osmometers. *Clin Ophthalmol* 2017;11:945–50.
12. Rocha G, Gulliver E, Borovik A, Chan CC. Randomized, masked, in vitro comparison of three commercially available tear film osmometers. *Clin Ophthalmol*. 2017;11:243–8.
13. Baenninger PB, Voegeli S, Bachmann LM et al. Variability of tear osmolarity measurements with a point-of-care system in healthy subjects-systematic review. *Cornea*. 2018;37:938–45.
14. Ganesalingam K, Ismail S, Sherwin T, Craig JP. Molecular evidence for the role of inflammation in dry eye disease. *Clin Exp Optom*. 2019;102:446–54.
15. Baudouin C, Aragona P, Messmer EM, et al. Role of hyperosmolarity in the pathogenesis and management of dry eye disease: proceedings of the OCEAN group meeting. *Ocul Surf*. 2013;11: 246–58.
16. Czajkowski G, Kaluzny BJ, Laudencka A, Malukiewicz G, Kaluzny JJ. Tear meniscus measurement by spectral optical coherence tomography. *Optom Vis Sci*. 2012;89:336–42.
17. Masmali A, Alqahtani TA, Alharbi A, El-Hiti GA. Comparative study of repeatability of phenol red thread test versus Schirmer test in normal adults in Saudi Arabia. *Eye Contact Lens*. 2014;40:127–31.
18. Arita R. Meibography: a Japanese perspective. *Invest Ophthalmol Vis Sci*. 2018;59:48–55.
19. Nelson JD, Shimazaki J, Benitez-Del-Castillo JM, et al. The international workshop on meibomian gland dysfunction: report of the definition and classification subcommittee. *Invest Ophthalmol Vis Sci*. 2011;52: 1930–7.
20. Prokopich CL, Bitton E, Caffrey B, et al. Screening, diagnosis and management of dry eye disease: practical guidelines for Canadian optometrists. *Can J Optom*. 2014;76(suppl. 1):1–31.

21. Guillemin IBC, Chalmers R, Baudouin C, Arnould B. Appraisal of patient-reported outcome instruments available for randomized clinical trials in dry eye: revisiting the standards. *Ocul Surf.* 2012;10:84–99.

22. Yamaguchi M, Kutsuna M, Uno T, Zheng X, Kodama T, Ohashi Y. Marx line: fluorescein staining line on the inner lid as an indicator of meibomian gland function. *Am J Ophthalmol.* 2006;141:669–75.

23. Nichols KK, Foulks GN, Bron AJ, et al. The international workshop on meibomian gland dysfunction: executive summary. *Invest Ophthalmol Vis Sci.* 2011;52:1922–9.

24. Begley C, Caffery B, Chalmers R, Situ P, Simpson T, Nelson JD. Review and analysis of grading scales for ocular surface staining. *Ocul Surf.* 2019;17:208–20.

25. Tomlinson A, Bron A, Korb D, et al. The international workshop on meibomian gland dysfunction: report of the diagnosis subcommittee. *Invest Ophthalmol Vis Sci.* 2011;52:1930–7.

26. Cho P, Douthwaite W. The relation between invasive and noninvasive tear break-up time. *Optom Vis Sci.* 1995;72:17–22.

27. Bron AJ, Evans VE, Smith JA. Grading of corneal and conjunctival staining in the context of other dry eye tests. *Cornea.* 2003;22:640–50.

28. Sullivan BD, Crews LA, Sönmez B, et al. Clinical utility of objectives tests for dry eye disease: variability over time and implications for clinical trials and disease management. *Cornea.* 2012;31:1000–8.

29. Tucker NA, Codère F. The effect of fluorescein volume on lacrimal outflow transit time. *Ophthalmic Plast Reconstr Surg.* 1994;10:256–9.

30. Pandit RJ, Taylor R. Mydriasis and glaucoma: exploding the myth. A systematic review. *Diabet Med.* 2000;17:693–9.

31. Foster PJ, Devereux JG, Alsbirk PH, et al. Detection of gonioscopically occludable angles and primary angle closure glaucoma by estimation of limbal chamber depth in Asians: modified grading scheme. *Br J Ophthalmol.* 2000;84:186–92.

32. Campbell P, Redmond T, Agarwal R, Marshall LR, Evans BJW. Repeatability and comparison of clinical techniques for anterior chamber angle assessment. *Ophthalmic Physiol Opt.* 2015;35:170–8.

33. Dabasia PL, Edgar DF, Murdoch IE, Lawrenson JG. Noncontact screening methods for the detection of narrow anterior chamber angles. *Invest Ophthalmol Vis Sci.* 2015;56:3929–35.

34. Bailey IL, Bullimore MA, Raasch TW, Taylor HR. Clinical grading and the effects of scaling. *Invest Ophthalmol Vis Sci* 1991;32:422–32.

35. Johnson TV, Ramulu PY, Quigley HA, Singman EL. Low sensitivity of the Van Herick method for detecting gonioscopic angle closure independent of observer expertise. *Am J Ophthalmol.* 2018;195:63–71.

36. Sun X, Dai Y, Chen Y, et al. Primary angle closure glaucoma: what we know and what we don't know. *Prog Retin Eye Res.* 2017;57:26–45.

37. Browning DJ, Scott AQ, Peterson CB, Warnock J, Zhang Z. The risk of missing angle neovascularization by omitting screening gonioscopy in acute central retinal vein occlusion. *Ophthalmology.* 1998;105:776–84.

38. Dabasia PL, Edgar DF, Garway-Heath DF, Lawrenson JG. A survey of current and anticipated use of standard and specialist equipment by UK optometrists. *Ophthalmic Physiol Opt.* 2014;34:592–613.

39. Gordon MO, Beiser JA, Brandt JD, et al. The ocular hypertension treatment study: baseline factors that predict the onset of primary open-angle glaucoma. *Arch Ophthalmol.* 2002;120:714–20.

40. Johnson M, Kass MA, Moses RA, Grodzki WJ. Increased corneal thickness simulating elevated intraocular pressure. *Arch Ophthalmol.* 1978;96:664–5.

41. Doughty MJ, Zaman ML. Human corneal thickness and its impact on intraocular pressure measures: a review and meta-analysis approach. *Surv Ophthalmol.* 2000;44:367–408.

42. Brandt JD, Beiser JA, Kass MA, Gordon MO. Central corneal thickness in the Ocular Hypertension Treatment Study (OHTS). *Ophthalmology.* 2001;108:1779–88.

43. Emara BY, Tingey DP, Probst LE, Motolko MA. Central corneal thickness in low-tension glaucoma. *Can J Ophthalmol.* 1999;34:319–24.

44. Chihara E. Assessment of true intraocular pressure: the gap between theory and practical data. *Surv Ophthalmol.* 2008;53:203–18.

45. Belovay GW, Goldberg I. The thick and thin of the central corneal thickness in glaucoma. *Eye (Lond)* 2018;32:915–23.

46. Medeiros FA, Weinreb RN. Is corneal thickness an independent risk factor for glaucoma? *Ophthalmology.* 2012;119:435–6.

47. Sng CCA, Ang M, Barton K. Central corneal thickness in glaucoma. *Curr Opin Ophthalmol.* 2017;28:120–6.

48. Rozema JJ, Wouters K, Mathysen DGP, Tassignon MJ. Overview of the repeatability, reproducibility, and agreement of the biometry values provided by various ophthalmic devices. *Am J Ophthalmol.* 2014;158:1111–20

49. Read SA, Collins MJ. Diurnal variation of corneal shape and thickness. *Optom Vis Sci.* 2009;86:170–80.

50. Aghaian E, Choe JE, Lin S, Stamper RL. Central corneal thickness of Caucasians, Chinese, Hispanics, Filipinos, African Americans, and Japanese in a glaucoma clinic. *Ophthalmology.* 2004;111:2211–9.

51. Hollands H, Johnson D, Hollands S, Simel DL, Jinapriya D, Sharma S. Do findings on routine examination identify patients at risk for primary open-angle glaucoma? The rational clinical examination systematic review. *JAMA.* 2013;309:2035–42.

52. Heijl A, Leske MC, Bengtsson B, Hyman L, Bengtsson B, Hussein M. Reduction of intraocular pressure and glaucoma progression: results from the Early Manifest Glaucoma Trial. *Arch Ophthalmol.* 2002;120:1268–79.

53. Shaikh NM, Shaikh S, Singh K, Manche E. Progression to end-stage glaucoma after laser in situ keratomileusis. *J Cataract Refract Surg.* 2002;28:356–9.

54. Park SJK, Ang GS, Nicholas S, Wells AP. The effect of thin, thick and normal corneas on Goldmann intraocular pressure measurements and correction formulae in individual eyes. *Ophthalmology.* 2012;119:443–9.

55. Tonnu PA, Ho T, Newson T, et al. The influence of central corneal thickness and age on intraocular pressure measured by pneumotonometry, noncontact tonometry, the Tono-Pen XL, and Goldmann applanation tonometry. *Br J Ophthalmol.* 2005;89:851–4.

56. Cook JA, Botello AP, Elders A, et al. Systematic review of the agreement of tonometers with Goldmann applanation tonometry. *Ophthalmology.* 2012;119:1552–7.

57. Khan S, Clarke J, Kotecha A. Comparison of optometrist glaucoma referrals against published guidelines. *Ophthalmic Physiol Opt.* 2012;32:472–7.

58. Sood V, Ramanathan US. Self-Monitoring of intraocular pressure outside of normal office hours using rebound tonometry: initial clinical experience in patients with normal tension glaucoma. *J Glaucoma*. 2016;25:807–11.

59. Wang AS, Alencar LM, Weinreb RN, et al. Repeatability and reproducibility of Goldmann applanation, dynamic contour and ocular response analyzer tonometry. *J Glaucoma*. 2013;22:127–32.

60. Susanna BN, Ogata NG, Daga FB, Susanna CN, Diniz-Filho A, Medeiros FA. Association between rates of visual field progression and intraocular pressure measurements obtained by different tonometers. *Ophthalmology* 2019;126:49–54.

61. Schweitzer JA, Ervin M, Berdahl JP. Assessment of corneal hysteresis measured by the ocular response analyzer as a screening tool in patients with glaucoma. Clin Ophthamol 2018; 12:1809–13.

62. Lavanya R, Baskaran M, Kumar RS, et al. Risk of acute angle closure and changes in intraocular pressure after pupillary dilation in Asian subjects with narrow angles. *Ophthalmology*. 2012;119: 474–80.

63. van Minderhout HM, Joosse MV, Grootendorst DC, Schalij-Delfos NE. Adverse reactions following routine anticholinergic eye drops in a paediatric population: an observational cohort study. *BMJ Open*. 2015;5:e008798.

64. Nucci P, de Pellegrin M, Brancato R. Atlantoaxial dislocation related to instilling eyedrops in a patient with Down's syndrome. *Am J Ophthalmol*. 1996;122:908–10.

65. Gaynes BI. Monitoring drug safety; cardiac events in routine mydriasis. *Optom Vis Sci*. 1998;75:245–6.

66. Enyedi LB, Dev S, Cox TA. A comparison of the Marcus Gunn and alternating light tests for afferent pupillary defects. *Ophthalmology*. 1998;105: 871–3.

67. Chang DS, Xu L, Boland MV, Friedman DS. Accuracy of pupil assessment for the detection of glaucoma. *Ophthalmology*. 2013;120:2217–25.

68. Kawasaki A, Moore P, Kardon RH. Long-term fluctuation of relative afferent pupillary defect in subjects with normal visual function. *Am J Ophthalmol*. 1996;122:875–82.

59. Lam BL, Thompson HS. A unilateral cataract produces a relative afferent pupillary defect in the contralateral eye. *Ophthalmology*. 1990;97:334–8.

70. Hrynchak P, Hutchings N, Jones D, Simpson T. A comparison of cup-to-disc ratio evaluation in normal subjects using stereo biomicroscopy and digital imaging of the optic nerve head. *Ophthalmic Physiol Opt*. 2003;23:51–9.

71. Grey RH, Hart JC. Screening for sight threatening eye disease. Stereoscopic viewing of the retina needed to identify maculopathy. *Br Med J*. 1996;312:440–1.

72. Fingeret M, Medeiros FA, Susanna Jr R, Weinreb RN. Five rules to evaluate the optic disc and retinal nerve fiber layer for glaucoma. *Optometry*. 2005;76: 661–8.

73. Bradnam MS, Montgomery DM, Moseley H, Dutton GN. Quantitative assessment of the blue-light hazard during indirect ophthalmoscopy and the increase in the 'safe' operating period achieved using a yellow lens. *Ophthalmology*. 1995;102:799–804.

74. Bartnik SE, Copeland SP, Aicken AJ, Turner AW. Optometry-facilitated teleophthalmology: an audit of the first year in Western Australia. *Clin Exp Optom*. 2018;101:700–3.

75. Kitzmann AS, Fethke NB, Baratz KH, Zimmerman MB, Hackbarth DJ, Gehrs KM. A survey study of musculoskeletal disorders among eye care physicians compared with family medicine physicians. *Ophthalmology*. 2011;119:213–20.

76. Jonas JB, Budde WM, Panda-Jonas S. Ophthalmoscopic evaluation of the optic nerve head. *Surv Ophthalmol*. 1999;43:293–320.

77. Henderson AD, Biousse V, Newman NJ, Lamirel C, Wright DW, Bruce BB. Grade III or grade IV hypertensive retinopathy with severely elevated blood pressure. *West J Emerg Med*. 2012;13:529–34.

78. Fujimoto JG, Huang D. Introduction to optical coherence tomography. In: Huang D, Duker JS, Fujimoto JG, et al, eds. *Imaging the Eye from Front to Back with RTVue Fourier-Domain Optical Coherence Tomography*. New Jersey: SLACK Inc.; 2012:1–22.

79. Hatef E, Khwaja A, Rentiya Z, et al. Comparison of time domain and spectral domain optical coherence tomography in measurement of macular thickness in macular edema secondary to diabetic retinopathy and retinal vein occlusion. *J Ophthalmol*. 2012:354783.

80. Pichj F, Sarraf D, Arepalli S, et al. The application of optical coherence tomography angiography in uveitis and inflammatory eye diseases. *Prog Retin Eye Res*. 2017;59:178–201.

81. Jones-Odeh E, Hammond CJ. How strong is the relationship between glaucoma, the retinal nerve fibre layer and neurodegenerative diseases such as Alzheimer's disease and multiple sclerosis? *Eye (Lond)*. 2015;29:1270–84.

82. Sridhar MS, Martin R. Anterior segment optical coherence tomography for evaluation of cornea and ocular surface. *Ind J Ophthalmol*. 2018;66:367–72.

83. Vincent SJ, Alonso-Caneiro D, Collins MJ. Optical coherence tomography and scleral contact lenses—clinical and research applications. *Clin Exp Optom*. 2018;102:224–41.

84. Pierro L, Gagliardi M, Iuliano L, Ambrosi A, Bandello F. Retinal nerve fiber layer thickness reproducibility using seven different OCT instruments. *Invest Ophthalmol Vis Sci*. 2012;53:5912–20.

85. Khan H, Asrar A, Ikram B, et al. Comparison of image quality between swept source and spectral domain OCT in media opacification. *Pak J Ophthalmol*. 2016;32:128–33.

86. Staurenghi G, Sadda S, Chakravarthy U, Spaide RF, International Nomenclature for Optical Coherence Tomography (IN-OCT) Panel. Proposed lexicon for anatomic landmarks in normal posterior segment spectral-domain optical coherence tomography: the IN-OCT consensus. *Ophthalmology*. 2014;121:1572–8.

87. Stanga PE, Sala-Puigdollers A, Caputo S, et al. In vivo imaging of cortical vitreous using 1050-nm swept-source deep range imaging optical coherence tomography. *Am J Ophthalmol*. 2014; 157:397–404.

88. Kim KE, Park KH. Macular imaging by optical coherence tomography in the diagnosis and management of glaucoma. *Br J Ophthalmol*. 2018; 102:718–24.

89. Hood DC, De Cuir N, Blumberg DM, et al. A single wide-field OCT protocol can provide compelling information for the diagnosis of early glaucoma. *Transl Vis Sci Technol*. 2016;5:4.

90. Leung CK, Yu M, Weinreb RN, et al. Retinal nerve fiber layer imaging with spectral-domain optical coherence tomography: a prospective analysis of age-related loss. *Ophthalmology*. 2012;119:731–7.

91. Kashani AH, Chen CL, Gahm JK, et al. Optical coherence tomography angiography: A comprehensive review of current methods and clinical applications. *Prog Retin Eye Res*. 2017;60:66–100.

92. Daien V, Le Pape A, Heve D, Carriere I, Villain M. Incidence, risk factors, and impact of age on retinal detachment after cataract surgery in France: a national population study. *Ophthalmology.* 2015;122:2179–85.

93. Silva PS, El-Rami H, Barham R et al. Hemorrhage and/or microaneurysm severity and count in ultrawide field images and early treatment diabetic retinopathy study photography. *Ophthalmology.* 2017;124:970–6.

94. The Eye Disease Case-Control Study Group. Risk factors for idiopathic rhegmatogenous retinal detachment. *Am J Epidemiol.* 1993;137:749–57.

95. Ogawa A, Tanaka M. The relationship between refractive errors and retinal detachment—analysis of 1,166 retinal detachment cases. *Jpn J Ophthalmol.* 1988;32:310–5.

96. Mitry D, Singh J, Yorston D, et al. The predisposing pathology and clinical characteristics in the Scottish retinal detachment study. *Ophthalmology.* 2011;118:1429–34.

97. Bullimore MA, Brennan NA. Myopia control: why each diopter matters. *Optom Vis Sci.* 2019;96:463–5.

98. Duncan EM, Cassie H, Pooley J, et al. Areas for improvement in community optometry: flashes and floaters take priority. *Ophthalmic Physiol Opt.* 2018;38:411–21.

99. Kinori M, Hashem F, Granet DB. The retinal lesion is moving! *J Pediatr Ophthalmol Strabismus.* 2017;54:128.

100. Mackenzie PJ, Russell M, Ma PE, Isbister CM, Maberley DA. Sensitivity and specificity of the optos optomap for detecting peripheral retinal lesions. *Retina.* 2007;27:1119–24.

101. Cheng SC, Yap MK, Goldschmidt E, Swann PG, Ng LH, Lam CS. Use of the Optomap with lid retraction and its sensitivity and specificity. *Clin Exp Optom.* 2008;91:373–8.

102. Ahn HM, Rim TH, Chung EJ. Diagnostic availability of ultra-wide-field fundus imaging in Korean patient with retinal break. *J Korean Ophthalmol Soc.* 2016;57:1254–9.

103. Ly A, Nivison-Smith L, Hennessy M, Kalloniatis M. The advantages of intermediate-tier, inter-optometric referral of low risk pigmented lesions. *Ophthalmic Physiol Opt.* 2017;37:661–8.

Chapter | 8

Variations in appearance of the normal eye

David B. Elliott and Konrad Pesudovs

The vast majority of patients examined in optometry practice have normal, healthy eyes. This chapter presents information about some of the subtle variations that occur in the normal eye and presents changes that commonly occur with normal ageing. To discriminate between ocular disease and the normal eye, it is essential to be familiar with the range of presentations that is considered to represent 'normal.' A brief description and collection of photographs of these normal variations is presented here to supplement the information provided in atlases of ocular disease. In addition, more photographs, online quizzes, and video clips are provided on the accompanying website. The variations in younger adult eyes are mainly caused by differences in ocular size and pigmentation and the occasional presence of embryological remnants. We thank Kelly Gibbons (Wodonga Eye Care, Australia) for the optomap images and Jason Booth (Optometry, Flinders University, Adelaide, Australia) for some of the photographs.

8.1 Anterior eye variations

Concretions and pinguecula can be found in young adults, but are more common in older patients and are discussed in section 8.2.

8.1.1 Epicanthus

Bilateral inner canthal nasal folds are very common in Caucasian infants and South and South-East Asians. It can make a child appear strabismic.

8.1.2 Subconjunctival haemorrhage

Whilst a striking appearance, most subconjunctival haemorrhages (Fig. 8.1) are benign. These may be idiopathic or caused by trauma, a sudden increase in blood pressure resulting from heavy lifting, coughing or sneezing or blood thinning medication.[1] No treatment is required, with complete resorption occurring within 21 days. In a large haemorrhage the posterior edge should be identified to rule out retrobulbar haemorrhage. In multiple, recurrent presentations without cause, investigation for blood disorders is appropriate.

8.1.3 Conjunctival epithelial inclusion cyst

These small benign fluid-filled cysts which are easily visible on slit-lamp examination (Fig. 8.2). They occur when conjunctival cells find their way under the basement membrane,

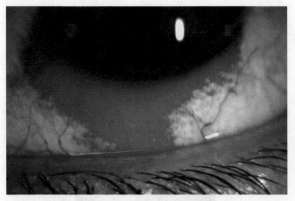

Fig. 8.1 Subconjunctival haemorrhage.

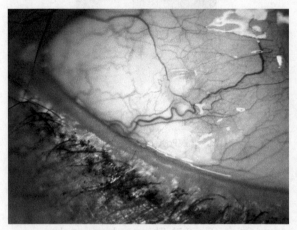

Fig. 8.2 Conjunctival epithelial inclusion cyst.

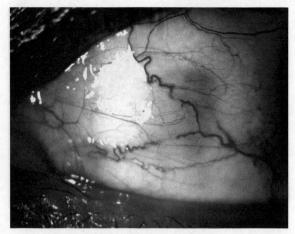

Fig. 8.3 Scleral hyaline plaque.

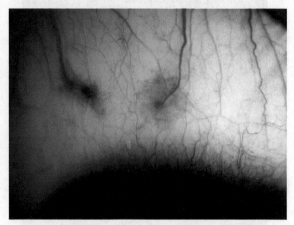

Fig. 8.4 Axenfield nerve loops.

proliferate, and create a fluid-filled sphere. They may be idiopathic or commonly seen after trauma or surgery. No treatment is required for small cysts. Larger cysts may cause foreign body sensation that may be alleviated by lubrication. Surgical removal may be considered for very large cysts.[2]

8.1.4 Scleral hyaline plaque

A scleral hyaline plaque (Fig. 8.3) represents a localised hyaline degeneration of the sclera that occurs anteriorly to the medial rectus insertion. The sclera is thinned in this area enabling visibility of the uvea, hence the blue appearance. This condition is asymptomatic and of no consequence.[3]

8.1.5 Axenfield (intrascleral) nerve loops

The long posterior ciliary nerves travel within the sclera from the posterior segment before turning to branch into

the ciliary body.[4] The loops formed by these nerves as they turn into the ciliary body are sometimes visible as grey or purple-grey patches, possibly raised, possibly associated with pigment, typically associated with large veins, and located 3 mm posterior to the limbus (Fig. 8.4). These are an entirely normal finding that should be differentiated from congenital conjunctival melanosis.

8.1.6 Congenital conjunctival melanosis

Relatively common, bilateral, benign, flat, pigmented areas of conjunctiva, typically near the limbus in young, heavily pigmented eyes (Fig. 8.5 and online), which sometimes are called complexion-associated conjunctival melanosis.[5] The pigmentation is darkest at the limbus with decreasing intensity away from it. It should be differentially

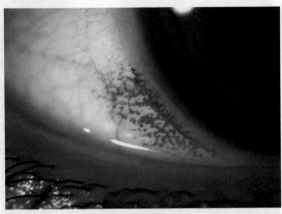

Fig. 8.5 Conjunctival melanosis.

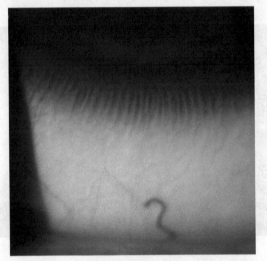

Fig. 8.6 Limbal palisades.

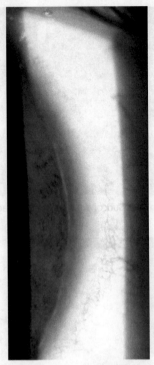

Fig. 8.7 Posterior embryotoxon.

diagnosed from the typically unilateral conjunctival naevus (or 'freckle').

8.1.7 Palisades of Vogt

Limbal epithelial folds that are arranged radially. They are more easily seen in young heavily pigmented eyes and are most prominent in the lower limbus (Fig. 8.6 and online). They house limbal epithelial stem cells, which produce epithelial cells to maintain the normal corneal epithelium or replace it in the event of injury.[6]

8.1.8 Posterior embryotoxon

Posterior embryotoxon occurs when the junction between the posterior cornea and the trabeculum

(Schwalbe's line) is thickened, making it more prominent and visible through the cornea on slit-lamp examination (Fig. 8.7). This may be a complete or partial white ring, usually most visible at 3 and 9 o'clock. Posterior embryotoxon occurs in 8% to 30% of normal eyes, so as an isolated finding is of no concern. However, posterior embryotoxon is also associated with a number of anterior segment syndromes including Axenfeld-Rieger syndrome.[7]

8.1.9 Pigment changes in the iris

Little or no pigment gives 'blue eyes.' With increasing amounts of pigment, the iris is seen as green, hazel, or brown. People with blue irises have greater light scatter than those with more pigmented irides and may suffer more from disability glare in situations such as driving at night.[8] Variations in pigment can produce wedge-shaped sections of hyper- or hypopigmentation (heterochromia, Fig. 8.8 and online) in one or both eyes. Hyperpigmented spots (naevi or 'iris freckles,' Fig. 8.9 and online) are common, but should be monitored using photography for changes owing to the slight risk of malignant melanoma.

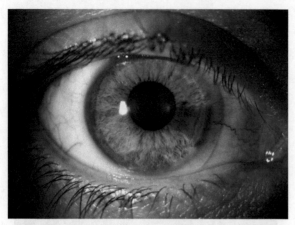

Fig. 8.8 A section of iris hyperpigmentation (heterochromia).

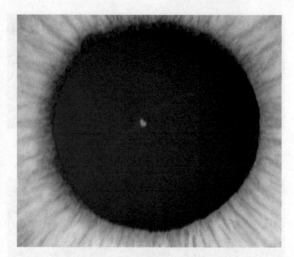

Fig. 8.10 Persistent pupillary membrane.

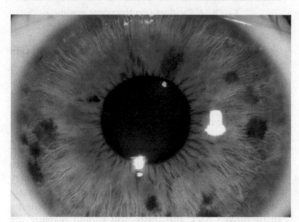

Fig. 8.9 Iris naevi.

8.1.10 Persistent pupillary membrane

These are strands of the embryonic pupillary membrane that remain into adulthood. One end of the strand inserts into the iris colarette and the other is either attached to the anterior lens capsule or floats in the anterior chamber (Fig. 8.10 is a common example, while Fig. 8.11 is rare).

8.2 Anterior eye changes in older patients

See online quiz 8.1 and additional online photographs. With increasing age, there is progressive loss of tone and bulk of the eyelids, a loss of tear film stability, a reduction in corneal sensitivity, decreased cell density, and increased variation in cell size (polymegethism) and

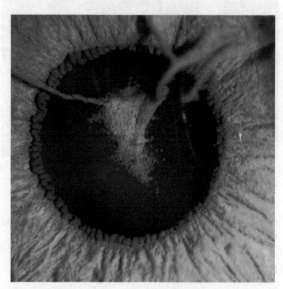

Fig. 8.11 A large persistent pupillary membrane.

shape (pleomorphism) in the corneal endothelium. In the iris, the crypts disappear, especially near the pupil and the pupillary ruff appears eroded and, as novice retinoscopists and ophthalmoscopists will readily confirm, the pupil gets smaller with age (pupillary miosis).

8.2.1 Dermatochalasis

Dermatochalasis is benign, bilateral drooping of excess upper lid tissue with age that gives the appearance of tired or sleepy looking eyes (Figs. 8.12 and 8.13, and online). Cosmetic surgery is sometimes requested. Blepharoplasty

279

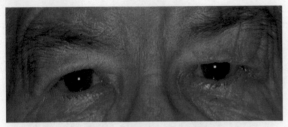

Fig. 8.12 Dermatochalasis.

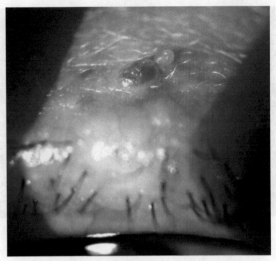

Fig. 8.14 Papilloma on the upper eyelid.

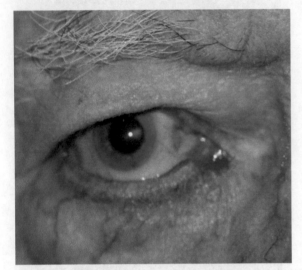

Fig. 8.13 Ectropian with rosacea exposure and slight dermatochalasis.

or blepharoptosis repair can improve functional vision and may be recommended if the patient reports problems.[9]

8.2.2 Ectropion and entropion

The eyelid is either turned outward (ectropion, see Fig. 8.13) or inward (entropion) owing to loose lids so that the inferior lid margin or puncta are not in contact with the eye. The patient may complain of epiphora or be symptomless. They are common complaints, found in about 4% of older patients and are often associated with dry eye and chronic blepharitis.[9]

8.2.3 Seborrheic keratosis

Seborrheic keratosis is one of the most common benign eyelid tumours in the elderly. Hyperkeratinised, waxy, light grey-brown plaques are found over the eyelids and face and appear to be stuck onto the skin. Typically benign, but their natural history of gradually increasing in

size, thickness, and/or pigmentation leads to fears of skin cancer and cosmetic concerns.[10]

8.2.4 Papilloma

Papilloma, the most common benign lesion of the eyelid, is often known as a 'skin tag.'[11] They are avascular, epithelial lesions of variable size, shape, and colour (amelanotic to black) with a roughened surface reflecting the redundant epithelial cell growth (Fig. 8.14). Over time, they grow and become attached to the eyelid surface by a stalk (pedunculated, see online figure), so that the papilloma can be moved back and forth. You should reassure the patient and photograph the lesion, which can be removed for cosmetic reasons.

8.2.5 Xanthelasma

Bilateral, flat, light brown/yellow, triangular lipid masses with a nasal base, xanthelasma are typically found on the inner upper eyelids of elderly patients and especially females (Fig. 8.15 and online). They usually have a familial aetiology, but can be linked with atherosclerosis and high cholesterol and any initial diagnosis of xanthelasma should be referred for further investigation.[12] They often reoccur if removed, so the patient should be warned of this if considering cosmetic removal.

8.2.6 Corneal arcus (previously termed 'arcus senilis')

Commonly found, corneal arcus is a bilateral, 1.0 to 1.5 mm wide, greyish-white ring or part ring occurring in

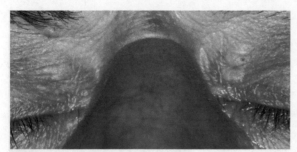

Fig. 8.15 Xanthelasma.

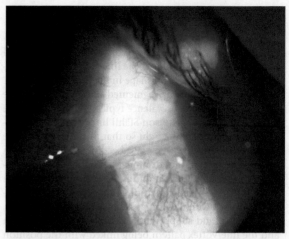

Fig. 8.17 Solitary hard concretion in the lower palpebral conjunctiva.

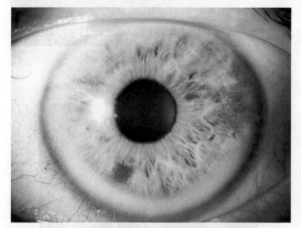

Fig. 8.16 A near-complete corneal arcus.

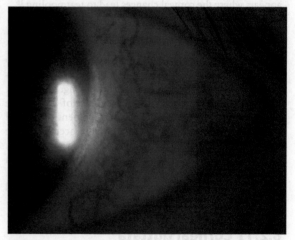

Fig. 8.18 Limbal girdle of Vogt seen in indirect illumination.

the periphery of corneas of older patients that is separated from the limbus by a thin ring of clear cornea, the lucid interval of Vogt (Fig. 8.16 and online). It is called a corneal arcus rather than a corneal ring as it initially presents as arcs in the inferior and superior poles of the perilimbal cornea before spreading to form a complete ring. The inner edge is typically more diffuse than the sharper outer edge. Its prevalence increases significantly with age after 50 years.[13] It is caused by lipid being deposited in the corneal stroma, having permeated from the limbal blood vessels, which become more permeable with age. Corneal arcus may be a sign of systemic hyperlipidaemias if seen in younger adults and any patient with arcus who is below the age of 50 years should be referred for further investigation.

8.2.7 Concretions

Typically concretions are asymptomatic, small (1 to 3 mm), yellow-white calcium lesions found in the palpebral conjunctiva of the upper and lower eyelid.[14] They can be found in young adults, but are more common in

elderly patients. The majority are superficial, hard, and single (Fig. 8.17 and online).[14] A small percentage of concretions can cause symptoms, likely from corneal irritation.

8.2.8 Limbal girdle of Vogt

The limbal girdle of Vogt is a common, bilateral degenerative condition producing a narrow band of white, crystal-like opacities along the nasal or temporal limbus, typically found in older female eyes (Fig. 8.18 and online). Two types are described: type I has a perilimbal clear zone similar to corneal arcus and contains numerous holes, whereas type II has neither holes nor a clear zone.

8.2.9 Hudson-Stähli line

The Hudson-Stähli line is a common, corneal orangey-brown iron deposition line found close to where the lid margins meet when blinking. The line is generally horizontal, possibly with a slight V-shape in the middle (Fig. 8.19). It can be continuous or segmented and, although some texts suggest that the prevalence typically matches the age of the patient, many Hudson-Stähli lines are faint and difficult to see under white light so that this high prevalence seems unlikely. However, they become more visible in cobalt blue (see online) or ultraviolet light.[15] For this reason you may first notice it during a slit-lamp examination using fluorescein and cobalt blue illumination. Its aetiology is unclear, with the iron possibly arising from the tears, perilimbal blood supply, and/or caused by UV radiation and the line/vortex pattern being linked with the position of eyelid closure or the growth and repair patterns of the corneal epithelium.[15] Similar corneal iron deposition can occur in orthokeratology patients where the pigment line appears where the corneal changes lead to tear pooling.[16]

8.2.10 Crocodile shagreen

Crocodile shagreen is a polygonal pattern of white or grey opacity in the cornea with an appearance similar to crocodile skin (Fig. 8.20). Peripheral crocodile shagreen is most common with a reported clinical incidence of 13%.[17] The pattern is probably related to the arrangement of corneal fibrils allowing opacities to preferentially occur in some locations. Peripheral shagreen tends to progress towards, but never reaching, the central cornea. It can vary from faint to striking, and whereas the latter may be of concern, vision seems unaffected. No treatment is required, and referral is not appropriate.

8.2.11 Corneal guttata

Corneal guttata are small excrescences of abnormal basement membrane and collagen fibrillar material from distressed corneal endothelium. They occur in the periphery of all corneas where they are termed Hassall-Henle

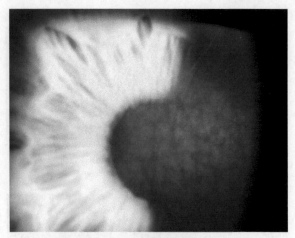

Fig. 8.20 Crocodile shagreen.

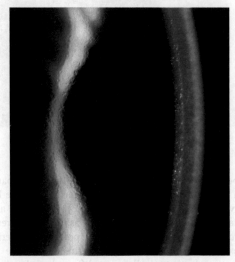

Fig. 8.21 Corneal guttata seen on the right in direct illumination as *white dots* of increased backscatter in the corneal endothelium and on the left as a '*beaten copper metal*' appearance in retro-illumination against the iris.

bodies or 'warts' and the prevalence of frank central corneal guttata in those aged over 55 is about 9%, with smoking doubling their likelihood.[18] Guttata are often accompanied by a fine pigment dusting, and the endothelial layer is said to take on a beaten metal appearance when viewed with specular reflection or retro-illumination (Fig. 8.21). Identification of central corneal guttata may be important in patients undergoing cataract and refractive surgery, as mild corneal guttata has been associated

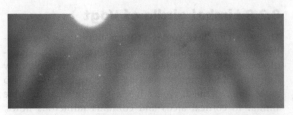

Fig. 8.19 A Hudson-Stähli line seen in front of the blurred iris.

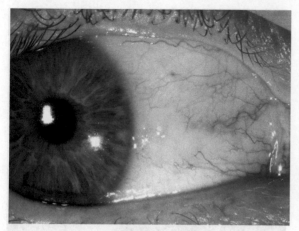

Fig. 8.22 Pinguecula.

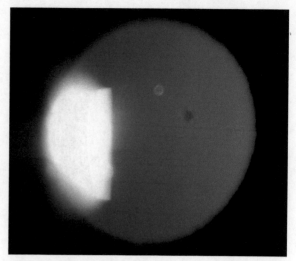

Fig. 8.23 Mittendorf dot (the *black dot* seen slightly superior nasally from the pupil centre).

with increased risk of complications after surgery.[19,20] The transition from a simple observation of corneal guttata to a diagnosis of Fuchs endothelial dystrophy occurs when the guttata are accompanied by corneal thickening as evidenced by signs of oedema: striae, folds, or clouding. Corneal guttata are a benign clinical finding, as is early Fuchs endothelial dystrophy.

8.2.12 Pinguecula

A pinguecula is a degenerative thickening of the bulbar conjunctiva adjacent to the limbus (Fig. 8.22 and online) and often found nasally. Although it is seen in adult patients who work outdoors and do not wear sunglasses, its prevalence increases with age and it is very common in the elderly.[21] During blinking, pingueculae can lift the lids away from the surrounding conjunctiva, leading to a local area of drying and hyperaemia for which artificial tears can be helpful. Given their minimal impact on the patient, and a likelihood to recur, surgical excision is rarely considered. Pinguecula can increase in size with age, so the mainstay of treatment is preventative with UV blockers in glasses and/or sunglasses.

8.3 Lens and vitreous variations

Vitreous floaters can be found in young adults, particularly the large eyes of moderate to high myopes (section 8.10), but are more common in older patients and are discussed in section 8.4.

8.3.1 Mittendorf dot

A Mittendorf dot is seen as a small black dot in fundal retro-illumination (Fig. 8.23 and online) and a white dot

on the posterior capsular surface in direct illumination. It is usually displaced nasally or inferior nasally and it is a remnant of the attachment of the hyaloid canal to the posterior lens surface. The hyaloid artery provides nutrients to the developing lens in the growing foetus and is typically fully regressed before birth (but see video 8.1 which shows a full hyaloid artery in a young adult). It runs from the ophthalmic artery at the optic disc to the crystalline lens where it spreads over both surfaces of the lens in a capillary net or tunica vasculosa lentis.

8.3.2 Epicapsular stars

Epicapsular stars are small, light brown or tan star-shaped deposits on the anterior lens surface (Fig. 8.24 and

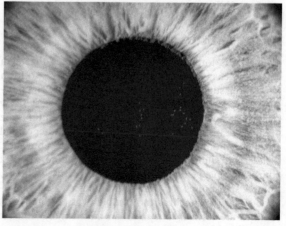

Fig. 8.24 Epicapsular stars.

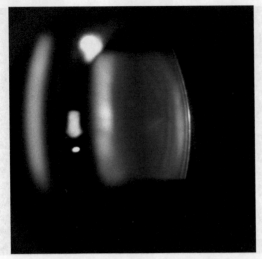

Fig. 8.25 Zones of discontinuity in a posterior lens optical section. The arc to the left is the cornea.

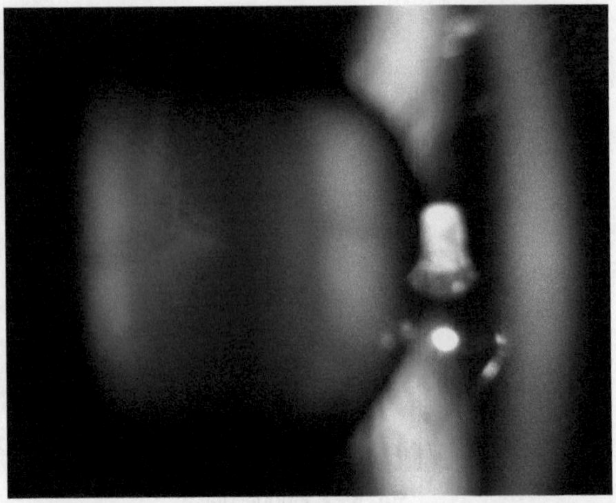

Fig. 8.26 An inverted Y-suture in the posterior lens seen by optical section in the left part of the image. To the right is the blurred anterior lens, iris, and cornea.

online) that are remnants of the tunica vasculosa lentis (section 8.3.1). They can be bilateral or unilateral and single or multiple.

8.3.3 Zones of discontinuity (or Wasserspalten)

The slit-lamp appearance of the normal adult lens shows a series of zones of clear media in both the anterior and posterior lens cortex delineated by a curved line of reflected light (Fig. 8.25 and online). These zones are discontinuities between lens fibres and watery layers (hence the name 'Wasserspalten' in German) and are caused by reflections from the rough surfaces.[22,23]

8.3.4 Y-sutures

The lens is formed by the meeting of fibres that arch over the lens equator and join with other fibres to form branching suture lines that take on an upright 'Y' appearance anteriorly and an inverted 'Y' appearance posteriorly (Fig. 8.26 and online) in the foetal lens. The sutures are visible because of the large amount of light scatter caused by the non-uniform shape and size of the lens fibre ends. These lens sutures become progressively more complex during distinct periods of lens growth. In early childhood, simple star sutures are formed. In adolescence and adulthood, star (9 branches) and complex star (12 branches) sutures are formed, but these are much more difficult to see.[22]

8.4 Lens and vitreous changes in older patients

See online quiz 8.2 and additional online photographs. The lens continues to grow and thicken with age, leading to a gradual reduction in anterior chamber depth and volume. There is increased light scatter owing to an increased number of cortical layers and the production of large aggregates in the lens nucleus.[23] Pigments that absorb blue wavelength light and fluoresce also increase with age, leading to progressive lens yellowing and fluorescence. In addition, the prevalence of cataract increases substantially.

8.4.1 Posterior subcapsular cataract

The posterior subcapsular (PSC) cataract presents at the back of the lens just in front of the posterior capsule. In the age-related type, vacuoles are found in the early stages (Fig. 8.27 and online). Later, there is a posterior migration of epithelial cells from the lens equator to the posterior pole, where they form the balloon or bladder cells of Wedl. Large particle scattering is increased by many organelles in the epithelial cells. To categorise a cataract as PSC, an optical section technique is required, although PSC cataract is best viewed through a dilated pupil using retro-illumination.

A PSC cataract typically presents earlier than do the other morphological types, at about age 55 years. Some are associated with diabetes, other ocular diseases, such as

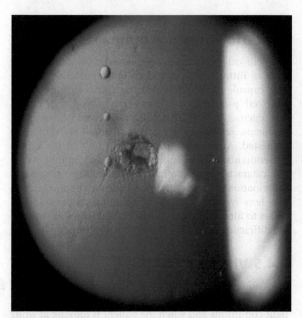

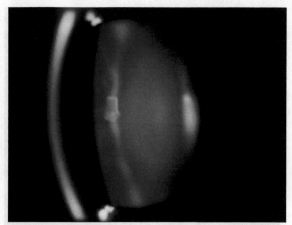

Fig. 8.28 Nuclear cataract seen by optical section of LOCS III grade[24] ~NC3.0, NO 3.0. The blurred blue arc to the left is the out-of-focus cornea (blue owing to Rayleigh light scatter).[24] Some cortical opacities are seen as bright spots of light scatter in the anterior cortex.

Fig. 8.27 Posterior subcapsular cataract and several vacuoles seen in fundal retro-illumination. The LOCS III grade[24] is ~ P2.2.

retinitis pigmentosa and uveitis, after ocular trauma, and found as a side effect of systemic drugs such as corticosteroids.[25] PSC cataracts can cause a dramatic reduction in vision with pupil constriction because they are generally centrally positioned within the pupil. These cataracts can hide behind the corneal and lens reflexes when viewed through an undilated pupil and be missed. Clinicians have been successfully sued for missing PSC cataracts in patients with no symptoms at the time of the eye examination, but who subsequently had holidays ruined owing to poor vision in a brighter, sunnier climate.

8.4.2 Nuclear cataracts

Nuclear cataracts present as a homogenous increase in light scatter in the lens nucleus and can be associated with an increased yellowing turning to brunescence (Fig. 8.28 and online), which is indicative of blue light absorption.[24] The use of a slit-lamp optical section technique is the only accurate way of detecting and assessing nuclear cataract, and it is best performed with a dilated pupil, although is still possible undilated. Nuclear cataract typically presents in the very old age persons. However, it is possible for nuclear cataract to present in patients in their 50s or even 40s. The early presentation can easily be missed with undilated pupil examination because the nucleus typically shows little brunescence at this age. This presentation

is typically associated with index myopia so a thorough examination of the lens is indicated by a large myopic shift in older age groups.[26]

8.4.3 Cortical cataract

Cortical cataracts are wedge-shaped opacities found in the anterior and/or posterior lens cortex. Vision is only affected if the cortical spokes enter the pupillary area, and it therefore varies depending on pupil size. Cortical opacities are most often found in the inferior-nasal part of the lens, which may reflect UVB radiation involvement in their aetiology.[27] Opacification is caused by the scattering of light when it meets irregular interfaces between regions of different refractive index and some cortical cataracts cause astigmatic changes.[26] Cortical opacities are best seen using retro-illumination, when they appear black against the red fundal glow (Fig. 8.29 and online). The brightest reflection from the fundus is obtained when the illuminating beam strikes the optic nerve head, so that typically the illumination system is placed on the temporal side of the biomicroscope. The slit-lamp illumination of beam size, shape, and position can be altered to avoid the cortical opacities on its way to the fundus. Some slit lamps allow a half-moon shape illumination beam that can be placed inside the edge of the pupil. In some cases you may need to view the opacities with the illumination in two positions. Retro-illumination gives an overall view of the cataract, although note that the depth of focus is usually not sufficient to provide an assessment of both the anterior and posterior lens at the

285

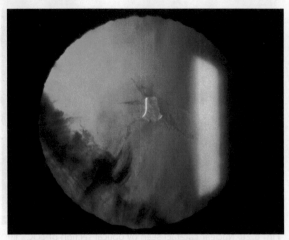

Fig. 8.29 Cortical cataract seen in fundal retro-illumination with LOCS III grade[24] ~C3.5. The rectangular image in the centre is the reflection of the slit-lamp mirror.

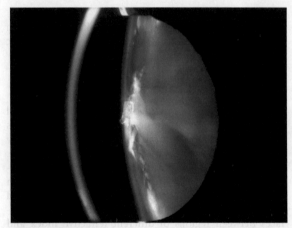

Fig. 8.30 Cortical cataract seen in direct illumination. Compare its appearance with that of cortical cataract in retro-illumination in Fig. 8.29.

8.4.4 Intraocular lenses and posterior capsular remnants

You will often examine a patient who is pseudophakic with an intraocular lens and an intact posterior capsule. This capsule can thicken or form a scaffold for residual lens cell proliferation. If posterior capsular opacification encroaches on the pupillary area and causes visual problems, referral for YAG laser capsulotomy should be suggested. After YAG capsulotomy, a hole in the capsular remnants will be visible (Fig. 8.31 and online). As for PSC cataracts, capsular remnants are best seen using retro-illumination from the fundus. A wide variation in intraocular lens types may be seen including yellow coloured lenses to filter blue light and multifocal lenses incorporating diffraction grooves or multiple optical zones.

8.4.5 Vitreous floaters

See online video 8.1. Vitreous floaters cast a shadow on the retina and are most obvious to the patient in bright light conditions and when the patient is looking at white walls, snow, and so forth. They are common in myopes and with increasing age.[28] Patients typically report seeing black flecks floating in their vision. Some patients mistake them for flies or spiders moving out of the corner of their eye and are very relieved when these symptoms are explained. Vitreous floaters can often be most easily seen with the retro-illumination view provided by a direct

same time, particularly with higher magnification, so that separate assessments are required. The cataracts appear white in direct illumination (Fig. 8.30) and are often associated with water clefts, which are optically clear wedges that can be seen with slit-lamp biomicroscopy. Using optical sections to view cortical cataracts is much less useful as it can show large amounts of light scatter owing to backward light scatter and reflections that do not cause vision loss, and an overall view of the cataract is only possible by mentally combining the views of the many optical sections.

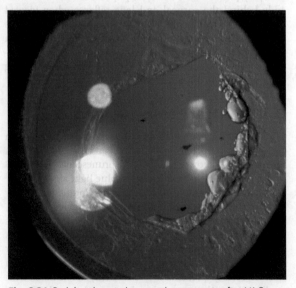

Fig. 8.31 Peripheral posterior capsular remnants after YAG capsulotomy has removed central capsular remnants.

ophthalmoscope. Otherwise use the slit-lamp biomicroscope and direct illumination through a dilated pupil to view the anterior vitreous and fundus biomicroscopy to view the posterior vitreous. To look more carefully for floaters, it can be useful to ask the patient to look up, down, and then straight ahead and watch for any floaters moving in your view.[28]

8.4.6 Posterior vitreous detachment

With ageing, liquefaction and shrinkage (syneresis) of the vitreous occurs and this leads to posterior vitreous detachment (PVD). PVD is common after the age of 50 years, with increasing prevalence with age and myopia and is accelerated after cataract surgery.[29] Many PVDs are asymptomatic, but symptoms are classically a sudden onset of flashes of light, owing to tugging on the vitreo-retinal adhesion, and floaters. Recent onset floaters (especially if > 10) may indicate blood or pigment in the vitreous indicating the presence of a retinal tear and or small vessel injury.[30] After the vitreous detaches from the optic nerve head, it can be seen as a ring-like vitreous floater known as a Weiss ring (Fig. 8.32 and online). PVDs can be detected using ocular coherence tomography (OCT, section 7.11) and binocular indirect ophthalmoscopy through a dilated pupil.

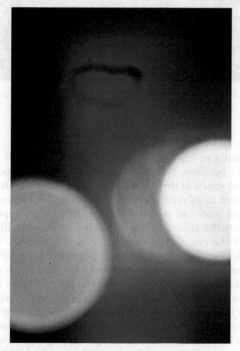

Fig. 8.32 A Weiss ring photographed using fundus biomicroscopy.

8.5 Optic nerve head variations

See online quiz 8.3 and additional online photographs.

8.5.1 Optic nerve head size and shape

The optic nerve head or disc comes in a variety of shapes and sizes (Figs. 8.33 to 8.35 and online quiz 8.3; note that relative size is affected by the degree of magnification of the book figures). Discs have been shown to be smaller in Caucasians compared to other ethnic groups who were all similar (African, Chinese, Filipino, Hispanic).[31] Disc size is larger in myopes beyond −8 D (section 8.10) and smaller in hyperopes greater than +4 D.[32] Oval discs are often found with corneal astigmatism and the direction of the longest optic disc diameter can indicate the axis of astigmatism (Fig. 8.35).[33] Malinserted discs also appear oval (Fig. 8.36) and are more commonly found in myopes (section 8.10.2)

8.5.2 Optic cupping

The central proportion of the nerve head usually contains a depression called the 'cup.' This is often associated with an area of pallor owing to the lamina cribrosa reflecting through in the absence of axons and their associated capillaries. However, in some cases the cup can extend beyond the area of pallor, so that this should not be used as an

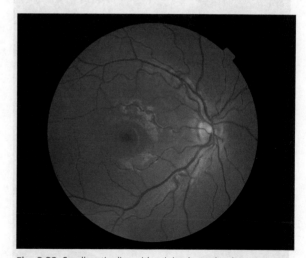

Fig. 8.33 Small optic disc with minimal cupping in a young Caucasian patient. There is also some arterial vessel tortuosity, visible nerve fibre layer, and macular pigment. The arc-like features around the macular area are reflections from the camera flash.

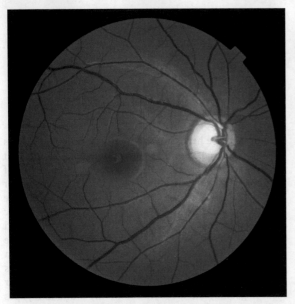

Fig. 8.34 Large optic disc and large cupping (CD ratio ~0.65), choroidal crescent, visible nerve fibre layer, and macular pigmentation. There are reflections in and around the macular from the camera flash.

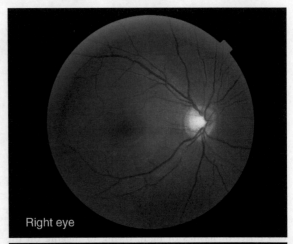

Right eye

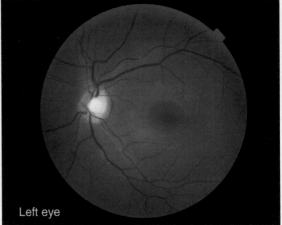

Left eye

Fig. 8.36 Optic disc malinsertion with the nasal side raised and the blood vessels nasally displaced in both eyes.

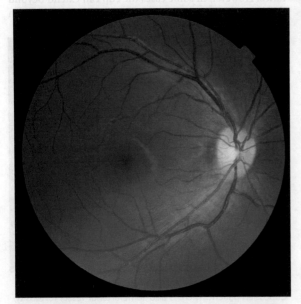

Fig. 8.35 An oval optic disc of a young British Asian patient, with a 0.30 vertical CD ratio, visible nerve fibre layer, and macular pigment.

indicator of cup size during 2D evaluations such as provided by direct ophthalmoscopy. Rather the kinking of blood vessels as they pass over the edge of the cup should be used as an estimate of the cup position. As discussed above, discs can vary considerably in size, yet approximately the same number of axons (about one million) leave the eye via the optic nerve head. Therefore, large optic discs typically have larger cupping because of the absence of axons in the middle of the disc as the neurons leave the retina in the larger rim tissue of larger discs (compare Figs. 8.33 and 8.34). The physiological cup-to-disc (CD) ratio is normally less than 0.60, but is relative to the size of the disc so that smaller cupping should be seen in a small-sized disc and larger cupping is expected in large discs. An increased vertical CD ratio of 0.2 is typical of large discs (1.8 to 2.0 mm) compared with small discs

(1.1 to 1.3 mm).[34] The vertical CD ratios indicated for the photographs presented here are based on the 2D diagrams. The optic nerve heads and cups of the two eyes are typically mirror images of each other and the differential diagnosis of many optic nerve head anomalies is provided by an intereye comparison.

8.5.3 Spontaneous venous pulsation

See online video 8.2. Spontaneous venous pulsation is present in about 90% of adult eyes with careful observation and most obvious at the point of entry of the central retinal vein into the optic nerve.[35] It is caused by the intracranial pressure pulse which acts on the central retinal vein as it passes through the subarachnoid space where it leaves the optic nerve. It can be useful to record its presence because its cessation is a sensitive marker of raised intracranial pressure and can help in the differential diagnosis of true papilloedema (it is absent) from pseudopapilloedema (it is present).[35] Venous pulsation is best seen with high magnification and mydriasis.[35]

8.5.4 Lamina cribrosa

Seen in about 30% of eyes, the lamina cribrosa appears as grey dots at the bottom of the optic cup (Figs. 8.37, 8.38 and online).[36] It is a sieve-like connective and glial tissue that is continuous with the scleral canal. It is more visible in larger discs and larger cups.[36] Visualising lamina cribrosa may well simply represent normal anatomy as in Figs. 8.37 and 8.38, but in larger cups where glaucoma is suspected, lamina cribrosa may be highly visible (see online) with greater depth shown using OCT.[37]

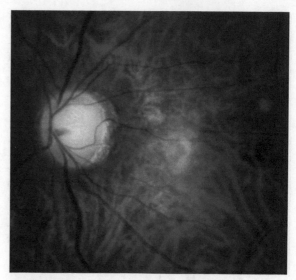

Fig. 8.38 Tigroid fundus in a young myopic patient with a visible lamina cribrosa in a large optic disc and cup (CD ratio ~0.55).

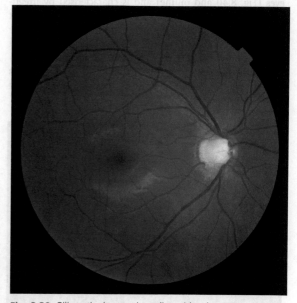

Fig. 8.39 Cilio-retinal artery in a disc with a large cup (CD ratio 0.7).

8.5.5 Cilio-retinal artery

This is found in about 15% to 20% of normal eyes, is seen as an artery that hooks out of the temporal edge of the disc and runs towards the macula (Fig. 8.39 and online). Its shape gives it the nickname of the 'Shepherd's crook.'

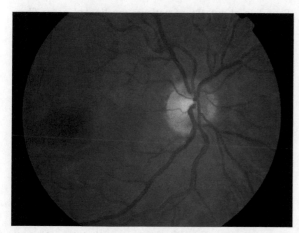

Fig 8.37 Lamina cribrosa in a relatively small (CD ratio ~ 0.25) but deep cup.

It is derived from the short posterior ciliary system or choriocapillaris rather than the central retinal artery and it becomes most relevant after a central retinal artery occlusion, when it saves the retina around its distribution. Of course, the cilio-retinal artery can itself become occluded.

8.5.6 Retinal nerve fibre layer striations

These nerve fibre layer striations are brightest at the superior and inferior poles, where the nerve fibre layer is thickest. They are best seen in young patients, particularly those with heavily pigmented fundi (see Figs. 8.33 through 8.35 and online). The striations are caused by the tubes of astrocytes that surround the retinal ganglion cell axon. New imaging techniques have made assessment of the retinal nerve fibre layer a valuable tool in the assessment of glaucoma.[38]

8.5.7 Peripapillary atrophy

Peripapillary atrophy (PPA) can be categorised into zone alpha and beta. Zone alpha is present in nearly all normal eyes (Fig. 8.40 and online) and is characterised by irregular hyper- and hypopigmented areas in the retinal pigment epithelium (RPE), either on their own or surrounding zone beta PPA. It is often not recorded if present on its own as it is so common. Zone Beta PPA is found adjacent (bordering) to the disc and is present in about 15% of normal eyes (Fig. 8.41 and online). The RPE and choriocapillaris are lost

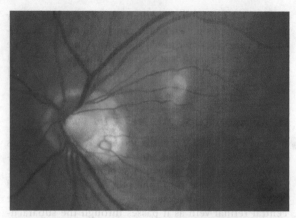

Fig. 8.41 Peripapillary atrophy (PPA). There appears to be a ring of beta zone, with temporal alpha zone. The image is slightly more washed out compared with those from younger patients owing to light scatter from early cataract. Drusen are visible in the macular region.

and all that is visible are the large choroidal vessels and sclera. PPA is most commonly found at the temporal edge of the disc in a crescent shape. It should be differentially diagnosed from high myopic atrophy and malinserted optic discs. PPA may also be associated with glaucoma, where it occurs adjacent to extensive disc damage often at the superior or inferior poles of the disc and is typically beta zone PPA.[39] PPA may also be associated with atrophic age-related macular degeneration (AMD) whereby it is continuous with the atrophic retinal changes. PPA associated with glaucoma, and AMD can be easily differentiated from normal PPA by its shape and location and the presence of other disease features.[39]

8.5.8 Myelinated nerve fibres

Found in about 1% of patients myelinated nerve fibres represent myelin sheathing of the optic nerve fibres that extends beyond the lamina cribrosa and present a superficial, white, feathery opacification that hides any underlying retinal blood vessels. They are usually continuous with the optic nerve head (Fig. 8.42 and online), although small discrete patches of myelinated nerve fibres can appear (Fig. 8.43) and may mimic a cotton wool patch. They are typically benign, although they may cause visual field loss at threshold. In most cases, myelinated nerve fibres remain unchanged over time. However, it can be part of a syndrome of extensive myelinated nerve fibres, optic disc hypoplasia, axial myopia, and amblyopia.[40]

8.5.9 Optic disc drusen

Optic disc drusen is a familial, typically bilateral condition, found in up to 2.4% of patients, becoming more

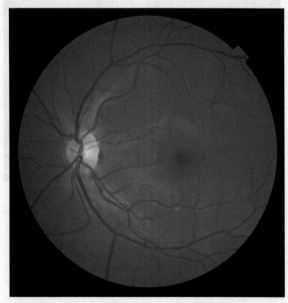

Fig. 8.40 Peripapillary atrophy (PPA) zone alpha.

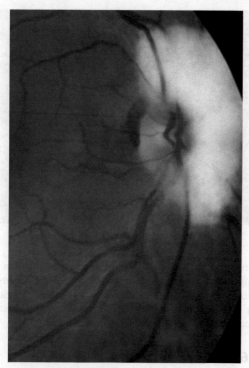

Fig. 8.42 Myelinated nerve fibres.

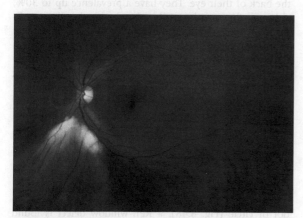

Fig. 8.43 Myelinated nerve fibres separate from the optic nerve head (Optomap).

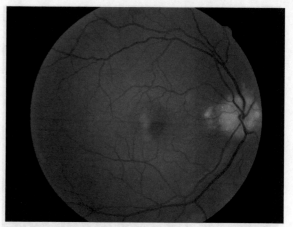

Fig. 8.44 Drusen in the optic nerve head.

and online). They are typically found in small discs with little or no cupping, and this appearance can mask signs of early glaucoma. Although typically benign they can shear blood vessels and/or nerve fibres, leading to haemorrhages (2% to 10%) and visual field loss (up to 87%), some of which can be progressive, so that visual field monitoring is essential. Acute vision loss can occur with ischaemic optic neuropathy and vascular occlusion.[41]

8.6 Fundus variations

The colour of the fundus is determined by the choroidal blood supply and the amount of pigmentation in the choroid and overlying retinal pigment epithelium. The retinal veins are typically dark red/purple and the retinal arteries are about two-third the thickness and a brighter red, with a slight reflex along the centre of the vessel. The arterioles and venules should have a smooth course and cross at oblique angles without nipping or compressing the venule.

8.6.1 Fundus pigmentation

Fundus pigmentation typically mimics skin pigmentation. Compare the British Asian fundi in Figs. 8.34 and 8.39 with the Caucasian fundi in Figs. 8.33 and 8.45. With a lightly pigmented and/or thin (typically myopic) RPE, the choroidal vessels and choroidal pigmentation can be seen (section 8.10).

8.6.2 Macular pigmentation

The macula lutea area contains a yellow-brown pigment, although the amount is highly variable between individuals,

obvious with age.[41] In children, the drusen may be buried in the nerve head and not seen ophthalmoscopically (but visible with OCT) and the disc appears swollen, so that the condition is sometimes called pseudopapilloedema. They are golden, autofluorescent, glowing, calcific globular deposits that sit in front of the lamina cribrosa (Fig. 8.44

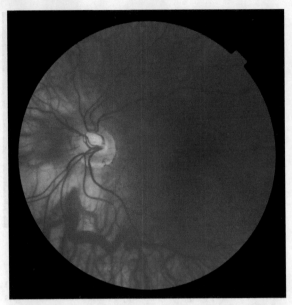

Fig. 8.45 Tilted disc syndrome and highly visible choroidal blood vessels in a young, highly myopic and astigmatic Caucasian patient. The disc is tilted inferior nasally with situs inversus.

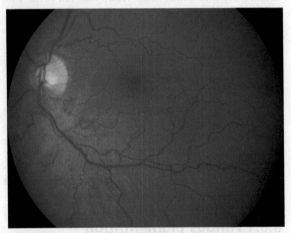

Fig. 8.46 Tortuous retinal arteries in a young Caucasian patient.

and is most obvious in highly pigmented eyes (Figs. 8.33 and 8.35 and online). A bright reflex may be seen at the foveola in younger patients, as the ophthalmoscope light is reflected back from the foveal pit.

8.6.3 Congenital vascular tortuosity

Most commonly bilateral and involving both arteries and veins and all quadrants (Fig. 8.46 and online). Acquired

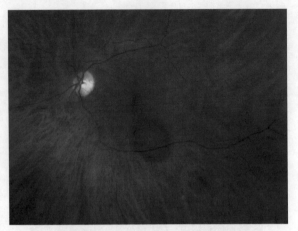

Fig. 8.47 A choroidal naevus (optomap).

tortuosity, particularly of veins, is less common than the congenital condition, but should be considered because it is connected with a variety of ocular and systemic diseases. For this reason, eyes with very tortuous vessels, ideally, should be photographed and monitored.

8.6.4 Choroidal naevus

A commonly found localised area of choroidal pigmentation that can be described to patients as a freckle on the back of their eye. They have a prevalence up to 30%, although they can be easily missed with the direct ophthalmoscope given its limited field of view. They appear grey as your view of a choroidal naevus is filtered through the RPE and sensory retina (Figure 8.47 and online). Naevi can be flat or raised, with drusen often appearing on the surface with age. They vary in size, although the vast majority are less than two disc diameters. All naevi should be routinely monitored, preferably using multimodal imaging as they can rarely transform into a malignant melanoma.[42]

8.6.5 RPE window defect

A fairly common, benign, yellow-white, well-circumscribed dot or circle (Fig. 8.48), a RPE window defect is found throughout the retina, but particularly in the mid-peripheral fundus (two disc diameters either side of the equator of the eye). It is caused by the absence of melanin in the RPE in a localised area. It is typically not associated with surrounding RPE hyperplasia (increase in the number of RPE cells) as would be seen with a chorioretinitis. It is easily differentiated from the red-brown retinal hole, which often has a surrounding cuff of retinal oedema or RPE hyperplasia. RPE window defects can enlarge with age, but this is of no concern.

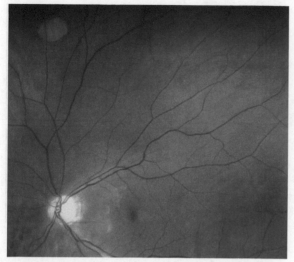

Fig. 8.48 A retinal pigment epithelium (RPE) window defect (optomap)

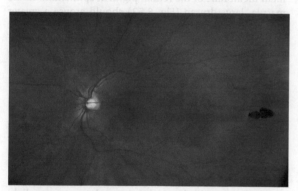

Fig. 8.49 Congenital hypertrophy of the retinal pigment epithelium (CHRPE)

8.6.6 Congenital hypertrophy of the retinal pigment epithelium

Pronounced as 'chirpy', these are congenital, unilateral, flat, typically round or oval patches of pigment ('birthmarks') found in the peripheral retina (Fig. 8.49). Typically darker than naevi (although they can be grey, brown, or black) with sharply defined edges, they consist of a layer of hyper-pigmented RPE cells over a thickened Bruch's membrane. They are found in about 1.2% of the optometric popula-tion (although many would not be seen with the limited view provided by a direct ophthalmoscope). About one-half have a depigmented halo just inside the border (this gives rise to the alternative name of halo naevi) and about one-half contain hypopigmented lacunae, which are areas

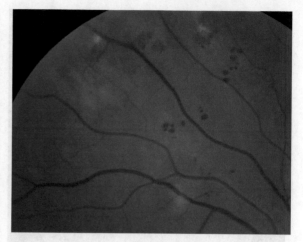

Fig. 8.50 Bear tracks in the peripheral retina

of chorioretinal atrophy.[43] Increasing atrophy may lead to slight enlargement of the lesion. A group of small pigment patches in an isolated quadrant of the peripheral fundus are known as 'bear tracks' (Fig. 8.50) given their character-istic clustering. Although commonly referred to as a type of congenital hypertrophy of the retinal pigment epithe-lium (CHRPE), bear tracks do not show haloes or lacunae and histolopathologically differ from CHRPE. Both are benign features and cause no problem other than the pos-sible loss of the overlying retinal receptors with associated visual field loss. As with choroidal naevi, CHRPE need to be differentially diagnosed from malignant melanoma and require regular monitoring with multimodal imaging and photography.[42]

8.7 Fundus changes in older patients

8.7.1 Macular pigmentary changes

Pigmentary changes occur at the macula with age, with increased disorganisation of the RPE and areas of depig-mentation and pigment clumping (Fig. 8.51, compared with maculae from young adults, Figs. 8.33 through 8.35). These changes need not cause losses of visual function, but can progress to early age-related maculopathy.

8.7.2 Drusen

Drusen are small, circular yellow or yellow-white dots, commonly seen around the macula (Figs. 8.51 and 8.52), disc, and more in the periphery (Fig. 8.53). They consist of

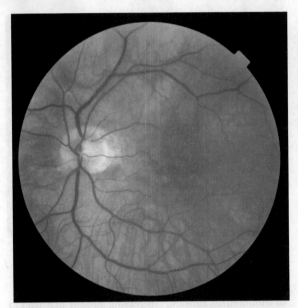

Fig. 8.51 Pigmentary changes and small drusen in the macular area, with zone beta PPA at the disc.

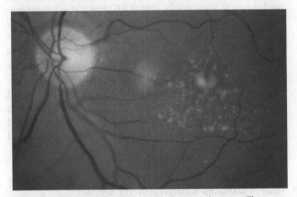

Fig. 8.52 Soft confluent drusen in the macular area. The purple area is a light scatter artefact. The image has reduced contrast due to light scatter from cataract.

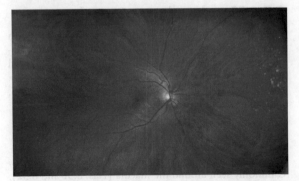

Fig. 8.53 Drusen in the peripheral retina (optomap).

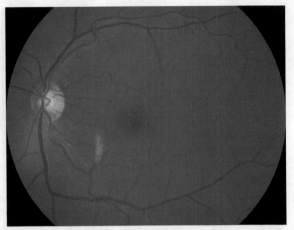

Fig. 8.54 Arteriosclerotic changes in retinal vessels, with 90 degree crossings.

deposits lying between Bruch's membrane and the basement membrane of the retinal pigment epithelium. In the macula, large drusen (Fig. 8.52) should arouse a greater level of concern because they indicate a greater level of RPE compromise and are associated with the development of exudative age-related maculopathy.[44] Peripheral drusen are of no concern (Fig. 8.53).

8.7.3 Retinal blood vessels

Changes to the retinal blood vessels can occur with normal ageing or can indicate early signs of hypertensive retinopathy.[45] The more significant the changes at an early age, the more likely the changes are early hypertensive changes. Arteriolar narrowing and hardening of the arteries occurs with increasing age and can cause a slight broadening of the reflex on the arterioles. Arteriosclerotic changes can lead to changes to the veins at artery–vein crossings, with 90-degree crossings and nipping of the vein on the distal side of the artery becoming increasingly common (Fig. 8.54).[45]

8.8 Peripheral fundus variations

The posterior pole is bordered by the superior and inferior temporal vascular arcades and includes the macula and optic nerve head. The mid-periphery extends anteriorly from the vascular arcades to the equator, which is defined by the posterior border of the vortex vein ampullae. The periphery extends anteriorly from the equator to the ora serrata, which is 4 to 5 disc diameters beyond the equator, at the termination of the choroid and retina.

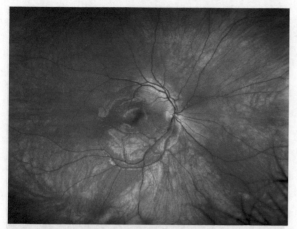

Fig. 8.55 An optomap image of a blonde fundus. The vortex vein ampullae are particularly obvious in the inferior and superior temporal quadrants. Eyelashes hide the inferior nasal ampulla.

8.8.1 Vortex vein ampullae

The vortex veins drain blood from the choroid, ciliary body, and iris. The ampullae, which are their dilated sacs, are red-orange octopus- or spider-shaped, often surrounded by pigment. The ampullae are found at the equator, with at least one per quadrant, typically in the four oblique meridians, and up to 10 in each eye. They are most easily seen in a lightly pigmented eye (Fig. 8.55).

8.8.2 Ciliary nerves and arteries

Two long posterior ciliary nerves bisect the superior and inferior fundus at the 3 and 9 o'clock positions in the fundus periphery and 10 to 20 short posterior ciliary nerves can be seen away from the horizontal meridian. They appear as faint, yellow-white short lines (Fig. 8.56), often with pigmented borders. The long posterior ciliary arteries run below the corresponding ciliary nerve in the temporal retina and above it in the nasal retina. The short posterior ciliary arteries may have pigmented margins.

8.8.3 Peripheral cystoid degeneration

Peripheral cystoid degeneration is the most prevalent of the benign peripheral retinal conditions whose extent increases with age. The cystoid area appears as a hazy grey zone of thickened retina near to the ora serrata and can extend to the equator. Red dots may appear with the cystoid degeneration, and strands in the vitreous may appear above it.

8.9 Peripheral fundus changes in older patients

8.9.1 Pavingstone degeneration

Pavingstone degeneration, a primary chorioretinal atrophy, with depigmented areas surrounded by RPE hyperplasia, is found in about 25% of patients over 20 years of age (Fig. 8.56), but increases with age. If the lesions coalesce, the underlying choroidal vessels may be seen. It is often bilateral with about 75% of lesions being found in the inferior nasal quadrant. It is thought to be caused by occlusion of some of the peripheral choriocapillaris vessels.

8.9.2 Peripheral pigmentary or tapetochoroidal degeneration

Peripheral pigmentary or tapetochoroidal degeneration has a granular pigment appearance between the equator and ora serrata that occurs in about 20% of patients after the age of 40 and becomes more prominent with age. It often has a honeycomb appearance and is associated with peripheral drusen. If the pigment takes on a reticular (Fig. 8.57)

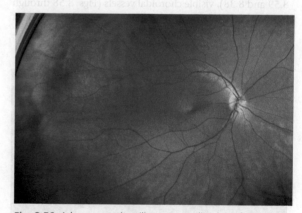

Fig. 8.56 A long posterior ciliary nerve splits the inferior and superior temporal retina. White without pressure is also seen in the temporal periphery of this myopic patient.

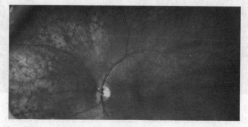

Fig. 8.57 Peripheral recticular degeneration (optomap).

or bone spicule appearance, differentiation from retinitis pigmentosa is required. It is a degenerative condition of the RPE, possibly associated with vascular compromise.

8.10 Myopic eyes

There has been a large increase in the prevalence of myopia and high myopia throughout the world, particularly in East Asian countries.[46] The majority of myopia is caused by an increased axial length, so myopic eyes are big eyes. The anterior angle is typically deeper in myopes and the vitreous is more liquefied and degenerative the higher the myopia. Therefore, there is a higher prevalence of vitreous floaters and a greater likelihood of PVD at an earlier age. If the RPE is pulled away from the disc in long myopic eyes, a crescent-shaped section of the choroid (choroidal blood vessels and pigment) can be seen. If both the RPE and choroid are pulled away from the disc, a white scleral crescent can be seen. These crescents are typically seen along the temporal edge.[47] The optic disc is typically larger in high myopia (more than –8 D) often with a larger CDR. The retina of the large myopic eye is relatively thin. This leads to a greater prevalence of tessellated/tigroid fundi (Figs. 8.58, 8.59 and 8.38), visible choroidal vessels (Figs. 8.58 through 8.61), chorioretinal atrophy (Fig. 8.61), white without pressure (Fig. 8.56) and lattice degeneration (Fig. 8.62).[46]

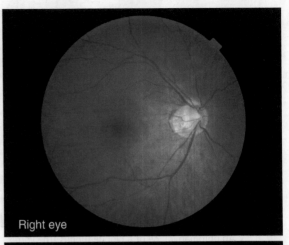

Right eye

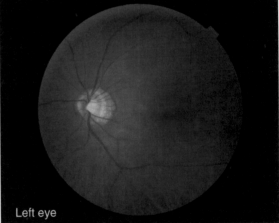

Left eye

Fig. 8.59 Optic disc malinsertion with the nasal side raised, blood vessels nasally displaced and temporal peripapillary atrophy (PPA) in both eyes in a myopic patient with tessellated fundi.

8.10.1 Tessellated or tigroid fundus

The thin myopic RPE allows the red choroidal vessels and heavily pigmented choroid to be seen and can give a tessellated or tiger stripe appearance (see Figs. 8.38 and 8.58).[46]

8.10.2 Optic disc malinsertion and tilted disc syndrome

Optic disc malinsertion which can be seen with the 3D view of fundus biomicroscopy and OCT, is caused by the insertion of the optic nerve at an acute angle.[48] The malinsertion is almost always bilateral and the malinserted discs are mirror images of each other, typically elevated nasally, tilting downwards temporally and with a temporal scleral and/or

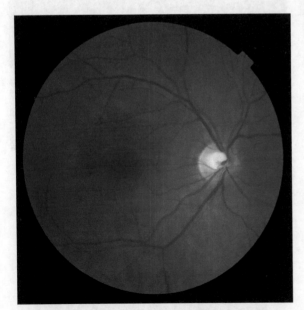

Fig. 8.58 A tessellated fundus from a moderately myopic patient, with the choroidal vessels visible through the thin myopic retina.

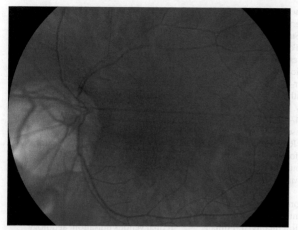

Fig. 8.60 Malinserted disc in high myopia with myopic atrophy.

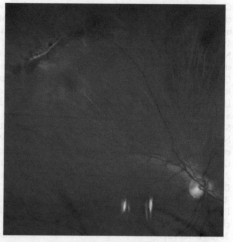

Fig. 8.62 Lattice degeneration in a patient with myopia (optomap).

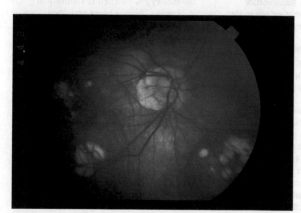

Fig. 8.61 Highly myopic fundus with visible choroid, areas of chorioretinal atrophy and disc peripapillary atrophy (PPA).

choroidal crescent or PPA. Malinserted discs are more common in myopes, with scleral crescents and in American Asians.[48] Photographs from the right and left eyes of a patient with malinserted discs are shown in Figs. 8.36 and 8.59 and online. A malinserted disc in a highly myopic eye is shown in Fig. 8.60.

Tilted disc syndrome is more rare, with the disc or discs commonly tilted inferior nasally with a nasal staphyloma (bulging of the sclera) and situs inversus, where the temporal blood vessels first course towards the nasal retina before sharply changing course (see Fig. 8.45). Tilted discs are thought to be caused by an incomplete closure of the embryonic foetal fissure, similar to the aetiology of a coloboma. The condition is typically benign, although the area of nasal staphyloma can produce a temporal visual field defect and it may be associated with macular complications in later years.[49] Tilted discs are associated with corneal astigmatism and myopia, and the direction of the longest optic disc diameter can indicate the axis of corneal astigmatism.[33]

8.10.3 Pathological myopia

In addition to the physiological changes discussed above, myopia changes can become pathological and high myopia is an increasing cause of low vision and blindness, particularly in East Asian countries.[46] Changes include chorioretinal atrophy, staphyloma, choroidal neovascularization, and retinal detachment (section 7.12.1). A large increase in pathological myopia is likely given the current high prevalence of high myopia in children and young adults and the increase in pathological myopia with age.[46]

References

1. Cronau H, Kankanala RR, Mauger T. Diagnosis and management of red eye in primary care. *Am Fam Physician*. 2010;81:137–44.
2. Thatte S, Jain J, Kinger M, Palod S, Wadhva J, Vishnoi A. Clinical study of histologically proven conjunctival cysts. *Saudi J Ophthalmol*. 2015;29:109–15.
3. Horowitz S, Damasceno N, Damasceno E. Prevalence and factors associated with scleral hyaline plaque: clinical study of older adults in southeastern Brazil. *Clin Ophthalmol*. 2015;9:1187–93.
4. Stevenson TC. Intrascleral nerve loops. A clinical study of frequency and treatment. *Am J Ophthalmol*. 1963;55:935–9.

5. Gloor P, Alexandrakis G. Clinical characterization of primary acquired melanosis. *Invest Ophthalmol Vis Sci.* 1995;36:1721–9.

6. Nowell CS, Radtke F. Corneal epithelial stem cells and their niche at a glance. *J Cell Sci.* 2017;130:1021–5.

7. Rao A, Padhy D, Sarangi S, Das G. Unclassified Axenfeld-Rieger syndrome: a case series and review of literature. *Semin Ophthalmol.* 2018;33:300–7.

8. Nischler C, Michael R, Wintersteller C, et al. Iris color and visual functions. *Graefes Arch Clin Exp Ophthalmol.* 2013;251:195–202.

9. Damasceno RW, Avgitidou G, Belfort Jr R, Dantas PE, Holbach LM, Heindl LM. Eyelid aging: pathophysiology and clinical management. *Arq Bras Oftalmol.* 2015;78:328–31.

10. Jackson JM, Alexis A, Berman B, Berson DS, Taylor S, Weiss JS. Current understanding of seborrheic keratosis: prevalence, etiology, clinical presentation, diagnosis, and management. *J Drugs Dermatol.* 2015;14:1119–25.

11. Jang SM, Lee H, Baek SH. Clinical characteristics of benign eyelid tumors. *J Korean Ophthalmol Soc.* 2016;57:174–80.

12. Nair PA, Singhal R. Xanthelasma palpebrarum – a brief review. *Clin Cosmet Investig Dermatol.* 2017;11:1–5.

13. Vurgese S, Panda-Jonas S, Saini N, Sinha A, Nangia V, Jonas JB. Corneal arcus and its associations with ocular and general parameters: the Central India Eye and Medical Study. *Invest Ophthalmol Vis Sci.* 2011;52:9636–43.

14. Haicl P, Janková H. Prevalence of conjunctival concretions. *Cesk Slov Oftalmol.* 2005;61:260–4.

15. Every SG, Leader JP, Molteno AC, Bevin TH, Sanderson G. Ultraviolet photography of the in vivo human cornea unmasks the Hudson-Ståhli line and physiologic vortex patterns. *Invest Ophthalmol Vis Sci.* 2005;46:3616–22.

16. Cho P, Chui WS, Mountford J, Cheung SW. Corneal iron ring associated with orthokeratology lens wear. *Optom Vis Sci.* 2002;79:565–68.

17. Ansons AM, Atkinson PL. Corneal mosaic patterns—morphology and epidemiology. *Eye (Lond).* 1989;3:811–5.

18. Zoega GM, Fujisawa A, Sasaki H, et al. Prevalence and risk factors for cornea guttata in the Reykjavik Eye Study. *Ophthalmology.* 2006;113:565–9.

19. Moshirfar M, Feiz V, Feilmeier MR, Kang PC. Laser in situ keratomileusis in patients with corneal guttata and family history of Fuchs' endothelial dystrophy. *J Cataract Refract Surg.* 2005;31:2281–6.

20. Zhu DC, Shah P, Feuer WJ, Shi W, Koo EH. Outcomes of conventional phacoemulsification versus femtosecond laser–assisted cataract surgery in eyes with Fuchs endothelial corneal dystrophy. *J Cataract Refract Surg.* 2018;44:534–40.

21. Asokan R, Venkatasubbu RS, Velumuri L, Lingam V, George R. Prevalence and associated factors for pterygium and pinguecula in a South Indian population. *Ophthalmic Physiol Opt.* 2012;32:39–44.

22. Kuszak JR, Peterson KL, Sivak JG, Herbert KL. The interrelationship of lens anatomy and optical quality. II. Primate lenses. *Exp Eye Res.* 1994;59:521–35.

23. van den Berg TJTP. Intraocular light scatter, reflections, fluorescence and absorption: what we see in the slit lamp. *Ophthalmic Physiol Opt.* 2018;38:6–25.

24. Chylack Jr LT, Wolfe JK, Singer DM, et al. The lens opacities classification system III. The longitudinal study of cataract study group. *Arch Ophthalmol.* 1993;111:831–6.

25. Vasavada AR, Mamidipudi PR, Sharma PS. Morphology of and visual performance with posterior subcapsular cataract. *J Cataract Refract Surg.* 2004;30:2097–104.

26. Pesudovs K, Elliott DB. Refractive error changes in cortical, nuclear, and posterior subcapsular cataracts. *Br J Ophthalmol.* 2003;87:964–7.

27. Rochtchina E, Mitchell P, Coroneo M, Wang JJ, Cumming RG. Lower nasal distribution of cortical cataract: the Blue Mountains Eye Study. *Clin Exp Ophthalmol.* 2001;29:111–5.

28. Milston R, Madigan MC, Sebag J. Vitreous floaters: etiology, diagnostics, and management. *Surv Ophthalmol.* 2016;61:211–27.

29. Degirmenci C, Afrashi F, Mentes J, Oztas Z, Nalçaci S, Akkin C. Evaluation of posterior vitreous detachment after uneventful phacoemulsification surgery by optical coherence tomography and ultrasonography. *Clin Exp Optom.* 2017;100:49–53.

30. Gishti O, Nieuwenhof R, van den, Verhoekx J, Overdam K van. Symptoms related to posterior vitreous detachment and the risk of developing retinal tears: a systematic review. *Acta Ophthalmol.* 2019;97:347–52.

31. Lee RY, Kao AA, Kasuga T, et al. Ethnic variation in optic disc size by fundus photography. *Curr Eye Res.* 2013;38:1142–47.

32. Wang Y, Xu L, Zhang L, Yang H, Ma Y, Jonas JB. Optic disc size in a population based study in northern China: the Beijing Eye Study. *Br J Ophthalmol.* 2006;90:353–56.

33. Jonas JB, Kling F, Gründler AE. Optic disc shape, corneal astigmatism, and amblyopia. *Ophthalmology.* 1997;104:1934–7.

34. Crowston JG, Hopley CR, Healey PR, Lee A, Mitchell P. The effect of optic disc diameter on vertical cup to disc ratio percentiles in a population based cohort: the Blue Mountains Eye Study. *Br J Ophthalmol.* 2004;88:766–70.

35. Jacks AS, Miller NR. Spontaneous retinal venous pulsation: aetiology and significance. *J Neurol Neurosurg Psychiatry.* 2003;74:7–9.

36. Healey PR, Mitchell P. Visibility of lamina cribrosa pores and open-angle glaucoma. *Am J Ophthalmol.* 2004;138:871–2.

37. Park, SC, Brumm J, Furlanetto RL, et al. Lamina cribrosa depth in different stages of glaucoma. *Invest Ophthalmol Vis Sci.* 2015;56:2059–64.

38. Townsend KA, Wollstein G, Schuman JS. Imaging of the retinal nerve fibre layer for glaucoma. *Br J Ophthalmol.* 2009;93:139–43.

39. Jonas JB. Clinical implications of peripapillary atrophy in glaucoma. *Curr Opin Ophthalmol.* 2005;16:84–88.

40. Bass SJ, Westcott J, Sherman J. OCT in a myelinated retinal nerve fiber syndrome with reduced vision. *Optom Vis Sci.* 2016;93:1285–91.

41. Hamann S, Malmqvist L, Costello F. Optic disc drusen: understanding an old problem from a new perspective. *Acta Ophthalmol.* 2018;96:673–84.

42. Kaur G, Anthony SA. Multimodal imaging of suspicious choroidal neoplasms in a primary eye-care clinic. *Clin Exp Optom.* 2017;100:549–62.

43. Coleman P, Barnard NA. Congenital hypertrophy of the retinal pigment epithelium: prevalence and ocular features in the optometric population. *Ophthalmic Physiol Opt.* 2007;27:547–55.

44. Khan, KN, Mahroo OA, Khan RS, et al. Differentiating drusen: drusen and drusen-like appearances associated with ageing, age-related macular degeneration, inherited eye disease and other pathological processes. *Prog Retin Eye Res.* 2016;53:70–106.

45. Fraser-Bell S, Symes R, Vaze A. Hypertensive eye disease: a review. *Clin Exp Ophthalmol.* 2017;45:45–53.

46. Verkicharla PK, Ohno-Matsui K, Saw SM. Current and predicted demographics of high myopia and an update of its associated pathological changes. *Ophthalmic Physiol Opt.* 2015;35:465–75.

47. Moghadas Sharif N, Shoeibi N, Ehsaei A, Mallen EA. Optical coherence tomography and biometry in high myopia with tilted disc. *Optom Vis Sci.* 2016;93:1380–86.

48. Marsh-Tootle WL, Harb E, Hou W, et al. Optic nerve tilt, crescent, ovality, and torsion in a multi-ethnic cohort of young adults with and without myopia. *Invest Ophthalmol Vis Sci.* 2017;58:3158–71.

49. Cohen SY, Dubois L, Nghiem-Buffet S, et al. Spectral domain optical coherence tomography analysis of macular changes in tilted disk syndrome. *Retina.* 2013;33:1338–45.

Chapter | 9

Physical examination procedures

Patricia Hrynchak

9.1 Blood pressure measurement

Hypertension, the most common cause of mortality in the developed world, is a major contributing factor in stroke, myocardial infarction, coronary artery disease, heart failure, abdominal aortic aneurysm, and peripheral arterial disease.[1,2] Hypertension affects about 25% of adults and over 50% of people aged 65 and older in Canada and the United Kingdom and over 60 million Americans, with varying prevalence throughout the world.[3-6] The number of people with hypertension is increasing globally. This increase in hypertension is associated with increased dietary salt intake and obesity and with reduced fruit and vegetable consumption and physical activity.[7]

Systemic hypertension can be classified as primary (which has no known cause, 90% to 95%) or secondary (where the causative factor could be renal or endocrine disease or congenital narrowing of the aorta, 5% to 10%).[1] Early hypertension is often asymptomatic, but in acute cases, the patient may complain of headaches, including suboccipital pulsating headaches that occur early in the morning and subside during the day.[8] Headache, shortness of breath, epistaxis, or severe anxiety can occur in hypertensive urgencies (>180/110).[9] Awareness, treatment, and control of hypertension have been steadily improving; however, only 49% of men and 55% of women have overall control of their hypertension.[7]

9.1.1. The evidence base: when and how should blood pressure be measured

Blood pressure (BP) should be measured when fundus features suggest hypertension. These include hypertensive retinopathy, choroidopathy, optic neuropathy, arterial and venous occlusive disease, embolic events, and arteriolar macroaneurysm formation.[10] Wong and Mitchell proposed a simplified classification of hypertensive retinopathy that combined the Keith–Wegener–Barker classification of stage I and II into a 'mild' category (Table 9.1).[11] However, not all patients with hypertension develop retinopathy.[12] Even after 10 years, 70% of patients show either no retinopathy or only slight constriction and arteriolosclerosis.[1] In addition, the inter-rater reliability of detection and classification of hypertensive retinopathy with ophthalmoscopy has been shown to be poor.[12,13] Barnard showed that referral made on fundus signs alone resulted in a 78% false–positive rate in patients between 45 and 64 years of age.[14] BP should also be measured when there is a positive family history because with this history the risk of developing hypertension is increased two to four times.[15] A history of cardiovascular disease, cerebrovascular disease, obesity, physical inactivity, heavy alcohol intake, smoking, diabetes mellitus, and hyperlipidaemia are indicators that BP measurement may be useful. The presence of unexplained headaches, particularly pulsating, suboccipital headaches that subside during the day, particularly in an

Table 9.1 Simplified classification of hypertensive retinopathy as proposed by Wong and Mitchell[11]

Grade of retinopathy	Retinal signs	Systemic associations
None	No detectable signs	None
Mild	Generalised arteriolar narrowing, focal arteriolar narrowing, arteriovenous nicking, opacity ('copper wiring') of arteriolar wall, or a combination of these signs	Modest association with risk of clinical stroke, subclinical stroke, coronary heart disease, and death
Moderate	Haemorrhage (blot, dot, or flame-shaped), microaneurysm, cotton-wool spot, hard exudate, or a combination of these signs	Strong association with risk of clinical stroke, subclinical stroke, cognitive decline, and death from cardiovascular causes
Malignant	Signs of moderate retinopathy plus swelling of the optic disc	Strong association with death

older patient, may suggest acute hypertension and thus the need for BP measurement.[8]

It can be useful to measure BP in a patient who is being treated for hypertension, depending on the patient. For example, if a patient is taking medication regularly and having their BP regularly monitored, then there would be little need for you to measure BP. If, however, the patient stopped taking their medication 6 months ago owing to an adverse reaction and has not seen their physician to follow up, it would be prudent to take a BP reading and advise the patient accordingly even in the absence of abnormalities on the ocular fundus examination.

It can also be useful to measure BP in patients with ocular hypertension, glaucoma suspects, and patients with glaucoma. High BP is associated with high intraocular pressure. Hypotension (i.e., low BP) should be considered in patients with normal tension glaucoma or in patients with glaucoma who are experiencing progressive loss of visual field despite treatment adherence.[16] This is hypothesised to be as a result of impaired ocular perfusion pressure (the difference between the mean arterial BP and the intraocular pressure) especially at night when BP drops and intra-ocular pressure is raised.[16] In addition, some patients with hypertension may be over-treated, which can result in impaired ocular perfusion pressure.[16] Ambulatory BP monitoring in these patients might be helpful in determining if there are significant nocturnal dips that are contributing to the disease.[17] A survey by Wolffsohn et al. found that the majority of primary care physicians would appreciate receiving a report of their patients' BP if it was found to be over 140/90.[12] The usefulness of routine BP screening as an add-on to the eye examination of older patients needs further research. The negative aspects of false–positive results need to be considered (section 1.3).

Most devices for measuring BP occlude a blood vessel in an extremity (usually the arm, wrist, or finger) with an inflatable cuff then measure the BP either by detection of

Korotkoff sounds or oscillometrically.[18] In the auscultatory method a stethoscope is used on the brachial pulse to detect Korotkoff phase I sound (the systolic BP) and the cessation of the Korotkoff phase V sounds (the diastolic pressure) on the deflation of the cuff. In this method the sphygmomanometer used to measure the pressure can be mercury, aneroid, or electronic with a digital display. Mercury sphygmomanometers have largely gone out of use owing to concerns about toxicity of mercury for users, personnel, and the environment.[19] Aneroid devices are inexpensive and portable but the bellow-and-lever system used to measure pressure is subject to jolts and bumps, which can lead to false readings.[19] Aneroid devices require regular calibration and should be checked against a mercury sphygmomanometer every 6 months.

An alternative to the auscultatory method are automated (oscillometric) sphygmomanometers, which are very simple and easy to use (Fig. 9.1). They detect the variation in pressure oscillations caused by arterial wall movement under the cuff to measure systolic, diastolic, and mean arterial BP.[20] Canadian, US, European, and Australian Guidelines for diagnosis and measurement of hypertension recommend using validated automated (oscillometric) upper arm devices over auscultation for in-office and at-home measurements.[2,21-23] Oscillometric measurements improve the repeatability of the measurements, are closer to ambulatory measurements, and the results are lower than conventional methods.[21,23] Ambulatory measurements may be better predictors of cardiac outcomes than conventional methods.[21] Patients are usually left alone in the room and multiple measures are taken one to two minutes apart. This has the advantage of not taking up clinician time. These devices should not be used in patients who have arrhythmia. Thresholds for conventional sphygmomanometry should not be applied to automated readings. The definition of hypertension when using these devices is the same as for ambulatory methods at normal being <135/85.[24,25]

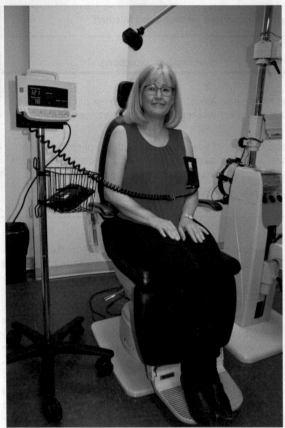

Fig. 9.1 A patient undergoing an automated (oscillometric) sphygmomanometer assessment of blood pressure.

9.1.2 Automated oscillometric blood pressure measurement

1. Have the patient remain seated quietly with feet on the floor and back against a chair (see Fig. 9.1) for at least 5 minutes before BP readings are measured. Caffeine and other stimulants, and smoking and exercise should have been avoided for 30 minutes prior to the BP reading.[9] There should be no acute anxiety, stress, or pain, and there should not be bowel or bladder discomfort.

2. Describe the procedure to the patient: "I am now going to measure your blood pressure. This involves wrapping a cuff around your arm and inflating it. You will feel the pressure on your arm increase, but you shouldn't experience any pain. Please stay silent during the test."

3. Ask the patient to remove any clothing covering the arm and ensure that any rolled up sleeve does not excessively constrict the arm.

4. Ask the patient to bend their arm slightly with the palm turned upwards and rest it on the chair armrest or nearby table. The arm should be at heart level.

5. Select a BP cuff that encircles at least 80% of the arm to ensure accuracy.[9] Typically two cuff sizes are required: large and regular adult (Fig. 9.2). A too small cuff will result in an artificially elevated reading.

6. Locate the brachial artery along the inner upper arm by palpation. Wrap the cuff smoothly and snugly around the arm, centering the bladder over the brachial artery (the artery arrow on the cuff should be pointing at the artery). The lower margin should be 2.5 to 3 cm above the antecubital crease (bend of the elbow).

7. Check that the cuff fits snugly, but is not too tight or too loose. If it is difficult to insert a finger under the cuff edge, it is too tight; if you can insert more than one finger, it is too loose.

8. Set the device to take measurements at 1- or 2-minute intervals. You should verify the first measurement and then leave the patient alone while the device automatically takes the subsequent readings. Depending on the device three to six readings are taken and then averaged, usually discounting the first reading.

9.1.3 Recording

Record the patient's position and the time and the arm used for the measurement. Record the cuff size if it was not the regular adult cuff that was used. Record the pulse rate and record the systolic and diastolic reading in mmHg.

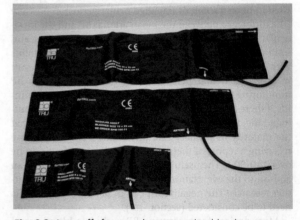

Fig. 9.2 Arm cuffs for use when measuring blood pressure using an automated (oscillometric) sphygmomanometer: large and regular adult and child size.

Examples:

120/80 right arm seated @ 2:30 pm. Pulse 70 bpm
132/84, left arm, seated @ 9.30 am, large adult cuff.
Pulse 72 bpm

9.1.4 Interpreting the results

The classification of hypertension, which is based on two properly measured seated BP readings on each of two or more separate office visits, is shown in Fig. 9.3, although research suggests that ambulatory measurements better predict who should be placed on treatment.[9,25] Individuals who are suspected to be in the elevated classification should be referred to a general physician for health-promoting lifestyle modifications. These modifications include weight control, increase in physical activity, a reductions in salt intake and alcohol consumption, and smoking cessation. Stage 1 and 2 hypertension (i.e., systolic BP above 130mmHg and diastolic BP above 80mmHg, see Fig. 9.3) should be referred to a general physician for further investigation and to consider treatment with pharmacological interventions. Cardiovascular disease risk and concomitant disorders, such as diabetes, will inform the decision to treat hypertension and to what level.[2,21] A hypertensive emergency occurs when the systolic BP is greater than 210 mmHg and the diastolic greater than 130 mmHg. There is evidence of progressive or impending target-organ damage and the BP must be lowered immediately but carefully to prevent end-organ damage from lowering the BP too quickly. This treatment normally requires hospitalisation. A hypertensive urgency is an increase in diastolic BP to greater than 120 to 130 mmHg without end-organ damage which can be treated in office or in the emergency room with oral medications over several hours

to lower the BP. This usually occurs in patients who discontinue their treatment after achieving normal BP.[11,26]

9.1.5 Most common errors

1. Not preparing and positioning the patient correctly. The pressure in the arm increases as the arm is lowered from the level of the heart (phlebostatic axis); conversely, raising the arm above this position lowers the pressure measurement.
2. Using the wrong cuff size: Typically two cuff sizes are required in optometric practice: large adult and regular adult. Child size cuffs are also available (see Fig. 9.2), but unlikely to be used in optometric practice.

9.2 Carotid artery assessment

Carotid artery (Fig. 9.4) occlusive disease may result in stroke and the resultant neurological disability or loss of life.[27]

9.2.1 The evidence base: when and how to assess the carotid artery

Ocular signs and symptoms that suggest carotid artery stenosis include transient monocular loss of vision (amaurosis fugax), retinal emboli (Hollenhorst plaques), retinal vascular occlusions, peripheral retinal haemorrhages with dilated and tortuous veins (hypoperfusion retinopathy also called venous stasis retinopathy),[28] with more rare signs including microrubeosis iridis, ocular ischaemic syndrome, anterior ischaemic optic neuropathy, normal tension, and neovascular glaucoma and asymmetric diabetic retinopathy.[27,29] Additionally, light-induced transient vision loss can be present in carotid artery stenosis.[30]

Amaurosis fugax is a sudden onset, painless loss of vision in one eye that is classically described as a curtain

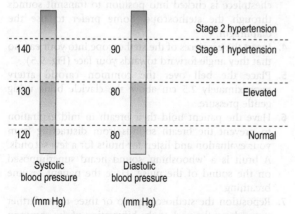

140	90	Stage 2 hypertension
		Stage 1 hypertension
130	80	Elevated
120	80	Normal
Systolic blood pressure	Diastolic blood pressure	
(mm Hg)	(mm Hg)	

Fig. 9.3 Classification of hypertension in adults.[2] Normal BP is systolic BP less than 120mmHg and diastolic BP less than 80mmHg. It is defined as 'elevated' when systolic BP is between 120-129mmHg and diastolic less than 80mmHg.

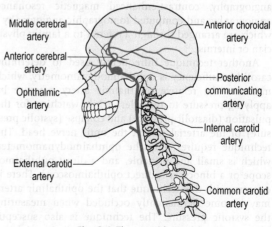

Fig. 9.4 The carotid artery.

coming down over the vision. The vision loss generally lasts longer than one minute.[28] This can result from an embolism from the carotid artery or heart or from transient hemodynamic insufficiency to the retina.[31,32] Systemic symptoms include transient ischemic attacks (TIA) in the form of transient weakness, numbness, or paralysis. Systemic factors that are additive to the risk of carotid artery disease include hypertension, hyperlipidaemia, diabetes mellitus, coronary artery disease carotid bruit, and smoking.[27]

It is important to determine if the patient has already sought medical care and if and what investigations have already been done or are being planned. It is not uncommon to determine that the patient has already seen their physician and that a carotid ultrasound or other investigations are being arranged. The patient is then presenting to determine if any additional information can be gained through a dilated fundus examination.

Because ocular signs and symptoms alone can be poor or unreliable predictors of carotid artery occlusive disease (studies show a range of 0% to 100%), the additional information gained by the detection of a carotid bruit can be helpful when referring the patient with ocular signs to have carotid artery imaging studies performed.[28,29] However, screening for asymptomatic stenosis is not recommended because the prevalence is low and there is a risk of harm with treatment.[33,34]

Auscultation for a systolic bruit is a simple, rapid technique that is helpful in the diagnosis of significant carotid stenosis (abnormal narrowing). A bruit is the sound of turbulence in blood flow when the normal laminar flow is disrupted by the stenosis. While the presence of a bruit can be heard when there is 25% to 30% occlusion, it may be absent if there is nearly total occlusion of the artery.[35] Clinically relevant stenosis is considered to be 70% or higher, although this varies from study to study.[35] More sensitive testing for carotid stenosis includes duplex ultrasonography, magnetic resonance angiography, contrast-enhanced magnetic resonance angiography, and computed tomographic angiography , which are arranged through a referral to a family physician or internist.[35]

Another technique infrequently used to determine carotid insufficiency is ophthalmodynamometry, which measures the relative ophthalmic artery pressure by applying pressure to the sclera while watching for the pulsation (diastolic pressure) and collapse (systolic pressure) of the arterial tree at the optic nerve head. The technique requires only the ophthalmodynamometer, which is small and portable, and a direct ophthalmoscope or a binocular indirect ophthalmoscope. There is concern with this technique that the ophthalmic artery may become permanently occluded when measuring the systolic pressure. The technique is also susceptible to error with patient cooperation being crucial and

may require an assistant to read the values. In addition, a clear ocular media is required for adequate visualisation of the retinal vasculature. The results are dependent on the intraocular pressure and are compared with the patient's brachial BP to determine if the values are within normal limits (the diastolic should be within 45% to 60% of the diastolic BP and the systolic should be within 57% to 70% of the brachial artery BP).

Palpating the carotid arterial pulse is a straightforward technique requiring no equipment that gives the examiner an indication of the strength of the blood flow through the arteries. However, if the examiner palpates the vessels too high on the neck the carotid sinus may be compressed. This may result in an increase in vagal tone, reflex bradycardia, a reduction in BP, and even syncope. Cardiac standstill is possible but very rare. Vigorous examination of the carotid arteries can also rarely cause embolisation of plaque and result in a cerebral stroke, especially in older patients. As a result, palpation of the arteries should be performed with care, always unilaterally and after substantial training. The technique is not described here.

9.2.2 Carotid auscultation procedure

1. Explain the test to the patient: "I am now going to use a stethoscope on your neck to check your blood circulation."
2. For the right carotid artery assessment, stand to the right of the patient and ask the patient to look to their left. For the left carotid artery assessment, stand to the left of the patient and ask the patient to look to their right. Adjust the headrest on the examination chair so that the patient's head is resting backwards with the chin slightly elevated.
3. Adjust the stethoscope so that the bell side of the chestpiece is clicked into position to transmit sounds through the stethoscope. Some prefer to use the diaphragm.
4. Insert the earpieces of the stethoscope into your ears so that they angle forward towards your face (Fig. 9.5).
5. Place the bell over the common carotid artery approximately 2.5 cm above the clavicle bone using gentle pressure.
6. Have the patient hold their breath in mid expiration to prevent the breath sounds from distracting from your evaluation and listen for bruits for a few seconds. A bruit is a 'whooshing' sound heard superimposed on the sound of the pulse. Have the patient resume breathing.
7. Reposition the stethoscope two or three times farther upwards on the neck to the bifurcation of the common carotid artery and then the internal carotid artery. Listen for bruits.
8. Repeat the procedure on the contralateral side.

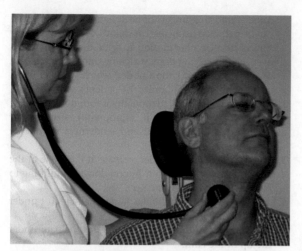

Fig. 9.5 Using the stethoscope to listen for carotid bruits.

9.2.3 Recording

Bruits are recorded as present or absent. Additionally, if the artery is occluded by approximately 50% a soft, early systolic bruit may be heard and if it is occluded by approximately 75% a systolic and early diastolic bruit may be heard.

Examples:

Carotid pulse: R 3+	L3+
Carotid bruit: R absent	L absent
Carotid pulse: R 1+	L2+
Carotid bruit: R soft, systolic bruit	L absent

9.2.4 Interpreting the results

In a systematic review of the utility of a carotid bruit, McColgan et al. found a pooled sensitivity of 53% and specificity of 83% for a clinically relevant stenosis of greater than 70%.[35] In a subgroup analysis of symptomatic patients, the pooled sensitivity was 59% and specificity was 85%.[35] Picket et al. conducted a meta-analysis of the relationship between the presence of a carotid bruit and the subsequent occurrence of TIA, stroke, and death from stroke.[34] The rate ratio for TIA in patients with a bruit was 4.0, for stroke was 2.49, and for death from stroke was 2.71. In another meta-analysis, Picket et al. found that the odds ratio in patients with a bruit for having a myocardial infarction was 2.15 and for cardiovascular death it was 2.27.[36] Therefore, referral should be made for an appropriate medical assessment in the presence of a carotid bruit. Note that the absence of a carotid bruit does not however rule out carotid stenosis because the artery could be nearly entirely occluded resulting in the absence of turbulent flow sounds. An evaluation of symptoms,

ocular and other systemic risk factors, and current and previous medical care for carotid disease should be considered when deciding on referral for further assessment.

9.2.5 Most common errors

1. Interpreting as abnormal a bruit found in children or young adults. These are a result of the vessel elasticity in this age group and are benign.
2. Producing an iatrogenic bruit by placing too much pressure on the artery. Moving the bell over the skin; moving your fingers on the chestpiece or breathing on the tubing can also produce confusing sounds.

9.3 Lymphadenopathy in the head–neck region

The lymph nodes are situated along the course of the lymphatic vessels. They are bean-shaped organs containing large numbers of leukocytes and phagocytes that filter out infectious and toxic material and destroy it. When infection occurs, the nodes become enlarged and often painful and inflamed because of the production of anti-inflammatory lymphocytes and plasma cells.[37]

The lymphatic system of the head and neck is important in infections of the eye (Fig. 9.6), particularly the preauricular lymph nodes which receive lymph from the upper eyelid, the outer half of the lower eyelid, and the lateral canthus. They are located 1 cm anterior and slightly inferior to the tragus of the external ear at the temporomandibular joint. The submandibular lymph nodes lie in close proximity to the submandibular gland and drain lymph from the medial portion of the upper and lower eyelids, the medial canthus, and the conjunctiva. They also drain lymph from the submental nodes that

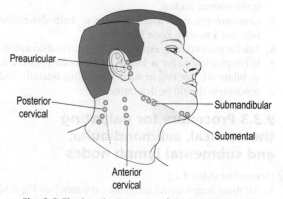

Fig. 9.6 The lymphatic system of the head and neck.

are located under the tip of the chin. The mental nodes also drain anterior aspects of teeth, tongue, and lower lip; if an oral infection is present, they may be enlarged and this should not be mistaken for a sign of an ocular infection. The superior cervical nodes are located inferior to the ear and superficial to the sternocleidomastoid muscle. They receive lymph from the occipital nodes as well as the preauricular and post-auricular nodes.[37] The skin and orbicularis oculi muscles drain into the deep cervical nodes near the internal jugular vein (see Fig. 9.6).

9.3.1 The evidence base: when and how to perform lymph node palpation

The presence of lymphadenopathy in the head and neck region can provide information about the differential diagnosis of a red eye and this technique should be performed on every red eye work-up where infection is part of the differential diagnosis.[38,39] Assessment of the lymphatic system by palpating the nodes is a quick and easy way of gaining information to aid in the differential diagnosis of a red eye. There are no alternative tests and no complications or contraindications to performing this technique other than being gentle with patients who have node tenderness.

9.3.2 Palpating the preauricular lymph nodes

(See online video 9.1.)
1. Wash your hands thoroughly.
2. Stand in front of the seated patient.
3. Place the index and middle fingers of each hand in front of the tragus of the patient's external ears.
4. Slowly move your fingers in a circular motion to slide the patient's skin over the underlying bony structures of the temporomandibular joint and search for swollen lymph nodes. They will feel like a small pebble or bean under the patient's skin. A slight depression of the joint is the normal finding.
5. Compare the right and left sides to help determine whether a swollen node is present.
6. Ask the patient if they experience any pain or discomfort.
7. If lymphadenopathy is found, its laterality (right, left, or bilateral), size (big or small), mobility, warmth, and tenderness should be determined.

9.3.3 Procedure for palpating the cervical, submandibular, and submental lymph nodes

(See online video 9.2.)
1. All these lymph nodes are in the neck area (see Fig. 9.6) and should be palpated using the tips of your index,

middle, and ring fingers of both hands (the submental can be palpated using just one hand). Slowly move your fingers in a circular motion to slide the patient's skin over the underlying bony structures and/or muscle and search for swollen lymph nodes, which will feel like a small pebble or bean under the patient's skin.
2. In each case, if lymphadenopathy is found, its laterality (right, left, or bilateral if appropriate), size (big or small), mobility, warmth, and tenderness should be determined.
3. To assess the cervical nodes, palpate at the angle of the jaw and slowly move your fingers down, continuing to palpate to the base of the neck.
4. To assess the submandibular nodes, palpate just under the edge of the jawbone.
5. To assess the submental lymph nodes, palpate under the tip of the chin.

9.3.4 Recording

Record if the nodes are palpable (positive, +ve) or not (negative, −ve). The preauricular node is commonly abbreviated as PAN. If swollen nodes (lymphadenopathy) are found, describe their laterality (right, left, or bilateral), size (big or small), and mobility (mobile or non-mobile) and indicate whether warmth and tenderness are present.
Examples:

−ve PAN and neck lymph nodes.
+ve bilateral PAN small, mobile, non-tender, without overlying warmth.
+ve right PAN, large, tender, and warm.

9.3.5 Interpreting the results

In the absence of disease there should be no palpable lymph nodes. Palpable lymph nodes (lymphadenopathy) are seen in the following conditions:
1. Viral and adenoviral conjunctivitis: visible preauricular lymphadenopathy in up to 50% of cases,[38,39] often greater on the side of the more involved eye and accompanied by ear, nose, and throat symptoms.[39] It is more prevalent in viral than bacterial conjunctivitis.[38]
2. Severe bacterial lid conditions, such as preseptal cellulitis or infection in the medial canthal region: preauricular or submental lymphadenopathy.
3. Parinaud's oculoglandular conjunctivitis: often visible preauricular lymphadenopathy.
4. Chlamydial conjunctivitis or trachoma: preauricular lymphadenopathy.
5. Following the resolution of an ocular infection (several weeks).

The presence of preauricular lymphadenopathy will therefore help rule in one of the above conditions when it is present, although if it is not present the condition cannot be reliably ruled out.[40,41] An awareness of the areas that the nodes drain is also important to rule out other causes of enlargement of the nodes. For example, if the submental and the submandibular nodes are swollen the infection could be in the area drained by the submental nodes, such as infections of the teeth, tongue, and lower lip. This should be ruled out in the case history.

9.3.6 Most common error

Pushing too hard with patients who have lymphadenopathy because they may experience tenderness.

References

1. Hurcomb PG, Wolffsohn JS, Napper GA. Ocular signs of systemic hypertension: a review. *Ophthalmic Physiol Opt.* 2001;21:430–40.

2. Whelton PK, Carey RM, Aronow WS, et al. 2017 Guideline for the prevention, detection, evaluation, and management of high blood pressure in adults: a report of the American College of Cardiology/American Heart Association Task Force on Clinical Practice Guidelines. *Hypertension.* 2018;71: e13–e115.

3. Daskalopoulou SS, Khan NA, Quinn RR, et al. The 2012 Canadian hypertension education program recommendations for the management of hypertension: blood pressure measurement, diagnosis, assessment of risk and therapy. *Can J Cardiol* 2012;28:270–87.

4. NICE clinical guideline CG 217. *Hypertension: Clinical Management of Primary Hypertension in Adults.* National Institute of Health and Clinical Excellence. 2011. Available at: www.guidance.nice.org.uk/CG217.

5. Meetz RE, Harris TA. The optometrist's role in the management of hypertensive crises. *Optometry.* 2011;82:108–16.

6. Kearney PM, Whelton M, Reynolds K, Whelton PK, He J. Worldwide prevalence of hypertension: a systematic review. *J Hypertens.* 2004;22:11–9.

7. Forouzanfar MH, Liu P, Roth GA, et al. Global burden of hypertension and systolic blood pressure of at least 110 to 115 mm Hg, 1990–2015. *JAMA.* 2017 317:165–82.

8. Headache Classification Subcommittee of the International Headache Society. The International classification of headache disorders: 2nd edition. *Cephalalgia.* 2004;24(suppl 1):9–160.

9. Chobanian AV, Bakris GL, Black HR, et al. Seventh report of the joint national committee on prevention, detection, evaluation and treatment of high blood pressure. *Hypertension.* 2003;42: 1206–52.

10. DellaCroce JT, Vitale AT. Hypertension and the eye. *Curr Opin Ophthalmol.* 2008;19:493–8.

11. Wong TY, Mitchell P. Hypertensive retinopathy. *N Engl J Med.* 2004;351: 2310–7.

12. Wolffsohn JS, Napper GA, Ho SM, Jaworski A, Pollard TL. Improving the description of the retinal vasculature and patient history taking for monitoring systemic hypertension. *Ophthalmic Physiol Opt.* 2001;21:441–9.

13. Figueiredo Neto JA, Palácio GL, Santos AN, Chaves PS, Gomes GV, Cabral TS. Direct ophthalmoscopy versus detection of hypertensive retinopathy: a comparative study. *Arq Bras Cardiol.* 2009;95:215–21.

14. Barnard NA, Allen RJ, Field AF. Referrals for vascular hypertension in a group of 45–64-year-old patients. *Ophthalmic Physiol Opt.* 1991;11:201–5.

15. Blaustein B. *Ocular Manifestations of Systemic Disease*: Chapter 3 Cardiovascular Disease. New York: Churchill Livingstone; 1994:32.

16. Levine RM, Yang A, Brahma V, Martone JF. Management of blood pressure in patients with glaucoma. *Curr Cardiol Rep.* 2017;19:109.

17. Bowe A, Grünig M, Schubert J, et al. Circadian variation in arterial blood pressure and glaucomatous optic neuropathy—a systematic review and meta-analysis. *Am J Hypertens.* 2015;28:1077–82.

18. Beevers G, Lip GY, O'Brien E. ABC of hypertension. Blood pressure measurement. Part I-Sphygmomanometry: factors common to all techniques. *Br Med J.* 2001;322:981–5.

19. World Health Organization. *Affordable Technology: Blood Pressure Measuring Devices for Low Resource Settings.* WHO library; 2005.

20. Skirton H, Chamberlain W, Lawson C, et al. A systematic review of variability and reliability of manual and automated blood pressure readings. *J Clin Nurs* 2011;20:602–14.

21. Nerenberg KA, Zarnke KB, Leung AA, et al. Hypertension Canada's 2018 guidelines for diagnosis, risk assessment, prevention and treatment of hypertension in adults and children. *Can J Cardiol.* 2018;34:506–25.

22. Piepoli MF, Hoes AW, Agewall S, et al. 2016 European guidelines on cardiovascular disease prevention in clinical practice: the sixth joint task force of the European society of cardiology and other societies on cardiovascular disease prevention in clinical practice (constituted by representatives of 10 societies and by invited experts) developed with the special contribution of the European association for cardiovascular prevention & rehabilitation (EACPR). *Atherosclerosis.* 2016;252:207–74

23. Gabb GM, Mangoni AA, Anderson CS, et al. Guideline for the diagnosis and management of hypertension in adults—2016. *Med J Aust.* 2016;205:85–9.

24. Myers MG, Godwin M. Automated office blood pressure. *Can J Cardiol.* 2012;28:341–6.

25. Hodgkinson J, Mant J, Martin U, et al. Relative effectiveness of clinic and home blood pressure monitoring compared with ambulatory blood pressure monitoring in diagnosis of hypertension: systematic review. *Br Med J.* 2011;342:d3621.

26. Lou BP, Brown GC. Update on the ocular manifestations of systemic arterial hypertension. *Curr Opin Ophthalmol.* 2004;15:203–10.

27. Lyons-Wait VA, Anderson SF, Townsend JC, De Land P. Ocular and systemic findings and their correlation with hemodynamically significant carotid artery stenosis: a retrospective study. *Optom Vis Sci.* 2002;79:353–62.

28. McCullough HK, Reinert CG, Hynan LS, et al. Ocular findings as predictors of carotid artery occlusive disease: is carotid imaging justified? *J Vasc Surg.* 2004;40:279–86.

29. Lawrence PF, Oderich GS. Ophthalmologic findings as predictors of carotid artery disease. *Vasc Endovascular Surg.* 2002;36:415–24.

30. Kaiboriboon K, Piriyawat P, Selhorst JB. Light-induced amaurosis fugax. *Am J Ophthalmol.* 2001;131:674–6.

31. Hayreh S, Zimmerman MB. Amaurosis fugax in ocular vascular occlusive disorders: prevalence and pathogeneses. *Retina.* 2014;34:115–22.

32. Hoya K, Morikawa E, Tamura A, Saito I. Common carotid artery stenosis and amaurosis fugax. *J Stroke Cerebrovasc Dis.* 2008;17:1–4.

33. Jonas DE, Feltner C, Amick HR, et al. Screening for asymptomatic carotid artery stenosis: a systematic review and meta-analysis for the US preventative service task force. *Ann Intern Med.* 2014;161:336–446.

34. Pickett CA, Jackson JL, Hemann BA, Atwood JE. Carotid bruits and cerebrovascular disease risk: a meta-analysis. *Stroke* 2010;41:2295–302.

35. McColgan P, Bentley P, McCarron M, Sharma P. Evaluation of the clinical utility of a carotid bruit. *QJM.* 2012;105:1171–7.

36. Pickett CA, Jackson JL, Hemann BA, Atwood JE. Carotid bruits as a prognostic indicator of cardiovascular death and myocardial infarction: a meta-analysis. *Lancet.* 2008;371: 1587–94.

37. Gardner M. *Basic Anatomy of the Head and Neck.* Philadelphia: Lea and Febiger; 1992. pp. 183–6.

38. Azari AA, Barney NP. Conjunctivitis: a systematic review of diagnosis and treatment. *JAMA.* 2013;310:1721–9.

39. Jhanji V, Chan TC, Li EY, Agarwal K, Vajpayee RB. Adenoviral keratoconjunctivitis. *Surv Ophthalmol.* 2015;60:435–43.

40. Uchio E, Takeuchi S, Itoh N, et al. Clinical and epidemiological features of acute follicular conjunctivitis with special reference to that caused by herpes simplex virus type 1. *Br J Ophthalmol* 2000;84:968–72.

41. Aoki K, Kaneko H, Kitaichi N, et al. Clinical features of adenoviral conjunctivitis at the early stage of infection. *Jpn J Ophthalmol* 2011;55: 11–5.

Subject Index

311